ORAL FACIAL GENETICS

ORAL FACIAL GENETICS

Edited by

Ray E. Stewart, D.M.D., M.S.

Associate Professor, Department of Dentistry and Division of Medical Genetics, UCLA/Harbor General Hospital, Torrance, California; Dental Director, UCLA Craniofacial Anomalies Clinic, Los Angeles, California

Gerald H. Prescott, D.M.D., M.S.

Associate Professor of Medical Genetics and Perinatal Medicine; Co-director, Prenatal Diagnostic Clinic, University of Oregon Health Sciences Center, Portland, Oregon

with 660 illustrations

The C. V. Mosby Company

Saint Louis   1976

Library of Congress Cataloging in Publication Data

Stewart, Ray E   1942-
   Oral facial genetics.

   Bibliography: p.
   Includes index.
   1. Teeth—Diseases—Genetic aspects. 2. Mouth
—Diseases—Genetic aspects. 3. Oral manifestations
of general diseases. 4. Facial manifestations
of general diseases. 5. Mouth—Abnormalities
and deformities—Genetic aspects. I. Prescott,
Gerald H., joint author. II. Title. [DNLM:
1. Face—Growth and development. 2. Mouth—Growth
and development. 3. Mouth diseases—Familial and
genetic. 4. Tooth diseases—Familial and genetic.
5. Oral manifestations. WU140 S851o]
RK305.S73   617'.522   76-21322
ISBN 0-8016-4810-6

CB/CB/B   9 8 7 6 5 4 3 2 1

CONTRIBUTORS

DAVID BIXLER, Ph.D., D.D.S.
Professor and Chairman of Oral Facial Genetics and Professor of Medical Genetics, Indiana University Schools of Dentistry and Medicine, Indianapolis, Indiana

JOSEPH J. BONNER, Ph.D.
Research Fellow, Division of Biology, California Institute of Technology, Pasadena, California

JAROSLAV CERVENKA, M.D., C.Sc.
Associate Professor of Human Genetics, Department of Oral Pathology, Division of Human and Oral Genetics, University of Minnesota School of Dentistry and Graduate School, Minneapolis, Minnesota

M. MICHAEL COHEN, Jr., D.M.D.
Associate Professor, Departments of Oral and Maxillofacial Surgery, Orthodontics, and Pediatrics, University of Washington Schools of Dentistry and Medicine, Seattle, Washington

GORDON H. DIXON, D.D.S.
Fellow in Oral-Facial Genetics and Craniofacial Anomalies, UCLA/Harbor General Hospital, Torrance, California

DAVID G. GARDNER, D.D.S., M.S.D.
Professor and Chairman, Division of Oral Pathology, The University of Western Ontario; Consultant to Children's Psychiatric Research Institute; staff member, University Hospital, London, Ontario, Canada

ROBERT J. GORLIN, D.D.S., M.S.
Professor and Chairman, Department of Oral Pathology, University of Minnesota School of Dentistry; Professor of Pathology, Pediatrics, Obstetrics, Gynecology, Otolaryngology, and Dermatology, University of Minnesota School of Medicine, Minneapolis, Minnesota

RONALD J. JORGENSON, B.S., D.D.S.
Associate Professor of Oral Medicine and Assistant Professor of Pediatrics (Genetics), Medical University of South Carolina; Instructor of Medicine, The Johns Hopkins University, Baltimore, Maryland; Section of Clinical Genetics, College of Dental Medicine, Medical University of South Carolina, Charleston, South Carolina

ROSARIO H. YAP POTTER, D.M.D., M.S.D., M.S.
Associate Professor of Dentistry, Oral-Facial Genetics, and Statistics, Indiana University School of Dentistry, Indianapolis, Indiana

GERALD H. PRESCOTT, D.M.D., M.S.
Associate Professor of Medical Genetics and Perinatal Medicine; Co-director, Prenatal Diagnostic Clinic, University of Oregon Health Sciences Center, Portland, Oregon

G. R. RIVIERE, D.D.S., Ph.D.
Assistant Professor, Sections of Pedodontics, Oral Biology, and the Dental Research Institute, University of California at Los Angeles School of Dentistry, Los Angeles, California

JOHN J. SAUK, Jr., D.D.S., M.S.D.
Associate Professor, Division of Human and Oral Genetics, University of Minnesota School of Dentistry, Minneapolis, Minnesota

v

BURTON L. SHAPIRO, D.D.S., M.S., Ph.D.

Professor and Chairman, Department of Oral Biology, University of Minnesota School of Dentistry, Minneapolis, Minnesota

HAROLD C. SLAVKIN, B.A., D.D.S.

Professor of Biochemistry, Laboratory for Developmental Biology, School of Dentistry, Department of Biochemistry and Nutrition, University of Southern California, Los Angeles, California

M. ANNE SPENCE, Ph.D.

Associate Professor in Residence, Departments of Psychiatry and Biomathematics, University of California at Los Angeles, Los Angeles, California

RAY E. STEWART, D.M.D., M.S.

Associate Professor, Department of Dentistry and Division of Medical Genetics, UCLA/Harbor General Hospital, Torrance, California; Dental Director, UCLA Craniofacial Anomalies Clinic, Los Angeles, California

CARL J. WITKOP, Jr., D.D.S., M.S.

Professor, Division of Human and Oral Genetics, University of Minnesota School of Dentistry, Minneapolis, Minnesota

FOREWORD

The extraordinary proliferation of information in medical genetics within the past two decades has been surpassed only by the even more rapid accumulation of knowledge in genetics applied to facial and oral diseases of interest to dentistry as well as medicine. This advancement was inevitable when it became apparent that so many of the oral diseases that at one time had been considered as being due to happenstance were in reality genetic phenomena with a reasonably predictable occurrence as established through the tracking of their transmission patterns.

This book is a pioneer effort, compiling the detailed information currently available concerning the genetic factors and mechanisms that influence disturbances in craniofacial development: disturbances in the tooth, in the formation of enamel, dentin, and cementum, and in the pulp and periodontal structures; immunological and mucocutaneous disorders; errors of metabolism and blood disorders; cytogenetic anomalies; cleft lip and cleft palate; and other facial dysmorphogenic syndromes. It thoroughly documents the application of advanced technology in medical genetics to our understanding of these oral and facial diseases.

The editors have acted wisely in selecting recognized authorities, all of whom have special interest and expertise in their particular areas of contribution to this book. Each has a research-oriented background in genetics along with clinical experience.

This book will be of interest to both students and practitioners of dentistry and medicine, as well as to researchers and clinicians in the broad fields of basic and applied genetics. It is not intended as a basic text of genetic principles, but neither does it presume a profound genetic background for an understanding of the diseases considered. It is a landmark contribution that will fill a recognized void and that will serve well in stimulating further interest and further exploration of oral facial genetics.

William G. Shafer, B.S., D.D.S., M.S.
Distinguished Professor and Chairman,
Department of Oral Pathology,
Indiana University School of Dentistry,
Indianapolis, Indiana

PREFACE

"Necessity is the mother of invention" is an axiom that applies well to the original idea of writing this book. During our years as postdoctoral students and fellows in medical genetics, and more recently as teachers and clinicians, we have been acutely aware of the need for a textbook or other reference that dealt specifically with genetic diseases affecting oral and facial structures.

An extensive literature has developed over the past two decades that documents the accumulation of knowledge in genetics as applied to diseases affecting oral and facial structures. This information, up to now, has been scattered throughout the medical and dental literature, making anything but a cursory review extremely difficult and time consuming. We hope that this book will provide students and practitioners of dentistry and medicine, as well as people involved in basic and applied genetic research, with a comprehensive overview of the subject.

It was not our intent to produce a basic text of genetic principles, since there are several excellent books currently available to fill this need. Instead, we have attempted to provide a comprehensive review of oral facial diseases that are either directly or indirectly affected by genetic influences, the understanding of which does not require an extensive genetic background.

We wish to express our sincere thanks to our colleagues who contributed to this effort and without whom this work would not have been possible. We are particularly indebted to those friends, colleagues, and teachers who have, over the years, instilled in us the curiosity and incentive to undertake this project. At the risk of omitting many persons to whom we are indebted, we feel that a select few deserve special mention. In particular, we would like to acknowledge Dr. Donald R. Porter, Dr. Everett Lovrien, Dr. Fred Hecht, and Dr. David Rimoin for their support and guidance before and during this project.

Our special thanks go to Mrs. Sheryl Turner and Mrs. Lorene Pickett, who typed the many drafts, revisions, and volumes of correspondence that this project generated.

Last, but not least, we wish to express our sincere thanks and appreciation to our wives and families who have persevered and encouraged us throughout this project.

Ray E. Stewart
Gerald H. Prescott

CONTENTS

ORAL FACIAL GENETICS

1

Genetic control mechanisms during early oral facial development

HAROLD C. SLAVKIN
JOSEPH J. BONNER

In multicellular organisms a remarkably ordered program of changes is demonstrable during the development of the mature animal from the fertilized egg: a great range of functions is simultaneously orchestrated to produce the harmonious pattern that is characteristic of normal development. It is now possible to recognize two major classes of processes during embryogenesis and the subsequent developmental stages of animal development: (1) *cell differentiation* describes the emergence of functionally and morphologically distinct cell types and (2) *histogenesis, organogenesis,* and *morphogenesis* describe the association of cell types into precise patterns to form tissues, organs, and interrelated organ systems. Many features of cell differentiation can now be discussed in biochemical terms. Numerous levels of regulation have now been described. In contrast, spatial and temporal patterns associated with constituents of the developing organisms remain largely a mystery to which genetics, molecular biology, and developmental biology have not as yet made striking contributions.

It is often convenient to consider animal development in terms of the evolution of a program or a series of coordinated programs comparable to contemporary computer programs that employ a common information store. In attempting to analyze this process during embryogenesis, three essential phases should be considered: (1) the establishment of the program during the maturation of the egg in the oocyte (the limited amounts of material at this stage of development have made it difficult to obtain reliable qualitative or quantitative data); (2) a phase for the selection or expression of different subprograms from the master program (genotype), which will be expressed by discrete populations of cells (phenotypes) within the forming embryo (often called *determination* in classical embryology); and (3) a final phase, which represents a series of maturation processes in which predetermined programs are expressed among interdependent populations of cells, tissues, and organs.

During animal development numerous biological features are remarkable. For ex-

We wish to acknowledge our appreciation to the untiring efforts of Ms. Kari Chandler for typing the manuscript and for her attention to the numerous details in the references cited. We wish also to thank Mr. Pablo Bringas, Jr., for his excellent drawings and for the preparation of the scanning and transmission electron photomicrographs for this chapter. The research derived from our laboratory was supported by research grants DE-02848, DE-03569, and DE-03513, and training grant DE-00094 from the National Institute of Dental Research, United States Public Health Service.

ample, two types of development have been observed. A *mosaic type of development* has been described, which is characteristic of insects and has several interesting implications. In many insects the pronucleus is situated at one pole of the egg. After fertilization, the pronucleus undergoes repeated divisions, but *without any discrete cellular divisions*. A cluster of pronuclei forms at one end of the egg. These pronuclei then migrate to different parts of the egg, and only after this nuclear migration is completed do cell walls form. Many years ago a significant observation was made that an injury to a particular region of the unfertilized egg could give rise to a specific and predictable defect in the insect that developed from it. The implications of this observation are many, but one of the conclusions to be drawn is that some of the information for the development of the insect organism was localized within the cytoplasm of the egg. A strikingly different course of events was observed in *vertebrate development*. After fertilization of the vertebrate egg, the nucleus undergoes a series of rapid doublings and divisions, but in this instance, each division is accompanied by segregation of the daughter nuclei followed by cytoplasmic cleavage. These cleavages result in the formation of an aggregate of nucleated cells called a *morula*. During the early stages of morula formation, the cells appear to have a high degree of cytological and biochemical *equivalence* in that if some cells are removed, the remaining cells can form a normal, albeit smaller, embryo resulting in a viable organism. During embryogenesis in vertebrate development (for example, mouse and man), the forming organism clearly possesses a more flexible set of mechanisms during early stages of embryogenesis (that is, morulation) than do organisms such as insects, which exhibit mosaic development.

Much of our current knowledge of the mechanisms involved in cell differentiation, development, and regulative molecular biology has been derived from investigations into the control of protein synthesis in both prokaryotic and eukaryotic cell systems. It is clearly recognized now that the same basic mechanisms apply to mammalian as well as bacterial cells, namely that the genetic information for protein synthesis is carried in the DNA and that this inherited genetic information is transcribed into messenger RNA. Messenger RNA is in turn translated into polypeptide chains on ribosomes by a process that also involves activating enzyme systems, specific cations, energy, transfer RNAs, and other factors. Such a mechanism for protein synthesis obviously provides numerous levels at which regulation could be applied. In this chapter we will consider regulation at various levels of vertebrate development and indicate the major controls that have been found to be operant during these critical developmental stages with particular reference to the mammalian craniofacial complex. There is appreciable evidence to indicate that during cell differentiation, histogenesis, organogenesis, and morphogenesis, regulative controls of generalized importance to normal development also apply at discrete stages of craniofacial development.

Investigations into gene regulation in prokaryotic cells have described two forms of regulatory controls, the *positive* function of factors that stimulate the transcription of DNA by RNA polymerase, and *negative* or repressor factors of transcription. However, when considering differential gene regulation during craniofacial development in mammals, a number of perplexing and significant features must be considered. Unlike the genome of bacterial cells, the eukaryotic nucleus contains a hundred to a thousand times more genetic information than the prokaryotic cell. Furthermore, in prokaryotic cells only a few genes are present in DNA as multiple copies, whereas in eukaryotic cells a considerable proportion of the genome consists of *repetitious* copies of genes throughout the total DNA, and the remainder of the DNA consists of *unique* sequences of genes present in far greater numbers than those found in the entire DNA of many bacteria!

Another major feature of eukaryotic cells that is extremely important when considering genetic regulation during early craniofacial development is the fact that the DNA is

Table 1-1. Complexity of the genetic apparatus in bacterial and animal cells*

	Bacteria	*Man*
DNA	0.02×10^{-12} gm/cell	7×10^{-12} gm/cell
	Single copy of genes	Frequent, multiple, repeated gene sequences
Protein	Small concentration of acidic protein	Histone (basic) proteins, 1 gm/gm DNA
		Nonhistone proteins (acidic) 0.1 to 1.5 gm/gm DNA
RNA	Nascent mRNA	Up to 0.15 gm/gm DNA—nascent mRNAs and other RNA types (rRNAs and tRNAs)
Gene regulation	Discrete alterations with single stimuli	Simple stimuli can generate multiplicity of cascading effects

*Bacterial cells serve as an example of prokaryotic cells; human cells serve as an example of eukaryotic cells.

permanently associated with large amounts of basic and acidic proteins (that is, histones and nonhistone chromosomal acidic proteins, respectively) (Table 1-1). In the last several years an appreciable body of knowledge has become available that clearly indicates that these chromosomal proteins serve as gene regulators in eukaryotic cells. It is postulated that the interactions between chromosomal proteins and DNA can restrict or make *unavailable* gene sequences, whereas, in other developmental phases, chromosomal proteins can unmask and make *available* unique sequences of polynucleotides (structural genes), making them available for transcription. If all somatic cells within the developing embryo contain the same genetic information, and if during replication each daughter cell inherits the same genetic information, at what level of biological regulation is cell diversity determined and subsequently maintained?

Numerous levels of regulatory controls are operant during mammalian embryogenesis, development, maturation, and senescence. It has become reasonable to anticipate that, in addition to the transcriptional controls within the cell nucleus, there are additional and equally complex forms of regulatory gene controls functioning in the extranuclear cytoplasm of the cell. Humoral factors, extracellular matrix environments, cell surface ligand–molecule interactions, plasma cell membrane–intracytoplasmic interactions, and a variety of cytoplasmic-nuclear interactions are current areas of great interest related to problems in the regulation of normal mammalian craniofacial developmental biology. In the following sections we shall attempt to review but a few of the salient structural and functional constituents in the early regulation of oral facial genetics and discuss their respective roles in normal and abnormal craniofacial developmental biology.

CELL ARCHITECTURE: A CLUE TOWARD UNDERSTANDING CELL DIVERSITY

Despite the fact that all somatic cells within the same animal contain an identical genetic inheritance, eukaryotic cells within the organism demonstrate a myriad of sizes, shapes, and cytological and biochemical makeups. The study of morphology teaches us the diversity of living forms; so too, biochemistry, molecular biology, immunology, and genetics impress us with the unity of life. During the last two decades developmental biologists have addressed themselves increasingly to the solution of the mechanisms of the genetic control of differentiation. The logical dilemma can be simply stated as follows: If visible differentiation of cells merely reflects the emerging differences in their protein content, and if the code for all proteins is spelled out by genetic messages reaching the cytoplasm from the nucleus, then *how can cells ever become different if all cells contain precisely the same genes?*

In an attempt to resolve this dilemma, an appreciable number of investigations have provided evidence in support of the proposition that although all somatic cells contain all the genetic information for making all the proteins found in the organism, not all of the potential instructions or messages inscribed in the DNA are actually transcribed and sent to the cytoplasm for processing.*

The preponderance of available evidence indicates that the type of specific genetic messages that are transmitted is influenced by the cytoplasmic environment in which the nucleus is located.* In turn, the cytoplasmic environment is influenced by the microenvironment in which the cell finds itself.†

*See references 11, 13, 21, 30, 46, 50, 79, 84, 105, 111.

*See references 7, 13, 14, 20, 21, 30, 50, 53, 61, 73, 75, 79, 105.
†See references 1, 11, 18, 30, 32, 36, 40, 42, 44, 51, 52, 61, 67, 73, 95, 106.

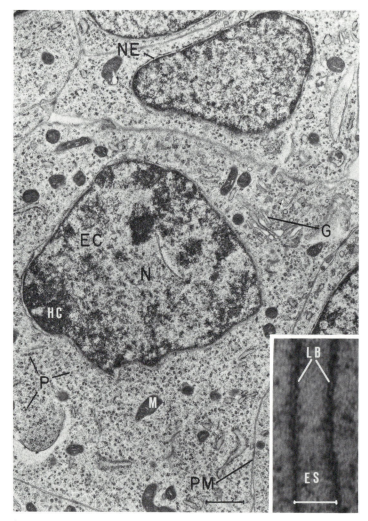

Fig. 1-1. Survey electron photomicrograph of embryonic oral epithelial cells from 16-day mouse fetus demonstrating ultrastructural characteristics of this cell type. Within nuclear envelope, *NE,* surrounding the nucleus, *N,* appears characteristic euchromatin, *EC,* and heterochromatin, *HC.* Cytoplasm contains numerous polysomes, *P,* few mitochondria, *M,* and Golgi apparatus, *G.* Higher-magnification inset displays typical lipid bilayer, *LB,* of plasma membrane, *PM,* with extracellular space, *ES,* between adjacent cell outer surfaces. Bar line in figure is 1.0 μm; bar line in inset is 0.1 μm.

For example, the ultrastructure of an embryonic epithelial cell in the oral cavity (Fig. 1-1) is different in appearance when compared to the differentiated epidermis of the gingiva (Figs. 1-2 and 1-3). The embryonic cell reflects diversity in terms of structure and in terms of functions such as growth, cell division, the formation of transient intercellular contacts, and the synthesis of gene products (that is, proteins), which become part of the extracellular matrix environment. In contrast, mature differentiated epidermal cells within the gingiva are limited as a protein-synthesizing cell type forming keratin, and they are spatially localized through permanent intercellular junctions that become highly specialized (Figs. 1-2 to 1-5), providing the tissue strength and durability required for function in the oral cavity. Each of these cell types possesses an identical genotype, although each cell type through differential gene regulation has expressed a myriad of structural and functional differences. How are these differences stabilized and maintained?

Replication and transcription

For the purposes of our discussions, embryonic differentiation is considered as cellular changes in macromolecular synthesis and composition, patterned in time and space, and resulting in specialized cell functions, forms, and intercellular organizational units

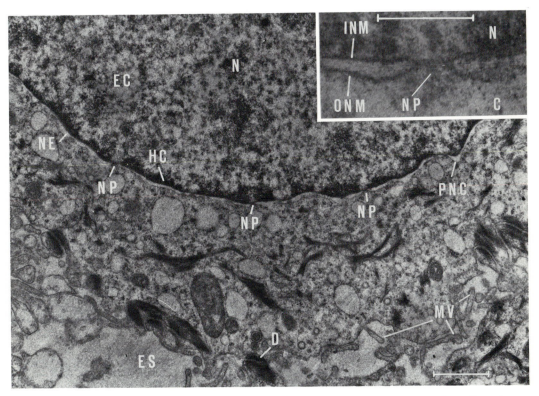

Fig. 1-2. Epithelial cell from adult mouse periodontium contains variety of nuclear, *N,* and cytoplasmic, *C,* ultrastructural components. Cellular periphery has numerous microvilli, *MV,* which extend into extracellular space, *ES.* Plasma membranes of adjacent cells are bound together by specialized intercellular junctions called desmosomes, *D.* Condensed on surface of inner nuclear membrane is heterochromatin, *HC,* and dispersed throughout nucleus is euchromatin, *EC. Inset:* Nuclear envelope, *N,* is composed of two membranes, outer nuclear membrane, *ONM,* and inner nuclear membrane, *INM,* with perinuclear cistern, *PNC,* separating membranes. Nuclear envelope has many pores, *NP,* which are functional in transport of macromolecules. Bar line in figure is 1.0 μm; bar line in insert is 0.5 μm.

(for example, tissues and resulting organs).[11, 54] There is now ample evidence that these changes cannot be ascribed to gross differences in the genotype of cells within the same forming organism[13, 20, 50]; rather, cell differentiation is predominantly due to differences in gene expression in genetically equipotential genomes. Therefore mechanisms must exist that specify which genes are to be expressed at particular times during embryonic development. Identification of these mechanisms and their respective modes of action is a major objective of research in craniofacial developmental biology.

Morphologically we can locate the entire genome of each somatic cell within the nucleus,[68] the most conspicuous of all intracytoplasmic organelles. Within its membranous boundary all the necessary molecular elements for replication and transcription are con-

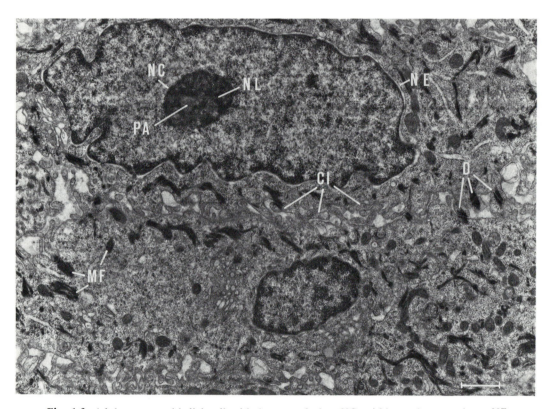

Fig. 1-3. Adult mouse epithelial cell with large nucleolus, *NC,* within nuclear envelope, *NE.* Several internal ultrastructural features, nucleolonema, *NL,* and pars amorpha, *PA,* of nucleolus can be observed. Adjacent cells in this tissue have intercellular interdigitation, *CI,* and many desmosomes, *D,* associated with microfilaments, *MF,* which are continuous within cell interior. Bar line is 1.0 μm.

Fig. 1-4. Survey of ultrastructural complexities of intercellular interdigitation, *CI,* specialized intercellular junctions called desmosomes, *D,* and associated microfilaments, *MF,* which anchor plasma membrane forming desmosome with cytoplasm. Bar line is 1.0 μm.

Fig. 1-5. Electron-dense area between two cell membranes, *PM,* of desmosome, *D,* is called intermediate dense plaque, *IDP,* which is continuous with extracellular space, *ES.* Microfilaments, *MF,* anchor specialized junction with cytoplasm, *C.* Bar line is 0.1 μm.

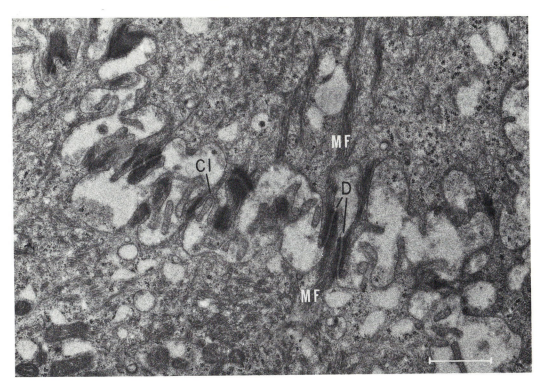

Fig. 1-4. For legend see opposite page.

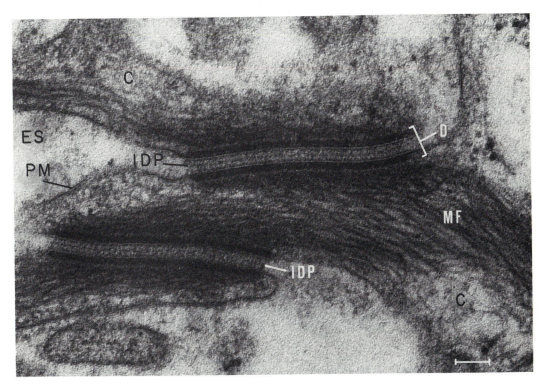

Fig. 1-5. For legend see opposite page.

tained (Figs. 1-2 and 1-3). In conventional-light microscopic preparations the nucleus stains basophilic, with a dense basophilic inclusion called the nucleolus. In transmission electron-microscopic preparations the general area of the nucleus consists of two types of chromatin material, heterochromatin and euchromatin.[19, 100, 105] Chromatin consists of chromosomal DNA, acidic and basic chromosomal proteins (that is, the histones and the *nonhistone chromosomal proteins,* respectively), replicases, transcriptases, and polymerases integrated with the appropriate mixture and amounts of enzyme substrates and ligands. Electron-microscopic, radiographic, hydrodynamic, optical, biochemical, radioisotopic tracer, and immunological investigations have all provided unequivocal data to demonstrate that chromatin is the fundamental structure of genetic inheritance.*

The nucleus synthesizes copies of the total inherited DNA during mitosis for cell replication and is also capable of synthesizing specific transcripts of the DNA for transcription in the form of either messenger RNA (mRNA), ribosomal RNA (rRNA), or transfer RNA (tRNA).[20]

The molecular processes of replication and transcription are compartmentalized and restricted to certain areas within the nucleus (Figs. 1-2 and 1-3). DNA replication is believed to occur along the inner surfaces of the nuclear membrane when the DNA is in the heterochromatic state.[18] DNA in the euchromatic state is thought to be actively synthesizing RNA but is dormant for DNA synthesis.[18] The nucleolus, the centralized electron-dense area of the nucleus, is active in the synthesis and assembly of ribosomal RNA.[20, 46, 55, 58]

The products of transcription are ribonucleic acids. A relatively small percentage of newly synthesized RNA is transported through the nuclear membrane specifically in the areas of the nuclear membrane pores (Fig. 1-2). The nuclear pores are characteristic membrane structural components specialized for the passage of ribonucleoprotein macromolecules between the nucleus and the cytoplasm.[79] Proteins synthesized in the cytoplasm also are transported through the nuclear pores into the nucleus.

Ultrastructural morphology of nuclei within intact cells reveals two types of chromatin on the basis of electron density and condensation. Electron-microscopic and biochemical studies of isolated chromatin depleted of the lysine-rich histones demonstrate that the fundamental structure consists of a flexible chain of spherical particles about 125 Å in diameter connected by DNA filaments.[46, 63] Isolated chromatin is essentially a fiberlike structure consisting of highly condensed regions, which appear coiled, and naked regions, which appear stretched.[63] The condensed regions are transcriptively inactive, whereas the stretched regions are active.[84]

Translation

The smallest unit of translation is the ribosome (Figs. 1-6 and 1-7). Using transmission electron microscopy, ribosomes appear as small, electron-dense, spherical structures in the cytoplasm. They appear as free, discrete particles or associated with an intracellular membrane system called the *rough endoplasmic reticulum* (RER) where they appear clustered in chains of four or more. This functional unit is called a polysome. Each ribosome within the polysome is attached to the same mRNA molecule.[20] The polysomes, either free in the cytoplasm or clustered in the rough endoplasmic reticulum, possess different protein synthesizing capacities. Proteins synthesized on the free polysomes (Fig. 1-6) are functionally active within the cell,[72] whereas proteins synthesized on the RER (Fig. 1-7) are often secreted by the cell.[33] For example, the enzymes that metabolize glucose are intracellular polypeptides, whereas extracellular macromolecules such as collagen are synthesized and secreted by the cell into the extracellular matrix microenvironment. Collagen is synthesized on the RER.*

---

*See references 5, 13, 14, 19, 21, 46, 50, 63, 70, 80, 84, 100.

---

*See references 17, 20, 31, 33, 62, 96, 98, 102, 108.

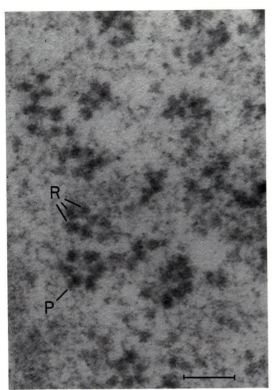

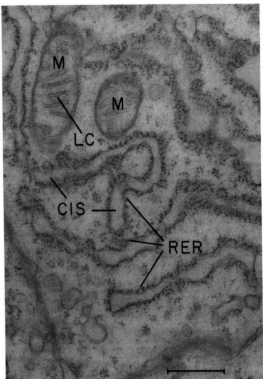

Fig. 1-6. High-magnification survey electron photomicrograph of mouse embryonic polysomes, *P,* showing characteristic rosette pattern of ribosomes, *R,* which are usually interconnected by an mRNA molecule. Bar line is 0.1 µm.

Fig. 1-7. Representative example of rough endoplasmic reticulum, *RER.* Proteins are synthesized on clusters of ribosomes bound to intracellular membrane system (reticulum), and then newly synthesized proteins pass through membrane and enter cisternae, *CIS.* Within cisternae, newly synthesized proteins are modified posttranslationally. Usually many mitochondria, *M,* are dispersed throughout area of RER, providing energy for protein synthesis. *LC,* Mitochondrial lamellar cristae. Bar line is 0.5 µm.

When proteins are synthesized for secretion, other subcellular organelles are often associated with the process. After the proteins have been synthesized by the ribosomes of the RER, the newly formed proteins are then transported into the cisternae of the RER. The proteins are transported through the cisternae and then enter the smooth endoplasmic reticulum (SER). While the proteins are in transit they can be chemically modified (glycosylated or phosphorylated) by specific glycosyltransferase enzymes located on the inner surface of the SER; this is an example of posttranslational modification.[31, 33] The enzymatically modified proteins enter the Golgi apparatus (Fig. 1-8), where they are concentrated, and the final gene products are packaged in condensing vacuoles, which evolve into secretory granules. The secretory granules empty their contents into the extracellular space by a process of reverse pinocytosis at the cell surface (Fig. 1-9). Additional enzymes in the vacuoles and granules and within the plasma cell membrane can further modify the newly synthesized gene product.

Self-replicating intracellular structures

The process of differentiation is characterized by the appearance of tissue-specific proteins at specific times during embryogenesis. Although such generalizations are most applicable to numerous synthetic events that accompany embryonic cell differentiation, some ubiquitous and important intracellular organelles are inherited as preexisting structures.

Maternal mitochondrial inheritance. Eukaryotic cells contain a class of cytoplasmic DNA molecule that is found only within the mitochondria. The mitochondrial DNA replicates within this important organelle and is also transcribed into a small number of mRNAs that code for a small number of polypeptides (perhaps four).[10, 35, 43] The syn-

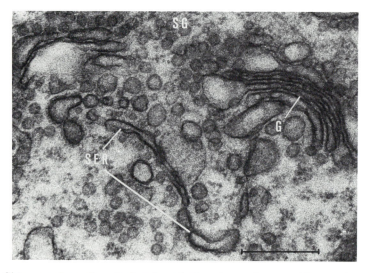

Fig. 1-8. Cisternae of rough endoplasmic reticulum is continuous with smooth endoplasmic reticulum, *SER,* and Golgi apparatus, *G.* Enzymes localized in membranes of SER further modify proteins originally synthesized on RER; Golgi concentrates proteins into condensing vacuoles or secretion granules, *SG,* which are eventually secreted by cell. Bar line is 0.5 μm.

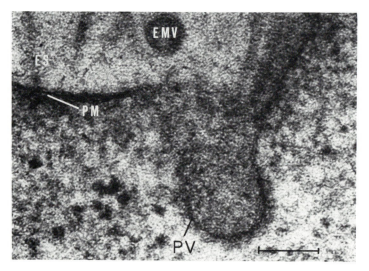

Fig. 1-9. Protein products are secreted into extracellular space, *ES,* at plasma membrane surface by process of reverse pinocytosis, which is characterized by fusion of membrane of pinocytotic vesicles, *PV,* with plasma membrane, *PM.* Often vesicles, *EMV,* can be observed in extracellular space; vesicles contain variety of macromolecules (for example, enzymes, RNAs, inorganic ions). Bar line is 0.1 μm.

thesis of the vast majority of mitochondrial proteins, both structural and functional, is under the control of genes located in the nuclear DNA.

A most interesting contemporary question in genetics deals with the mechanism for the inheritance of the mitochondrial genome (mtDNA).[35] Evidence is now available that in fungi, amphibians, and mammals, the mitochondrial genome of an individual organism is derived solely from the maternal parent in contrast to chromosomal nuclear genes, which are inherited biparentally.[35] Although it is not necessarily surprising that mtDNA is inherited maternally in mammals, it could not be predicted a priori, since the

middle piece of the mammalian spermatozoan, which contains the mitochondria, usually enters the ovum at fertilization and then scatters throughout the egg cytoplasm. Subsequently, these paternally derived mitochondria are partitioned (often asymmetrically) throughout the cells during mitosis. However, the mechanism now established is that mtDNA is essentially derived through maternal inheritance. This results from a preponderance of maternal mtDNA in the zygote. One can estimate that 10^6 molecules of mtDNA are inherited from the maternal contribution or the ovum.

The evidence is convincing that maternally inherited mitochondria and the centriole are

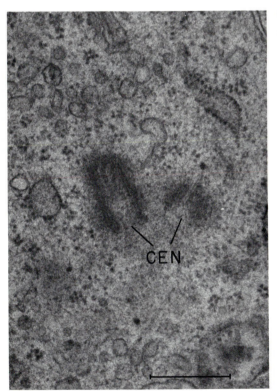

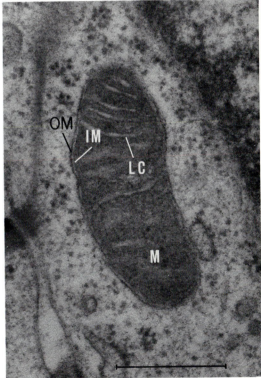

Fig. 1-10. Oblique section through centriole, *CEN,* in embryonic epithelial cell from fetal rabbit incisor tooth organ. There are two microtubular arrays perpendicular to each other. Because of plane of section, tubular ultrastructure is not apparent. Bar line is 0.5 μm.

Fig. 1-11. This mitochondrion, *M,* is located within mouse embryonic oral epithelial cell. Mitochondrion has several interesting ultrastructural characteristics: outer membrane, *OM,* and inner membrane, *IM.* Inner membrane system forms lamellar cristae, *LC,* which contain many enzymes operant in oxidative phosphorylation and production of ATP. Bar line is 0.5 μm.

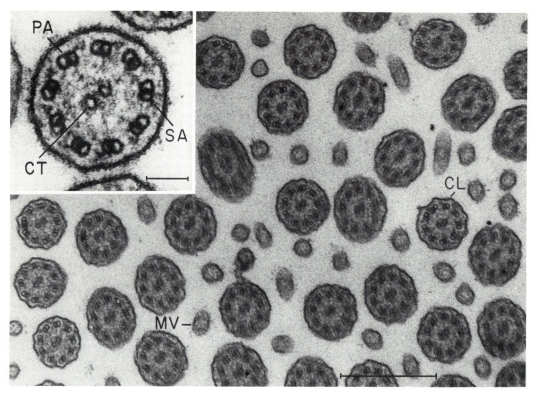

Fig. 1-12. Cross-sectional area of cilia, *CL,* from oral cavity of embryonic mouse. Within plasma membrane can be seen characteristic 9 + 2 microtubule array. There are nine pairs, *PA,* of microtubules, which have figure-8 appearance, often with small side arms, *SA;* these nine pairs of microtubules surround internal structure containing two central tubules, *CT.* Small circular bodies, *MV,* are cross-sectional areas through microvilli often associated with cilia. Bar line in figure is 0.5 μm; bar line in inset is 0.1 μm.

genetically distinct and independent units within the cell (Figs. 1-10 and 1-11). The mitochondria function to generate adenosine triphosphate (ATP), which supplies the energy to accommodate most enzymatic processes within the cell. The centriole serves as the organizer for microtubule formation. Microtubules are essential components of the mitotic spindle and the cilia in the cell (Figs. 1-12 and 1-13). Both mitochondria and centrioles possess a small amount of DNA. The mitochondrion has the molecular tools for replication, transcription, and translation of its genome, albeit on a small scale. The mitochondrial genome has encoded within its mtDNA sequence a few proteins necessary for many mitochondrial structural elements.[43] It has been suggested that millions of years ago mitochondria and the centriole were possibly unicellular organisms (like bacteria) that began a symbiotic relationship with a primitive eukaryotic cell.[48] The symbiosis evolved into the present obligatory-dependent relationship. All four structures, nucleus, cytoplasm, mitochondria, and centriole, are totally and mutually interdependent for the maintenance of the cell and its differentiated state. The genetic uniqueness of the nucleus, mitochondria, and centriole clearly expand the scope of studying genetic controls and mechanisms for inheritance. Dependencies among genetically different subcellular organelles are just now beginning to be explored and appreciated.

Structural elements of the cell

Cell structure and function are dependent on organized unit elements, which have spe-

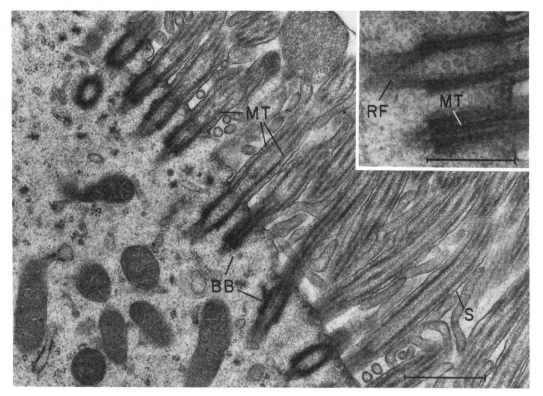

Fig. 1-13. Transverse section through same cilia as in Fig. 1-12 showing basal body, *BB,* which is organizer for microtubule, *MT,* formation, which is continuous with shaft, *S,* of cilium. At base of basal body are often seen microfilaments or root filaments, *RF,* which run into cellular interior. Bar line in figure is 1.0 μm; bar line in inset is 0.5 μm.

cific structural properties. These structural components provide the cell with unique properties of size and shape that further express cell diversity.

Intracellular filaments are called microfilaments and microtubules (Figs. 1-4, 1-5, 1-12, and 1-13). Often these structural elements extend from one side of the cell to the other anchored in the cell membrane. These elements are contractile, contain actin and myosin, and provide the ability to maintain and alter cell shape and cell mobility.[64, 68] Specialized cell processes such as cilia (Figs. 1-12 and 1-13) have an organized tubular system that functions in maintaining the cilia length and waving activity.[66]

In addition to the obvious importance of the genome in the determination of cellular development and function, the plasma membrane and the outer cell surfaces of eukaryotic cells function in crucial ways in the control of embryonic cell differentiation, histogenesis, organogenesis, and the general morphogenesis of the forming organism. In addition to its role of maintenance of the intracytoplasmic integrity and serving as the physical boundary between the cell and the immediate microenvironment (Fig. 1-1), the membrane also provides a selective, semipermeable boundary permitting limited passive diffusion and regulating active transport of nutrients from the extracellular environment into the cell.[1, 15, 47, 54] The molecular composition of the membranes serves to provide each cell with a complex lexicon of developmentally significant information encoded within the structure of the limiting plasma membranes of somatic cells. The fundamental structure of the membrane is a lipid bilayer (Fig. 1-1) resulting from interactions between choline phospholipids, glycolipids, phospholipids, proteins, and glycoproteins. In addition to the actual structural constituents of the plasma membrane, some proteins extend across the bilayer. These molecules generally are glycoproteins with unique carbohydrates (hexoses such as galactose, mannose, and glucosamines) located on the outer cell surfaces (Fig. 1-14). The configuration and unique carbohydrate sequences associated with these surface molecules provide the basis for all types of cell-to-cell communication, including cell migrations, cell recognition, cell-substratum interactions, and specific cell aggregation into tissues and organ systems.[54] Recent advances in membrane biology have demonstrated that the plasma membrane contains developmentally significant in-

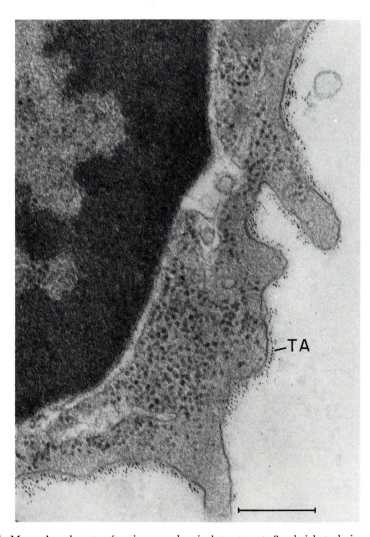

Fig. 1-14. Mouse lymphocyte after immunochemical treatment. Sandwich technique was used to visualize cell surface transplantation antigens, *TA,* H-2K, and H-2D. Visualization technique first binds antibody to cell surface transplantation antigen, then second antibody, which has been conjugated to ferritin (electron-dense macromolecule), is bound to transplantation antigen-antibody complex. Ferritin molecules are small dots along cell periphery visualized in electron microscope. Bar line is 1.0 μm.

formation mediated by cell surface molecules such as glycosyltransferases, histocompatibility antigens (H-2 in mice and HL-A in man), hormone receptors, differentiation alloantigens (theta markers on thymocytes), and other functionally and structurally significant surface molecules (Figs. 1-14 and 1-15).

GENETIC REPLICATION, MITOSIS, CELL SURFACES, AND THE EXTRACELLULAR ENVIRONMENT

The process by which external factors elicit changes in embryonic cells resulting in tissue-specific protein synthesis is called *embryonic induction.*[30] The regulation of gene activity has been elegantly illustrated in a large number of prokaryotic systems. The genetic fine structure in the genome of viruses and bacteria has provided a technology with which to explore the more complex eukaryotic cells in animal systems. This technology has been most helpful in providing models designed to explain the control of transcriptional patterns of RNA synthesis during cell proliferation within forming embryos. Furthermore, regulatory mechanisms have been proposed to explain the process of translation whereby the genetic information carried in mRNA serves as a template for subsequent polypeptide synthesis. However, the details of the cellular mechanisms controlling cell division, DNA replication, transcription, and translation in vertebrate animal systems, particularly in vivo, remain relatively obscure. Defining the systems that specifically control selective gene expression presents one of the most challenging and fundamental problems in craniofacial biology.

With genetic analysis at the molecular level at present somewhat impeded in vertebrate animal cells, the genetic apparatus must be

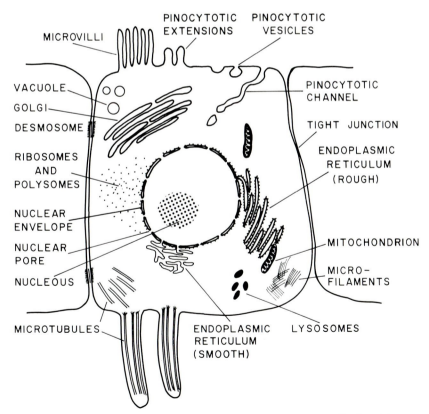

Fig. 1-15. Illustrated summary of cellular ultrastructural elements usually found in many cell types. Diagram is not drawn to scale.

analyzed essentially in terms of its biochemical constitution. Recent advances in cellular and molecular biology have permitted appreciable progress in the identification of the sequences in the DNA that represent structural genes and in the determination of the distribution in the total genome of other sequences of genetic information. Major advances have been made in the characterization of different components of the animal cell genome as demonstrated by their unique rates of renaturation. Before further exploring some of this recent information, it is a prerequisite to briefly review the salient features of DNA.

Almost all of the inherited material in eukaryotic cells is contained in the polynucleotide sequences of the DNA located within the nucleus. Smaller, albeit important, amounts of DNA are contained within the mitochondria (mtDNA) and the centriole. Replication of the DNA in all three of these organelles is a prerequisite for mitosis. Many cellular and environmental factors are known to affect the rates of DNA synthesis. The actual factors that control DNA synthesis are not yet defined; however, this important problem is the subject of extensive investigation.[44, 73, 76, 111] Elucidation of the molecular processes that control the rates and duration of DNA synthesis is essential for the comprehension of overgrowth and undergrowth as a cause of many oral facial anomalies.

DNA is a large polymeric molecule composed of individual subunits called nucleotides. Each nucleotide has a carbohydrate residue called deoxyribose, a phosphate group, and either a purine or pyrimidine base, all covalently linked. The deoxyribose and the phosphate portion of the nucleotide form the repeating backbone structure of the DNA helix; the purines (adenine and guanine) and pyrimidines (thymidine and cytosine) follow a defined sequence along the helix. The sequence of nucleic acid bases that comprise the DNA macromolecule determines the genetic information (Table 1-2).

The nucleic acid bases have characteristic properties to pair with each other through specific hydrogen bonds. Adenosine always pairs to thymidine; guanine pairs with cyto-

Table 1-2. Genetic information: base pairings of nucleic acid biosynthesis

$DNA \rightarrow DNA$	$DNA \rightarrow RNA$
A-T	A-U
G-C	G-C
C-G	C-G
T-A	T-A

DNA contains genetic information determined by the precise sequence of purines, adenosine (A) and guanine (G), and pyrimidines, cytosine (C) and thymidine (T), nucleotide bases. DNA forms the template from which other nucleic acid molecules of precise structure can be synthesized. The purine of the DNA chain will pair only with other purine bases. The obligatory base pairings are described above in this table. The constraints of base pairing specifics allow specific genes to determine the nucleotide or base sequences in synthesized complementary molecules of DNA or RNA. Replication defines DNA-directed synthesis of complementary DNA molecules as during cell division in which the mother cell will produce two identical daughter cell progeny (DNA → DNA). The *transfer* of information from DNA to RNA involves no change of language (nucleotide → nucleotide) and is called *transcription*. *Translation* describes the transfer of information from RNA to a polypeptide (protein) and involves *new* language (nucleotide → amino acid). In addition, isolated RNA molecules can be used to serve as a template to synthesize a reversed transcript of DNA (cDNA). RNA → DNA is mediated by an enzyme called RNA-dependent DNA polymerase or *reverse transcriptase*.

sine. Adenosine and thymidine are associated by two hydrogen bonds, whereas cytosine and guanine base pair with three hydrogen bonds. These diagnostic characteristics clearly demonstrate how a polymer (polynucleotide) made from a sequence of nucleic acid bases can be biochemically constructed from inherited or acquired genetic information. The specific sequence of hydrogen bonds, either two or three together, along a linear sequence of nucleotides, is the precise method by which DNA stores information ionically in the hydrogen bond (Fig. 1-16).

The property of nucleic acid base pairing demonstrates an additional characteristic of profound importance in understanding genetics. Base pairing permits a polynucleotide to pair with another polynucleotide molecule

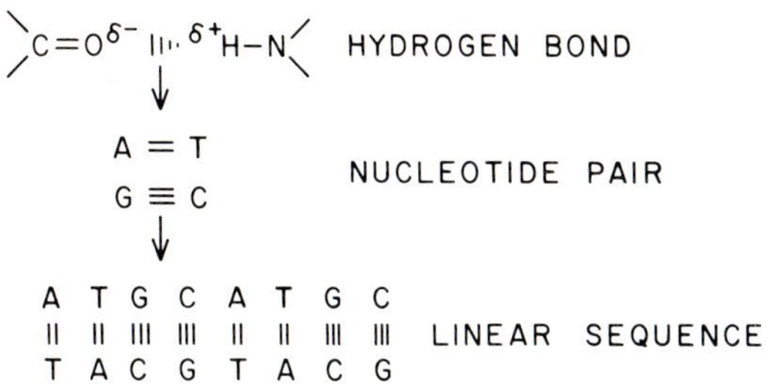

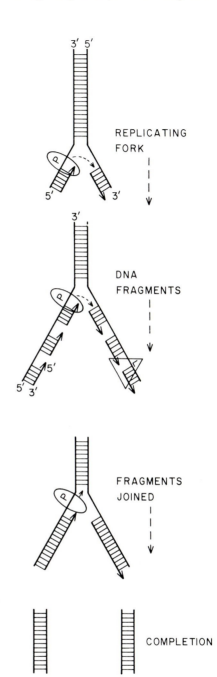

$$\text{C}=\text{O}^{\delta-} \text{ III} \cdot \cdot \delta^{+} \text{H}-\text{N} \quad \text{HYDROGEN BOND}$$

$$\text{A} = \text{T}$$
$$\text{G} \equiv \text{C} \quad \text{NUCLEOTIDE PAIR}$$

$$\text{A T G C A T G C}$$
$$\text{II II III III II II III III} \quad \text{LINEAR SEQUENCE}$$
$$\text{T A C G T A C G}$$

Fig. 1-16. Representation of hydrogen bond, the type of binding energy by which nucleotide bases pair. Oxygen atom, *O,* with slightly negative, δ⁻, charge is attracted to slightly positive, δ⁺, charge on hydrogen atom, *H.* Adenine, *A,* and thymidine, *T,* pair with two of these bonds, guanine, *G,* and cytosine, *C,* with three hydrogen bonds. DNA and RNA are linear sequences of nucleotide pairs. Hydrogen bonding pattern stores genetic information ionically.

complementary to itself or to act as the template replicating itself. Two complementary DNA molecules (polynucleotides) form the unique structure of the double helix DNA molecule. Replication occurs when the double helix separates, and single nucleotides pair with each of the two DNA strands resulting in nucleotides that are covalently joined together by DNA polymerase (Fig. 1-17). A necessary condition for DNA replication is that the DNA molecule must have two free ends, a 5′ (phosphate) end, and a 3′ (hydroxyl) end. During replication, DNA polymerase migrates in the 5′ → 3′ direction. The DNA polymerase synthesizes a short sequence of DNA on one strand of the double helix, then jumps the replicating fork and synthesizes another short sequence on the other complementary strand (Fig. 1-17). The short sequences are then joined together by DNA ligase III.

The DNA polymerases and DNA ligases are actually classes of enzymes because many different enzymes have been isolated that have the same apparent function. These enzymes are functionally dependent on a variety of substrates and ligands. The enzyme dependence on substrates and ligands infers still another possible group of factors that may affect or control DNA synthesis: the nucleotide triphosphates (dATP, dTTP, dCTP, dGTP),

Fig. 1-17. Illustration of DNA replication. Replicating fork forms when double helix unwinds and polymerase, *P,* attaches to 5′ end. Enzyme translocates in 5′→3′ direction, synthesizing short segment of DNA, then polymerase jumps replicating fork and synthesizes another short segment of DNA on sister strand of replicating DNA double helix. DNA short fragments are subsequently joined together by DNA ligase, *L.* Process continues until DNA molecule is completely replicated.

ATP as an energy source, divalent cations (Ca++, Mg++), and the DNA template.

The DNA-synthesizing enzymes are proteins synthesized on the polysomes in the cytoplasm. An important experimental question is concerned with the dependence of DNA synthesis on protein synthesis. Does the inhibition of protein synthesis by specific compounds, such as puromycin, inhibit DNA synthesis? No! DNA synthesis is initiated irrespective of potein synthesis. This observation implies that the enzymes necessary for initiating DNA synthesis are usually present before DNA replication.[73]

Polymerases and almost all enzymes are dependent on an energy source for their respective functions. The energy necessary to drive the chemical reactions is usually supplied in the form of a high-energy phosphate bond in adenosine triphosphate (ATP). ATP is generated through the complex molecular processes of glycolysis and oxidative phosphorylation in mitochondria. Mitochondria depleted of a carbon energy source stop producing ATP. If cells are grown in vitro and if the carbon energy source is depleted from the culture medium, the cells reinitiate growth and DNA synthesis. Although the presence or absence of glucose determines whether DNA synthesis will or will not occur, the concentration of glucose, within limits, has no effect on the rates of DNA synthesis. The interpretation of this and ancillary data is that glucose in the cell medium does affect DNA synthesis, but it does not control DNA synthesis. Additional experimentation on nutritional factors, such as amino acids and vitamins, has provided the same types of conclusions. Nutrients are necessary for DNA synthesis but generally have no regulatory control over differential DNA synthesis.[73]

Polymerases require cations (Ca++, Mg++) for enzymatic functions. On removal of divalent ions, the enzymes cease to function. An experiment designed to test the removal of the divalent cations from the medium with a chelating agent (EDTA) demonstrated that DNA synthesis stopped but RNA and protein synthesis continued. The inhibition was reversed by adding zinc to the medium.

These observations demonstrated that the divalent ion concentrations within the cell have the capacity to affect enzyme function and possibly control enzyme activity.[73]

The ionic and nutrient composition of the cytoplasm is greatly affected by the extracellular matrix environment. If all the surfaces of a cell are free or open to the environment, then the passage of molecules through the membrane can occur unhindered. But if a cell growing in vitro is bordered on all sides by other cells, growth and DNA synthesis is inhibited. The phenomenon is called *density-dependent inhibition,* a property not characteristic of cancer cells. Normal cells growing in vitro on artificial tissue culture dishes stop growing when the surface of the dish is saturated or confluent with cells, even if the culture medium has an adequate supply of nutrients. The molecular nature of density-dependent inhibition of cell growth is not understood. An explanation may be that the nutrients in the culture medium, which are necessary for growth, no longer have free access to the cell. Most cell surfaces would be blocked by contact with other cells and by contact with the solid substrate on which the cells are growing. An alternative explanation is that there may be an interaction of specific cell surface molecules on one cell with complementary cell surface molecules on a neighboring cell, which has the effect of inhibiting cell growth. It is, in essence, a sensing mechanism that allows the cells to determine whether they have a neighbor and whether the neighbor cell properties are conducive to optimal cell function.[3, 15, 36, 51]

The presence of these cell surface molecules has been hypothesized and tested in a variety of ways. The lectin concanavallin A (Con A) is a plant protein that binds to specific carbohydrate moieties on the outer cell surface.[15, 54] The carbohydrate is attached covalently to cell surface glycoproteins. Con A, when bound to a cell in culture, inhibits growth of the cells. Sulfated polysaccharides bound to cell surfaces also inhibit cell growth. Trypsin, a proteolytic enzyme that removes glycoproteins from cell surfaces, stimulates cell growth in vitro. Therefore most cell biologists concur that substances that specifically interfere with cell surface properties have the effect of stimulating or suppressing cell growth, depending on the type of treatment.[73] The identification and structure of these specific cell surface molecules is yet to be determined.

The integration of the basic cellular functions of metabolism, ion flux, and nutritional requirements with specific environmental cues mediated through the cell surface is probably the primary manner in which cell growth, DNA replication, and mitosis are controlled. The physical separation of any one cellular function or the chemical inhibition of a cellular function undoubtedly affects the cellular growth. Ultimately, the genes are responsible for cell growth. Within the genes is coded the information necessary for the synthesis of the many proteins functioning in the process of cell growth and cell division.[6, 15, 52, 69]

GENE REGULATION AND TRANSCRIPTION

The control mechanism for differential gene expression in animal cells is not entirely clear. The nucleus contains the genome of the cell. Each somatic cell nucleus is equivalent in terms of the content of inherited genetic information. The nuclear membrane surrounding the nucleus compartmentalizes the cell with definitive effects on the transport of unstable nuclear RNA transcripts from the nucleus to the cytoplasm. Most of the synthesized heterogeneous nuclear RNA in mammalian cell nuclei is unstable, and the kinetics of turnover have been studied in numerous laboratories throughout the world.[20] The differential transport of this population of heterogeneous and somewhat unstable nuclear RNA from the nucleus to the cytoplasm is a critical step in regulation. The spectrum of mRNA transcripts that are selectively transported to the cytoplasm for subsequent translation into polypeptides, which serve as enzymes, structural intracellular proteins, secreted extracellular matrix macromolecules, cell surface glycoproteins, or chromosomal proteins, must be responsible for the basic

biochemical differences that exist among tissues throughout the forming embryo.

The process of differentiation is that set of reactions which enables somatic cells, each containing identical nuclear DNA sequences, to express phenotypically distinct patterns of constitutive proteins. The differences in gene activity that initiate and maintain distinct cell protein profiles at different stages of embryonic development in mammals and in different tissues throughout the forming embryo, involve regulatory mechanisms. Regulation obviously operates at the levels of DNA replication, gene activation, RNA transcription, selective modification and transport of RNA molecules from the nucleus into the cytoplasm, differential stabilities of the mRNAs, and the fidelity of translation and subsequent posttranslational modifications of the polypeptide gene product. Normal craniofacial development requires, therefore, that the pattern of protein molecules characteristic for each of the tissue types associated with processes such as primary palate formation and tooth development (that is, epithelial-mesenchymal interactions), involves a dynamic equilibrium representing the summation of regulation at all levels cited.[18, 29, 37, 69, 90]

Defining the unit of gene expression

Defining the unit of gene expression is a most important issue in contemporary molecular biology. Recent advances have identified the sequences of polynucleotides that represent structural genes.* These investigations have also made significant progress in determining the nature and distribution of other sequences of polynucleotides.

Conventional genetic studies have demonstrated that a mutation at a particular point on the gene could alter the structure of all the protein molecules coded by it. The data available clearly support the generalization that related protein species (globin, enamel protein, elastin, type I collagen, myosin, actin, dentin, phosphoprotein, and types II, III,

---

*See references 8, 13, 14, 19-21, 38, 46, 50, 55, 60, 65, 70, 77, 80, 84, 100, 105, 111.

Table 1-3. Transcriptional activity of nonrepeated DNA base sequences in mammalian embryonic development*

Source of RNA	Percentage of DNA hybridized
Blastocyst	0.8 to 1.0
Organogenesis (10 to 12 days in mouse embryo)	7.0
Parturition (newborn mouse)	10.0 to 12.0

*See references 7, 13, 14, 38, 46, 70, 80, 84, 100, 105, and 107 for further details.

and IV collagen) are coded for by a single structural gene in the haploid genome.[46] Hybridization experiments using purified mRNAs with DNA support this conclusion.[13, 14, 20, 80] With the exception of the histone mRNAs, which have been demonstrated to be repeated some 500 to 1000 times in the genome, all specific mRNA species appear to be derived either from nonrepeated sequences or infrequently repeated sequences.[13, 14, 20, 21, 46] This information must be considered tentative, however, since so few species of mRNA have been isolated. At this time it would be reasonable to assume that most structural genes are either not repeated at all or that they are represented only a few times in the genome.[46, 100]

How many genes are contained within the total genome in man? Estimates of the number of genes in any eukaryotic cell type can at best be only imprecise. In man this estimate would suggest that the number is in the order of 50,000 genes.[8] A theoretical estimate of the number of genes in man in the haploid genome would be three million.[8, 46, 100, 111] This speculative estimate will have to suffice until it becomes technically possible to determine whether all of the repetitive and nonrepetitive sequences in the genome code for proteins, or whether only a certain percentage of the total sequences actually code for a specific species of protein (Table 1-3).

Localization of specific genes

Minimum estimates of the number of active genes can be derived by examining the nature of the sequences represented in the cellular population of mRNAs. This number is substantial. For example, at the 600-cell stage of development in sea urchin embryos, the sequence complexity corresponds to about 13,000 genes.[8, 13, 14] This calculation is made by determining the amount of polysomal associated mRNAs per cell. It is reasonable to project that a somewhat larger number of genes would be expressed in later stages of embryonic development and still later in the mature adult tissues (Table 1-9).

The complexity of the genome in higher organisms argues strongly for the anticipation of an equally complex regulation for transcription in the genome of mammalian embryos (Table 1-3). Genome complexity can be defined as the number of distinct DNA base sequences present in the haploid sperm complement of a species.[46] The complexity of the genome is further increased by the relative size of the genome. The average mammalian cell nucleus contains 6×10^{-12} grams of DNA per somatic cell, which is equivalent to 4.5 to 5.0×10^9 nucleotide pairs.* On the basis of reassociation kinetics of sheared, single-stranded DNA from various higher organisms, it has been repeatedly shown that the genome contains various classes of reiterated or repeated sequences and nonrepeated, unique, or single-copy DNA base sequences.[84, 111]

Before continuing this discussion we will digress and briefly emphasize that much of the nomenclature and many of the functional attributes ascribed to sequences of DNA are *operational conventions* based on the currently available technology. Defining the units of gene expression and localizing specific structural genes are distinctions that are as yet only *operational*. The considerations that suggest the functional and structural heterogeneity in chromatin within the animal cell nucleus are (1) limited transcription as measured by RNA-DNA hybridization (for example, total isolated cellular RNA hybridized at saturation to less than

*See references 8, 13, 14, 20, 21, 38, 46, 49, 50, 65, 70, 80, 84, 100, 105, 107, 111.

10% of nuclear DNA), suggesting a severe restriction in DNA transcription, (2) thermal denaturation profiles of DNA and circular dichroic spectral analyses of DNA (for example, both criteria indicate two different general structural conformations), and (3) electron-microscopic studies of isolated nuclei, chromatin, and native DNA, which have demonstrated variable fiber widths and variability in regions of extended and coiled chromatin (that is, extended and condensed regions).* In addition, the reassociation profiles of a number of different DNAs according to the C_0t nomenclature have recently provided a laboratory method to study the relationship between the second-order reassociation kinetics of any population of nucleotide sequences and the size of the genome.[13, 14] For example, the AT-rich satellite sequence of DNA isolated from the total mouse genome on cesium chloride gradients has been shown to reassociate approximately 10^6 times faster than the major component of the mouse genome.[80] The estimate is derived from highly reproducible comparisons between the percent of reassociated material per C_0t (defined as moles × seconds per liter). By conventional definition, the AT-rich DNA fractions contain nucleotide sequences that were present in one million copies per genome.[8, 80] The relationship between genome size and complexity, as seen in reassociation kinetic studies, holds only for sequences that are present once per genome; the unique, nonrepeated sequences are assumed to contain the structural genes.[46] Using this convention, therefore, investigations have determined that the reiterated DNA base sequences constitute from 10% to 60% of the total mammalian genome.[80] To date, the available data indicate that there are three classes of base sequence reiteration frequency in the mammalian genome.

The *first class* contains a rapidly renaturing fraction equal to 6% to 9% of the genome.[46] This fraction reassociates 10^6 times faster than one would expect for base sequences that appear only once in the genome.[13, 14, 46, 50, 111] These are called highly repetitive sequences and apparently do not transcribe into RNA species in any tissues at any stage of development. These sequences appear to be located morphologically within the centromere and telomere regions of mammalian chromosomes.[46]

The *second class* of rapidly reassociating DNA sequences equals 20% to 25% of the total genome.[80] The *third class* comprises 60% to 70% of the genome and consists of sequences that renature at a rate that is consistent with the second-order kinetics predicted for the entire mammalian genome, assuming that each sequence is present only once per haploid genome.[80] These are called the nonrepeated, unique, or single-copy DNA base sequences (Tables 1-3 and 1-4).

Clearly it is evident to the nonspecialist that the kinetics of reassociation can only begin to approximate the frequency of sequence reiteration in the mammalian genome and the average number of repetitions. These values are not absolutes, and much depends on the stringency of the conditions and methods prevailing during reassociation and during hybridization experiments. Hybridization establishes the degree of complementarity between base sequences needed for reaction and defines experimentally how closely related sequences must be to constitute a family. What defines the function of such a family? How long is a repeating unit? What is the degree of repetition? Is there interspersion among nonrepetitive and repetitive sequences? It must be emphasized that the relatively low RNA concentrations that can be isolated and characterized for each species of mRNA, the short reaction times, the relatively nonspecific reassociation conditions, the methods for obtaining different C_0t values of DNA, the thermal stability of RNA/DNA and DNA/DNA hybrids, the concentration of salts and organic solvents in the reaction mixtures, and the definition of the nucleic acid fragment size are but a few of the technical difficulties associated with interpreting the data obtained in a qualitative manner. The experimental limitations imposed by the complexity of the

---

*See references 13, 19, 38, 46, 50, 65, 70, 84, 105.

mammalian genome must be carefully considered when appreciating the advances of cellular, molecular, and developmental biology.[8, 21, 55, 75, 85]

Recent advances in gene regulation

The understanding of the control processes underlying mammalian development will ultimately be derived from the accumulation of information from various mammalian experimental systems, the studies of comparative and experimental embryology, and the contributions of genetics and molecular and developmental biology. Because of the small size of the mammalian egg, the difficulties of obtaining large numbers of embryos for experimentation, the problems associated with culturing preimplantation embryos, and the limitations of available techniques, the biochemical basis of embryogenesis in mammals has not yet been studied in the same detail that has characterized the biochemistry of prokaryotes. However, considerable progress in understanding mechanisms of differential gene activity in the preimplantation and early postimplan-

Table 1-4. Nuclear and polysomal heterogeneous RNA associated with poly(A) sequences in preimplantation mammalian embryos

RNA source	Percentage associated with poly(A)
2-day nuclear RNA	5.5 to 16.3
4-day nuclear RNA	8.2 to 8.8
6-day nuclear RNA	7.5 to 11.6
2-day polysomal RNA	62.0 to 81.0
4-day polysomal RNA	55.0 to 96.0
6-day polysomal RNA	60.0 to 77.5

Messenger RNAs are generally associated with poly-(A) sequences. Nuclear and polysomal mRNAs containing poly(A) sequences were prepared from embryos labeled in vitro with tritiated uridine in the presence of actinomycin D sufficient to inhibit rRNA synthesis. The data are expressed as the percentage of radioactive labeled mRNA associated with poly(A) as defined by molecules adhering to a nitrocellulose acetate filter (Millipore filter method) or by an assay using poly(U) fiberglass. See references 7, 46, 49, 50, 61, 65, 80, 84, 105, 107, and 111.

tation embryo has been made (Tables 1-3 and 1-4).[80]

The molecular details of RNA synthesis have been established in bacteria, and the process is similar to DNA synthesis (Fig. 1-18). There is one important exception: RNA synthesis has specific start and stop signals. The start signal on the DNA is recognized by a 90,000 dalton protein called the sigma (σ) factor, which initially binds

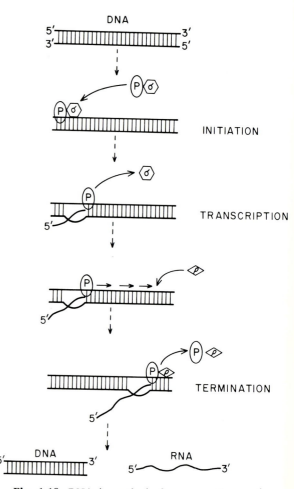

Fig. 1-18. RNA is synthesized as copy of one of DNA template strands. Sigma (σ)-RNA polymerase, *P,* complex binds to initiation site on DNA molecule. After RNA synthesis commences in $5' \rightarrow 3'$ direction, sigma is released. RNA polymerase transcribes along DNA strand until reaching rho (ρ) factor (termination signal), then polymerase-rho complex and newly synthesized RNA molecule are released from rewound DNA.

to the RNA polymerase core enzyme, after which the complex binds to the DNA. The DNA sequence unwinds, and RNA synthesis is initiated on only one of the DNA strands in a 5′ → 3′ direction. The sigma factor then dissociates from the transcribing complex. Transcription continues until the polymerase reaches a stop signal, mediated by a protein called the rho (ρ) factor.[111] The RNA molecule is displaced by the rewound DNA double helix. The molecular system of RNA synthesis in animal cells is probably similar to that described for bacteria, but the start and stop signals may be much more complex.

Some of the regulatory mechanisms involved in the process of cell differentiation in craniofacial embryonic development include (1) activation of structural genes in chromatin,* (2) qualitative changes in RNA transcriptional products brought about either by specificity of initiation site of each transcriptional unit or by RNA polymerase activity differences,† (3) the cleavage, selection, and maturation of potential mRNAs from the intranuclear pool of unstable HnRNAs,‡ (4) the differential transport of potential mRNAs containing poly(A)-rich segments from the nucleus to the cytoplasm, which can be mediated by hormones§ (for example, hydrocortisone induction of glutamine synthetase in embryonic retinal cells,[54, 77] insulin induction of crystallin synthesis in lens epithelium, hormonal regulation of ovalbumin synthesis,[61, 65] or thyroxin induction of collagenase during tadpole tail metamorphosis) or by physiological conditions in the immediate extracellular matrix microenvironment‖ (for example, changes in anions or cations,[39, 73] macromolecules that serve as constituents of the protein matrices,[41] types of collagen,¶ vascularization,

mineralization, and calcification, proteoglycans, or glycosaminoglycans,[41] and (5) the functional half-life of mRNA in the cell, including the differential stability and storage of mRNA molecules in the cytoplasm.[20, 46]

Recent advances in molecular biology suggest that nonhistone chromosomal proteins (acidic chromosomal proteins) determine the specificity in chromatin of RNA synthesis in eukaryotic cell differentiation.[5] The relevant experiments that formulated this suggestion have included (1) fractionation of chromatin into three constituents (DNA, histones, and nonhistone chromosomal acidic proteins), (2) reconstitution of homologous and heterologous chromatins by dialysis of the required components from 6M urea and 2M NaCl into 0.2M NaCl, (3) transcription of native and reconstituted chromatin with bacterial RNA polymerase, and (4) characterization of the nucleotide sequences in the synthesized RNA transcript by RNA/DNA hybridization methods.* The nonhistone proteins were found to be organ specific and to demonstrate both greater diversity and more demonstrable tissue specificity than histones.[5, 50, 84, 105]

The discovery of RNA-dependent DNA polymerase (reverse transcriptase) in RNA viruses suggested a method for measuring concentrations of specific mRNAs.[49, 61, 69] It is also interesting to note that reverse transcriptase has been demonstrated in various RNA virus–induced tumors,[49, 82] leukemia, and within "normal" embryonic avian, mammalian, and primate tissues[82] in the apparent absence of RNA viruses.[93] Type C viruses have been clearly implicated as a cause of certain types of cancer. RNA viruses contain an enzyme called RNA-dependent DNA polymerase, which functions to transcribe the viral RNA into the genome of the host cell DNA. Recent evidence suggests that RNA tumor virus (type C viruses) genes have been maintained as stable endogenous genetic elements in primates, including man, for 40 million years.[93] This evidence raises the possibility that RNA viruses can transmit

---

*See references 5, 13, 19, 21, 49, 50, 70, 80, 100, 105, 107.
†See references 7, 9, 20, 43, 46, 53, 55, 56, 60, 61, 65, 71, 73, 79, 84, 101, 111, 114.
‡Heterogeneous nuclear RNAs; see references 20, 46, 55, 58, 65, 72.
§See references 2, 27, 34, 60, 61, 78.
‖See references 1, 3, 6, 15, 18, 40, 42, 44, 45, 47, 51, 52, 54, 67, 75, 76, 81, 86, 92, 106.
¶See references 16, 17, 31, 62, 98, 102, 108.

---

*See references 5, 13, 14, 21, 38, 46, 49, 50, 60, 61, 63, 65, 70, 80, 84, 100, 105, 111.

themselves between the inherited DNA of different species (for example, mouse, cat, pig, old-world primates, new-world primates, and man) and can also carry genetic messages from cell to cell within the same organism during embryogenesis as well as during postnatal development and maturation.[49, 92, 93]

The discovery of reverse transcriptase activity challenged the central dogma of DNA → RNA. Isolated RNA species could be experimentally used as a template to synthesize a DNA copy in vitro (cDNA). Conditions were determined to isolate various specific mRNAs that could also stimulate the reverse transcriptase to copy the isolated mRNA into a base pair specific DNA transcript (Table 1-5). For example, it was possible to isolate globin mRNA and, with the reverse transcriptase, to make a complementary DNA product synthesize in vitro from radioactive nucleic acid precursors. This technique provided an extremely sensitive probe for globin mRNA.[49] The cDNA probe was then used to measure the concentrations of globin-specific sequences in chromatin transcripts. In this erythropoietic system, the nonhistone acidic chromosomal proteins were demonstrated to be required for the activation and expression of the globin genes in native and reconstituted chromatin.[46]

Three classes of nuclear DNA sequences

were previously discussed. The most highly repetitive sequences fall into a distinct class of simple-sequence, noncoding DNA satellites that appear to occur in long uninterrupted segments of the genome. In contrast, moderately repetitive DNA sequences appeared to occur in short segments intimately interspersed with unique sequences. The structural genes for most proteins, such as collagens,[62] keratin,[38] elastin, globin, ovalbumin,[61, 65] actin, or myosin, are to be found in the unique sequences. The genes for ribosomal RNA (rRNA) and histones are moderately repetitive sequences and occur as tandem repeats in the DNA. Recently, Kemp[38] demonstrated that unique and repetitive sequences in multiple genes for feather keratin are present in the avian genome. The mRNA coding for embryonic chick feather keratin polypeptides has been obtained in a pure form and transcribed into cDNA using reverse transcriptase from an avian virus.[38] The kinetics of reassociation, reannealing, and hybridization of cDNA indicated that there were 25 to 35 different keratin mRNA species in the chick embryonic feather and a total of 100 to 240 keratin genes in the chick genome.[38] Each keratin gene contained both a unique and a repetitive sequence. Current evidence suggests that the repetitive sequences contain the

Table 1-5. Molecular properties of isolated eukaryotic messenger RNAs

Cell	Protein	Coding length*	mRNA length†	Poly(A) length‡
Rabbit blood cell	Globin	430	550 to 650	40
Mouse myeloma	Light Ig	660	1200 to 1300	200
Mouse myeloma	Heavy Ig	1350	1800	150 to 200
Chick oviduct	Ovalbumin	1164	1670 to 2640	Not known
Calf lens epithelia	α A2-crystallin	520	1460	200
Calf lens epithelia	γ-crystallin	1260	2000	Not known
Silk gland epithelia	Fibroin	14,000	16,000	100
Sea urchin	Histone f2a1	310	370 to 400	None
Chick feather epithelia	Keratin	300 to 400	500 to 800	∼ 200

*The coding lengths represent the number of nucleotides required to specify for each protein and were estimated from the number of amino acids and the molecular weight of the protein.
†The lengths of mRNA were determined experimentally; where more than one value is presented, there were independent determinations.
‡The poly(A) length varies with the age of the mRNAs (generally in terms of minutes to hours).
See references 20, 38, 46, 49, 60, 61, 65, 70, 80, 84, and 105 for details of procedures.

keratin genes with coding sequences and that the unique sequences correspond to unactivated or untranslated regions.[38]

TRANSLATIONAL CONTROLS AND PROTEIN SYNTHESIS

As a start toward defining the mechanisms that control gene expression during early craniofacial development, it is both useful and necessary to quantitate each of the parameters that govern the concentration of a specific gene product within a specific population of cells. Gene products are proteins defined by the primary sequence of amino acids that constitute the molecule. Estimates of the rate of synthesis and degradation of the specific protein and its mRNA are imperative. Analysis of these parameters (1) under steady-state conditions, (2) when the specific protein concentrations change during normal differentiation and cell interactions, and (3) when the specific protein concentrations are altered due to teratogens (for example, corticosteroids and the induction of cleft lip and palate in mammals), all provide valuable clues concerning the rate-limiting steps in transcription and translation and how these steps may be controlled (Figs. 1-18 to 1-20).

Consider for a moment the exact molecular details involved in the complex series of events that are responsible for protein synthesis (Fig. 1-20). Ribosomes are composed of two smaller subunits, one 30S and the other 50S in size.[20, 58] The subunits are dissociated when not actively synthesizing a polypeptide, but when protein synthesis is initiated, the subunits come together in a stepwise manner. The primary event is the activation of the tRNAs with the appropriate amino acid. The tRNA polynucleotide chain is folded into a cloverleaf form with one of the loops containing the three-lettered *anticodon*, which is a sequence of three nucleotide bases that are complementary to the *codon* on the mRNA. Each amino acid has a unique set of codons and a unique set of tRNA molecules to which they become covalently bound (Table 1-6). The amino acids attach through their carboxyl groups to the 3′ terminal adenosine of tRNA molecules by high-energy covalent bonds. There is a specific group of proteins, the amino acyl synthetases, which catalyze the reaction of the tRNA to the amino acid. Each amino acid has its own synthetases and tRNA with which it can combine. After the tRNA and the amino acid are bound, the unit is activated. The tRNA activation step is believed to be one of the points in the molecular process of protein synthesis that has the possibility of being a rate-limiting control step.

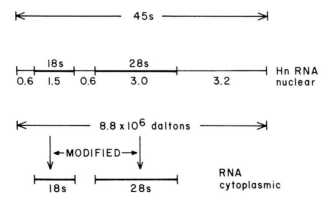

Fig. 1-19. Example of nuclear modification of heterogenous nuclear RNA (HnRNA). In this case ribosomal RNA (rRNA) is initially synthesized as single 48s HnRNA molecule, which is enzymatically modified into two RNA molecules, 18s and 28s in size.

Protein synthesis cannot proceed without tRNA activation. The activated tRNA then moves to the ribosome and positions the amino acid so that it can be incorporated into the growing polypeptide chain.[20]

All mRNA chains have a common initial codon that signifies protein synthesis initiation.[111] The codon is AUG or GUG. The 30S ribosomal subunit and an initiation factor, a protein called F3, recognizes the initiation

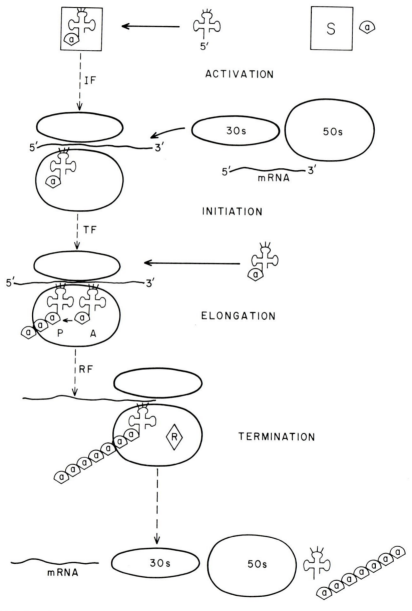

Fig. 1-20. Proteins are synthesized through complex series of macromolecular reactions. Transfer RNA (tRNA) is activated by synthetase, *S,* which covalently binds amino acid, Ⓐ, to tRNA, ⌘. Ribosomal subunits 30s and 50s complex in stepwise manner with mRNA and tRNA and several initiation factors, *IF.* Polypeptide is elongated by sequential addition of amino acids in order specified in codon-anticodon interaction of mRNA and tRNA, enzymatically catalyzed by translocation factors, *TF.* Polypeptides are terminated and ribosomal complex is disaggregated by releasing signal, *R,* and releasing factors, *RF.*

Table 1-6. The genetic code: examples of the biochemical language

DNA (codons)	→mRNA (codons)	→tRNA (anticodons)	→Amino acids
AAA	UUU	AAA	phe
AAC	UUG	AAC	leu
GAA	CUU	GAA	leu
ACC	UGG	ACC	try
GGT	CCA	GGU	pro
CCG	GGC	CCG	gly

The complementarity between DNA, mRNA, and tRNA codons and anticodons that are specific for amino acids is shown. There are two or more codons for some of the amino acids as indicated for leucine.

codon and binds to it.[58] The necessity of the formation of an initiation complex introduces another translational rate-limiting control step. If the initiation codon is masked, then the initiation complex can be recognized neither by the initiation factor nor by the ribosomal subunit.[33, 111]

In bacteria and animal cells the first amino acid on a growing polypeptide chain is N-formyl-methionine. Its tRNA anticodon recognizes the AUG or GUG initiation codon; a reaction catalyzed by two or more initiation factors and the energy from the high-energy phosphate bond is GTP. Subsequently, the 30S subunit, the activated N-formyl-methionine-tRNA, and the mRNA are complexed. The 50S ribosomal subunit binds to the complex, and protein synthesis is in progress.[111] Each ribosome has two functional sites: A (amino acyl) and P (peptidyl). The activated tRNA binds to the A site only when the codon on the mRNA and the anticodon on the tRNA are complementary. The activated tRNA translocates to the P site during the process of polypeptide chain elongation; this is the addition of tRNA's amino acid to the growing polypeptide chain. After the amino acid is transferred from the tRNA to the ribosome, the tRNA is rejected from the P site. These transfer steps all require additional proteins called transfer factors and energy in the form of GTP.

The codons on the mRNA are read in the $5' \rightarrow 3'$ direction. The message is continuously read until the chain termination signal is reached. Two conditions are necessary for chain termination, (1) the termination codon and (2) a protein-releasing factor. The newly formed polypeptide chain is then released from the ribosome.

In numerous cell types associated with the formation of the developing craniofacial complex, proteins are involved as extracellular macromolecules and participate in the architecture of those extracellular matrices which subsequently mineralize and calcify (chondrogenesis, amelogenesis, dentinogenesis, and osteogenesis). Extracellular proteins are generally glycosylated with the exception of albumin. After the release of the polypeptides from the ribosomes, often associated with the rough endoplasmic reticulum (RER), polypeptides accumulate in the RER cisternae and are transported to the Golgi apparatus, where a multienzyme complex (xylose transferase, glycosyltransferases, galactosyltransferases) is involved with glycosylation. The glycosylated proteins are subsequently packaged for export in secretory vesicles or granules, possibly sulfated and/or phosphorylated, and then secreted from the cell by reverse pinocytosis characteristic of merocrine-type secretory cells (acinar cells in the salivary glands, odontoblasts and dentin formation, chrondroblasts and cartilage formation, fibroblasts and collagen fibril formation, osteoblasts, and osteoid formation).

Posttranscriptional control of protein synthesis in bacteria seems to be confined to the possible existence of messenger or cistron-specific initiation factors and their modification after phage infection.[111] In animal cells, however, where the site of transcription is physically separated by the nuclear membrane surrounding the nucleus from the translational protein synthesizing apparatus in the cytoplasm, there is the possibility of more complex forms of control.*

---

*See references 9, 10, 20, 26, 31, 33, 43, 55, 56, 72, 79.

Studies of translational control require extreme accuracy. For example, these experiments require that both the quantitative yield of protein be assayed and the efficiency of translation or the fidelity of the translational process be determined. Therefore the specific mRNA must be isolated in a pure form, the concentration of functional mRNA available for translation must be defined, the number of complete polypeptides released from each polysomal mRNA per minute must be experimentally determined, and the rate of polypeptide synthesis per unit of time can then be calculated on a per-cell basis. This is extremely difficult to do for many reasons. One principle that has emerged from the study of RNA metabolism in animal cells is that all of the major classes of RNA species (mRNA, rRNA, and tRNA) are initially synthesized in the nucleus (Fig. 1-19) as largely precursor molecules and undergo a complex process of nucleolytic cleavage before becoming functional in the cytoplasm.[20] Only a small percentage of the initially synthesized heterogeneous nuclear RNAs are stable and are transported into the cytoplasm.*

Despite these requirements, recent advances in cellular and molecular biology have provided investigators with sensitive radioimmunoassays with which to detect specific polypeptides synthesized in small amounts and radioactively labeled cDNA probes with which to detect specific mRNA molecules. For example, it has recently been demonstrated that the absolute rate of a specific polypeptide synthesis is controlled primarily by the cellular concentration of that specific mRNA.[33, 61, 65] It has also been found that certain hormones that bind to specific intracellular receptors stimulate translational efficiency.† Estrogen-stimulated ovalbumin synthesis in chick oviduct reaches a level of 6×10^5 molecules/minute/cell and can be accounted for by a single ovalbumin gene per haploid genome being transcribed at 35% of maximal efficiency.[65] The essential point appears to be that animal cells, unlike bacteria,

exhibit an adaptation that allows a high degree of specialization in the synthesis of a single polypeptide that is crucially dependent on the stability of the mRNA. The half-life of mRNA in animal cells is about a thousand times longer than that typical for bacterial mRNA. In contrast, the differences in translational efficiency are threefold higher in bacteria. The reader is encouraged to further explore this fascinating problem area* and to judiciously consider the steroidal controls on cellular proliferation during organogenesis throughout the forming mammalian embryo,[65] intercellular interactions associated with tissue morphogenesis,† cranial neural crest migrations,[37, 112, 113] the formation of unique extracellular organic matrices, and the formation of the peripheral and central nervous systems[83] and their respective influences on translational efficiency.

EXTRACELLULAR MATRIX INFLUENCES ON GENE EXPRESSION

The discussion presented so far within this chapter has introduced the general themes of selected types of developmental investigations designed to explore the regulation of gene expression in mammalian embryonic cells. Although the genetic code itself is now well understood, the actual mechanisms permitting differential gene expression remain somewhat obscure. How is gene expression controlled? It should be apparent that numerous questions remain unanswered concerning this problem. If each somatic cell nucleus contains identical biparentally inherited concentrations of DNA, how is cell diversity achieved in the early stages of embryogenesis? What regulates the timing of embryogenesis? What initiates and terminates gastrulation? Transcription and translation describe the processes by which specific structural genes are expressed into specific polypeptides. What regulates which genes are expressed and when? All osteoblasts, for example, contain the same genetic material

---

*See references 20, 46, 50, 55, 80, 105, 111.
†See references 33, 46, 60, 61, 65, 77.

*See references 1, 11, 20, 25, 27, 33, 34, 46, 50, 61, 65, 73, 80.
†See references 1, 4, 36, 37, 42, 69, 93.

and can be identified on the basis of their various intracellular metabolic patterns (receptors to parathyroid hormone, synthesis of bone phosphoprotein, synthesis of bone type I collagen, nuclear polarity, distribution of the RER and Golgi apparatuses, the release of matrix vesicles associated with nucleation of mineralization, and the calcium pump making available amorphous calcium ions to participate in the formation of calcium hydroxyapatite crystals). What determines the shape and other macroscopic characteristics of the occipital bone, maxilla, mandible, temporal bone, frontal bone, femur, tibia, ulna, or ethmoid processes? In addition to the synchronous expression of structural genes during development in specific cell populations, what regulates cell-to-cell interactions, cell migrations, cell density, histogenesis, organogenesis, morphogenesis, and the general features of the organism?

Cell migrations

Understanding those processes which shape the embryo requires the synthesis of evidence derived from many different investigations.* These studies include three-dimensional reconstructions from serial sections of embryos, tritiated-labeled thymidine autoradiography, cell aggregations, organ dissociation studies, heterologous tissue recombinations, cell sorting experiments, time-lapse cinephotomicrography, transmission electron microscopy, freeze-etching, and, more recently, scanning electron microscopy of early stages of embryonic development (Fig. 1-21). It is evident that the highly regulated cell and tissue movements are controlled by intercellular contacts, specialized intercellular junctions, and the intimate interactions among and between cells and their immediate extracellular matrix substratum. Soluble hormones, growth factors, relatively insoluble macromolecules within the extracellular organic matrices, cell surface proteases and protease inhibitors, cell surface receptor

*See references 1, 3, 4, 6, 11, 15, 26, 27, 32, 36, 37, 39-42, 44, 47, 51, 52, 54, 59, 66, 67, 73, 75, 91, 96, 106, 112, 113.

molecules, and cell surface differentiation alloantigens each mediate many of the temporal and spatial aspects of cell migrations and the resulting morphogenesis.* Molecules located in the plasma membrane of cells can serve as receptors that can be mobile in a fluid surface membrane.[6, 15, 54] Molecules that can bind specifically and reversibly to carbohydrate-containing sites located on the outer cell surfaces of the plasma membrane have been demonstrated to induce changes in the membrane and associated changes in the regulation of cell proliferation.[6, 15, 54]

Studies conducted on amphibian, avian,

*See references 6, 15, 37, 40, 44, 47, 51, 52, 54, 66, 67, 75, 112, 113.

Table 1-7. Cranial neural crest cell derivatives

Structures or tissues	Derivatives
Connective tissues	Intramembranous bones (osteoblasts)
	Dental papilla (odontoblasts)
	Visceral cartilage (chondroblasts)
	Sclera and choroid optic coats
	Anterior trabecular cartilage
	Meckel's cartilage (mandibular)
	Maxillary processes
	Hyoid arch cartilages
	Corneal mesenchyme
Sensory ganglia	Trigeminal (V)
	Geniculate (VII)
	Superior (root IX)
	Jugular (root X)
Parasympathetic (cholinergic) ganglia	Ciliary
	Ethmoid
	Sphenopalatine
	Submandibular
	Enteric system
Accessory cells	Glial cells
	Schwann sheath cells
Pigment cells	Melanophores in iris

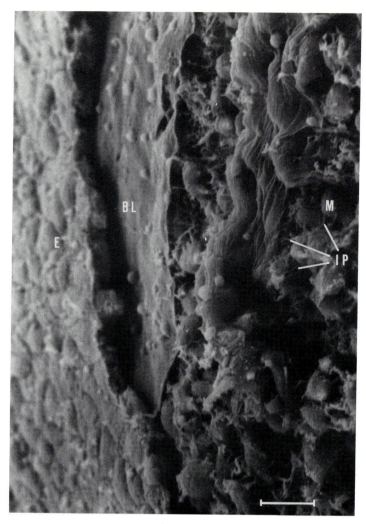

Fig. 1-21. Scanning electron photomicrograph of epithelial-mesenchymal interface in 11-day embryonic oral-nasal epithelium. Photomicrograph clearly demonstrates separation of epithelium, *E,* and mesenchyme, *M,* by basal lamina, *BL.* Epithelium is single layer of squamous cells, whereas mesenchyme cells are densely packed along basal lamina. There are many intercellular projections, *IP,* radiating out from mesenchymal cells. Bar line is 10.0 μm.

and rodent embryos have shown that facial mesenchyme and derived skeletal and connective tissues are of cranial neural crest origin.[37] Bone, cartilage, periodontal ligament, dentin, and gingival dermis are but a few of the numerous derivatives (Table 1-7) of cranial neural crest cells.[95] The cranial neural crest cells initiate their migrations from the dorsal aspect of the neural tube at about the time of neural tube closure.[37, 112, 113] The crest cells migrate in relatively cell-free spaces beneath the basal lamina-coated un-

dersurface of the surface ectoderm.[37] Are the crest cells predetermined before their extensive migrations? What determines their path of migration? Do they divide while in migration? Do the migrating crest cells synthesize and secrete extracellular macromolecules? These are but a few of the questions to which craniofacial biologists are currently seeking answers. Aberrations in cranial neural crest cell migrations can lead to a significant number of craniofacial anomalies expressed as malformations of the eyes, brain, and face as well as the dentition, palate, and pharynx.[37]

Failure of the crest cells to migrate results in characteristic brain-eye-face malformations.[37] Environmental hazards such as radiation, corticosteroids, and various other teratogens introduced into the forming mammalian embryo at the time of initial crest cell migrations often results in defects of the frontonasal processes such as clefts of the primary palate. It becomes imperative to attempt to define the time of teratogen administration and the timing of crest cell migration. Subtle differences involving only several hours produce profound craniofacial defects. What is being affected, and what is causal to the production of the malformation? is a question that should be asked when studying a patient with a craniofacial malformation.

Cell-to-cell and cell-to-matrix interactions

During early embryonic craniofacial development, one can easily observe that the cells that were clonal derivatives of a single cell, the zygote, continued to differentiate along divergent pathways. In this section the discussion is limited to how molecules of the cell surface of the plasma membrane interact with molecules associated with dissimilar cell surfaces and/or with relatively insoluble macromolecules associated with the extracellular matrix microenvironment. We will limit this discussion to recent developments in immunogenetics and morphogenesis.[6, 25] Our thesis suggests that the immunogenetics of outer cell surfaces reflects the phenotype of the cell, which can be experimentally explored to decipher the mechanisms that influence differential gene expression.

Cranial neural crest cells are the progenitor cells for facial ectomesenchyme.[37, 112, 113] The primary and secondary palate, Meckel's cartilage in the mandible, the dental papilla and odontoblasts, which secrete dentin matrix, the mesenchyme of the epidermis, which forms the lips, the sensory ganglia associated with the innervation of the oral facial region of the forming embryo, and many other derivatives result from crest cells. It is apparent that specific regions in the dorsal neural tube regions give rise to specific populations of crest cells that have spatially and temporally specific migratory pathways.[37, 112] However, the available data do not support the notion that the cranial neural crest cells are predetermined.[112, 113] It does not seem plausible that the entire program of morphogenesis is contained within the genome in the form of instructions for the destination of each premigratory crest cell.[36, 37, 50, 95, 112]

After fertilization, up to the eight-cell stage of mammalian embryogenesis, the individual blastomeres can regenerate an entire organism.[6, 11, 30] At more advanced stages, single cells from the inner surface of blastocysts can be experimentally repositioned in extremely different locations and acquire different characteristics.[6, 11, 30] Tooth organs consist of two different tissue types, (1) ectodermally-derived enamel organ epithelium and (2) cranial neural crest–derived ectomesenchyme dental papilla.[29, 86-99] During early odontogenesis, dental papilla mesenchyme can instruct nonoral, nontooth epithelium to differentiate into ameloblasts and secrete enamel matrix.[95] Embryonic chick feather mesenchyme can instruct embryonic mouse skin epithelium to form a feather, and mouse skin mesenchyme can instruct chick epithelium to form a hair follicle.[54, 95] These examples and numerous others clearly indicate that the development of complex organisms requires epigenetic mechanisms in addition to genetic factors to design and orchestrate embryogenesis.*

Two cells are considered to be *differentiated* when it can be determined that each cell contains identical genetic information, yet each cell synthesizes different proteins. Recent observations indicate that the exterior surfaces of differentiated cells contain information affecting both genotypic and phenotypic characteristics.[6, 54] During the actual assembly of cells into morphogenetic units, in addition to genetic determination, the epigenetic mechanisms mediated by cell

---

*See references 11, 30, 32, 40, 42, 51, 59, 67, 69, 73, 75, 87, 94, 95, 97-99.

position, time, cell densities, extracellular macromolecules, and ion concentrations are operant and provide additional modes of developmental instructions.[6, 54, 95] Immunogenetic studies of cell surface molecules and the new analyses of extracellular macromolecular heterogeneity are providing fresh insights into many important developmental questions.[4, 25, 54]

Gene products have been specifically located on the outer cell surfaces,[6, 25, 54, 95] which imparts phenotypic diversity to the cell surfaces of different populations of cells. Cell functions, such as cell division, can be modified by cell surface alterations of surface glycoproteins and exogenous molecules.[15] Phenotypically diversified cell types can recognize self and nonself in vitro and reassociate specifically according to phenotype (for example, heart, cartilage, skin, liver, brain).[54] Furthermore, if cells are synthesizing and secreting a specific gene product and are then repositioned to a different microenvironment (various macromolecular substrata), the phenotype can be altered to a different expression of a different set of structural gene products.* These findings are providing new avenues with which to explore the influence of epigenetic effects on gene expression.†

Extracellular matrix macromolecules

Throughout embryogenesis cells synthesize and secrete macromolecules. Hyaluronate, glycosaminoglycans, proteoglycans, collagen, elastin, keratin, albumin, various hormones, and many other molecules are synthesized and secreted by specific populations of cells at defined stages of development. The orchestration of synthesis and secretion must be precise and exquisite to prevent aberrations and resulting malformations. Recent advances in collagen and glycosaminoglycan biochemistry should provide the reader with a set of fresh insights into this fascinating research area.

---

*See references 30, 40, 42, 51, 75, 96.
†See references 4, 6, 11, 15, 25, 30, 32, 36, 39, 40, 42, 44, 45, 54, 59, 67, 71, 73, 74, 83, 91, 104, 106, 112, 113.

Collagen heterogeneity. Until 1969 it had been assumed that all collagens associated with vertebrate tissues consisted of a polymeric molecule containing two $\alpha1$ chains and one $\alpha2$ polypeptide chain. These three polypeptide chains were assembled to form the tropocollagen macromolecule. We now realize that there is considerable molecular heterogeneity in both polypeptide chain distribution and the amino acid sequence of the α chains.[88, 96, 102]

The most common type of collagen to be found in vertebrate tissues consists of two $\alpha1$ chains, each chain having an identical amino acid sequence, called $\alpha1$ (I), and a third polypeptide chain called $\alpha2$, which differs from the other two chains in amino acid sequence. The intact tropocollagen molecule is designated as $[\alpha1\ (I)]_2\ \alpha2$ or type I collagen. The ratio of $\alpha1:\alpha2$ polypeptide chains is 2:1. Combining results obtained by various tissue extraction schemes, solubility characteristics of these macromolecules, carboxymethyl cellulose column chromatography, sodium dodecyl sulphate polyacrylamide gel electrophoresis, cyanogen bromide degradation, immunological methods to produce specific antibodies directed against specific antigenic determinants in procollagen molecules, and several other methods have provided the developmental biologist with definitions for collagen heterogeneity (Table 1-8).

It is now evident that there are many different structural genes for collagen in vertebrate cells.[16, 17, 62, 96, 108] In addition to type I collagen requiring two different structural genes, type II collagen is found in cartilage and is designated as $[\alpha1\ (II)]_3$.[96] Cartilage collagen polypeptide chains are each identical yet genetically different from those chains that assembled to form type I collagen. A third type of collagen has recently been identified in embryonic human dermis, bovine periodontal ligament and cementum, aorta, and uterine leiomyoma, called $[\alpha1\ (III)]_3$.[16, 17] This is called type III collagen. Finally, a type IV collagen has been identified, which is found in basement membranes and basal lamina associated with many different types of epithelia, $[\alpha1\ (IV)]_3$.[96] These four different

Table 1-8. Collagen heterogeneity

Tissues	Collagen molecules	Collagen types	Developmental processes
Bone, cementum, dentin, gingival dermis, periodontal ligament, and skin dermis	$[\alpha 1 \ (I)]_2 \ \alpha 2$	Type I	Cementogenesis, fibrogenesis, osteogenesis, and dentinogenesis
Cartilage	$[\alpha 1 \ (II)]_3$	Type II	Chondrogenesis
Aorta, cementum, embryonic dermis, periodontal ligament, and uterine leiomyoma	$[\alpha 1 \ (III)]_3$	Type III	Fibrogenesis and cementogenesis
Basement membranes	$[\alpha 1 \ (IV)]_3$	Type IV	Basal lamina formation

Table 1-9. Regulation of collagen biosynthesis, intracellular transport, secretion, and extracellular fibril formation

Processes	Enzymes
Selection of structural genes	
Transcription	RNA polymerases
Translation of mRNAs into polypeptides*	
Hydroxylations	Peptidyl proline hydroxylase and peptidyl lysine hydroxylase
Molecular assembly	
Helix formation	
Glycosylations	Galactosyl transferase and glucosyl transferase
Procollagen-tropocollagen conversion	Procollagen peptidase(s)
Cross-linking	Lysyl oxidase

*Available data suggest that there are at least five different collagen structural genes in the mammalian genome.

collagen macromolecules require five different structural genes for their respective biosynthesis (Table 1-9).

It was historically assumed that mesenchymal cells or fibroblasts synthesized and secreted collagen. In light of our new understanding of collagen heterogeneity, one can enquire as to which cells secrete which types of collagen. Can one cell type express several different types of collagen? Can a single cell synthesize genetically distinct molecular species such as types I and II collagens? What epigenetic factors induce modulations in collagen synthesis? Do different molecular species of collagen function in differentiation, histogenesis, organogenesis, and morphogenesis? Might aberrations in transcription, translation, hydroxylation, glycosylation, collagen peptidase activity, or lysyl oxidase activity be determinants in craniofacial anomalies?

During embryonic tooth formation the inner enamel epithelium synthesizes and secretes both types I and IV collagen.[98, 108] The fibroblasts within the periodontal ligament appear to synthesize both types I and III collagen.[16] Chondroblasts in tissue culture appear to synthesize types I and II collagen.[45] An appreciable literature indicates that collagenase-labile molecules are prerequisite for normal differentiation, many different types of tissue interaction, and morphogenesis.[42, 45, 86, 91, 96] Recently, an intracellular form of collagen has been isolated and characterized, called *procollagen*. After transcription, the three polypeptide chains are translated on polyribosomes that contain additional peptide extensions attached distally as the NH_2-terminal telopeptides.[32] These telopeptides serve as registration peptides and provide the mechanism for each major collagen chain to be aligned with one another by disulfide bonds.[82] The amino acid composition of the registration peptides is not homologous to that of collagen; it is 3% glycine, 1% proline, six residues per thousand of half cystine, and detectable amounts of tryptophan.[88] Procollagen is the precursor form of tropocollagen.[102] After translation, helix assembly, glycosylation, and intracellular transport to the cell surface, the registration peptides are enzymatically cleaved by collagen peptidase during secretion of the the molecules into the extracellular matrix environment.[102] The extracellular macromolecule is approximately 300,000 daltons; each polypeptide chain is about 100,000 daltons. The intracellular procollagen molecule is approximately 450,000 daltons. In situ it requires approximately 20 to 30 minutes to transcribe the specific mRNAs, translate the messenger into polypeptide chains, hydroxylate the proline and lysine amino acid residues, form the triple helix, glycosylate the serine amino acids, package and transport the procollagen to the cell surface, digest the registration peptide with collagen peptidase, and secrete the tropocollagen into the environment, where it then participates in fibril formation and intramolecular and intermolecular crosslinks (Table 1-9). Although there appear to be few posttranslational modifications of most proteins after peptide bond formation, collagen biosynthesis has at least six posttranslational enzymatic alterations of the primary structure and at least three interchain and intermolecular interactions involving conformational changes and covalent bond formation before the protein is functional.[17, 31, 45, 62, 88]

In light of these findings it becomes most pertinent to study in detail such disorders as dermatosparaxis disease in cattle,[102] amelogenesis and dentinogenesis imperfecta, osteolathyrism, osteogenesis imperfecta,[62] Ehlers-Danlos disease,[62] Marfan's syndrome, and homocystinuria in man in an attempt to determine the basic defect in each. It is important to appreciate that different birth defects resulting from collagen aberrations may all manifest with similar clinical features, such as severe skeletal deformities, hyperextensibility of joints, and fragility of the connective tissues, especially in the joints, skin, eyes, and vascular system; however, the biochemical mechanisms that result in these lesions may be much different from one another.

Glycosaminoglycans. The extracellular matrix contains a variety of complex macromolecules, that serve crucial functions in cell differentiation and morphogenesis.[88] Many of these molecules are comprised of polysaccharides covalently linked to protein. Some confusion has existed in the literature regarding the nomenclature of acid mucopolysaccharides. The new terminology refers to "acid mucopolysaccharides" as *glycosaminoglycans (GAGs)*.[41, 88] GAGs are comprised of amino sugars (glycosamino-) and uronic acids (glycurono-) joined in long chains (-glycans).[41] Thus glycosaminoglycans consist of linear carbohydrate chains covalently linked to a protein core to form macromolecules called *proteoglycans*.[88] The substances classed as glycosaminoglycans include hyaluronic acid, chondroitin 4- and 6-sulfates, dermatan sulfate, heparin sulfate, and heparin and keratan sulfate (Table 1-10). Glycosaminoglycans possess structural heterogeneity and are polyanions by virtue of the numerous carboxylate groups, sulfate groups, or both, that are present in the molecule.[41] The polyanionic character of these molecules largely determines the nature of the interactions between proteoglycans and collagen, other glycoproteins, and ions within the extracellular matrix environment.[41] Substances that stain metachromatically are polyanionic and of high molecular weight. Cationic dyes (that is, toluidine blue and methylene blue) stain GAGs metachromatically and can be used diagnostically along with other criteria to assay for excess intracellular or extracellular glycosaminoglycan accumulation.

The major precursors of glycosaminoglycan synthesis are uridine nucleotide sugars. The individual sugars (mannose, glucose, galactose, xylose, fructose) are sequentially transferred by glycosyltransferases (a multienzyme complex located within the Golgi apparatus) from their UDP derivatives to growing glycosaminoglycan chains.[45] Unlike proteins and nucleic acid biosynthesis, the ordering of the sugar sequence in GAG is not specified by a template (mRNA or DNA) but rather by the specificity of the individual enzymes that are membrane-bound

Table 1-10. Glycosaminoglycans: nomenclature and composition

Compounds	Abbreviations	Monosaccharides—repeating units	Linkage to protein
Hyaluronic acid	HA	D-Glucosamine and D-Glucuronic acid	
Chondroitin	Ch	D-Galactosamine and D-Glucuronic acid	-GlcUA-Gal-Gal-Xyl-Ser
Chondroitin 4-sulfate	C-4-S	D-Galactosamine and D-Glucuronic acid	-GlcUA-Gal-Gal-Xyl-Ser
Chondroitin 6-sulfate	C-6-S	D-Galactosamine and D-Glucuronic acid	-GlcUA-Gal-Gal-Xyl-Ser
Dermatan sulfate	DS	D-Galactosamine and L-Iduronic acid or D-Glucuronic acid	-GlcUA-Gal-Gal-Xyl-Ser
Heparin sulfate	HS	D-Glucosamine and D-Glucuronic acid or L-Iduronic acid	-GlcUA-Gal-Gal-Xyl-Ser
Heparin	Hep	D-Glucosamine and D-Glucuronic acid or L-Iduronic acid	-GlcUA-Gal-Gal-Xyl-Ser
Keratan sulfate I*	KS-I	D-Glucosamine and D-Galactose	-GLcNAc-Asp
Keratan sulfate II*	KS-II	D-Glucosamine and D-Galactose	-GalNac-Ser/thr | Gal-NANA

*Although keratan sulfates are not glycosaminoglycans per se, they are glycoproteins that share many properties with GAG.

in the Golgi apparatus and which catalyze transfer of the monosaccharide to the growing chain.

Significant advances in understanding glycosaminoglycan synthesis have been derived from studies of chondrogenesis.[45] The core protein and glycosyl transferase enzymes are translated into proteins by membrane-bound ribosomes in the rough endoplasmic reticulum. The initiation of GAG chains and synthesis of the linkage region occurs in the cisternae of the rough endoplasmic reticulum.[45] Chondroitin chain formation proceeds while the membrane-associated macromolecule is transported from the rough into the smooth endoplasmic reticulum and Golgi apparatus.[45] Sulfation occurs in the Golgi region.[45] The product is packaged in secretory vesicles derived from the Golgi apparatus, which are subsequently secreted by reverse pinocytosis into the extracellular matrix.

At least a dozen different mucopolysaccharidoses have been described.[41] Hunter's, Hurler's and Sanfilippo's syndromes, the Maroteaux-Lamy syndrome, β-glucuronidase deficiency, and Morquio's syndrome illustrate many of the salient features of these genetic defects in glycosaminoglycan biosynthesis and secretion. Such patients are moderately dwarfed, present grotesque facial features, joint stiffness, deafness, mental retardation, corneal clouding, and often vascular diseases.[41] Recent research in the molecular biology of GAG-related genetic diseases indicates that the critical deficiency in Hunter's syndrome is probably a sulfatase, which can be treated by the Hurler corrective factor, which is a heat-labile protein molecule of 65,000 daltons.[41] This factor has been found to also demonstrate α-L-iduronidase activity and can be transferred from normal to abnormal fibroblasts in tissue culture under defined conditions.[41] Despite this controversial observation, the accumulation of glycosaminoglycans during embryogenesis and growth is a major molecular lesion in development that remains somewhat obscure.

IMMUNOGENETICS AND CRANIOFACIAL ANOMALIES

Immunogenetics provides methods for answering questions concerning the structural organization of the outer cell surface and genetic and epigenetic controls. Recent advances have resulted from studies designed to establish a direct relationship between specific genes and identifiable cell surface gene products.[6] The methods using alloimmunization (immunization within the same species but using genetically defined strains of animals) provided opportunities to identify polymorphic antigens localized on the cell surfaces with particular genes. These cell surface alloantigens have been identified with serological methods, immunochemistry, and the use of immunoelectron microscopy. A number of genetically different antigens can be recognized on the surfaces of differentiated cells (for example, theta, histocompatibility alloantigens, and TL antigen on thymocytes).[6] The qualitative or quantitative representation of these alloantigens can be used to characterize the phenotype of individual cell types. The antigens are arranged on the surface in a mosaic pattern. Epigenetic influences modulate their expression. Therefore one can predict that early stages of craniofacial development might proceed on the basis of cell recognition mediated by progressively changing patterns of the cell surface molecules (that is, differentiation alloantigens).

Embryonic cells possess mechanisms for mutual recognition and selective adhesion. Cell recognition functions in integrating and ordering different cells within the embryo, and it enables cells with different surface specificities and affinities to aggregate into tissues.[54] These specificities reside in the cell surface and are expressed during development. As cells divide and diversify, discrete molecules, complementary to the cell pheno-

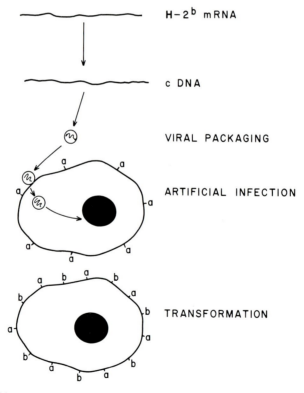

$H-2^b$ mRNA

c DNA

VIRAL PACKAGING

ARTIFICIAL INFECTION

TRANSFORMATION

Fig. 1-22. Graphic representation of future mechanism for genetic engineering. In this case, cell that has $H-2^a$ cell surface molecules is transformed into $H-2^{a/b}$ haplotype cell. From $H-2^b$ mRNA molecule is made cDNA molecule by using enzyme reverse transcriptase. cDNA is packaged into a viral assembly, and artificial virus is used to infect cell. cDNA is incorporated into infected cell's genome, resulting in modified genotype expressing new phenotype on cell surface.

type, are localized on the surface, resulting in differential cell affinities and adhesiveness.

In mice both the T locus and the H-2 locus have been implicated as containing genes controlling embryogenesis by coding for differentiation alloantigens located on the cell surface.[6, 54] Both the T locus and the major histocompatibility locus (H-2) are located in the IX murine chromosome linkage group[6] (Fig. 1-22). The T locus and the H-2 locus have been directly linked to congenital anomalies in mice including craniofacial anomalies such as microcephaly, anophthalmia, adontia, microphthalmia, and otocephaly. Recent immunogenetic observations have suggested that cleft lip and palate susceptibility traits in congeneic strains of mice are associated with the major H-2 locus.[11, 78] Corticosteroid-induced cleft palate frequency in congeneic hybrids demonstrated that the H-2 haplotype specificity of the mother significantly determined either resistance or susceptibility to craniofacial anomalies[11] (Table 1-11).

Recent studies have demonstrated a resemblance between the mouse (H-2) region and the human major histocompatibility region (HL-A).[110] As in the mouse, the human locus includes two loci that determine serologically detectable HL-A antigens.[6] Both mouse and human histocompatibility antigens are located on the cell surfaces. HL-A is not sex-linked and, therefore, resides on one of twenty-two autosomal chromosomes.[110] The HL-A system consists of two loci designated LA and FOUR, which are analogous to the D and K regions of the mouse H-2 system.[110] Pedigree data have demonstrated that LA and FOUR loci are closely linked and that each of these two loci has a distinct set of alleles that appear to be codominant.[110] Two or more alleles at a single locus occurring with an appreciable frequency in one animal population represent genetic polymorphism. There are at least thirty HL-A antigens.[110] Terasaki has postulated that antibodies produced by the mother against incompatible HL-A antigens of the developing fetus may have deleterious effects resulting in congenital malformations.[103] Since 1971, the statistical association between HL-A antigens and numerous congenital anomalies has been unequivocally established.[110]

SUMMARY

How is gene expression controlled and what determines the distribution of molecules in and among differentiating cells are two of the most important questions in craniofacial developmental biology. An answer to the first question would explain how various cell types within a forming organism synthesize different proteins and thereby products of different enzyme-controlled reactions. At present little can be stated on the second question, since most of the available data are as yet descriptive. This introductory chapter to oral facial genetics has attempted to present salient and selected problems in craniofacial developmental biology.

Table 1-11. Cleft palate frequency in four inbred, H-2–defined strains of mice

Strain	H-2 haplotypes	Number of litters	Viable fetuses at day 17	Cortisone (2.5 mg day 1)	Percent cleft palate
A/J	H-2[a]	10	72	2.5	99
A/J	H-2[a]	6	40	0*	4
B6	H-2[b]	6	34	2.5	25
B6	H-2[b]	5	41	0*	ND†
B10	H-2[b]	8	50	2.5	22
B10	H-2[b]	5	31	0*	ND
B10.A	H-2[a]	11	86	2.5	81
B10.A	H-2[a]	4	27	0*	ND

*Sterile saline injected.
†Not detected.

Obvious limitations necessitated a format designed to provide the reader with an orientation to many of the major questions being explored in this field. Transcription is probably the level at which gene expression is principally controlled during development.[11] At the level of transcription, it now seems useful to regard genes as functioning in two classes whose transcription is regulated in different ways: (1) those genes potentially active in all somatic cell types which are present in multiple copies in the genome and whose transcription is limited in some manner other than by template availability and (2) those genes which are expressed in only a limited number of cell types, genes which are present in only one or a few copies per genome, and whose transcription is limited by template availability. Genes in the second class include enamel protein, five different collagen structural genes, globin, ovalbumin, and keratin, whereas genes in the first class would constitute all of the housekeeping genes essential for intracellular metabolism and cell division. If unique genes are regulated by the availability of template, one must predict that gene-specific molecules interact with these structural genes and activate gene function. Recent data indicate that the nonhistone acidic chromosomal proteins are, in principle, capable of fulfilling this function as regulators

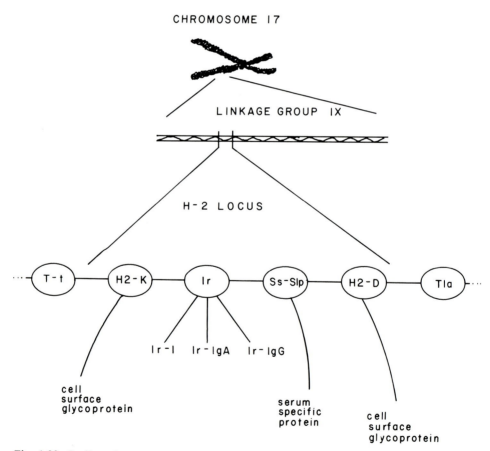

Fig. 1-23. Outline of components of H-2 locus in mouse. K and D cell surface glycoproteins are antigens about 60,000 daltons in molecular size. *Ir* region elicits and controls immune response against series of known immunological determinants. *Ss-Slp* region codes for many components of complement found in serum. *H-2* locus is bordered on one side by *T-t* locus and on other side by *Tla* locus.

of gene activity in eukaryotic cells.[5, 19, 21]

Embryonic development can be visualized as a series of interactions between a nucleus and a changing cytoplasmic environment, rate-limiting steps associated with transcription and translation, cell surfaces and extracellular matrix macromolecules, and the obscure parameters of spatial, temporal, and positional information.[104] Understanding these interdependent parameters should provide significant advances in our abilities to prevent craniofacial anomalies.

In addition to providing more understanding into human biology and improving the diagnosis and treatment of genetic diseases, an increased understanding of the reproductive process also has profound social and political significance for the human condition.[22, 23, 26, 85] Recent advances in somatic cell hybridization,[71, 74] gene transplantation[24, 28, 49] (Fig. 1-23), RNA viral transformation,[82] hormonal induction of ovulation, artificial insemination, nuclear transplantation,[53, 79] cloning methods, amniocentesis, enzyme therapy,[81] contraceptive technology, and genetic counseling[57] now present an awesome responsibility to the biomedical professional community.[85] The potential hazards of genetic and population engineering necessitate an enlightened social awareness and confrontation with complex ethical issues.[109] Although as yet remote, the possible hazards to society of genetic engineering or mass screening to detect persons with specific mutant genes as a technique of disease prevention are serious issues now demanding the enquiry of an informed public and the biomedical professional community. Clearly there is an immediate and imminent requirement for an improved knowledge of genetics among scientists, physicians, dentists, pharmacists, nurses, and clients to improve the quality and perceptions of health care delivery.

REFERENCES

1. Agarwal, M. K.: Intercellular interactions in eukaryotic homeostasis, Differentiation **2:** 371, 1974.
2. Agarwal, M. K.: Chromatographic demonstration of mineralocorticoid-specific receptors in rat kidney, Nature **254:**623, 1975.
3. Aidley, D. J.: The physiology of excitable cells, New York, 1971, Cambridge University Press.
4. Auerbach, R.: Development of immunity. In Lash, J., and Whittaker, J. R., editors: Concepts of development, Stamford, Conn., 1974, Sinauer Associates, pp. 261-271.
5. Barrett, T., Maryanka, D., Hamlyn, P. H., Gould, H. J.: Nonhistone proteins control gene expression in reconstituted chromatin, Proc. Natl. Acad. Sci. U.S.A. **71:**5057, 1974.
6. Bennett, D., Boyse, E. A., and Old, L. J.: Cell surface immunogenetics in the study of morphogenesis. In Silvestri, L. G., editor: Cell interactions, Amsterdam, 1972, North-Holland Publishing Co., pp. 247-263.
7. Bernstein, R. M., and Mukherjee, B. B.: Cytoplasmic control of nuclear activity in preimplantation mouse embryos, Dev. Biol. **34:**47, 1973.
8. Bishop, J. O.: The gene numbers game, Cell **2:**81, 1974.
9. Bock, R. M.: The multiple relations of tRNA to metabolic control. In Hay, E. D., King, T. J., and Papaconstantinou, J., editors: Macromolecules regulating growth and development, New York, 1974, Academic Press, Inc., pp. 181-190.
10. Boell, E. J., and Greenfield, P. C.: Mitochondrial differentiation during animal development. In Weber, R., editor: The biochemistry of animal development, New York, 1975, Academic Press, Inc., pp. 337-387.
11. Bonner, J. T.: On development, the biology of form, Cambridge, Mass., 1974, Harvard University Press.
12. Bonner, J. T., and Slavkin, H. C.: Cleft palate susceptibility linked to histocompatibility-2 (H-2) in the mouse, Immunogenetics **2:**213, 1975.
13. Britten, R. J., and Davidson, E. H.: Gene regulation for higher cells: a theory, Science **165:**349, 1969.
14. Britten, R. J., et al.: Studies of the molecular organization of genetic material. In Motulsky, A. G., and Lenz, W., editors: Birth defects, New York, 1974, American Elsevier Publishing Co., Inc., pp. 21-31.
15. Burger, M. M.: Role of the cell surface in growth and transformation. In Hay, E. D., King, T. J., and Papaconstantinou, J., editors: Macromolecules regulating growth and development, New York, 1974, Academic Press, Inc., pp. 3-23.
16. Butler, W. T., Birkedal-Hanse, H., and Taylor, R. E.: Proteins of the periodontium: the chain structure of the collagens of bovine

cementum and periodontal ligament. In Slavkin, H. C., and Greulich, R. C., editors: Extracellular matrix influences on gene expression, New York, 1975, Academic Press, Inc., pp. 371-378.

17. Chung, E., Kinsey, R. W., and Miller, E. J.: Biosynthesis of type III collagen: relative insolubility of the molecules synthesized in the presence of a lathyrogen. In Slavkin, H. C., and Greulich, R. C., editors: Extracellular matrix influences on gene expression, New York, 1975, Academic Press, Inc., pp. 285-292.

18. Croissant, R., Guenther, H., and Slavkin, H. C.: How are embryonic preameloblasts instructed by odontoblasts to synthesize enamel? In Slavkin, H. C., and Greulich, R. C., editors: Extracellular matrix influences on gene expression, New York, 1975, Academic Press, Inc., pp. 515-521.

19. Cummings, E. D.: The role of heterochromatin. In Motulsky, A. G., and Lenz, W., editors: Birth defects, New York, 1974, American Elsevier Publishing Co., Inc., pp. 44-52.

20. Darnell, J. E., Jelinek, W. R., and Molloy, G. R.: Biogenesis of mRNA: genetic regulation in mammalian cells, Science **181:**1215, 1973.

21. Davidson, E. H., and Britten, R. J.: Molecular aspects of gene regulation in animal cells, Cancer Res. **34:**2034, 1974.

22. Dubos, R. J.: Medical utopias. In Beecher, H. K., editor: Disease and the advancement of basic science, Cambridge, Mass., 1960, Harvard University Press, pp. 391-404.

23. Dubos, R. J.: A God within, New York, 1972, Charles Scribner's Sons.

24. Dutrillaux, B.: New techniques in the study of human chromosomes. In Motulsky, A. G., and Lenz, W., editors: Birth defects, New York, 1974, American Elsevier Publishing Co., Inc., pp. 59-72.

25. Edelman, G. M.: Variability symmetry and periodicity in the structure of immunoglobins. In Silvestri, L. G., editor: Cell interactions, New York, 1972, American Elsevier Publishing Co., Inc., pp. 73-90.

26. Edwards, R. G.: Advances in reproductive biology and their implication for studies on human congenital defects. In Motulsky, A. G., and Lenz, W., editors: Birth defects, New York, 1974, American Elsevier Publishing Co., Inc., pp. 92-104.

27. Filburn, C. R., and Wyatt, G. R.: Developmental endocrinology. In Lash, J., and Whittaker, J. R., editors: Concepts of development, Stamford, Conn., 1974, Sinauer Associates, pp. 321-348.

28. Gray, J. W., et al.: Chromosome measurement and sorting by flow systems, Proc. Natl. Acad. Sci. U.S.A. **72:**1231, 1975.

29. Guenther, H. C., Croissant, R. D., Schonfeld, S. E., and Slavkin, H. C.: Enamel proteins: identification of epithelial specific differentiation products. In Slavkin, H. C., and Greulich, G. R., editors: Extracellular matrix influences on gene expression, New York, 1975, Academic Press, Inc., pp. 287-397.

30. Hamburgh, M.: Theories of differentiation, New York, 1971, American Elsevier Publishing Co., Inc.

31. Harwood, R., Grant, M. E., and Jackson, D. S.: Post-translational processing of procollagen polypeptides. In Peeters, H., editor: Protides in biological fluids, Oxford, England, 1975, Pergamon Press, Ltd., pp. 83-85.

32. Hay, E. D.: Cellular basis of regeneration. In Lash, J., and Whittaker, J. R., editors: Concepts of development, Stamford, Conn., 1974, Sinauer Associates, pp. 404-428.

33. Hogan, B. L. M.: Post-transcriptional control of protein synthesis. In Weber, R., editor: The biochemistry of animal development, vol. 3, Molecular aspects of animal development, New York, 1975, Academic Press, Inc., pp. 183-216.

34. Hsueh, A. J. W., Peck, E. J., and Clark, J. H.: Progesterone antagonism of the oestrogen receptor and oestrogen-induced uterine growth, Nature **254:**337, 1975.

35. Hutchison, C. A., III, Newbold, J. E., Potter, S. S., and Edgell, M. H.: Maternal inheritance of mammalian mitochondrial DNA, Nature **251:**536, 1974.

36. Johnson, K. E.: Gastrulation and cell interactions. In Lash, J., and Whittaker, J. R., editors: Concepts of development, Stamford, Conn., 1974, Sinauer Associates, pp. 128-148.

37. Johnston, M. C., and Pratt, R. M.: The neural crest in normal and abnormal craniofacial development. In Slavkin, H. C., and Greulich, R. D., editors: Extracellular matrix influences on gene expression, New York, 1975, Academic Press, Inc., pp. 773-778.

38. Kemp, D. J.: Unique and repetitive sequences in multiple genes for feather keratin, Nature **254:**573, 1975.

39. Klein, N. W.: Protein nutrition in growth regulation during early development. In Weber, R., editor: The biochemistry of animal development, vol. 3, Molecular aspects of animal development, New York, 1975, Academic Press, Inc., pp. 293-336.

40. Konigsberg, I. R., and Buckley, P. A.: Regulation of the cell cycle and myogenesis by cell-medium interaction. In Lash, J., and Whittaker, J. R., editors: Concepts of devel-

opment, Stamford, Conn., 1974, Sinauer Associates, pp. 179-196.

41. Lamberg, S. I., and Stoolmiller, A. C.: Glycosaminoglycans: a biochemical and clinical review, J. Invest. Dermatol. **63:**433, 1974.

42. Lash, J.: Tissue interactions and related subjects. In Lash, J., and Whittaker, J. R., editors: Concepts of development, Stamford, Conn., 1974, Sinauer Associates, pp. 197-320.

43. Leenders, H. J., et al.: Nuclear-mitochondrial interactions in the control of mitochondrial respiratory metabolism, Subcell. Biochem. **3:**119, 1974.

44. Levin, S., Pictet, R., and Rutter, W. J.: Control of cell proliferation and cytodifferentiation by factor reacting with the cell surface, Nature New Biol. **246:**49, 1973.

45. Levitt, D., Ho., P. L., and Dorfman, A.: Differentiation of cartilage. In Moscona, A. A., editor: The cell surface in development, New York, 1974, John Wiley & Sons, Inc., pp. 101-126.

46. Lewin, B.: Units of transcription and translation: the relationship between heterogeneous nuclear RNA and messenger RNA, Cell **4:**11, 1975.

47. Loewenstein, W. R.: Cell-to-cell connections. In Silvestri, L. G., editor: Cell interactions: third lepetit colloquim, New York, 1972, American Elsevier Publishing Co., Inc.

48. Margolis, L.: Origin of eukaryotic cells, New Haven, 1970, Yale University Press.

49. Marks, P. A., et al.: Isolation and synthesis of human genes. In Motulsky, A. G. and Lenz, W., editors: Birth defects, New York, 1974, American Elsevier Publishing Co., Inc., pp. 73-80.

50. McCarthy, B. J., and Janowski, M.: The structural basis of selective gene expression. In Hay, E. D., King, T. J., and Papaconstantinou, J., editors: Macromolecules regulating growth and development, New York, 1974, Academic Press, Inc., pp. 201-216.

51. McMahon, D.: A cell-contact model for cellular position determination in development, Proc. Natl. Acad. Sci. U.S.A. **70:**2396, 1973.

52. McMahon, D.: Chemical messengers in development: a hypothesis, Science **185:**1012, 1974.

53. Merrill, C. R., Grier, M. R., and Trigg, M. E.: Transduction in mammalian cells. In Motulsky, A. G., and Lenz, W., editors: Birth defects, New York, 1974, American Elsevier Publishing Co., Inc., pp. 81-91.

54. Moscona, A. A.: Surface specification of embryonic cells: lectin receptors, cell recognition and specific cell ligands. In Moscona, A. A., editor: The cell surface development, New York, 1974, John Wiley & Sons, Inc., pp. 67-100.

55. Nemer, M.: Molecular basis of embryogenesis. In Lash, J., and Whittaker, J. R., editors: Concepts of development, Stamford, Conn., 1974, Sinauer Associates, pp. 101-118.

56. Neubert, D., Gregg, C. T., Bass, R., and Merker, H.-J.: Occurrence and possible functions of mitochondrial DNA in animal development. In Weber, R., editor: The biochemistry of animal development, vol. 3, Molecular aspects of animal development, New York, 1975, Academic Press, Inc., pp. 388-466.

57. Niswander, J. D.: Genetics of common dental disorders, Dent. Clin. North Am. **19:**197, 1975.

58. Nomura, M.: Biosynthesis of bacterial ribosomes. In Hay, E. D., King, T. J., and Papaconstantinou, J., editors: Macromolecules regulating growth and development, New York, 1974, Academic Press, Inc., pp. 195-199.

59. Nossal, G. J. V.: The biological basis of histocompatibility and its implication for development and tissue grafting. In Motulsky, A. G., and Lenz, W., editors: Birth defects, New York, 1974, American Elsevier Publishing Co., Inc., pp. 105-113.

60. Ohno, S.: Single gene translational control of testerone "regulon." In Silvestri, L. G., editor: Cell interactions: third lepetit colloquium, New York, 1972, American Elsevier Publishing Co., Inc., pp. 105-113.

61. O'Malley, B. W., et al.: Hormonal control of oviduct growth and differentiation. In Hay, E. D., King, T. J., and Papaconstantinou, J., editors: Macromolecules regulating growth and development, New York, 1974, Academic Press, Inc., pp. 53-80.

62. Orkin, R. B. W., et al.: Function of the genetically distinct collagens. In Slavkin, H. C., and Greulich, R. C., editors: Extracellular matrix influences on gene expression, New York, 1975, Academic Press, Inc., pp. 795-798.

63. Oudet, P., Gross-Bellar, M., and Chambon, P.: Electron microscopic and biochemical evidence that chromatin structure is a repeating unit, Cell **4:**281, 1975.

64. Painter, R. G., Sheetz, M., and Singer, S. J.: Detection and ultrastructural localization of human smooth muscle myosin-like molecules in human non-muscle cells by specific antibodies, Proc. Natl. Acad. Sci. U.S.A. **72:**1359, 1975.

65. Palmiter, R. D.: Quantitation of parameters that determine the rate of ovalbumin synthesis, Cell **4:**189, 1975.

66. Pichichero, M. E., and Avers, C. J.: The evolution of cellular movement in eukaryotes: the role of microfilaments and microtubules, Subcell. Biochem. **2:**97, 1973.

67. Pitts, J. D.: Direct interaction between animal cells. In Silvestri, L. G., editor: Cell interactions: third lepetit colloquium, New York, 1972, American Elsevier Publishing Co., Inc., pp. 277-285.

68. Porter, K. R. and Bonneville, M. A.: Fine structure of cells and tissues, Philadelphia, 1968, Lea & Febiger.

69. Pratt, R. M., and Martin, G. R.: Epithelial cell death and cyclic AMP increase during palatal development, Proc. Natl. Acad. Sci. U.S.A. **72:**874, 1975.

70. Purdue, M. L.: Repeated DNA sequences in the chromosomes of higher organisms. In Motulsky, A. G., and Lenz, W., editors: Birth defects, New York, 1974, American Elsevier Publishing Co., Inc., pp. 32-43.

71. Ringertz, N. R.: Cell differentiation analyzed by somatic hybridization. In Moscona, A. A., editor: The cell surface in development, New York, 1974, John Wiley & Sons, Inc., pp. 273-282.

72. Rolleston, F. S.: Membrane-bound and free ribosomes, Subcell. Biochem. **3:**9, 1974.

73. Rubin, H.: Regulation of animal cell growth. In Cox, R. P., editor: Cell communication, New York, 1974, John Wiley & Sons, Inc., pp. 127-146.

74. Ruddle, F. H.: Cell fusion as a tool in the study of cellular biology. In Motulsky, A. A., and Lenz, W., editors: Birth defects, New York, 1974, American Eisevier Publishing Co., Inc., pp. 53-58.

75. Rutter, W. J., Pictet, R. L., and Morris, P. W.: Toward molecular mechanisms of developmental processes, Ann. Rev. Biochem. **42:**601-646, 1973.

76. Rytomaa, T.: Control of cell division in mammalian cells. In Balls, M., and Billett, F. S., editors: The cell cycle in development and differentiation, Cambridge, England, 1973, Cambridge University Press, pp. 457-472.

77. Sarkar, P. K., and Moscona, A. A.: Binding of receptor hydrocortisone complexes to isolated nuclei from embryonic neural retina cells, Biochem. Biophys. Res. Commun. **57:**980, 1974.

78. Saxen, I.: Effects of hydrocortisone on the development in vitro of the secondary palate in two inbred strains of mice, Arch. Oral Biol. **18:**1469, 1973.

79. Schjeide, O. A.: Nuclear-cytoplasmic transfers. In Schjeide, O. A., and deVellis, J., editors: Cell differentiation, New York, 1970, Van Nostrand Reinhold Co., pp. 169-198.

80. Schultz, G. A., and Church, R. B.: Transcriptional patterns in early mammalian development. In Weber, R., editor: The biochemistry of animal development, vol. 3, Molecular aspects of animal development, New York, 1975, Academic Press, Inc., pp. 48-90.

81. Scriber, C. R.: Enzyme therapy and induction in genetic disease: pox or pax. In Motulsky, A. G., and Lenz, W., editors: Birth defects, New York, 1974, American Elsevier Publishing Co., Inc., pp. 114-128.

82. Sherr, C. J., Benveniste, R. E., and Tadaro, G. J.: Type C viral expression in primate tissues, Proc. Natl. Acad. Sci. U.S.A. **71:** 3721, 1974.

83. Sidman, R. L.: Cell interactions in developing mammalian nervous system. In Silvestri, L. G., editor: Cell interactions: third lepetit colloquium, New York, 1972, American Elsevier Publishing Co., Inc., pp. 1-13.

84. Simpson, R. T.: Separation of transcribable and repressed chromatin. In Anfinsen, C. B., and Schechter, A. N., editors: Current topics in biochemistry, New York, 1974, Academic Press, Inc., pp. 135-186.

85. Singer, E.: Gene manipulation: progress and prospects. In Hay, E. D., King, T. J., and Papaconstantinou, J., editors: Macromolecules regulating growth and development, New York, 1974, Academic Press, Inc., pp. 217-240.

86. Slavkin, H. C.: The dynamics of extracellular and cell surface protein interactions. In Cameron, I. L., and Thrasher, J. D., editors: Cellular and molecular renewal in the mammalian body, New York, 1971, Academic Press, Inc.

87. Slavkin, H. C.: Intercellular communication during odontogenesis. In Slavkin, H. C., and Bavetta, L. A., editors: Developmental aspects of oral biology, New York, 1972, Academic Press, Inc., pp. 165-201.

88. Slavkin, H. C., editor: Proceedings of the Santa Catalina Colloquium: The comparative molecular biology of extracellular matrices, New York, 1972, Academic Press, Inc.

89. Slavkin, H. C.: Localization of H-2 histocompatibility alloantigens on mouse embryonic tooth epithelial and mesenchymal cell surfaces, J. Cell Biol. **60:**795, 1974.

90. Slavkin, H. C.: Research frontiers in oral biology—genetic alterations in craniofacial anomalies, J. Oral Surg. **32:**333, 1974.

91. Slavkin, H. C.: Tooth formation: a tool in developmental biology. In Melcher, A. H., and Zarb, G. A., editors: Oral science reviews, Copenhagen, 1974, Munksgaard.

92. Slavkin, H. C.: Isolation and characterization of calcifying and noncalcifying matrix

vesicles from dentine. In Montel, G., editor: International colloquium on physical chemistry and crystallography of paptites of biological interest, Paris, 1975, Centre National de la Recherche Scientifique, pp. 161-177.

93. Slavkin, H. C., Beierle, J., and Bavetta, L. A.: Odontogenesis: cell-cell interactions in vitro, Nature **217**:269, 1968.

94. Slavkin, H. C., Bringas, P., Cameron, J., et al.: Epithelial and mesenchymal cell interactions with extracellular matrix material in vitro, J. Embryol. Exp. Morphol. **22**:395, 1969.

95. Slavkin, H. C., and Croissant, R.: Intercellular communication during odontogenic epithelial-mesenchymal interactions. In Niu, M. C., and Segal, S., editors: The role of RNA in reproduction and development, Amsterdam, 1973, North-Holland Publishing Co.

96. Slavkin, H. C., Croissant, R. D., and Guenther, H.: The role of extracellular matrix macromolecules upon cell differentiation. In Peeters, H., editor: Protides of the biological fluids, vol. 22, Oxford, England, 1975, Pergamon Press, Ltd., pp. 23-32.

97. Slavkin, H. C., Flores, P., Bringas, P., and Bavetta, L. A.: Epithelial-mesenchymal interactions during odontogenesis. I. Isolation of several intercellular matrix low molecular weight methylated RNAs, Dev. Biol. **23**:276, 1970.

98. Slavkin, H. C., et al.: Epithelial-specific extracellular matrix influences on mesenchyme collagen biosynthesis in vitro. In Slavkin, H. C., and Greulich, R. C., editors: Extracellular matrix influences on gene expression, New York, 1975, Academic Press, Inc., pp. 237-251.

99. Slavkin, H. C., et al.: Matrix vesicle heterogeneity: possible morphogenetic functions for matrix vesicles, Fed. Proc. **35**(2):127, 1976.

100. Stubblefield, E.: Organization of DNA and proteins in mammalian chromosomes. In Hay, E. D., King, T. J., and Papaconstintinou, J., editors: Macromolecules regulating growth and development, New York, 1974, Academic Press, Inc., pp. 165-180.

101. Suzuki, D. T.: Developmental genetics. In Lash, J., and Whittaker, J. R., editors: Concepts of development, Stanford, Conn., 1974, Sinauer Associates, pp. 349-379.

102. Tanzer, J. L., Church, R. L., Yaeger, J. A., and Park, E.-D.: The multistep pathway of collagen biosynthesis: pro-collagen intermediates. In Slavkin, H. C., and Greulich, R. C., editors: Extracellular matrix influences on gene expression, New York, 1975, Academic Press, Inc., pp. 785-794.

103. Terasaki, P. I., Mickey, M. R., Yamazaki, J. N., and Vredeye, D.: Maternal-fatal incompatibility. I. Incidence of HL-A antibodies and possible association with congenital anomalies, Transplantation **9**:538, 1970.

104. Thomas, L.: The lives of a cell, New York, 1974, The Viking Press, Inc.

105. Thompson, E. B.: Gene expression in animal cells. In Anfinsen, C. B., and Schechter, A. N., editors: Current topics in biochemistry, New York, 1974, Academic Press, Inc., pp. 187-218.

106. Tiedemann, H.: Substances with morphogenetic activity in differentiation of vertebrates. In Weber, R., editor: The biochemistry of animal development, vol. 3, Molecular aspects of animal development, New York, 1975, Academic Press, Inc., pp. 258-292.

107. Tobler, H.: Occurrence and developmental significance of gene amplification. In Weber R., editor: The biochemistry of animal development, vol. 3, Molecular aspects of animal development. New York, 1975, Academic Press, Inc., pp. 91-144.

108. Trelstad, R. L., and Slavkin, H. C.: Collagen synthesis by the epithelial enamel organ of the embryonic rabbit tooth, Biochem. Biophys. Res. Commun. **59**:443, 1974.

109. Van-Renssilaer, P.: Bioethics: bridge to the future, Englewood Cliffs, N.J., 1971, Prentice-Hall, Inc.

110. Vladutiu, A. O., and Rose, N. R.: HL-A antigens: association with disease, Immunogenetics **1**:305, 1974.

111. Watson, J. D.: Molecular biology of the gene, ed. 2, New York, 1970, W. A. Benjamin, Inc.

112. Weston, J. A.: The migration and differentiation of neural crest cells. In Abercrombie, M., Brachet, J., and King, T. J., editors: Advances in morphogenesis, vol. 8, New York, 1970, Academic Press, Inc., pp. 41-114.

113. Weston, J. A.: Cell interaction in neural crest development. In Silvestri, L. G., editor: Cell interactions: third lepetit colloquium, New York, 1972, American Elsevier Publishing Co., Inc.

114. Wright, W. E., and Hayflick, L.: Contributions to cytoplasmic factors to in vitro cellular senescence, Fed. Proc. **34**:76, 1975.

ADDITIONAL RECOMMENDED READING

Balazs, E. A., editor: Chemistry and molecular biology of the intercellular matrix, vol. 1, Collagen, basal laminae, elastin, New York, 1970, Academic Press, Inc.

Balazs, E. A., editor: Chemistry and molecular biology, vol. 2, Glycosaminoglycans and proteoglycans, New York, 1970, Academic Press, Inc.

Balazs, E. A., editor: Chemistry and molecular biology, vol. 3, Structural organization and function of the matrix. New York, 1970, Academic Press, Inc.

Bekhor, I.: Consideration of the molecular biology of developing systems. In Slavkin, H. C., and Bavetta, L. A., editors: Developmental aspects of oral biology, New York, 1972, Academic Press, Inc., pp. 11-34.

Bekhor, I., Anne, L., Kim, J., Lapeyre, J.-N., and Stambaugh, R.: Organ discrimination through organ specific non-histone chromosomal proteins, Arch. Biochem. Biophys. **161**:11, 1974.

Biwas, B. B.: Chromatin and ribonucleic acid polymerases in the eucaryotic cell, Subcell Biochem. **3**:27, 1974.

Bonner, J. T.: On development: the biology of form, Cambridge, Mass., 1974, Harvard University Press.

Clegg, K. B., and Denny, P. C.: Synthesis of rabbit globin in a cell-free protein synthesis system utilizing sea urchin egg and zygote ribosomes, Dev. Biol. **37**:263, 1974.

Coggin, J. H., Jr., and Anderson, N. G.: Embryonic and fetal antigens in cancer cells. In King, T. J., editor: Developmental aspects of carcinogenesis and immunity, New York, 1974, Academic Press, Inc., pp. 173-186.

Daniel, Jr., J. C., editor: Methods in mammalian embryology, San Francisco, 1971, W. H. Freeman & Co.

Denny, P. C.: Interactions of translational control mechanisms during salivary gland development. In Slavkin, H. C., and Greulich, R. C., editors: New York, 1975, Academic Press, Inc.

Dostal, M., and Jelinek, R.: Sensitivity of embryos and intraspecies differences in mice in response to prenatal administration of corticoids, Teratology **8**:245, 1973.

Eisenstein, R., Sorgente, N., Soble, L. W., Miller, A., and Kuettner, K. E.: The resistance of certain tissues to invasion: penetrability of explanted tissues by vascularized mesenchyme, Am. J. Pathol. **73**:765, 1973.

Golditch, M., Barnes, P., and Schneir, M.: Rabbit palatal mucosa sialoglycoproteins: solubilization and in vitro biosynthesis, Arch. Oral Biol. **19**:65, 1974.

Grabb, W. C., Rosenstein, S. W., and Bzoch, K. R., editors: Cleft lip and palate: surgical, dental and speech aspects, New York, 1971, Little, Brown & Co.

Gurdon, J. B.: The control of gene expression in animal development, Cambridge, Mass., 1974, Harvard University Press.

Hamburgh, M.: Theories of differentiation, New York, 1971, American Elsevier Publishing Co., Inc.

Hard tissue growth, repair and remineralization, Ciba Foundation Symposium II (new series),

New York, 1973, American Elsevier Publishing Co., Inc.

Johnston, M. C., Bhakdinaronk, A., and Reid, Y. C.: An expanded role of the neural crest in oral and pharyngeal development. In Bosma, J. F., editor: Oral sensation and perception development in the fetus and infant, NIH 73-546, Bethesda, Md., 1973, U.S. Department of Health, Education, and Welfare, pp. 37-52.

Kalter, H.: Interplay of intrinsic and extrinsic factors. In Wilson, J. G., and Workany, J., editors: Teratology: principles and techniques, Chicago, 1965, The University of Chicago Press, pp. 57-80.

Koch, W. E.: Tissue interaction during the in vitro odontogenesis. In Slavkin, H. C., and Bavetta, L. A., editors: Developmental aspects of oral biology, New York, 1972, Academic Press, Inc., pp. 151-164.

Kollar, E. J.: Histogenetic aspects of dermal-epidermal interactions. In Slavkin, H. C. and Bavetta, L. A., editors: Developmental aspects of oral biology, New York, 1972, Academic Press, Inc., pp. 126-150.

Lapeyre, J.-N., and Bekhor, I.: Effects of 5-bromo-2'-deoxyuridine and dimethyl sulfoxide on properties and structure of chromatin, J. Mol. Biol. **89**:137, 1974.

Lash, J., and Whittaker, J. R., editors: Concepts of development, Stamford, Conn., 1974, Sinauer Associates.

Ledoux, L., editor: Informative molecules in biological systems, New York, 1971, American Elsevier Publishing Co., Inc.

Monroy, A., and Tsanev, R., editors: Biochemistry of cell differentiation: Federation of European Biochemical Societies, seventh meeting, Varna, Bulgaria, New York, 1973, Academic Press, Inc.

Moscona, A. A., editor: The cell surface in development, New York, 1974, John Wiley & Sons, Inc.

Needham, J.: Biochemistry and morphogenesis, Cambridge, Mass., 1966, Harvard University Press.

Nimni, M. E.: Metabolic pathways and control mechanisms involved in the biosynthesis and turnover of collagen in normal and pathological connective tissues, J. Oral Pathol. **2**:175, 1973.

Niu, M. C., and Segal, S. J., editors: The role of RNA in reproduction and development, proceedings of the A.A.A.S. Symposium, Dec. 28-30, 1972, New York, 1973, American Elsevier Publishing Co., Inc.

Noden, D. M.: The migratory behavior of neural crest cells. In Bosma, J. F., editor: Oral sensation and perception development in the fetus and infant, NIH 73-546, Bethesda, Md., 1973, U.S. Department of Health, Education, and Welfare, pp. 9-33.

Padilla, G. M., Cameron, I. L., and Zimmerman, A., editors: Cell cycle controls, New York, 1974, Academic Press, Inc.

Paul, J., editor: Biochemistry series one, vol. 9, Biochemistry of cell differentiation, Baltimore, 1974, University Park Press.

Pourtois, M.: Morphogenesis of the primary and secondary palate. In Slavkin, H. C., and Bavetta, L. A., editors: Developmental aspects of oral biology, New York, 1972, Academic Press, Inc., pp. 81-108.

Reinert, J., and Ursprung, H.: Origin and continuity of cell organelles, New York, 1971, Springer-Verlag New York, Inc.

Reynolds, J. J., and Minkin, C.: Bone studies in vitro: use of calcitonin as a specific inhibitor of bone resorption. In Taylor, S., editor: Calcitonin 1969, London, 1970, Heinemann Medical Books, p. 168.

Ross, B. B. and Johnston, M. C.: Cleft lip and palate, Baltimore, 1972, The Williams & Wilkins Co.

Roth, S.: A molecular model for cell interactions, Q. Rev. Biol. 48:541, 1973.

Schjeide, O. A., and Vellis, J. E., editors: Cell differentiation, New York, 1970, Van Nostrand Reinhold Co.

Schraer, H., editor: Biological calcification: cellular and molecular aspects, New York, 1970, Appleton-Century-Crofts, Educational Division/ Meredity Corp.

Slavkin, H. C., editor: The comparative molecular biology of extracellular matrices, New York, 1972, Academic Press, Inc.

Slavkin, H. C.: Embryonic tooth formation: a tool for developmental biology. In Melcher, A. H., and Zarb, G. A., editors: Oral science reviews, vol. 4, Copenhagen, 1974, Munksgaard.

Slavkin, H. C.: Biological regulatory mechanisms related to dentofacial deformities. In Bell, W. H., Profitt, W. R., Epker, B. N., and White, R. P., Jr., editors: The correction of dental facial deformities, Philadelphia, W. B. Saunders Co. (In press.)

Slavkin, H. C.: Current concepts in dermal-epidermal interactions. In Stahl, S. S., editor: Periodontal surgery—a current evaluation, Springfield, Ill., Charles C Thomas, Publisher. (In press.)

Slavkin, H. C., and Bavetta, L. A., editors: Developmental aspects of oral biology, New York, 1972, Academic Press, Inc.

Slavkin, H. C., and Greulich, R. C., editors: Extracellular matrix influences on gene expression, New York, 1975, Academic Press, Inc.

Smith, H. H., editor: Evolution of genetic systems, New York, 1972, Gordon & Breach, Science Publishers, Inc.

Stanbury, J. B., Wyngaarden, J. B., and Fredrickson, D. S., editors: The metabolic basis of inherited disease, New York, 1972, McGraw-Hill Book Co.

Temin, H. M., and Kang, C.-Y.: RNA-directed DNA polymerase activity in uninfected cells. In King, T. J., editor: Developmental aspects of carcinogenesis and immunity, New York, 1974, Academic Press, Inc., pp. 137-144.

Tenehouse, H. S., Gold, R. J. M., and Kachra, Z.: Biochemical marker in dominantly inherited ectodermal malformation, Nature 251:431, 1974.

Ursprung, H., editor: The stability of the differentiated state: results and problems in cell differentiation, vol. 1, New York, 1968, Springer-Verlag New York, Inc.

Ursprung, H., editor: Nucleic acid hybridization in the study of cell differentiation, New York, 1972, Springer-Verlag New York, Inc.

Warren, K. B.: Differentiation and immunology: symposia of the International Society for Cell Biology, vol. 7, New York, 1968, Academic Press, Inc.

Weber, R., editor: The biochemistry of animal development, vol. 3, The molecular aspects of animal development, New York, 1975, Academic Press, Inc.

Weiss, L.: The cell periphery, metastasis and other contact phenomena, Frontiers in biology, vol. 7, New York, 1967, John Wiley & Sons, Inc.

Weiss, P. A.: Dynamics of development: experiments and inferences: selected papers on developmental biology, New York, 1968, Academic Press, Inc.

White, E., and Trump, G. N.: Immunological determinants in development. In Slavkin, H. C., and Bavetta, L. A., editors: Developmental aspects of oral biology, New York, 1972, Academic Press, Inc., pp. 35-54.

2

Genetic factors in craniofacial morphogenesis

RAY E. STEWART

Chapter 1 provided a detailed discussion of current knowledge of the factors that direct and control embryogenesis and early craniofacial development at a molecular and cellular level. Specific attention was devoted to the numerous levels of regulation and major control mechanisms that are known to be operant during critical developmental stages. In general, genetic control of early developmental stages (cell differentiation, histogenesis, organogenesis, and morphogenesis) is mediated primarily through the regulation of gene expression at the level of RNA transcription. As development progresses through the later stages of embryogenesis, fetal development, postnatal growth, maturation, and senescence, additional regulatory mechanisms such as humoral factors, extracellular matrix environments, cell surface ligand-molecule interactions, and a variety of cytoplasmic-nuclear interactions come into play as important control factors.

As was pointed out in Chapter 1, one of the major challenges facing developmental biologists and experimental embryologists consists of identifying both the intrinsic and extrinsic control mechanisms and understanding the manner in which these mechanisms relate with one another to orchestrate the overall development of the organism.

This chapter will be an extension of the previous chapter in that it will deal with mechanisms controlling craniofacial development; however, it will approach the problem in a slightly broader sense, that is, at a structural rather than cellular level. By reviewing the nature of the specific control processes that function during specific stages of human development, it is hoped that a clearer overall picture of the relative roles of each of these factors during development will emerge.

OVERVIEW OF DEVELOPMENT

For an organism to develop normally from fertilization through the various complex stages that culminate in harmonious development involves the processes of *differentiation* and *growth,* both of which are highly coordinated, rigorously organized, and closely controlled.

Differentiation describes the appearance of functionally and morphologically distinct cell types, as in early gastrulation with the development of three distinct germ layers—ectoderm, endoderm, and mesoderm. With the emergence of distinct cell types, the embryo undergoes continued differentiation as well as *growth,* during which time the embryo acquires definitive species-specific form *(morphogenesis)* and organizes and develops the fundamental architecture of its organs *(organogenesis),* which later, during the fetal period, undergo a maturation process at the histological level *(histogenesis).*

Growth may be defined as an increase in spatial dimension and body mass. The human conceptus has the potential to grow from a single cellular unit of approximately 150 μm in diameter weighing a fraction of a milligram to a term neonate consisting of millions of cells and hundreds of cell types with a total birth length of over 50 cm and an average birth weight of approximately 3000 gm. This dramatic metamorphosis is the result of three types of growth processes, *multiplicative* growth resulting from a simple increase in cell number, *auxetic* growth or an increase in the size of individual cells, and *accretionary* growth due to an increase in the amount of nonliving intercellular material.

An organism undergoes various stages of development beginning as a zygote through birth, maturation, and senescence. For the sake of this discussion, these stages have been arbitrarily divided into various periods of development that are marked by the appearance of certain phenotypic characteristics or by the onset of specific physiological phenomena (Table 2-1).

The factors that regulate and effectively direct development at all stages fall into three main categories: (1) intrinsic genetic factors, (2) epigenetics factors, and (3) environmental factors.

The roles that these individual factors play in craniofacial differentiation, growth, and development have been widely studied. Careful analysis of this work indicates that it is unlikely that few, if any, individual morphological characteristics of the adult craniofacial complex are determined solely by the effects of a single gene, epigenetic influences, or entirely due to environmental factors.

All too frequently, heredity and environment (nature versus nurture) are considered as though they worked against one another to produce a given phenotype. More appropriately, the phenotype of an organism should be considered the product of a close interaction between genetic and environmental factors where an alteration in either will frequently lead to abnormal development or, in extreme cases, death of the organism.

Evidence in support of the role of genetics in the causation of many abnormalities is overwhelming. In lower animals and to a lesser extent in man it has been possible to associate certain phenotypic abnormalities with specific gene mutations or with specific chromosomal abnormalities. Pedigree analyses demonstrating the genetic transmission of certain abnormalities through several generations in some families clearly support the role of single-gene mutations in the creation of these abnormalities. Other (polygenic) abnormalities are almost certainly due to the action of more than one abnormal gene and do not exhibit the clear-cut pattern of Mendelian segregation seen in monogenetic disorders. This cumulative data establishes incontrovertably the role of intrinsic genetic factors in many human developmental aberrations.

The role of environmental factors has also been clearly established throughout the various stages of development of the organism. Such factors as gravity, temperature, and the presence of various metabolic agents and nutritive substances may affect development at an early time as evidenced by the effect of these external factors on the early development of the unfertilized egg itself. Although the precise role of environmental variation in man is difficult to study in the prenatal period, it is well established that environmental differences such as the number of developing embryos, the age of the parents, the number of previous pregnancies, and the presence of certain teratogenic substances and viruses at certain critical times significantly

Table 2-1. Developmental periods

Prenatal	
Early embryonic period	Fertilization → 21 days
Midembryonic period	21 days → 35 days
Late embryonic period	35 days → 60 days
Fetal period	60 days → 9 months
Postnatal	
Infancy	Birth → 2 years
Childhood	2 years → 11 years
Adolescence	11 years → 15 years
Adulthood	15 years → 60 years
Senescence	60 years →

influence the course of development. The size to which the fetus grows during gestation is affected by such factors as the rate of growth of embryonic cells, the availability of nutrients, and the duration of growth, all of which are, to a certain extent, controlled by intrinsic genetic factors, and the final size of the fetus is largely controlled by intrinsic and epigenetic factors. The environment plays a definite role as demonstrated by the effects of maternal malnutrition resulting in a smaller-than-normal full-term fetus.

Attempts have been made by various investigators and clinicians to assign the quantitative and qualitative aspects of craniofacial structure primarily to one or another of these factors, and although a number of theories of craniofacial development have been proposed, none of them satisfactorily explains the dynamic processes involved. Many traits, such as tooth size or jaw size, that in the past have been treated as discrete entities, have more recently been shown to be continuously variable and multifactorial in nature, which would indicate the involvement of several genes acting in concert with epigenetic and environmental factors.

The role these various controlling factors play in craniofacial development becomes even more clear if their relative influences at various stages of prenatal and postnatal development are considered. That is to say, if the periods of prenatal and postnatal development are distilled into more precise periods and an attempt is made to identify the relative roles of the controlling factors at each of these periods, the problem becomes less complex. For example, it is clear that the role of intrinsic genetic factors in craniofacial development is variable at various stages or periods of development. Epigenetic and environmental factors play an increasingly important role, particularly in later stages of development, but they play only a minor and insignificant role during the early stages of embryogenesis. Epigenetic factors may originate in adjacent tissues or structures and have local influences such as the influence of the developing brain on cranial structure. They may, however, be produced by distant structures that have more generalized influences, as in the case of hormones produced by various endocrine glands. In the context of this discussion, environmental factors are those which originate from the external environment. In this case, general environmental influences such as trauma, teratogens, or local external pressures causing postural changes should be distinguished from local environmental influences such as muscle forces, nutrition, and oxygenation of tissues.

This innovative method of viewing the relative roles of control mechanisms in craniofacial development was originally proposed by van Limborgh,[44] who examined the role of genetic and environmental factors during the periods of embryonic development and prenatal and postnatal skull growth. He hypothesized that the initial morphological characteristics of individual bones within the craniofacial complex are determined primarily by intrinsic genetic factors. Subsequent development and spatial orientation within the craniofacial complex, van Limborgh suggests, is primarily influenced by epigenetic and environmental factors.

Overall development of the interrelated group of components comprising the craniofacial complex is an extremely dynamic process. Craniofacial differentiation, morphogenesis, growth, and development are affected by and dependent on multiple factors, which influence both the hard and soft tissues. The extent of the effect of each of these factors will vary, depending on the stage or period of development of the organism.

CRANIOFACIAL COMPONENTS AND THEIR DERIVATIVES

In considering the craniofacial complex it is beneficial to conceptualize the entire unit as being comprised of certain basic tissue types that have been variously derived from one or more of the three basic germ layers (ectoderm, endoderm, mesoderm). The basic tissue types include (1) dental tissues consisting of enamel, dentin, cementum, dental pulp, and periodontal membrane, (2) soft tissues consisting of epithelium, muscle, glandular tissue, nerves, and connective tissue, and (3) skeletal tissues consisting of bone, cartilage, and tendon.[36]

The skeletal portion of the craniofacial complex develops as a blend of the morphogenesis of three primary skull components. These elements, functioning as a unit, are variably affected by the factors that operate to control differentiation, morphogenesis, growth, and development of the craniofacial complex (Fig. 2-1). The three primary skeletal components are as follows:

1. The *neurocranium* may be divided into two discrete components having different origins and are themselves affected variously by intrinsic and extrinsic controlling factors.
   a. The *desmocranium* comprises the vault of the skull, or the calvarium, which evolved in response to the need for a protective mechanism for the increasing size of the brain and is formed from intramembranous bone.
   b. The *chondrocranium* makes up the cranial base, which is derived ontogenetically as the primitive cranial floor. It arises from a number of primordial cartilages that eventually grow by endochondral bone formation and eventually fuse to form a contiguous structure.
2. The second primary skeletal component is the *viscerocranium*, which has evolved from the primitive branchial arch structures. It develops by intramembranous bone formation. The pharyngeal arches also give rise to the muscles of mastication and facial expression as well as the maxilla and mandible.
3. The third primary skeletal component consists of the *dentition and supporting structures*, which are derived ontogenetically from ectodermal structures and developed embryologically from invaginations of the primitive oral ectoderm.

The craniofacial complex is thus a mosaic of individual components, each of which contributes to a dynamic process of growth in the proper amount and direction to attain and maintain the stability necessary for normal development.

Each of the three main craniofacial components exhibits different characteristics of differentiation, growth, development, maturation, and function, yet each of the units is so integrated with the other that coordination of growth is required for normal development to occur. Failure of initiation or disproportionate growth of any individual component results in abnormal craniofacial relationships. Although the neurocranium and viscerocranium both contain skeletal elements of intramembranous and endochondral origin, the bony elements of the masticatory apparatus are predominantly of intramembranous origin.

From an evolutionary standpoint it is of interest to note that the more recent developments in the mammalian skull, the membranous bones of the jaws and facial skeleton (viscerocranium), are more susceptible to developmental anomalies than are the older cartilaginous parts of the skull. Developmental defects of the face and jaws are relatively common, whereas defects of the

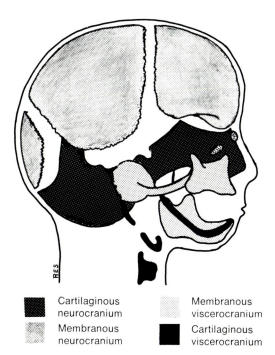

■	Cartilaginous neurocranium	▨	Membranous viscerocranium
▨	Membranous neurocranium	■	Cartilaginous viscerocranium

Fig. 2-1. Schematic diagram of lateral view of cranium with its various derivatives. Cartilaginous neurocranium, black stipple; cartilaginous viscerocranium, solid black; membranous neurocranium, gray stipple; membranous viscerocranium, white stipple.

skull base and of the nasal and otic capsules are relatively rare.

EARLY EMBRYONIC PERIOD

The early embryonic stage commences at fertilization and includes cleavage, blastocyst formation, formation of the extraembryonic membranes, and the development of the presomite embryo. The first 3 or 4 days after fertilization are occupied with transport down the fallopian tube and cleavage to form the morula. By 7 or 8 days after fertilization, implantation of the early blastocyst has begun. By 14 days, the early presomite embryo has formed a circular bilaminar disc with prechordal plate, primitive streak, Hensen's

node, notochordal process, and cloacal membrane (Fig. 2-2).

Certain specific changes occur in the region of Hensen's node that will eventually give rise to many of the primordia of the craniofacial complex. During the fourteenth day at the anterior pole of the primitive streak, the prechordal plate makes its appearance as a rapid proliferation of endodermal cells and comprises the future cephalic region. The appearance of the prechordal plate signals the earliest stages of development of the oral facial region. It is this region that later gives rise to the oral pharyngeal membrane. The third primary germ layer, the mesoderm, appears during the third week of development and converts the bilaminar germ disc into a trilaminar structure. The midline axis is defined by the formation of the notochord, an anterior proliferation of the primitive streak. The notochord ends at the prechordal plate and marks the site of the future pituitary gland development.

The three primary germ layers serve as a basis for the differentiating tissues and organ systems. From the ectoderm develop the cutaneous and neural elements of the embryo; from the mesoderm arrives the cardiovascular structure such as heart and blood vessels, bones, muscles, and connective tissue; and from the endoderm develops the lining epithelium of the gut between the pharynx and the anus, as well as the secretory cells of the liver and pancreas and the lining epithelium of the respiratory system.

Development of the ectoderm into its cutaneous and neural portions occurs by a proliferation of ectodermal cells that make up the neural plate. The neural plate overlies the notochord along the midline axis, which, through differential proliferation, gives rise to the neural tube, which is the site of the development of an additional group of ectodermally derived cells between the cutaneous ectoderm of the neural crest and the endoderm. These cells are commonly referred to as neural crest cells.

With respect to the early embryonic stage, which involves the differentiation of various cell types and the early development of pri-

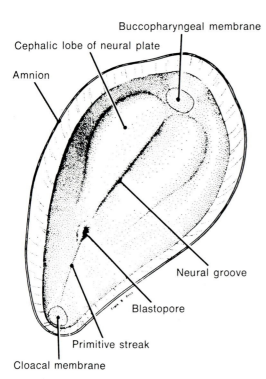

Buccopharyngeal membrane
Cephalic lobe of neural plate
Amnion
Neural groove
Blastopore
Primitive streak
Cloacal membrane

Fig. 2-2. Dorsal view of embryonic disc at approximately 3 weeks of development. At this time, embryo is trilaminar with all three embryonic tissue types being present. Expansion of embryonic disc at this time occurs mainly in cranial region; caudal end remains more or less unchanged. Growth and elongation of embryonic disc is direct result of continuous migration of mesenchymal cells from primitive streak. (Modified from Hamilton, W. J., and Mossman, H. W.: Human embryology, London, 1972, The Macmillan Press, Ltd.)

mordia of certain structures and organs in the craniofacial complex, we can surmise that these processes are controlled primarily by intrinsic genetic factors. These intrinsic genetic factors are also the primary sources of control for the metabolic processes of the cells through intracellular regulatory mechanisms and, furthermore, have direct control over the critical process of neural crest cell migration, which involves the movement of cells to predestined locations in the developing embryo beginning during the gastrula stage.[11a] Similarly, intrinsic genetic factors are probably the primary controlling factors in the early interaction or induction that occurs between adjacent cell groups and tissue types. Induction is an essential determinant of later stages of the embryonic development and is a process by which certain cellular groups mediate and direct the differentiation of adjacent cellular groups.[17a] An example of this phenomenon exists in the early development of the neural tube and vertebral column. Induction occurs between a condensation of cells along the primitive streak of the gastrula (the notochord) and adjacent tissues to form the somites, which are the structures from which a greater part of the axial skeleton and musculature will develop.

MIDDLE EMBRYONIC PERIOD

Late in the gastrula stage (21 days), the embryo passes from the early to the middle embryonic stage. This period is also sometimes referred to as the somite period in which the periaxial mesoderm lateral to the notochord divides into a series of segments or somites. The forty-two to forty-four paired somites appear sequentially in a cranial to caudal direction and set the pattern for regions of the body that will later develop and are identified as occipital, cervical, thoracic, lumbar, sacral, and coxal somite regions.

In the early somite stage (21 to 31 days) (Fig. 2-3), the cranial portion of the embryo develops the first of several ectodermally lined mesenchymal elevations. These elevations or processes arise from the rapid proliferation

of underlying mesenchyme, which has migrated into these regions. The facial processes surround the oral pharyngeal membrane, which lies in a central depression known as the stomodeum. With the differential growth of these mesodermal masses, the ectodermal grooves demarcating the facial processes soon become obliterated. Smooth contours develop, a characteristic feature of the later stages of embryogenesis. It is along these depressions or grooves separating the facial processes that facial clefts commonly develop.

By the seven-somite stage, closure of the neural tube has begun, and the cephalic enlargement of the embryo is marked. At the ten-somite stage, the three primary cerebral dilatations are obvious. Closure of the neural tube has progressed caudally beyond

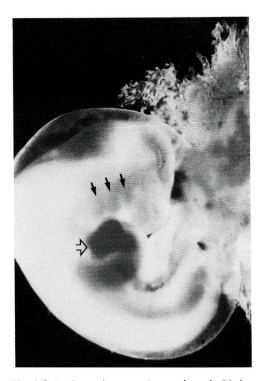

Fig. 2-3. Early somite stage (approximately 24 days of development) with early evidence of branchial arches, *filled arrows,* in cranial portion of embryo. Maxillary and mandibular processes of first branchial arch surround oropharyngeal membrane, which lies in central depression known as stomodeum. *Open arrow,* developing heart. (Courtesy D. W. Smith, Seattle, Wash.)

the region of formed somites and cranially to the midbrain region. The tube remains unclosed at the anterior and posterior neuropores.

The oropharyngeal membrane forms the floor of the stomodeum, which is bounded cranially by the anterior projecting edge of the neural plate (later the bulge of the forebrain) and caudally by the bulge of the pericardium. Laterally the stomodeum is bounded by swellings that have appeared in the angle between the neural plate and the pericardium, known as the mandibular process of the first branchial arch. These swellings, or facial processes, are the first signs of development of the face and viscerocranium. As successive arches appear, the pericardium is progressively removed from the caudal margin of the stomodeum.

By the thirty-fifth day of development (Fig. 2-4), the neural tube is nearly closed. Just before this time, a critical stage in craniofacial embryogenesis begins with the commencement of neural crest cell migration.

The role of neural crest cells in the development of skeletal and connective tissue derivatives of the craniofacial complex was discussed extensively in Chapter 1, where it was noted that these cells are derived from a condensation of ectodermal cells at the junction between the neural plate and surface ectoderm. These neural crest cells migrate extensively and give rise to numerous derivatives, including skeletal and connective tissue components of the craniofacial complex. Experimental evidence indicates that these cells migrate lateroventrally into the facial region. There, they interact with local cells and environment to form, among other things, bone, connective tissue, and cartilaginous derivatives.[29] Avail-

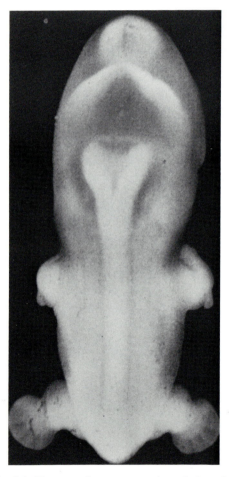

Fig. 2-4. Human embryo at approximately 5 weeks' development. Limbs are well along in development. Anterior portion of neural tube is nearing completion. (From Rugh, R., and Shettles, L.: From conception to birth, New York, 1971, Harper & Row, Publishers.)

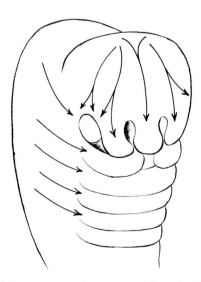

Fig. 2-5. Diagrammatic representation of origins and migration paths of neural crest cells, *arrows*, into facial region.

able information indicates that neural crest cells also migrate in a bipolar fashion (Fig. 2-5). At the completion of the cell migration, certain cell-to-cell interactions occur that permit the crest cells to differentiate according to the environment in which they find themselves. The source of the inductive influence that acts to produce the specific differentiation leading to the development of specific craniofacial structures is not well understood; however, cell interaction and tissue interaction are described and discussed in detail in Chapter 1.

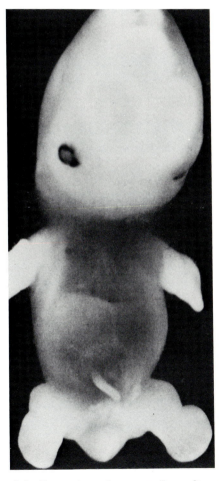

Fig. 2-6. Front view of same embryo shown in Fig. 2-4, illustrating prominent development of forebrain, optic placodes, and paddle-shaped hands and feet. (From Rugh, R., and Shettles, L.: From conception to birth, New York, 1971, Harper & Row, Publishers.)

At approximately 24 to 26 days, succeeding branchial arches appear, and the otic vesicles invaginate into head mesenchyme and are no longer visible through the ectoderm. During this time, an evagination of the forebrain, the optic vesicle, which is the precursor of the eye, makes its appearance beneath the head ectoderm (Fig. 2-6). Caudal to the first pharyngeal arch that borders the stomodeum is a wide first branchial cleft, which separates the mandibular and maxillary processes. Caudal to the maxillary process is the prominent second (hyoid) arch and the narrower second branchial cleft. The otic placode is an ectodermal thickening that lies dorsal to the second branchial cleft. This structure is the precursor of the membranous middle ear derivatives.

Development of the viscerocranium during this period is marked by a breakdown of the oropharyngeal membrane establishing continuity between the stomodeum and the primitive pharynx. The maxillary process grows toward the stomodeum from the dorsal end of the first arch. The stomodeum is bounded cranially by the frontal bulge of the forebrain, laterally by the maxillary process, and caudally by the mandibular processes, which approach each other and fuse at the midline to form the primitive lower jaw and lip.

Bilateral ectodermal thickenings, the olfactory placodes, appear above the lateral angles of the stomodeum. Proliferation of the mesenchyme near each placode causes the elevation of a horseshoe-shaped area of surrounding ectoderm. The margins of the placode are called the medial and lateral nasal folds. The nasal folds, together with the intervening convex frontal area, constitute the frontonasal process.

The control factors that operate during differentiation of the chondrocranium in the middle embryonic period continue to be strongly genetically determined and are subject to minimal environmental influence. After initial differentiation of specific cell types, the growth of the desmocranium and viscerocranium appear to be subject to diminishing intrinsic genetic determinants, whereas the influence of epigenetic and local environmental factors become stronger.

Both the findings in spontaneous malformations as well as the results of experiments carried out in normal embryos emphasize a close relationship between the development of the skull and the presence and the condition of the primordia of the other head structures (epigenetic factors). van Limborgh[43] points out that good examples of these relationships are those existing between eye and orbit. If there is no eye primordium, there will be no orbit. If there is only a single eye primordium, a single orbit will develop. If two eye primordia lie close together, as in holoprosencephaly, two contiguous orbits will develop. Orbits develop in their normal position only if the eye primordia, too, are normally located. If there is abnormal width between these primordia, as in hypertelorism, the orbits, too, will develop with abnormal space between. If there are three eye primordia, three orbits will develop. An abnormally large eye will result in large orbits, while small eye primordia result in small orbits.[4, 6, 46] These observations give evidence that the development of orbits, as well as their number, position, and size, depend entirely on the presence, number, position, and size of the eye primordia. There is nothing to indicate that orbits tend to differentiate independently.

A similar relationship between differentiation for many other parts of the mesenchymal embryonic skull primordium has also been established,[38] where adjacent structures of the head determine the presence, position, and form of skull parts. It is, therefore, logical to assume that these adjacent structures exert powerful morphogenetic influences on one another, and, since the development of the skull normally proceeds in a hereditary, species-specific pattern, we may class these influences in the category of local epigenetic factors.[43, 44]

Other experiments suggest that as development proceeds in the primitive condensed skull mesenchyme, intrinsic genetic factors are not entirely lacking; however, they are small in number, and determine general characteristics only, such as the potency to differentiate into connective tissue, dura, or bone. There is probably also a relationship between this potency of differentiation and age.

In conclusion, available data compel us to believe that the processes of viscerocranial and desmocranial differentiation are controlled mainly by local epigenetic factors originating from adjacent structures of the head and only minimally by a few intrinsic genetic factors. A role of minor importance may also be attributed to general epigenetic and environmental factors.

LATE EMBRYONIC PERIOD

At approximately 35 days, the embryo enters the late embryonic period. The occipital sclerotomal mesenchyme (occipital somites) concentrates around the notochord underlying the developing hindbrain. From this region, the mesenchymal concentration extends cephalically, forming the posterior portion of a floor for the developing brain. Conversion of this undifferentiated mesenchyme into cartilage constitutes the beginning of the chondrocranium or cranial base (Fig. 2-7).

The anterior end of the notochord approximates the level of the oropharyngeal membrane. Just cranial to the oropharyngeal membrane, Rathke's pouch, arising from the stomodeum, gives rise to the anterior lobe of the pituitary gland, which lies just cephalad to the termination of the notochord. In this region, *polar cartilages* develop that surround the pituitary gland, which will give rise to the sella turcica of the sphenoid bone.

Chrondrification centers forming around the anterior portion of the notochord are called the *parachordal cartilages*. A caudal extension of the parachordal cartilages incorporates the fused sclerotomes of the occipital somites, providing the anlagen for the basilar and condylar parts of the occipital bone.

Cranial to the pituitary gland, *trabecular cartilages* fuse to form the precursor of the body of the sphenoid bone. Laterally, the chondrification centers of the *orbitosphenoid*

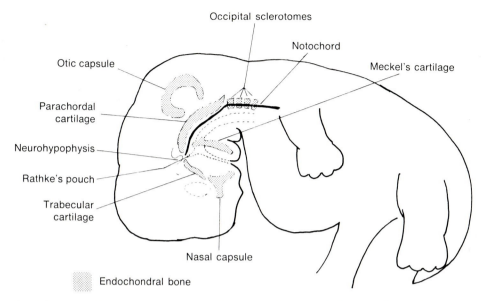

Fig. 2-7. Early development (seventh week) of cartilaginous skull primordium (chondrocranium). Chondrocranium develops from condensation of mesenchyme in specific regions, which eventually is reduced to thin layer of perichondrium that covers surface of developing islands of cartilage. Cartilaginous base of skull at this time consists of middle part, which is joined anteriorly with nasal capsule and laterally with optic capsules.

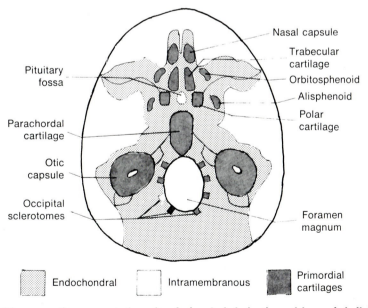

Fig. 2-8. Diagrammatic representation of endochondral derivatives of base of skull illustrating approximate locations of primordial cartilages, which fuse into single irregular and greatly perforated cranial base.

(lesser wing) and *alisphenoid* (greater wing) contribute to the sphenoid bone.

The condensed mesenchyme of the nasal and otic capsules chondrify to contribute to the cartilages of the cranial base. The cartilaginous *nasal capsules* ossify into the ethmoid and inferior nasal concha bones and remain cartilaginous in the midline as the nasal septum, which will be instrumental in midfacial growth. The *otic capsules* fuse with the parachordal cartilages to form the mastoid and petrous portions of the temporal bones. The otic capsules do not chondrify in humans (Fig. 2-8).

The initially separate cartilaginous centers of cranial base fuse into a single, irregular cranial base (Fig. 2-9). The early establishment of the blood vessels, cranial nerves, and spinal cord between the developing brain and its extracranial contacts before chondrification determines the presence of the numerous perforations (foramina) in the cartilaginous cranial base and in the subsequent osseous cranial floor.

Almost simultaneously with the formation of the chondrocranium begins the differentiation of the desmocranium. In the mesenchymal condensations of the calvaria and of the facial areas, centers of intramembranous ossification develop.

The mesenchyme, which gives rise to the vault of the neurocranium, is first arranged as a capsular membrane around the developing brain. The membrane later subdivides into two layers, an inner *endomeninges* and an outer *ectomeninges*. The endomeninges forms the two leptomeningeal coverings of the brain, the pia mater and the arachnoid. The ectomeninges differentiates into the dura mater, which remains unossified, covering the brain, and the outer superficial membrane with osteogenic properties that are realized in membranous bone formation. Despite their divergent fates, the two layers of the ectome-

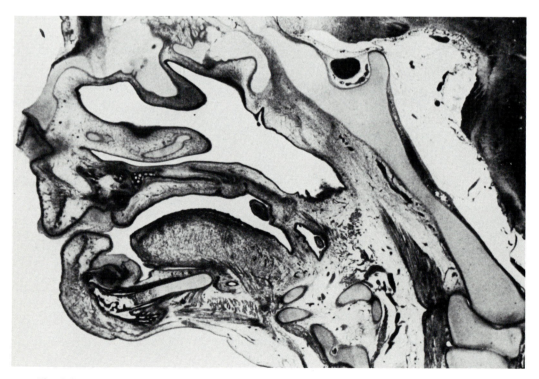

Fig. 2-9. Histological photomicrograph taken in parasagittal plane of human fetus illustrating cartilaginous cranial base before onset of ossification.

ninges remain in close apposition, except in regions where the venous sinuses develop. The dura mater and its septa, the falx cerebri and cerebelli and the tentorium cerebelli, show distinctly organized fiber bundles closely related and strongly attached to the sutural systems that later develop in the vault. The adult form of the neurocranium is the end result of the preferential direction of the forces set up by the growth of the brain along these dural fiber systems.

The vault of the skull, or calvaria, formed of intramembranous bone, is derived from several primary and secondary ossification centers that develop in the outer layer of the ectomeninges to form the individual calvarial bones. These centers, rather small in number, increase rapidly and soon take the shape of the bones to be formed in these areas, that is, the frontal bones, parietal bones, the interparietal (squamous) portion of the occipital, and the squamous portions of the temporals.

As the ossification centers grow, the quantity of condensed mesenchyme decreases. The narrow strips of connective tissue remaining between the bones become the sutures; the membranous layer of mesenchyme covering the bones forms the periosteum. Until this time, the genetic factors determining cell differentiation have played the predominant role in craniofacial development.

During the late embryonic period (Fig. 2-10), as the development of the face and viscerocranium is characterized mainly by changes in proportion and relative position, intrinsic genetic factors become less and less important while epigenetic factors increase in influence. The forebrain continues to expand, and the eyes, initially directed laterally, gradually become directed anteriorly. The nasal fossae are at first widely separated, but they come together as the intervening tissue. The primitive nasal septum becomes thinned, and the medial nasal folds fuse. At the same

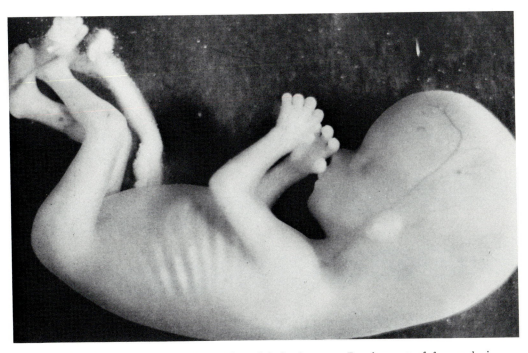

Fig. 2-10. Human embryo at about 10 weeks' development. Development of face and viscerocranium is nearly complete. Future development will consist mainly of changes in proportions and relative positions of structures. Eyelids have developed and fused and will not reopen until 4 or 5 months' gestation. (From Rugh, R., and Shettles, L.: From conception to birth, New York, 1971, Harper & Row, Publishers.)

time, a transverse groove appears, defining the upper limit of the external nose and separating it from the frontal prominence. The anterior nares become plugged with proliferated epithelium. The primitive external ear, which develops around the margins of the first ectodermal groove, is at first caudal to the developing face, but gradually it approaches and passes the level of the mouth.

FETAL PERIOD

By the beginning of the fetal period, which by convention begins at approximately 60 days of gestation, the embryo has acquired all of its basic morphological characteristics. For the remainder of its intrauterine existence, it will undergo maturation of its primordia, reorganize its spatial relationships, and begin to make functional use of some of its organ systems for its own needs (Fig. 2-10). Rapid and extensive growth characterizes the 7 months of fetal life with an increase from 30 to 330 mm, accompanied by an approximately tenfold increase in volume.

During late embryonic and early fetal periods, the primary embryonic posture is gradually modified by the growth of the nervous system with the development of the cervical pontine and midbrain flexures and the expansion of the forebrain (Fig. 2-11). As a result, the cranial base becomes flexed in the region of the pituitary fossa at the sphenooccipital junction, so that the developing face becomes tucked in under the cranium. The ventral surface of the developing brain stem similarly becomes flexed at the site of the pituitary fossa, resulting in a repositioning of the spinal cord from its posterior relationship to a more inferior one. Concomitantly, the exit of the spinal cord from the skull, the foramen magnum, changes from its posteriorly directed location to a vertical downward direction near the middle of the inferior surface of the skull. The downwardly directed foramen magnum is related to an upright (bipedal) posture and to an increased cranial capacity, both of which are features unique to man. A further consequence of the cranial flexure and a peculiarly hominid characteristic is the predominantly downward rather than forward displacement of the face during growth at the cranial base.

The growth of the cranial base is highly irregular in keeping with its shape, which it develops to accommodate the undulating ventral surface of the brain. The uneven growth of the different portions of the brain

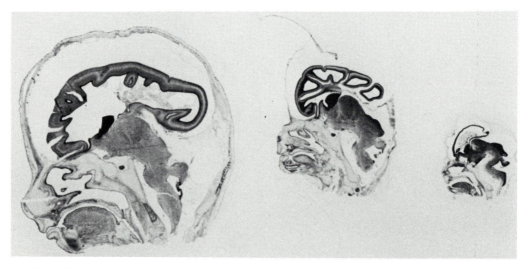

Fig. 2-11. Extent and direction of growth at cranial base that occurs in response to development of rapidly growing brain. (From Moss-Salentijn, L., Applebaum, E., and Lammé, A. T.: Orofacial histology and embryology: a visual integration, Philadelphia, 1972, F. A. Davis Co.)

is reflected in the related parts of the cranial base adapting as compartments or cranial fossae. The central ventral axis of the brain (the brain stem) undergoes conservative growth. It is related to the body of the sphenoid and basioccipital bones, which, by their slow growth, provide a comparatively stable base. Lateral, cranial, and caudal to this base, the frontal and temporal lobes of the neurocranium develop. The anterior, middle, and posterior fossae of the cranial floor, which contain the frontal and temporal lobes of the cerebrum, the cerebellum, expand rapidly as do these parts of the brain.

The integral relationship between the skeletal components and the rapidly developing brain is evidence of the relative importance of epigenetic factors, which increase markedly as the developing organism passes from the late embryonic period to the fetal period.

The expansion of the cranial base that occurs from the fetal period onward takes place as a result of a combination of growth processes, which includes interstitial, endochondral, and sutural or translational growth. Intrinsic growths of the cartilage remnants of the chondrocranium that persist between the bones are known as *synchondroses*. These cartilages contribute variably to cranial elongation and lateral expansion. The midsphenoidal synchondroses between the presphenoid and basisphenoid and between the body and wings of the sphenoid fuse shortly before birth (Fig. 2-12). The growth activity at the spheno-occipital synchondrosis is the major postnatal contributor to growth of the cranial base. It is the last of the synchondroses to fuse at approximately 17 to 20 years of age.

In addition to enlargement at the synchondroses, the cranial base undergoes selective appositional remodeling by resorption and deposition.[11] This process is characterized by activity on the part of the bone-forming cells, the osteoblasts, as well as bone-destroying cells, the osteoclasts, as described by Enlow.[9] Remodeling of bone allows preexisting spaces in the skull, such as the brain cavity and the orbits, to grow with the other structures, and

enables new cavities such as the paranasal sinuses to be formed.[17]

Marked resorption occurs in the floors of the cranial fossae, deepening these endocranial compartments. This deepening process is aided by the bodily displacement of the floors of the fossae as a result of sutural expansion of the lateral walls of the neurocranium. Parts of the sella turcica and the petrous portion of the temporal bone are exceptions to the generalized internal resorption of the cranial base in that some bone deposition may occur at these sites.

During the early stages of the fetal period, the initial centers of ossification in the facial region begin to develop and enlarge intramembranously within the condensed mesenchyme of the embryonic facial processes.

The ossification centers of the frontal bone, which forms the anterior part of the neurocranium, appear above the position of the future superciliary arches about the eighth week in utero. A variable number of secondary centers appear in each half and fuse before birth, but the left and right halves are separated by the frontal or metopic suture at birth. Obliteration of this suture commences about the second year and is complete at the fifth or sixth year, although in some cases the frontal bones remain separate throughout life.

In the frontonasal process, intramembranous single ossification centers appear for each of the nasal and lacrimal bones, and bilateral major and minor centers appear for the premaxillae. The embryonic maxillary facial processes develop numerous intramembranous ossification centers. Single centers appear for the maxillae and palatine bones, and two appear bilaterally for the vomer in the maxillary mesenchyme surrounding the cartilaginous nasal septum. The depths of the maxillary process develop intramembranous ossification centers for the greater wing of the sphenoid and for the pterygoid processes. Superficially, single centers appear for each of the squamous portions of the temporal and zygomatic bones. In the lower third of the face, the mandibular processes develop bilaterally from single intramem-

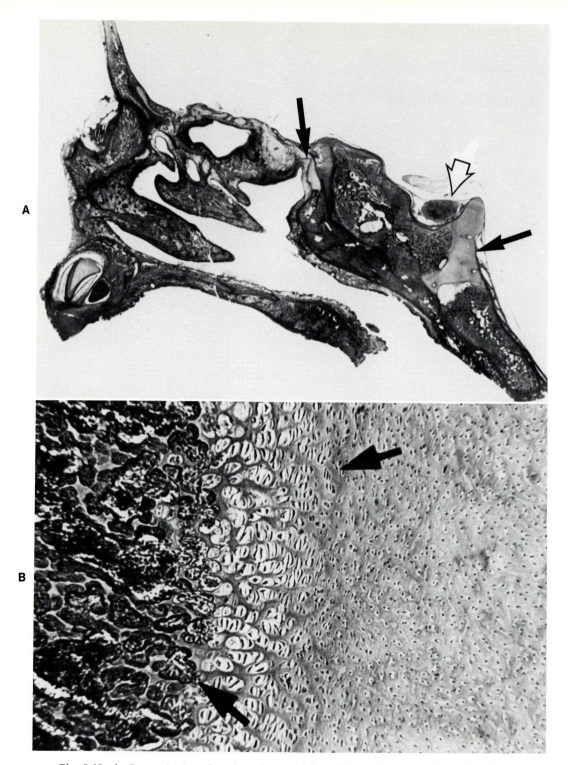

Fig. 2-12. A, Parasagittal section through cranial base illustrating progressive ossification of sphenoid and occipital bones and illustrating continued existence of endochondral growth centers at spheno-occipital and sphenoethmoidal synchondroses, *filled arrows. Open arrow,* pituitary fossa. **B,** Photomicrograph of higher magnification illustrating growth plate of the spheno-occipital synchondrosis showing various zones of transition between cartilage and bone. *Upper arrow,* hypertrophic zone; *lower arrow,* zone of calcification.

branous centers for the mandible and the tympanic portion of the temporal bone.

POSTNATAL PERIOD

A half century of controversy over the nature of the biological processes and the primary morphogenetic factors in postnatal craniofacial growth has been responsible for much interest in and investigation of the subject among clinicians and researchers alike. The problem goes beyond being one of simple academic or scholarly interest, since an understanding of these growth processes is fundamental to a rational and successful approach to treatment of individuals who present with acquired or congenital disturbances of growth in this region.

There are four mechanisms that have been held by various workers to provide self-sufficient explanations of the process of craniofacial growth with varying importance being attributed to the individual mechanisms depending on the investigator. These four mechanisms include (1) interstitial expansive forces generated by sutural tissues, (2) interstitial expansive forces generated by endochondral bone formation, (3) deposition and resorption of bone tissue, and (4) the action of periosteal and capsular functional matrices (epigenetic factors).

The first mechanism, that of the intrinsic forces of sutural growth, was introduced by Weinmann and Sicher,[45] who hypothesized that the primary factor in cranial growth was intrinsic expansion of the cranial sutures. Subsequent work, however, has shown that the sutures do not serve as primary growth centers. Sutural growth is compensatory and is reactive to growth changes occurring elsewhere in the craniofacial complex.

The second mechanism attributes the morphogenetic aspects of craniofacial growth to endochondral ossification at several cephalic cartilaginous areas. Perichondrial apposition and interstitial expansion of the cartilaginous tissues at these sites are said to serve as primary growth forces. Three principal cartilaginous areas have been proposed as serving these functions: the mandibular condyle, the nasal septum, and the basilar syn-

chondroses. Individuals who have been proponents of this as the primary process of craniofacial growth have compared these cranial cartilaginous areas to and made analogies in structure and function with the epiphyseal growth plates of the long bones elsewhere in the body. Numerous studies,[14, 19, 23] however, indicate that condylar cartilage is similar to articular cartilage in structure and is the site of secondary or compensatory growth rather than a primary growth site.

The work of Cleall and associates,[5a] using multiple injections of vital dyes, showed that the growth of the supraoccipital bone in rats from the time of birth consisted of deposition on the endochondral surface and resorption on the outer cranial surface despite a posterior movement of this bone in spatial relationship to the rest of the craniofacial complex.

The most recent theory of growth and development of the skull was conceived by van der Klaauw[40-42] and extended by Moss.[20, 21, 24, 26] They consider the growth of skeletal tissues to be secondary, compensatory, and mechanically obligatory responses to changes in the functional matrices. Moss[20] states that "the head is a composite structure, operationally consisting of a number of relatively independent functions: olfaction, respiration, vision, digestion, speech, audition, equilibration, and neural integration. Each function is carried out by a group of soft tissues which are supported and/or protected by related skeletal elements. Taken together, the soft tissues and skeletal elements related to a single function are termed a functional cranial component. The totality of all skeletal elements associated with a single function is termed a skeletal unit. The totality of soft tissues associated with a single function is termed a functional matrix." It may be demonstrated that the origin, growth, and maintenance of the skeletal unit depend almost exclusively on its related functional matrix; that is to say, functional matrices grow, and skeletal tissues respond.

Moss[26] believes there is little, if any, genetic control of skeletal tissue growth either of cartilage or bone but that the effects of genes are exerted directly on the functional matrices and secondarily or indirectly on the skeletal tissues themselves.

GENETIC ABNORMALITIES OF CRANIOFACIAL GROWTH

The role that heredity plays in the normal development of the craniofacial complex is never more evident than when an abnormality is produced, resulting in what has been referred to as "an experiment in nature." Numerous examples exist in which a single gene mutation results directly or indirectly in significant structural alterations in the head and face. A detailed analysis of the precise nature of the gene mutation often reveals the mechanisms by which a particular structure or group of structures affect overall craniofacial growth. For example, a number of aberrations in normal growth and development in the craniofacial complex have been attributed to abnormalities or deficiencies in the initial formation, migration, and subsequent development of cranial neural crest cells. These abnormalities can be divided into two broad categories, the first resulting from defects in neural crest cell formation and the second in defects in neural crest cell migration.

Deficiencies in the initial number of neural crest cells are frequently reflected in aberrant development in midfacial derivatives and are usually accompanied by defects in the forebrain and ocular structures. Experiments that artificially reduce the number of neural crest cells in avian embryos through the extirpation of small portions of the neural folds before crest cell migration result in characteristic brain-eye-face malformations.[6a] The facial defects involving the frontonasal processes were most common, whereas defects of derivatives of the maxillary processes and visceral arches were rare. Similar defects have been produced in mice by irradiating specific areas of the neural plate, thereby producing cell death limited to that region.[6a] The number of migrating cells is thereby significantly reduced, resulting in facial clefts and other frontonasal deficiency defects. The mass of the remaining neural plate is concomitantly reduced and presumably accounts for the associated brain and eye defects.

A group of human malformations similarly appear to be a result of variable deficiencies of the derivatives of neural crest cells. de Meyer and associates[6a] have described a spectrum of brain-eye-face malformations in which

Table 2-2. Types of holoprosencephaly*

Type of face	*Facial features*	*Cranium and brain*
Cyclopia	Single eye or partially divided eye in single orbit; arhinia with proboscis	Microcephaly; alobar holoprosencephaly
Ethmocephaly	Extreme orbital hypotelorism but separate orbits; arhinia with proboscis	Microcephaly; alobar holoprosencephaly
Cebocephaly	Orbital hypotelorism, proboscislike nose but no median cleft of lip	Microcephaly; usually has alobar holoprosencephaly
Median cleft lip	Orbital hypotelorism, flat nose	Microcephaly and sometimes trigonocephaly; usually has alobar holoprosencephaly
Bilateral cleft lip with median philtrum-premaxilla anlage	Orbital hypotelorism, bilateral lateral cleft of lip with median process representing philtrum-premaxillary anlage; flat nose	Microcephaly and sometimes trigonocephaly; semilobar or lobar holoprosencephaly

*Modified from de Meyer, W., Zeman, W., and Palmer, C. G.: The face predicts the brain; diagnostic significance of median facial anomalies for holoprosencephaly (arhinencephaly), Pediatrics **34:** 256, 1964.

the most consistent feature is a deficiency and variable degree of fusion of the cerebral hemispheres called *holoprosencephaly*. This group of malformation syndromes is listed in Table 2-2 in order of the degree of mesodermal deficiency resulting from the lack of neural crest cell formation and migration.

The second group of anomalies that results from an apparent hindrance of normal crest cell migration may be involved in the genesis of the midface cleft malformation, which is characterized by severe orbital hypertelorism, in which the two lateral facial primordia fail to fuse at the midline. This group of malformations, frequently referred to as frontonasal dysplasia, rarely have accompanying brain abnormalities or mental retardation. Other human malformations that have been attributed to defective neural crest cell migration include otocephaly, in which there is a failure of normal neural crest migration to the distal ends of the mandibular arch. In otocephaly the frontonasal derivatives are frequently intact. Treacher Collins syndrome (mandibulofacial dysostosis) is a malformation complex that involves coloboma of the eyelids, abnormal external ear development, micrognathia, and hypoplasia of the zygomaticomalar regions of the cranial skeleton. Treacher Collins syndrome has been produced in experimental animals by administering extremely high doses of vitamin A. Hypervitaminosis A results in an interruption in neural crest cell migration with the subsequent branchial arch anomalies.

Several other genetic diseases in humans have an effect on craniofacial development. These will be discussed in detail in Chapter 17. A few examples will be mentioned here to illustrate the indirect effects of gene mutation on craniofacial development.

Diseases that affect endochondral bone growth are generally reflected in the cranial base and produce what is described clinically as a "dished face" deformity and/or brachycephaly of the neurocranium. Conditions such as achondroplasia and other chondrodystrophies produce characteristic facial deformities by virtue of their effect on chondrocranial growth. Certain forms of class III dental malocclusion have also been shown to be related to defects of the chondrocranium.

The neurocranium is particularly susceptible to a number of genetic defects ranging from chromosomal to endocrine in etiology. The time of closure of the sutures is altered in many diseases leading to variable distortions of skull shape. In conditions such as cretinism, trisomy 21, and cleidocranial dysplasia, there is a delayed midline ossification of the frontal (metopic) and sagittal sutures of the calvaria, resulting in an anterior fontanelle that may remain open into adult life. The resulting brachycephalic skull in these conditions is typified by a broad forehead and hypertelorism.

Premature synostosis of various cranial sutures characterizes cases of acrocephalosyndactyly (Apert's syndrome) and craniofacial dysostosis (Crouzon's disease). The inability of the calvaria to grow normally in both of these conditions leads to skull distortion known as acrocephaly, oxycephaly, or turricephaly, all characterized by peaking of the vault of the skull. These skull anomalies invariably become worse during growth.

Defects of facial bones may occur as part of various genetic disorders. Among the more noteworthy anomalies are the scooped out facial appearance due to maxillary hypoplasia and a depressed nasal bridge in achondroplasia, Down's syndrome (trisomy 21), and anhidrotic ectodermal dysplasia. In mandibulofacial dysostosis (Treacher Collins syndrome), the sunken appearance of the midface occurs secondary to severe hypoplasia or absence of the zygomatic bones.

The combination of this direct and indirect evidence of the importance of the neural crest cells in normal craniofacial development provides strong evidence for the importance of the classical genetic mechanisms that involve DNA translation, transcription, and protein synthesis as a basic mechanism in craniofacial growth. The normal development of the craniofacial complex is organized and guided by an orderly and sequential turning on and off of the specific genes at specific places and times. Certain parts of the genetic material are activated at particular stages of the development, while other portions of the genome remain quiescent at those time only to become activated at some later stage in development. Normal development also depends on the inductive effect of one embryonic tissue on another. The phenotypic characteristics of a differentiated cell will depend both on its genotype and on the type and degree of gene repression and environmental influence that takes place in the course of differentiation. Disturbances in normal growth and development may result from defective genes or mutations, abnormal amounts of genetic material as in the case of aneuploidy or polyploidy or disturbances of the inductive patterns of embryonic tissues.

SUMMARY

The basic shape and, to a considerable degree, the size of individual bones are genetically determined. The various controlling factors that operate to give rise to the eventual structural phenotype of a give bone are not altogether clear; however, with regard to the intrinsic genetic factors, we can speculate that they operate through intracellular regulatory mechanisms in which the classical methods of RNA translation and transcription play an important role. Superimposed on the intrinsic genetic factors are epigenetic factors, such as nutritional, hormonal, and functional influences, which, due to the constant process of apposition and resorption occurring throughout life, enable the bone to respond to morphologically functional stresses. With respect to the general epigenetic and environmental factors, we can hypothesize that they affect the metabolic processes of the cells through stimulation or inhibition. The exact mechanism by which the functional forces produce structural bone changes is not clear, but it appears that forces are mediated through a piezoelectric effect.[1-3, 47] Bone, due to its crystalline nature, behaves as a crystal by generating a minute electric current that, when mechanically deformed, produces polar electric fields. These electric fields will, according to their charge, stimulate the activities of osteoblasts and osteoclasts to either resorb or deposit bone. These stress-induced electric currents may allow for the adjustments in bone structure that are made to meet new functional demands.

REFERENCES

1. Bassett, C. A. L.: Biologic significance of piezoelectricity, Calcif. Tissue Res. **1:**252-272, 1968.
2. Bassett, C. A. L., and Becker, R. O.: Generation of electric potentials by bone in response to mechanical stress, Science **137:**1063-1064, 1962.
3. Bassett, C. A. L., Pawluk, R. J., and Becker, R. O.: Effects of electric currents on bone in vivo, Nature **204:**652-654, 1964.
4. Bellaires, D. A.: Skull development in chick embryo after ablation of one eye, Nature **176:** 658-659, 1955.
5. Björk, A.: Facial growth in man, studied with the aid of metallic implants, Acta Odont. Scand. **13:**9-34, 1955.
5a. Cleall, J. F., Wilson, G. W., and Garnett, D. S.: Normal craniofacial skeletal growth of the rat, Am. J. Phys. Anthropol. **29:**225-242, 1968.
6. Coulombre, A. J., and Crelin, E. S.: The role of the developing eye in the morphogenesis of the avian skull, Am. J. Phys. Anthropol. **16:** 25-38, 1958.
6a. de Meyer, W., Zeman, W., and Palmer, C. G.: The face predicts the brain: diagnostic significance of median facial anomalies for holoprosencephaly (arhinencephaly), Pediatrics **34:** 256, 1964.
7. du Brul, E. L., and Laskin, D. M.: Preadaptive potentialities of the mammalian skull: an experiment in growth and form, Am. J. Anat. **109:**117-132, 1961.
8. Durkin, J. F., Irving, J. T., and Healey, J. D.: A comparison of the circulatory and calcification patterns in the mandibular condyle in the guinea pig with those found in the tibial epiphyseal and articular cartilages, Arch. Oral Biol. **14:**1365-1371, 1969.
9. Enlow, D. E.: The human face: an account of the postnatal growth and development of the craniofacial skeleton, New York, 1968, Harper & Row, Publishers.
10. Enlow, D. H.: A morphogenetic analysis of facial growth, Am. J. Orthod. **52:**283-299, 1966.
11. Hoyte, D. A. N.: Experimental investigations of skull morphology and growth. In Felts, W. J. L., and Harrison, R. J., editors: International review of general and experimental zoology, vol. 2, New York, 1966, Academic Press, Inc., pp. 345-407.
11a. Johnston, M. C., and Pratt, R. M.: The neural crest in normal and abnormal cranio-

facial development. In Slavkin, H. C., and Greulich, R. C., editors: Extracellular matrix influences on gene expression, New York, 1975, Academic Press, Inc.

12. Keith, A.: Human embryology and morphology, ed. 6, Baltimore, 1948, The Williams & Wilkins Co.

13. Koski, K.: Some characteristics of craniofacial growth cartilages. In Moyers, R. E., and Krogman, W. M.: Cranio-facial growth in man, Elmsford, N.Y., 1971, Pergamon Press, Inc.

14. Koski, K.: Cranial growth centers: facts or fallacies, Am. J. Orthod. **54:**566-583, 1968.

15. Koski, K., and Rönning, O.: Growth potential of subcutaneously transplanted cranial base synchondroses of the rat, Acta Odontol. Scand. **27:**343-357, 1969.

16. Kraus, B. S., Wise, W. J., and Frei, R. H.: Heredity and the craniofacial complex, Am. J. Orthod. **45:**172-217, 1959.

17. Krogman, W. M.: The growth of the head and face studied craniometrically and cephalometrically in normal and in cleft palate children, Symposium on Congenital anomalies of the face and associated structures, Springfield, Ill., 1961, Charles C Thomas, Publisher, pp. 208-236.

17a. le Douarin, N. M.: Extracellular factors controlling the migration and differentiation of the ganglioblasts of the autonomic nervous system. In Slavkin, H. C., and Greulich, R. C., editors: Extracellular matrix influences on gene expression, New York, 1975, Academic Press, Inc.

18. Moss, M. L.: Growth of the calvaria in the rat, Am. J. Anat. **94:**333-362, 1954.

19. Moss, M. L.: A functional analysis of human mandibular growth, J. Prosthet. Dent. **10:** 1149-1160, 1960.

20. Moss, M. L.: The functional matrix. In Kraus, B., and Reidel, R., editors: Vistas in orthodontics, Philadelphia, 1962, Lea & Febiger, pp. 85-98.

21. Moss, M. L.: Differential roles of periosteal and capsular matrices in orofacial growth, Trans. Eur. Orthod. Sec. (In press.)

22. Moss, M. L., and Bromberg, B.: The passive role of nasal septal cartilage in mid-facial growth, Plast. Reconstr. Surg. **41:**536-542, 1967.

23. Moss, M. L., and Rankow, R.: The role of the functional matrix in mandibular growth, Angle Orthod. **38:**95-103, 1968.

24. Moss, M. L., and Salentijn, L.: The primary role of functional matrices in facial growth, Am. J. Orthod. **55:**566-577, 1969.

25. Moss, M. L., and Salentijn, L.: The capsular matrix, Am. J. Orthod. **56:**474-490, 1969.

26. Moss, M. L., and Young, R.: A functional

approach to craniology, Am. J. Phys. Anthropol. **18:**281-292, 1969.

27. Moyers, R. E., and Krogman, W. M.: Craniofacial growth in man, Elmsford, N.Y., 1971, Pergamon Press, Inc.

28. Rönning, O., and Koski, K.: Obervations on the histology and histochemistry of growth cartilages in young rats, Dent. Pract. (Bristol) **17:**448-450, 1967.

29. Ross, R. B., and Johnston, M. C.: Cleft lip and palate, Baltimore, 1972, The Williams & Wilkins Co.

30. Sarnat, B. G.: Post-natal growth of the upper face: some experimental considerations, Angle Orthod. **33:**139-161, 1963.

31. Sarnat, B. G., and Laskin, D. M.: Cartilage and cartilage implants, Surg. Gynecol. Obstet. **99:**521-541, 1954.

32. Sarnat, B. G., and Wexler, M. R.: Growth of the face and jaws after resection of the septal cartilage, Am. J. Anat. **118:**755-767, 1966.

33. Schowing, J.: Influence inductrice de l'encéphale et de la chorde sur la morphogenese du squelette cranien chez l'embryon de poulet, J. Embryol. Exp. Morphol. **9:**326-334, 1961.

34. Scott, J. H.: The cartilage of the nasal septum: a contribution to the study of facial growth, Br. Dent. J. **95:**37-43, 1953.

35. Selman, A. J., and Sarnat, B. G.: Growth of the rabbit snout after extirpation of the frontonasal suture, Am. J. Anat. **101:**273-293, 1957.

36. Sperber, G. H.: Craniofacial embryology, Baltimore, 1973, The Williams & Wilkins Co.

37. Stenstrom, S. J., and Thilander, B. L.: Effects of nasal septal cartilage resections on young guinea pigs, Plast. Reconstr. Surg. **45:**160-170, 1970.

38. Tuchmann-Duplessis, H., David, G., and Haegel, P.: Illustrated human embryology, vol. 1, Embryogenesis, New York, 1972, Springer-Verlag New York, Inc.

39. van der Klaauw, C. J.: Cerebral skull and facial skull: a contribution to the knowledge of skull structure, Arch. Neerl. Zool. **7:**16-36, 1946.

40. van der Klaauw, C. J.: Size and position of the functional components of the skull: a contribution to the knowledge of the architecture of the skull, based on data in the literature, Arch. Neerl. Zool. **9:**1-176, 1948.

41. van der Klaauw, C. J.: Size and position of the functional components of the skull: a contribution to the knowledge of the architecture of the skull, based on data in the literature (continuation), Arch. Neerl. Zool. **9:**177-368, 1951.

42. van der Klaauw, C. J.: Size and position of the functional components of the skull: a con-

tribution to the knowledge of the architecture of the skull, based on data in the literature (conclusion), Arch. Neerl. Zool. **9**:369-560, 1952.

43. van Limborgh, J.: The regulation of the embryonic development of the skull, Acta Morphol. Neerl. Scand. **7**:101-102, 1968.

44. van Limborgh, J.: A new view on the control of the morphogenesis of the skull, Acta Morphol. Neerl. Scand. **8**:143-160, 1970.

45. Weinmann, J. P., and Sicher, H.: Bone and bones, St. Louis, 1947, The C. V. Mosby Co.

46. Weiss, P., and Amrpino, R.: The effect of mechanical stress on the differentiation of scleral cartilage in vitro and in the embryo, Growth **4**:245-258, 1940.

47. Yasuda, I.: On the piezoelectric activity of bone, J. Jap. Orthop. Surg. Soc. **28**:267-269, 1954.

3

The pedigree and its interpretation

RAY E. STEWART

In recent decades, recognition of the importance of genetics as a clinical science in dentistry has greatly increased as it has in the other health sciences. The incidence of diseases with infectious or environmental causes, which earlier accounted for the majority of major medical problems, has steadily declined due to the introduction and widespread use of antibiotics, vaccinations, and other wonder drugs (Fig. 3-1). The relative increase in the proportion of genetically determined diseases has made it essential for dentists and physicians to become familiar with the role of heredity in the cause of or predisposition to disease in man.[2]

The practice of dentistry and medicine is based primarily on an approach to disease that resolves the questions of, What is wrong with the patient? (diagnosis), What will happen to him? (prognosis), and What can be done about it? (treatment).[6]

In the course of developing a rational diagnosis, prognosis, and plan of management for the patient, the clinician is compelled to call on a body of background knowledge derived from basic sciences such as anatomy, physiology, biochemistry, and, increasingly, genetics.

A knowledge of genetics is essential (1) to recognize the probable presence of unobvious internal disease or dysmorphology based on the presence of other external signs or traits that are part of a hereditary syndrome and (2) to recognize early manifestations or mild expression of a genetic disease through an understanding of the usual mode of transmission for the disease in question and (3) to gain a knowledge of the family history of the individual under examination.

The rendering of an accurate diagnosis depends, in part, on a systematic method of gathering, recording, and interpreting information obtained from a thorough case history, the clinical examination, and laboratory tests. A complete case history should contain detailed medical, dental, family, and social histories, which, when combined with laboratory data, radiographic studies, and clinical examination, allows for the postulation of a differential diagnosis and the formulation of a comprehensive and rational plan for treatment.

Obtaining a complete family history as a part of the case history is one of the most important but, unfortunately, most frequently neglected steps in arriving at an accurate diagnosis. The procedure is of particular importance when the trait in question appears to be familial in its occurrence, thereby raising the possibility of a genetic cause.

Attitudes vary among busy practitioners toward taking a family history as part of the routine diagnostic procedure. Many believe that the information it reveals does not make it worth the time it takes to construct. A geneticist, on the other hand, believes that a complete pedigree should be done on every possible case of genetic interest. In fact, the

67

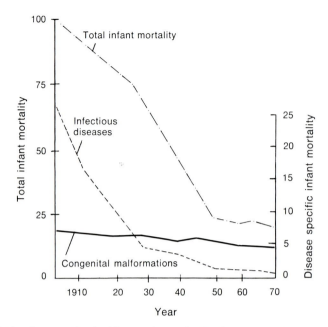

Fig. 3-1. Relative increase for incidence of genetically determined diseases. (Modified from Gordon, H.: J.A.M.A. **217:**1215, 1971.)

truth probably lies somewhere between these extremes, as we shall see.

The necessity for a dentist to be capable of recognizing and dealing with genetic disease is becoming increasingly important due to the number of recognized genetic traits and diseases that involve oral facial structures. Gorlin and Pindborg[3] list in excess of 150 syndromes, many of which are genetically determined and all having clinical manifestations in the head and neck region. McKusick[8] has cataloged in excess of 1900 genetic diseases, of which no fewer than 450, either directly or indirectly, affect structures in the craniofacial complex.

In this chapter I will discuss a simple and successful method for recording a family history and review some basic concepts necessary for interpretation of these data once they are available.

In man, that portion of the family history which deals with the distribution of particular characteristics or diseases in families is best studied by the *pedigree* method. The pedigree is a system of analyzing for a particular trait or traits that result from matings already made. Diagrams, commonly called family

trees, are constructed to symbolize individuals and illustrate relationships between them. Once the technique is mastered, a family history may be recorded much more lucidly and quickly in the form of a pedigree than in the usual paragraphic form. An experienced interviewer can construct an informative pedigree in a matter of a few minutes, with the added advantage of having the result be meaningful to anyone else reviewing the history.

The routine use of this procedure would not contribute greatly to the time needed for diagnosis or treatment planning of the majority of cases seen in a dental practice. As a basic minimum, the family history ought to include the following information:

1. A statement about the occurrence of any disease in the family that may be relevant to the patient's complaint
2. A statement about the patient's parents, siblings, and offspring, including age, sex, and health status
3. A statement concerning the presence or absence of consanguinity in the family

When the routine family history reveals the presence of more than one affected person in a family (kindred) or a history of consanguinity in a patient with an uncommon, non-infectious disease, the possibility of that disease having a genetic cause should be entertained and requires that the family history be examined in detail before arriving at a diagnosis and providing intelligent counseling. In addition to the obvious factors of genetic interest, the family history might also reveal certain nongenetic familial traits of interest and importance. The family's socioeconomic or cultural patterns should alert one to an increased risk to certain environmental pathogens or to the predisposition of a patient to a nutritional imbalance or to poor hygiene habits as a possible cause for the observed abnormalities.

It is important to differentiate *familial* and *genetic* traits. A trait or disease that occurs with a high frequency within a kindred does not necessarily have a genetic cause. An example of such a phenomenon is a condition of physical and mental retardation that accompanies endemic cretinism and is in fact caused by an environmental determinant resulting from the lack of iodine in the diet.

As with nomenclature, there is no universal agreement among geneticists concerning the use of pedigree symbols to represent individuals and their relationships within the family. In the United States, squares are used to represent males, and circles represent females. In the European literature, however, the pedigrees most commonly employ the symbols ♂ for males and ♀ for females. The sex symbols are connected similarly in both systems to indicate the relationship between the individuals.

For easier reference, individuals in a pedigree are frequently assigned numbers. Roman numerals in the left margin indicate the generation and increase from top to bottom. Arabic numerals, which are placed under or beside the individual symbols, increase from left to right within each generation. Using this system the propositus in the pedigree in Fig. 3-2 would be identified as III-5. It is important to remember that individuals within a generation are numbered irrespective of relationship, such that only II-2, II-4, II-5,

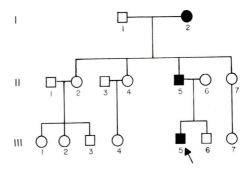

Fig. 3-2. Pedigree example showing use of various symbols to represent individuals and their relationships. Roman numerals in left margin indicate generation, and Arabic numerals under or beside each individual symbol represent their position within sibship and within generation.

and II-7 are siblings in the second generation.

To conserve space, certain shorthand methods are often used to represent uninformative progeny in a sibship rather than drawing them individually. Most commonly this is accomplished by entering a number inside a sex symbol. For example, ③ indicates three girls, and ②̄ indicates two boys. The symbol ⬦₇ would indicate seven siblings, sex unknown.

Couples producing offspring are joined by a horizontal line; □——○ indicates marriage; □- - -○ is commonly used to signify divorce or illegitimacy. Males are by convention placed on the left and the females on the right except in the case of multiple marriages. A double line, □══○, identifies a consanguineous mating. Frequently, uninformative or obviously normal spouses are omitted from the pedigree as in II-7 in Fig. 3-2, which should not be construed to imply parthenogenesis.

A line dropped vertically from the marriage line to a succeeding horizontal line or generation is called a *progeny line*. Short perpendicular lines attach the individual offspring to the progeny line with the order of birth being from left to right. A broken progeny line, ○┌┄┐□, indicates that the birth order is uncertain. A broken vertical line to one of the progeny is sometimes used to indicate doubtful legitimacy. Adoption is indicated by enclosing the individual symbol in brackets, [○].

Individuals in the pedigree who are affected with the disease or trait under study are indicated by inked-in symbols, ●, and those who are normal remain open, ○. Problems sometimes arise when multiple traits are being studied simultaneously. In such cases the sex symbol may be variously divided into segments with each segment representing a specific trait. When this technique is employed, a key is indispensable as a reference to the meanings of the various symbols.

Various other symbols are used less frequently but are often necessary in the construction of an extensive pedigree. These symbols are included in Table 3-1.

The interview procedure and recording of information necessary to construct the pedigree should follow an organized sequence. Most commonly, study of a particular trait in a family begins with an affected person referred to as the *proband, propositus* (female: proposita), or *index case,* who is indicated in the pedigree by an arrow, →. The patient's siblings are then recorded chronologically on the same line. All pregnancies,

including stillbirths, miscarriages, and abortions should be recorded. The parents, their siblings, and their offspring (the patient's first cousins) are then added. Husband and wife are usually placed at the adjacent ends of their respective sibships for the convenience of joining them by a marriage line. This process is extended to include three generations or further if information is available and pertinent.

Depending on the detail sought in a particular pedigree, the following information should be obtained for each individual entered in the pedigree:

1. Full name (including maiden name)
2. Residence location (county or city) or place of death
3. Age (birthdate) or age at death
4. Health status or cause of death
5. Consanguineous marriage
6. Number, ages, and sexes of offspring
7. Birth order in sibship
8. Marriage order for multiple marriages
9. Abortions and stillbirths for females
10. Illegitimacies where determined
11. Dates of marriages, divorces, and separations

In addition, a thorough pedigree should

Table 3-1. Frequently used pedigree symbols

□	Male	□——○	Marriage
[5]	Five males	□══○	Consanguineous marriage
○	Female	□╌─○──□	Double mating; illegitimacy or divorce
③	Three females		
◇	Sex unknown	□╌─┬╌─○	Illegitimacy
Ⓢ	Eight male and female siblings	□——⊥——○	No issue
■	Examined professionally; affected with trait	○══○	Identical twins
■	Not examined professionally; reported to have trait	○　FR　○	Fraternal twins
⊙	Clinically normal but a carrier		Smaller symbols
⊡	Examined professionally; normal for trait	⊘	Lived less than a day
□	Not examined; reported normal for trait	Ⓟ	Pregnancy
[□]	Adopted	⊞	Stillbirth
⊘	Male, deceased	●	Miscarriage

contain details of ethnic background, including race, religion, national origin, and family names for both maternal and paternal sides of the family. The information may be useful in several respects. Certain religious groups, such as the Mormons, keep detailed genealogical records including birth, death, and marriage data. The knowledge that some diseases are more prevalent in certain races or religious groups may be helpful in arriving at a differential diagnosis. Examples include Tay-Sachs disease in Ashkenazic Jews, sickle cell disease in Negroes, and pyruvate kinase deficiency in the Amish. Finally, this information may be helpful in establishing consanguinity when considering a diagnosis of a disease that is transmitted genetically as an autosomal recessive trait.

INTERPRETATION OF THE PEDIGREE

Once the pedigree is constructed, the information it contains must be analyzed and interpreted. Whenever possible, the pattern of transmission is determined for the trait or disease entity in question. Traits and rare diseases in man are often distributed in families in characteristic patterns that follow Mendel's laws.

Genetic traits are passed from generation to generation in all species, including *Homo sapiens,* according to principles that were first delineated by Mendel[9] in 1865 through hybridization experiments using the common garden pea. These principles, which have come to be called *laws* because of their universal application to all living organisms, demonstrate that the transmission of inherited traits is not always ambiguous but follows predictable patterns. The success of Mendel's experiments was due, in part, to his rigid selection of simple but constant characteristics or traits to be studied in which such factors as breeding could be completely controlled by the experimenter. His experiments resulted in the formulation of the following principles:

1. The law of dominance and recessiveness
2. The law of segregation
3. The law of random assortment

The law of dominance and recessiveness became apparent to Mendel when, during his experiments, he crossed two true-breeding plants differing in only one particular characteristic (for example, color of immature pods or length of stem) and noted that the first generation offspring (F_1 for filial 1) resembled only one of the parental types. For example, a cross of a true-breeding green pod plant with a true-breeding yellow pod plant resulted in 100% green podded F_1 offspring. A cross of F_1 green with another F_1 green ($F_1[gr] \times F_1[gr]$) plant resulted in both pod types (green and yellow) appearing in the F_2 generation in a ratio of 3:1, indicating that the factors determining yellow color were

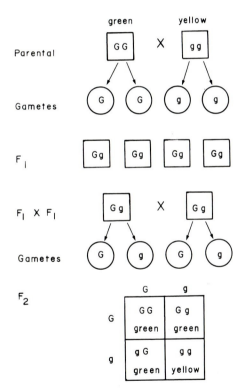

Fig. 3-3. Diagram illustrating Mendel's experiments using truebreeding plants, which produce homozygous green, *GG,* and yellow, *gg,* seed pods. Progeny of truebreeding parents resulted in F_1 generation of 100% heterozygous green, *Gg,* pod-producing plants. Backcross of $F_1 \times F_1$ heterozygotes (*Gg* × *Gg*) produces green and yellow F_2 offspring in ratio of 3:1. Mendel correctly concluded from these experiments that green trait is dominant to recessive yellow pod color trait.

still present in the F_1 plants but that their expression was somehow suppressed. Mendel concluded that the trait expressed in the F_1 offspring (green pod) was *dominant* over yellow pod color, which he called the *recessive* trait (Fig. 3-3).

By these experiments Mendel was able to establish the classical patterns of transmission of certain traits, which he correctly hypothesized were determined by a "pair of units" of which only one was derived from each parent. These units of inheritance are what we now call *genes*.

The gene pair, of which half is paternal and half is maternal in origin, which determines a particular trait, are referred to as *alleles*.

In his experiments Mendel noted that allelic pairs determining a particular trait were transmitted separately from one generation to the next. The phenomenon is called the *law of segregation*, which explains why the consistent ratios of phenotypes in the offspring are observed. By repeating the hybridization experiments, with various combinations of characteristics, Mendel observed that the different traits or alleles are transmitted independently of one another and reappear in random assortments or combinations in the offspring.

Although the majority of Mendel's work was done with the common garden pea, the principles he outlined form the basis for understanding the patterns of inheritance of single gene (monogenic) traits in man as well.

It is now a well established fact that human somatic cells contain a total of forty-six chromosomes consisting of twenty-two pairs of autosomes and two sex chromosomes. The sex chromosomes are conventionally designated X and Y, the normal female having an XX complement, the normal male XY.

A *gene* is simply defined as that portion of a chromosome which holds the DNA sequence and hence the coded information for a given polypeptide chain. The place on the chromosome where a particular gene is located is called a *locus*. There are corresponding loci on each of the chromosomes of a homologous pair that carry information for the same trait. If both chromosomes of a homologous pair contain the same information at a particular locus, the alleles are identical, and the individual is said to be *homozygous* for the trait. If the alleles are for variable forms of the trait, the individual is said to be *heterozygous* for the trait.

The specific pattern a trait follows depends on whether the responsible gene is located on an autosome or one of the sex chromosomes (X or Y). It also depends on whether the gene responsible for the trait is in the heterozygous state (single dose, or on only one of the alleles) or the homozygous state (double dose, or on both alleles of the allelic pair). Traits observable in a person heterozygous for a particular gene are called *dominant*, whereas those traits which are observable only in persons homozygous for the given gene are called *recessive*. Dominance and recessiveness are attributes of the trait, not the gene as is often implied by the use of the terms "dominant gene" or "recessive gene."

Following are brief descriptions of the classical modes of inheritance with an outline of the characteristics of each type:

A. Autosomal inheritance
  1. Autosomal dominant inheritance
    a. A gene that is located on an autosome and, regardless of the state of its allele, will result in the expression of a particular characteristic or disease, is called *autosomal dominant*. In a disease exhibiting simple autosomal dominant inheritance, the affected individual will in most cases be heterozygous for the trait and will produce gametes containing normal and abnormal alleles in a 1:1 ratio. If such a person were to marry a normal individual, there would be a 50% chance that each of the offspring would be affected (Fig. 3-4). It follows that, except in the case of a new mutation, which is extremely rare, each affected individual will have an affected parent. Autosomal dominant traits often show a wide range of variability. The degree of severity of a trait is referred to as its *expression*. The expression may be so reduced as to make the trait clini-

cally undetectable. This phenomenon results in apparent skip in generations and accounts for fewer than the expected 50% of children being clinically affected. If, for example, only 80 out of every 100 persons carrying a given dominant gene are clinically affected, the gene is said to have 80% *penetrance*. This range of variation in expression of gene action may be due to environmental influences or due to the effects of modifier genes. The following are general characteristics typical of a pedigree demonstrating autosomal dominant inheritance:

(1) Heterozygotes are affected.

(2) The transmission pattern is vertical (affected parent transmits to half of offspring).

(3) Affected males equal affected females.

(4) Male-to-male transmission is possible.

(5) There is wide variation in gene expression.

b. Examples of diseases following autosomal dominant transmission are hereditary opalescent dentin, missing or peg-shaped lateral incisors, osteogenesis imperfecta with dentinogenesis imperfecta, white sponge nevus, Peutz-Jeghers syndrome, hypocalcified type of amelogenesis imperfecta, and mandibulofacial dysostosis.

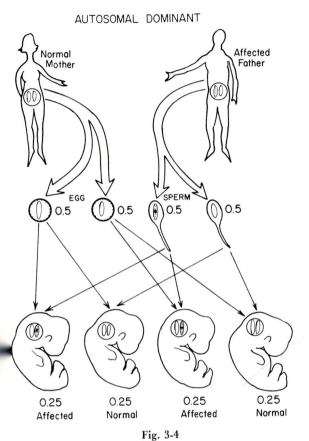

AUTOSOMAL DOMINANT

Fig. 3-4

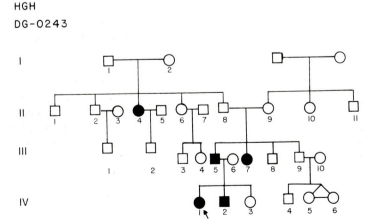

HGH
DG-0243

Fig. 3-5. Pedigree of kindred with hereditary opalescent dentin demonstrating features of autosomal dominant inheritance. Note vertical pattern of transmission and male-to-male transmission; both males and females are affected, and in general, half of offspring are affected.

c. Fig. 3-5 is a sample pedigree for autosomal dominant inheritance.

2. Autosomal recessive inheritance

a. As with dominant traits, autosomal recessive traits characteristically affect both males and females in equal numbers. In most cases, both parents appear clinically normal; however, both are heterozygous for the mutant gene and are commonly called *carriers*. Since related individuals are more likely to be heterozygous for the same rare mutant gene, one is apt to find evidence of a *consanguineous* mating in parents of individuals who are affected by recessive traits. In the case of a rare recessive trait, the elucidation of parental consanguinity may be the factor that leads the investigator to assign a genetic cause to the trait in question. Among the offspring of carrier parents, heterozygous for a mutant gene, the probability of

one child being homozygous for that gene is one in four (25%), and the chance that a sibling of an affected child will be similarly affected is also one in four irrespective of sex. The chance of an offspring being heterozygous (a carrier) for the trait is two in four (50%), and the chance of being free of the mutant gene is again one in four (25%) (Fig. 3-6). Autosomal recessive characteristics can be summarized as follows:

(1) Only the homozygote is affected.

(2) The pedigree pattern is horizontal (siblings are affected but not parents).

(3) Affected males equal affected females.

(4) Heterozygous (carrier) parents produce, on the average, 1 normal:2 carriers:1 affected.

(5) Consanguinity is common in rare recessive traits (the more rare the trait, the more frequently consanguinity is observed).

(6) There is little variation in clinical pattern of affected individuals.

(7) Often a defective enzyme system is involved.

b. Examples of autosomal recessive traits affecting oral facial structures are agranulocytosis, hypophosphatasia, acatalasia, acrocephalopolysyndactyly type (Carpenter), and Papillon-Lefèvre syndrome.

c. Fig. 3-7 is a sample pedigree for autosomal recessive inheritance.

B. Sex-linked inheritance

Some genetic traits are carried on one of the sex chromosomes, generally the X, and as a result are called sex-linked or, more properly, *X-linked* characteristics. The most prominent feature of X-linked inheritance is that male-to-male transmission does not occur. This results from the fact that the son gets only the father's Y sex chromosome and not the X, which carries the mutant gene. It follows that all female offspring of a hemizygous (having only one X chromosome) male will receive the mutant gene through his X chromosome.

In females, X-linked traits may be expressed either as dominant or recessive depending on whether the trait is clinically manifested in the homozygous state. In hemizygous males, on the other hand, sex-linked traits are regularly expressed.

AUTOSOMAL RECESSIVE

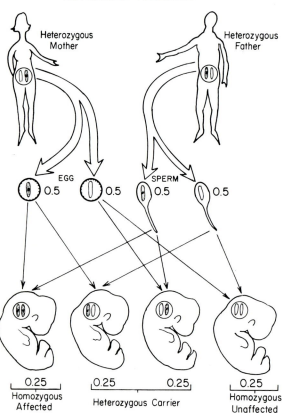

Fig. 3-6

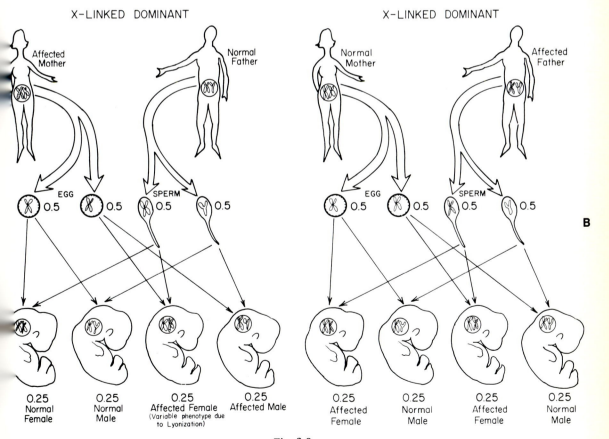

HGH
DG-0092

Fig. 3-7. Pedigree of family showing autosomal recessive inheritance of hereditary fructose intolerance, a metabolic disorder leading to intolerance of fructose from infancy and resulting in greatly reduced incidence of dental caries in affected individuals. Note horizontal transmission, both sexes affected, clinically normal parents, and consanguineous marriage of first cousins.

X-LINKED DOMINANT

X-LINKED DOMINANT

Affected Mother

Normal Father

Normal Mother

Affected Father

EGG 0.5 0.5   SPERM 0.5 0.5

EGG 0.5 0.5   SPERM 0.5 0.5

0.25 Normal Female

0.25 Normal Male

0.25 Affected Female (Variable phenotype due to Lyonization)

0.25 Affected Male

0.25 Affected Female

0.25 Normal Male

0.25 Affected Female

0.25 Normal Male

B

Fig. 3-8

1. X-linked dominant inheritance
   a. In X-linked dominant traits, heterozygous females and hemizygous males are affected. In a pattern resembling autosomal dominant transmission, an affected female transmits the trait to half of her sons and half of her daughters. An affected male, on the other hand, transmits the trait to all of his daughters and none of his sons. It is for this reason that X-linked dominant traits are observed in females about twice as frequently as in males (Fig. 3-8). X-linked dominant characteristics may be summarized as follows:
      (1) Hemizygous males and heterozygous females are affected.
      (2) An affected male transmits to all of his daughters and none of his sons (no male-to-male transmission).
      (3) An affected heterozygous female transmits to half of her offspring regardless of sex.
      (4) The pedigree resembles an autosomal dominant pedigree without male-to-male transmission.
      (5) There is a predominance of affected females (2:1).
   b. Examples of X-linked dominant traits having oral implications are vitamin D–resistant rickets, amelogenesis imperfecta (hypoplastic type), and orofaciodigital syndrome, type I.
   c. Fig. 3-9 is a sample pedigree for X-linked dominant inheritance.

2. X-linked recessive inheritance
   a. This particular type of disorder occurs almost exclusively in males. X-linked recessive traits are not expressed in the heterozygous female (carrier) except in extremely rare instances in which there is a random inactivation (Lyonization) of all of her normal X chromosomes, but she transmits the trait to half of her sons (Fig. 3-10, *A*). Among the offspring of a hemizygous affected male, none of the sons are affected, and all of the daughters will be heterozygous carriers for the trait (Fig. 3-10, *B*). Rarely, a homozygous, hence an affected female, may be produced when an affected male mates with a carrier female. X-linked recessive characteristics are summarized as follows:
      (1) The male hemizygote is affected; a female homozygote is affected; a female heterozygote (carrier) is clinically normal.
      (2) The transmission pattern is oblique: a heterozygous female transmits to half of her sons; half of her daughters are heterozygous carriers; maternal uncles may be affected.
   b. The most common examples of this type of inheritance are hemophilia A and color blindness. Other disorders that are transmitted as X-linked recessives and that have dental implications are amelogenesis imperfecta (hypomaturation type), anhidrotic ectodermal dysplasia,

HGH
DG–0491

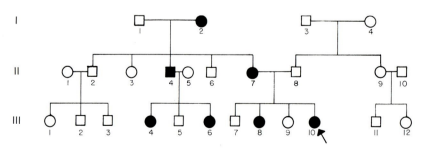

Fig. 3-9. Pedigree of kindred segregating for vitamin D–resistant rickets demonstrating typical X-linked dominant inheritance. Both sexes are affected; note absence of male-to-male transmission and preponderance of affected females (2:1).

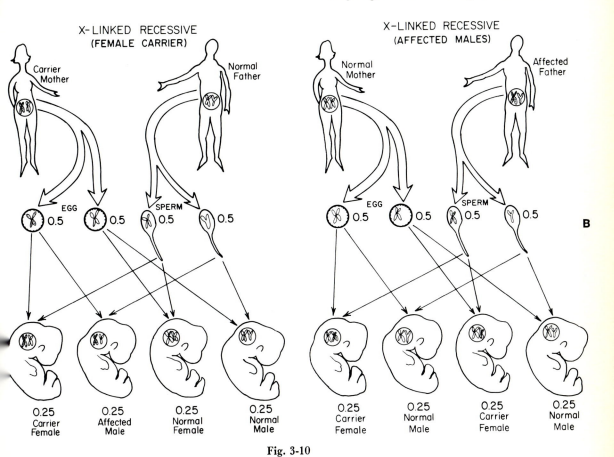

X-LINKED RECESSIVE
(FEMALE CARRIER)

Carrier Mother   Normal Father

EGG   SPERM
0.5   0.5   0.5   0.5

0.25   0.25   0.25   0.25
Carrier   Affected   Normal   Normal
Female   Male   Female   Male

X-LINKED RECESSIVE
(AFFECTED MALES)

Normal Mother   Affected Father

EGG   SPERM
0.5   0.5   0.5   0.5

B

0.25   0.25   0.25   0.25
Carrier   Normal   Carrier   Normal
Female   Male   Female   Male

Fig. 3-10

HGH
MG-1073

Fig. 3-11. Pedigree of kindred showing **X**-linked recessive inheritance in family segregating for hemophilia A. Only males are affected, and females are carriers.

congenitally missing teeth in certain families, and pseudohypoparathyroidism.

  c. Fig. 3-11 is a sample pedigree for X-linked recessive inheritance.

  3. Y-linked (holandric) inheritance

  a. At the present time there is conclusive evidence of only one specific gene being located on the Y chromosome. This gene results in a trait known as *hairy pinnae* (hairy ears). Holandric inheritance should be unmistakable on examination of a pedigree, since a father should pass the trait to all of his sons and none of his daughters (Fig. 3-12). The Y chromosome seems to play its major role as the determinant of "maleness" in man; however, a specific gene or genes for this trait has not been identified. The characteristics of holandric inheritance are summarized as follows:

  (1) Males are exclusively affected.

(2) A male transmits to all male offspring and to no female offspring.

  b. There are no known examples of dental traits following this mode of inheritance.

  c. Fig. 3-13 is a sample pedigree for Y-linked inheritance.

C. Polygenic (multifactorial) inheritance

The concept of action by multiple genes or polygenic inheritance is now one of the most important principles of genetics. This concept will be dealt with in detail in Chapters 4 and 5, but it will be mentioned briefly here to contrast it with monogenic inheritance. It differs from the classical Mendelian patterns of inheritance in its lack of gene specificity. The whole range of variation is observed in a graded series from one parental extreme to the other. An explanation of this wide range of variation is based on the action of many genes (polygenic) usually segregating independently but influencing the same phenotypic trait in a cumulative fashion; the gene action is said to be *continuously variable*. The most frequently encountered problems confronting dental practitioners involve this type of quantitative inheritance. Dental problems exhibiting a polygenic type of inheritance are malocclusion, dental caries, periodontal disease, and most forms of cleft lip and palate. The characteristics of polygenic traits are as follows:

1. The trait is expressed variably in siblings.
2. One or both parents and other relatives may be mildly or fully affected.
3. The genes are additive, giving a threshold effect.

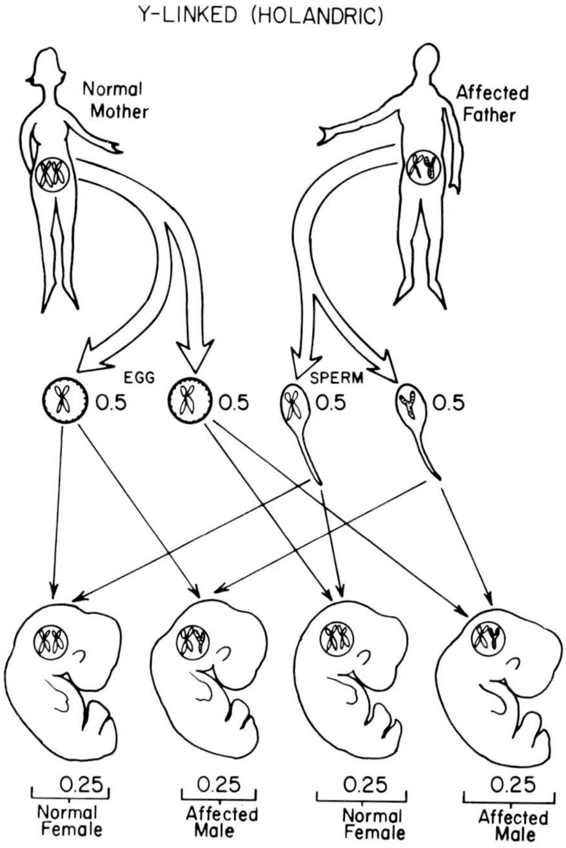

Y-LINKED (HOLANDRIC)

Normal Mother

Affected Father

EGG 0.5   0.5   SPERM 0.5   0.5

| 0.25 Normal Female | 0.25 Affected Male | 0.25 Normal Female | 0.25 Affected Male |

Fig. 3-12

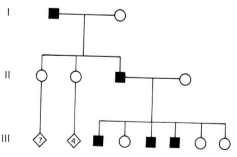

Fig. 3-13. Pedigree for family demonstrating Y-linked inheritance of hairy ears. Trait is transmitted from father to all his male offspring and none of his daughters.[7]

GENETIC COUNSELING

One of the most important aspects of the management of genetic disease is genetic counseling. Most cases involve studying the specific family pedigree to provide the patient and his family with information regarding the probability of recurrence within that family, as well as the *prognosis* of the affected individuals.

The information used in assessing risk falls into three main categories.[11]

Modular information is that which can be arrived at by rational use of genetic theory. The risk assessment may be precise in conditions caused by a single mutant gene, and a definite numerical probability for recurrence may be quoted.

Empirical information is obtained by the analysis of data obtained from sample surveys of populations, such as gene frequencies, mutation rates, and recombination values. This type of information is not extremely accurate, but it must often be relied on, especially in the case of most polygenic disorders.

Articular information is derived from an analysis of a particular pedigree. It should be stressed that accurate prognosis and counseling depends on an accurate diagnosis. Since various genes and some nongenetic causes may produce clinically similar disease patterns *(phenocopies),* it is essential that genetic counseling and the assessment of risks should always be preceded by a careful family history as well as a thorough clinical and laboratory examination of as many individuals in the kindred as possible.

The responsibility of the physician or dentist does not end when he has accurately diagnosed a genetic disease. It is incumbent on him to either relate the information regarding the diagnosis and prognosis to the patient or to refer the patient to a genetic counselor for this service.

Well established information on simple genetic control of specific traits, in addition to a knowledge of gene frequency within a population, is often adequate to provide a basis for detailed counseling.

When the genetics of a particular disease or trait is in doubt or possibly due to several genes (polygenic), counseling is necessarily less specific and less accurate. Under these circumstances useful risk figures must be derived from empirical information.

Genetic counseling is, indeed, an art as well as a science. Bixler[1] has outlined what he believes the requirements are for a person to become involved in counseling of patients on hereditary problems.

First, this person must have a working knowledge of human genetics. A complete understanding of the genetic modes of inheritance, gene interaction in families and human populations, and chromosomal abnormalities with all of their consequences are a few of the important subjects to be comprehended by the genetic counselor. With this armamentarium he can intelligently sort out and present facts and figures to his counselees. The second requirement for a genetic counselor is that he must possess a deep respect for the attitudes, sensitivities, and reactions of the people he is counseling. It is not enough to make a diagnosis and then present the bare facts of the problem. Only when the counselor is certain that the facts are understood and are not being distorted by his patients can he assume that he is doing a service. Feelings of guilt, fear, hostility, and resentment are not uncommonly encountered during counseling sessions. The counseling must be couched in tact and sensitivity, since no other area of human existence invokes a feeling of personal responsibility as in the matter of conception and the child bearing period. Finally, the genetic counselor must have a sincere desire to teach the truth to the fullest extent that it is known.

By careful attention to responses, the counselor can obtain the feedback necessary for evaluation of his success and communication, which is a technique used by all good teachers. The genetic counselor must be sure that the individuals affected with the hereditary conditions completely understand their risk for having similarly affected children. The decision on whether to have children is a practical consideration for the parents and hopefully will be reached after carefully weighing the information supplied by the counselor.

The decision of whether to have children is not the responsibility of the genetic counselor, and he should refrain from giving positive or negative intonations to his counseling.

To the question of whether a dentist should attempt to provide genetic counseling to his patients, the answer is an unqualified yes, providing that he meets the criteria outlined above. There are a growing number of programs in this country that are designed specifically to train dentists in the area of genetics. In most cases as part of this training the techniques and intricacies of genetic counseling are covered in detail. For dentists who are properly trained in this area, they are probably the most qualified individuals to provide counseling for genetic problems that relate to the head and neck.

If a dentist is to function adequately as a genetic counselor, it is imperative that he be certain of the diagnosis in his patient. He must also be familiar with the hereditary aspects of the condition in question. It is, for example, not sufficient to conclude that a patient has amelogenesis imperfecta and expect to provide effective genetic counseling on that basis. The dentist who intends to give counseling in such a case should be familiar with the heterogeneity that exists in heritable enamel defects and should know that the several forms of amelogenesis imperfecta show significantly different patterns of inheritance.

If there is any doubt concerning the qualifications of the individual, the accuracy of the diagnosis, or the genetic mode of inheri-tance, the dentist should refer his patient to a genetics clinic for counseling. Most major medical centers in the United States have a genetics clinic that offers counseling services, and in increasing numbers these clinics have a dental geneticist as a member of their staff.

REFERENCES

1. Bixler, D.: Genetic aspects of dental anomalies in children. In McDonald, R. E.: Dentistry for the child and adolescent, ed. 2, St. Louis, 1974, The C. V. Mosby Co., p. 403.
2. Fraser, F. C.: Taking the family history, Am. J. Med. **34:**585-593, 1963.
3. Gorlin, R. J., and Pindborg, J. J.: Syndromes of the head and neck, New York, 1964, McGraw-Hill Book Co.
4. Hecht, F., and Lovrien, E. W.: Genetic diagnosis in the newborn, Pediatr. Clin. North Am. **17:**1039-1053, 1970.
5. Levitan, M., and Montagu, A.: Textbook of human genetics, New York, 1971, Oxford University Press, Inc.
6. McKusick, V. A.: Genetics in medicine and medicine in genetics, Am. J. Med. **34:**594, 1963.
7. McKusick, V. A.: Human genetics, Englewood Cliffs, N.J., 1964, Prentice-Hall, Inc.
8. McKusick, V. A.: Mendelian inheritance in man, Baltimore, 1974, The Johns Hopkins University Press.
9. Mendel, G.: Versuche über Pflanzen-hybriden, Verh. Naturf. Verein Brünn. Royal Hort. Soc. **4:**3-47, 1866.
10. Motulsky, A. F. and Hecht, F.: Genetic prognosis and counseling, Am. J. Obstet. Gynecol. **90:**1227-1241, 1964.
11. Murphy, E. A.: The rationale of genetic counseling, J. Pediatr. **72:**121-130, 1968.
12. Prescott, G. H., and Bixler, D.: Implications of genetics in dental practice, Dent. Clin. North Am., pp. 57-68, March, 1968.

4

The genetics of common dental diseases

RAY E. STEWART

M. ANNE SPENCE

There are certain generalizations that can be made concerning the role of heredity in the three most common problems confronting the dental professional today—dental caries, periodontal disease, and malocclusion.

First, a large amount of heterogeneity in each of these entities exists. That is to say, the disorders that are traditionally relegated to the collective term *periodontal disease* are of a diverse nature with respect to cause, pathogenesis, prognosis, and treatment. Similarly, malocclusion may result from a mutation at a single gene locus resulting in abnormal endochondral bone growth in the cranial base manifesting as midfacial hypoplasia, as is the case in achondroplasia.[12] Alternatively, the malocclusion may result entirely from environmental factors as in the case of anterior open bite secondary to thumb-sucking.

Second, it is often difficult to distinguish a clear-cut difference between affected and normal individuals. Such is the case in many human traits, such as height, weight, and intelligence, in which no discrete variation exists, but in which there is a variation by imperceptible degrees over a wide range, with no sharp distinction between normal and abnormal phenotypes. In such cases the trait in question is said to be continuously variable.

Experimental and clinical evidence supports the concept that the phenotypic characteristics expressed by an individual are a result of combined genetic and environmental influences or are multifactorial. However, it is not always clear to what extent each of these factors is individually responsible for the observed phenotype. One can think of the different diseases and traits as a spectrum according to the relative roles played in their causation by heredity and environment. Such a concept is illustrated in Fig. 4-1. Various zones can be arbitrarily assigned as follows (modified from Fraser Roberts[5]):

A. Diseases or traits that occur only in persons with a certain genetic constitution, and always in these, without regard to environmental conditions (examples: achondroplasia, hemophilia, Papillon-Lefèvre syndrome).

B. Diseases or traits that occur only in persons having a certain genetic constitution, and in these not always but only when also influenced by certain environmental factors (examples: diabetes, cleft lip).

C. Diseases or traits that occur in persons with differing genetic constitutions but that differ in frequency and severity according to constitution and environment. Environmental factors play an important role but become effective only in certain genotypes (examples: essential hypertension, prognathism).

D. Diseases or traits that can occur in any arbitrary genetic constitution but whose severity and frequency depend on the constitution (examples: tuberculosis, dental caries).

E. Diseases or traits that can occur in every genetic constitution and whose frequency and

81

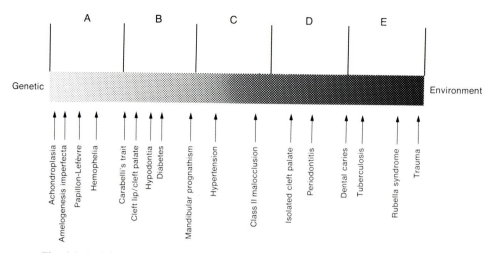

Fig. 4-1. Relative influence of genetic and environmental factors in various diseases.

severity depend almost exclusively on exogenous factors (examples: trauma, measles).

In the case of many abnormalities in tooth development such as peg-shaped or missing lateral incisors, supernumerary teeth, and taurodontism, extensive genetic contribution is substantiated by family studies through analysis of pedigrees and detailed clinical and radiographic examinations.

However, in attempting to determine the relative contributions of genetic versus environmental factors in traits that show extensive variability, as in the case of susceptibility or resistance of the teeth to dental caries, susceptibility of the supporting structures to periodontal disease, or predisposition toward the development of malocclusion, there is an even greater problem in identifying the relative significance of each. Epidemiological studies of populations, pedigree analysis of affected families, and data derived from twin studies have done much to improve our understanding of the role genetics plays in the underlying cause of these diseases.

Dental caries, periodontal disease, and malocclusion display certain characteristics that provide evidence for a significant genetic component in the cause of these disorders. These characteristics involve primarily reoccurrence within specific families at a rate significantly greater than the rate in the general population.[2] Also, these traits occur more

frequently in the general population than the rare genetic diseases.[2] However, no clear Mendelian segregation pattern of a single gene can be demonstrated to indicate a specific form of inheritance, such as autosomal dominant, recessive, or X-linked. It has been suggested that these traits fit the model of multifactorial inheritance. The specifics of this model are given here in some detail, and the data from the dental traits are discussed with respect to the model.

In Chapter 5 the transition for a quantitative trait from the segregation of one gene to the segregation of many genes is discussed. The multifactorial model proposed by Falconer[4] utilizes this assumption of many genes, each contributing a small and additive amount to the phenotype or trait of the individual. Therefore the number of genes a person has and not the specific genes is the important factor. Falconer's model also assumes that we are dealing with traits in which the environment plays a role, perhaps a major one, in the expression of the trait.

An example is presented in Fig. 4-2 for the height of 200 individuals. The trait measured, however, could be tooth size, as discussed in Chapter 5, or any other quantitative (measured) trait, for which individuals, when they are classified by their measurements, approximate a normal bell-shaped distribution. Given this characteristic dis-

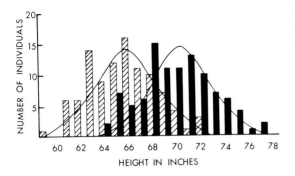

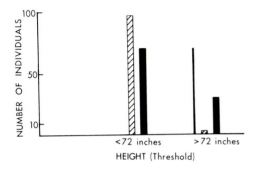

Fig. 4-2. *Top,* Distributions of two random samples of height are illustrated for 100 females (cross-hatched bars): mean = 66 inches, standard deviation = 3 inches, and 100 males (solid bars): mean = 70 inches, standard deviation = 3 inches. *Bottom,* Distribution of height for same 200 individuals when measurement was classified as greater than or less than 72 inches. See text for details.

tribution, the question arises as to how this model can be applied to traits such as malocclusion or periodontal disease that are classified in only two categories, usually present and absent, possibly with a few individuals in a category of borderline. The application to such data requires a third assumption: there are several observable categories for individuals; however, there is an underlying theoretical distribution for the trait that is continuous. The continuous trait is often characterized as being the liability or susceptibility to the trait. The reduction to two categories results because of a physiological threshold that must be achieved through the combined efforts of genes and environment before an individual can be classified as different from normal. There is no way to classify individuals for different amounts of

normality. In the example of height, this effect could be achieved if we had only one ruler approximately 72 inches long. All individuals would be classified as taller or shorter than the ruler, which is serving to define the threshold point on the height scale, but, in fact, we know that individuals are actually of many heights. The position of the threshold and the resulting dichotomy are indicated in the lower portion of Fig. 4-2.

Traits with a threshold have been called *quasicontinuous*[7] or *semicontinuous*.[10] For certain diseases, congenital malformation, or dental traits it is easy to imagine critical milestones in development that, if achieved, would produce a normal individual and if not achieved, would produce an affected individual. The threshold automatically converts the continuous developmental pathway to the all-or-none trait we observe.

Many of the traits considered to be multifactorial have distinct differences in the frequency of affected individuals in the two sexes.[2] This difference is thought to arise much as the specific example in Fig. 4-2 produces a lower frequency of tall women because the mean height of women is less than that for men and fewer women exceed the threshold. Likewise, genetic or environmental differences between the sexes could produce a shift in the mean of one distribution resulting in an altered frequency of affected individuals. For additional discussion of this concept of multifactorial inheritance, see Carter and Evans.[3]

After Falconer proposed the model, it was applied to a variety of traits, such as pyloric stenosis,[3] diabetes mellitus,[11] and schizophrenia.[6] It became apparent that one weakness of this particular model was that it could not be tested for goodness of fit to the data.[8] Therefore, many traits could be suggestive of multifactorial inheritance, but they could not be shown conclusively to be inherited in that way. This difficulty was circumvented when Reich and associates[10] proposed adding to the model at least a second threshold so that a minimum of three categories could be assigned. The additional threshold can arise by using the natural graded severity of the trait as was done by Reich and his colleagues. Suarez and Spence,[13] using degree of severity, found that the two-threshold model of multifactorial inheritance explained hypodontia better than the more traditional single-gene model. For other traits, where graded severity of the trait is less definable, sex differences can be utilized to provide the required second threshold.[9]

It is valid to ask the question, Why should an attempt be made to define a trait as multifactorial? There are several important reasons. First, this model provides a viable alternative for analysis to test the data for a single gene model. Second, it provides a method of assessing how much of the variation in the expression of the trait is determined by gene action and how much is determined by the environment. This could lead to direct experimentation to define specific environmental factors. Finally, a model that is shown to account for the existing data may be used to extrapolate to unknown situations to predict the risk of occurrence for individuals. A table of risk figures based on this model has been published for cleft lip and palate[1] and would provide a useful tool if similar estimates could be made concerning more common dental disorders.

DENTAL CARIES

Every dentist has had the experience of interviewing an exasperated patient or parent who attributes his susceptibility to dental caries to soft teeth that were inherited from his parents. The dentist must be careful to differentiate the familial problem, which is greatly influenced by environmental factors, such as diet and hygiene, from the hereditary one. Although most dentists tend to distinguish between these factors, the question frequently arises, How much of the caries process can be attributed to heredity? In the case of dental caries, the disease process itself is definitely not inherited but is infectious. Certain factors related to individual resistance or susceptibility to the caries process appear, however, to be significantly influenced by genetic factors.

Although there is no single gene trait that produces the disease of dental caries, there are several traits determined by a single gene that directly or indirectly affect the susceptibility or resistance of an individual to dental caries. An example of this phenomenon occurs in an inborn error of metabolism known as hereditary fructose intolerance. This is an autosomal recessive disorder that is manifested as a result of a genetic defect in the production of the enzyme fructose-1-phospho-aldolase. The intolerance to foods containing sugar (sucrose, fructose, etc.) by affected individuals leads to a diet that reduces the incidence of dental caries in affected individuals to almost zero. See Fig. 3-7 for a pedigree of a family with this metabolic disorder.

Similarly, individuals with certain single gene disorders exhibit a significantly altered susceptibility to carious destruction of the dentition. One such example is ectodermal dysplasia, which may be inherited as an autosomal dominant, X-linked, or autosomal recessive trait. In this disorder, decreased susceptibility is attributable to a hypoplastic morphology of the teeth with fewer pits and fissures and large interdental spaces allowing for self-cleaning and easier removal of plaque from the tooth surface. Several single gene disorders described in separate chapters in this book involve defective formation of enamel or dentin in which the affected teeth are associated with increased susceptibility to dental caries.

The role of heredity in relation to dental caries has been investigated in both man and experimental animals. It is apparent from these studies that genetics definitely plays a role in the cause of caries, although the relative importance of these factors is difficult to assess when compared with the combined influence of intrinsic and extrinsic or environmental factors.

There are enormous amounts of data to support the role of dietary factors as a cause of dental caries. It is, however, also clear from many of these studies that much individual variation in caries susceptibility exists even under closely controlled conditions. The widely quoted Vipeholm study,[29] for example, reported that some individuals consuming a diet known to be cariogenic showed no increase in carious lesions, whereas other individuals on low-carbohydrate, sugar-free diets developed several carious lesions in a year's time. These findings suggest that certain individuals possess some innate ability to respond to or resist some of the environmental influences predisposing to dental caries. The aim of much of the research in this area has been to elucidate the basis of genetic control of resistance and susceptibility and to attempt to identify the variable factors and demonstrate these differences by use of genetic and biostatistical methods.

Evidence of the existence of hereditary factors in the resistance or susceptibility to dental caries comes from four separate areas of research: (1) experimental animal studies, (2) human population studies, (3) human family studies, and (4) human twin studies.

Animal studies

More direct evidence concerning heritability of factors related to the production of resistance of susceptibility to dental caries has been derived experimentally from the results of studies on animals than from any of the human studies.

Hunt and associates[33] conducted selective breeding experiments on the Norway strain of laboratory rats under uniform environmental conditions in an effort to distinguish between genetic and environmental factors. They were able to develop genetically resistant and genetically susceptible strains after twenty-eight generations. The two groups were fed identical diets of coarse-particle rice. The caries-susceptible strain developed carious lesions within 70 days, whereas the caries-resistant strain required an average of 578 days. In another experiment,[32] these same workers demonstrated that placing caries-resistant or caries-susceptible newborns with opposite-strain foster mothers until weaning resulted in a caries index typical of the true prenatal strain. Similarly, when the oral flora of young rats was depressed by administration of penicillin, then inoculated with the feces from both parental strains, the original caries

indices of the resistant or susceptible strains were retained. These studies tend to discount the possibility that the variation in caries susceptibility was due to some factor mediated in the mother's milk or through fluctuations in the maternal oral-intestinal flora and suggested a strong genetic component in the resistance to dental caries in these animals.

Shaw and Griffiths[45] used the Harvard strain of laboratory rats to corroborate the findings of Rosen and co-workers by placing caries-susceptible offspring with caries-resistant mothers and vice versa until weaning. In both cases the caries activity was similar to that of the genotypic mothers. In a similar study in which susceptible or resistant-strain males were mated with opposite-strain females, the resultant offspring (F_1 generation) showed a caries activity approximately midway between the indices recorded for the susceptible and resistant genotypes.

In still another study using laboratory rats, Larson and Simms[38] used a double-mating technique to study heritable factors in dental caries. The double-breeding technique was accomplished by caging white Osborne-Mendel (O-M) females with both O-M strain and NIH black strains during the same mating period. The double mating technique provided an opportunity to compare O-M and O-M × NIH black crossbred strains from the same litter. Previous studies had shown that the O-M strain was significantly more caries-susceptible than NIH black on identical diets and that O-M × NIH black crosses resulted in offspring with caries activities somewhere between those of the susceptible O-M and resistant NIH black strains. The litters contained both O-M (white) and O-M × NIH black crosslinked (grey to black) offspring.

When the caries activities of the O-M and O-M × NIH black litter mates exposed to identical environmental conditions during the intrauterine, preweaning, and experimental periods were compared, a significant difference appeared. The O-M × NIH black crosses had significantly lower caries activity than the O-M strain, indicating strong heritable influence on the development of dental caries.

The morphological characteristics of teeth have been implicated as a possible contributing factor to the genetic influence on dental caries. Studies showing the positive correlation between increased susceptibility to caries and certain anatomic characteristics such as fissure depth and steepness of cusp inclination have been reported by several investigators.[26, 34, 37]

Human population studies

Studying various human populations for variation in incidence of a particular disease can also provide insight into the role of heredity in relation to the cause of that disease. Studies of individuals with differing levels of inbreeding offer potential for such investigations.

Japanese populations, which show a particularly higher level of inbreeding (5% of marriages are between cousins), have been studied.[20, 21, 44] In a study of 6739 offspring of cousin × cousin matings and age- and sex-matched controls, there was no evidence for an influence of inbreeding on dental caries rates. They concluded that "any genetic factors affecting caries prevalence are not recessive in nature, or if recessive genes play a role in caries susceptibility, their effects are overshadowed by environmental sources of variation not controlled for in this study."[42]

In a study[20] in the Hawaiian Islands, 9912 children with diverse racial backgrounds and admixture were examined. In this study, such variables as age, sex, birth order, maternal age, parental occupation, rural-urban residence, number of teeth present, and oral hygiene status were controlled.

Significant interracial differences in caries susceptibility were observed, however, none of this variability could be attributed to maternal factors, racial hybridity, or genetic recombination. The caries prevalence of offspring of interracial matings tended to be about midway between the prevalence observed between the parental racial types, suggesting an additive effect characteristic of polygenic inheritance.

Detailed analysis of caries susceptibility and prevalence in various populations has raised the possibility of several additional factors as mediating variability in caries susceptibility. Niswander[42] postulated that one could relegate the genetic control of resistance or susceptibility to dental caries to one or more of the following: (1) anatomical factors and arch form, (2) chemical composition of the tooth, (3) composition and consistency of saliva, and (4) dietary habits.

Turner and co-workers[47] measured titratable acidity and titratable alkalinity of fresh resting whole saliva in pairs of monozygotic twins and pairs of siblings and in individual children repeated a second time. They found titratable acidity in twins and retests more similar than siblings and retests or siblings and twins. Goodman and associates[25] reported differences between monozygotic and dizygotic twins in some salivary factors such as rate of flow, pH, amylase activity, and oral flora. The significance of these findings with respect to susceptibility to caries is not clear. In humans a relationship between caries susceptibility and the anatomic configuration and location of a tooth or teeth in the dental arch has been suggested; for example, the occlusal surfaces of molars with extensive pits and fissures are substantially more susceptible than any surfaces of an incisor tooth.[16]

The chemical structure of a tooth, more specifically the mineral content of the enamel, which normally reaches approximately 96%, is a potential factor in the susceptibility to dental caries. Although there are no studies to confirm that caries-susceptible individuals have a perceptibly diminished mineral content to their enamel when compared to caries-resistant individuals, the possibility of hypomineralization seems feasible. A variation in apatite structure of enamel between caries-resistant and susceptible teeth has been demonstrated in that the fluoride content (as fluoroapatite) of enamel of caries-free individuals is significantly higher. What is not so clear is whether these individuals have an increased ability to absorb exogenous fluoride ion or whether they have some genetic advantage that allows them to metabolize and incorporate endogenous fluoride.

Similarly, factors such as content and consistency of saliva, enzymes, bacterial inhibitors, and secretory factors, all of which are at least partially under genetic control, could hypothetically influence caries susceptibility. There is preliminary evidence that certain immunological mechanisms, some of which may be mediated as salivary antibodies, play a role in the pathogenesis of dental caries. Several investigators have suggested that salivary IgA and other antibodies could play a role in caries resistance[39]; however, a recent review by Sims[46] points out that the rationale of studies concerned with immunity to dental caries that were carried out in the lactobacillus era now appears faulty, which is to be expected, but the reasoning displayed in some recent publications is incredibly naive. They seem to infer that because serum antibodies are protective in diseases such as diphtheria or tetanus, they must necessarily be of consequence in dental caries. Practically all the work on immunity to bacterial diseases has been concerned with virulent, pathogenic organisms that produce toxins or possess antigenic components that enable them to resist the host's defenses and produce local or systemic infections. It is irrational to assume that the findings of these studies can be applied to the surface of an immunologically unreactive tissue at a site effectually external to the body.

Sims concludes that although antibodies specific for cariogenic bacteria are present in saliva in low concentrations, even an enormous increase would probably not result in an alteration of the progress of dental caries.

Finn[23] has pointed out that the time of tooth eruption has been shown to be governed by heredity in a number of studies. Although environmental factors such as premature primary extractions or disease may alter the eruption time in certain instances, overall the genetic factors seem to predominate.

Numerous investigators have made the observation that the permanent teeth of girls erupt earlier than those of boys, which points to the existence of a definite sex-linked variation associated with earlier maturation. Other studies have shown a sex difference in caries

incidence at early ages, which may be explained by this phenomenon.

By comparing monozygotic and dizygotic twins, Hatton[30] found that heredity has an important bearing on the time required for a primary tooth to erupt.

To associate time of tooth eruption with dental caries prevalence, Klein and Palmer[36] demonstrated that caries-immune families have a lesser number of erupted teeth. They attributed this difference in caries susceptibility to the difference in length of exposure to the oral environment.

Noteworthy also are the attempts that have been made to related blood group antigens and secretory status to prevalence of resistance to dental caries. It has been suggested that since blood groups are genetically transmitted, an antibody relationship against dental caries might exist. However, Witkop and associates[50] found no difference among the divisions of the ABO group and caries resistance or susceptibility among a group of Chileans. O'Roark and Leyschon,[43] using the same population, found that there was a significant relationship with caries status in only one age range in the MN blood group. All other ages and all other blood groups gave negative results. There is still insufficient confirmatory evidence to implicate any of the blood groups with the prevalence of dental caries. It would appear that the similarities of blood groups among monozygotic twin pairs as compared to dizygotic twin pairs and their similarities in dental caries are concomitant, but there is not necessarily a cause-and-effect relationship.

The presence of genetic factors that may relate to dietary preferences among individuals and populations that could be responsible for some of the variability reported in caries susceptibility was reported initially by Witkop,[51] who studied the hereditary ability or lack of ability to taste phenylthiocarbamide (PTC) when it is placed on the tongue. He found that 60% of all United States whites are tasters and 40% are nontasters. It was observed that tasters had a 25% lower DMF (observable caries experience) rate than nontasters.

More recent studies by Chung[18] reported an inverse relationship between the ability to taste phenylthiocarbamide and reduced numbers of dental caries in primary teeth. Similar studies reported by Mandel and Zengo[40] demonstrated a variation in the ability to taste sucrose between caries-resistant and susceptible individuals with the resistant group requiring a higher threshold (higher concentration) for perception.

Human family studies

Several reports have appeared in the literature that study the occurrence of dental caries in related individuals.

The first large-scale family study concerned with the dental caries experience of siblings was conducted by Kelin and Palmer[36] utilizing a group of 4416 unselected schoolchildren. Caries-immune children were defined as those who showed no evidence of clinical caries on an explorer examination. Caries-susceptible children were defined as those with six or more cavities at 10 years of age, with one additional cavity included for each additional year of age. The 306 siblings of the 148 immune children had a lower average caries score than the 182 siblings of the 117 susceptible children. This difference amounted to more than twice that found in the siblings of the resistant group and was statistically significant.

In another study on a group of 5400 persons, comprising 1150 families of Japanese ancestry residing in the United States, Klein[35] found among the children a definite reflection of the caries scores of their parents.

Böök and Grahnén[15] studied the families of forty caries-immune male conscripts for military training from whom the propositi were selected, consisting of a total of 202 related individuals. A control group of individuals was chosen comparable in as many respects as possible to the test group except in caries experience. This group comprised 114 individuals, including caries-susceptible inductees who constituted the propositi. Parents and siblings of caries-free adult individuals had a significantly lower dental caries index when compared with families of the control group. They concluded, from their analysis of these two groups, that there was a definite genetic factor or factors that appreciably determined resistance or susceptibility to dental caries.

In general, these family studies have shown a lower than expected caries experience among relatives of caries-free subjects. None of these studies, however, provides data to suggest a simply inherited trait for the control of susceptibility or resistance, nor do they support an explanation based simply on environmental factors. It would be more appropriate to postulate a complex multifactorial etiology with several genes affecting the individuals susceptibility to the disease.

Twin studies

The twin method, which uses monozygotic and dizygotic twin pairs to assess the relative effects of genetic and environmental factors on complex multifactorial traits, has been widely used in human genetics, specifically in the study of heritability factors in the cause of dental caries. The utility of this method is based on the fact that monozygotic twins have identical genotypes, whereas dizygotic twins share approximately 50% of their genes, as in the case of nontwin siblings. Therefore, discordance in phenotype, for example, caries experience, in monozygotic twins is attributable exclusively to environmental factors, whereas a combined genetic-environmental effect is responsible for any variability observed in dizygotic twins. The accuracy and reliability of this method is necessarily dependent on accurate determination of zygosity at a 95% to 99% probability. The data necessary to attain this level of probability often require information derived from detailed studies, such as blood group antigens and serum proteins, preferably from both parents and the twins; careful comparison of phenotypic traits, such as eye color, hair whorl, and general similarity of facial features; and dermatoglyphics for fingerprint ridge counts. Unfortunately, in few of the reported twin studies have the investigations been rigorous in their determination of zygosity. Finn[23] has reviewed the literature on twin studies and concludes that only a few have given sufficient information or adequate statistical analysis to offer a high degree of reliability.

Bachrach and Young[14] studied 130 pairs of identical and 171 pairs of fraternal twins, both of like and unlike sex, from 3 to 14 years old. Correlation coefficients indicated that although identical twins were more alike in total caries experience, the differences between the two twin types were not statistically significant.

In 1942 Dahlberg and Dahlberg[22] presented data on thirty-seven pairs of monozygotic twins and forty-four pairs of like-sexed and forty-five pairs of unlike-sexed dizygotic twins of 7 to 14 years of age, with an average age of 10 years. Corresponding teeth were compared for each twin pair. Statistical analysis for discordance revealed that 24% of the monozygotic twins were discordant, whereas 28% of the dizygotic twin pairs were discordant. When they considered the anterior and posterior segments separately there were small differences in concordance, especially between the monozygotic and like-sexed dizygotic twin pairs.

Horowitz and co-workers[31] studied forty-nine like-sexed pairs of twins, thirty monozygotic and nineteen dizygotic, utilizing the tooth surface as the unit of measurement. Examinations were both clinical and by radiography. Caries experience ratios were calculated from the observed number of DMF surfaces divided by the original number of surfaces available. The age range of the twins was from 18 to 55 years with a median of 24 years. Calculation of the intrapair variance ratios between the two types of twin pairs indicated that there was a statistically significant difference in dental caries scores and thus a measurable genetic component of susceptibility to dental caries. In determining the variance in anterior and posterior segments in each arch, the lower anterior teeth showed the greatest variance between the two twin types. Because of the age bracket of the twins, one can only speculate on the surface caries experience of the missing teeth in the other segments.

Mansbridge[41] examined ninety-six monozygotic and 128 pairs of like-sexed dizygotic twins of from 5 to 17 years of age, with an average age of approximately 9.5 years. Zygosity was established by similarities in physical characteristics, including fingerprints. Examinations of the teeth were made with mirror and explorer, and the condition of each surface of each tooth was recorded. One of each of the twin pairs was matched with a control child of the same age, sex, and number of erupted teeth. There were, therefore, a like number of unrelated pairs. When the concordance and discordance of corresponding teeth within each type of twin pair, between the twin pairs, and in the unrelated controls were calculated, Mansbridge found that the caries experience between the identical twin pairs showed greater resemblance than between fraternal twins. The unrelated children showed less resemblance than either type of twins.

Goodman and co-workers[25] examined thirty-eight pairs of like-sexed twins, nineteen monozygotic and nineteen dizygotic, from 14 to 38 years of age, with a median age of 19 years. Zygosity was determined serologically using fifteen markers. Dental caries were determined by clinical and radiological examination. Caries experience ratios were calculated utilizing the tooth surface as the unit of measurement. The mean intrapair variances were then calculated, and significance was determined between the twin types. The results were significant in that the monozygotic twins showed less variance.

Caldwell and Finn[17] studied intrapair differences of dental caries in monozygotic twins, dizygotic twins, and pairs of unrelated children from a home for the deaf and blind where the children had the same diet. According to their preliminary analysis, comparing tooth to tooth and surface to surface, it is apparent that identical twins are not identical as far as the distribution of dental caries is concerned. However, the identical twins have fewer differences than the fraternal twins, and the fraternal twins have fewer than the unrelated children.

In a later study, Finn and Caldwell[24] reported thirty-four sets of monozygotic and thirty-one sets of like-sexed dizygotic twins of 7 to 15 years of age, with a mean age of 19 years. Zygosity was determined serologically and by physical comparison. DMF surfaces and teeth, as determined by clinical and radiological examination, were used as the units of measurement. The coefficients of variance were calculated, based on both the absolute differences in the number of DMF teeth and surfaces and by comparison of the corresponding teeth and surfaces in the twin pairs. Monozygotic twins showed fewer DMF intrapair differences than did dizygotic twins and significantly fewer intrapair differences than did paired unrelated children.

The results of these twin studies are not altogether consistent. The observed differences may be due to a number of factors such as age, sampling methods, zygosity determination, and examination methods. The results do, however, support the role of heredity as a significant factor in the cause of dental caries. More well-designed and controlled investigations will be necessary if we are to refine estimates of the extent to which genes play a role, however.

Conclusion

Based on investigations of twins and families, it seems likely that genetic factors are responsible for a statistically significant portion of the variation in susceptibility to dental decay in man. Due to the multifactorial causation of caries it seems most likely that the genetic background is polygenic. Factors of saliva, oral flora, enamel formation and mineralization, tooth structure, and dietary habits must be considered (Fig. 4-3).

Although the resistance to dental caries is affected by genetic factors, from a practical point of view they have only a minor influence when compared to the environmental factors related to the caries phenomenon.

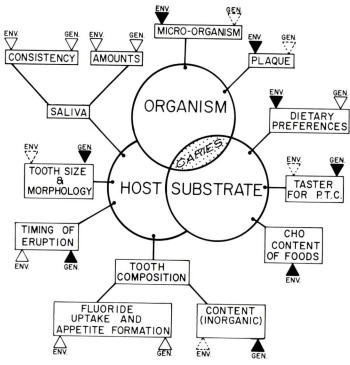

Fig. 4-3. Multifactorial etiology of dental caries, illustrating relationship between genetic and environmental factors affecting saliva, oral flora, enamel formation and mineralization, tooth shape and structure, and dietary habits. *Broken-line arrows,* minor contribution; *solid-line arrows,* moderate contribution; *filled arrows,* extensive contribution.

PERIODONTAL DISEASE

Although our knowledge of the exact role that genetics plays in the resistance or susceptibility to dental caries is somewhat limited, the genetic aspects of periodontal disease are even less clear.

As a pathological entity, periodontal disease is generally considered to be inflammatory with possible underlying systemic factors.

Many investigators believe that the variable clinical and histopathological findings that occur in periodontal disease indicate that there are probably many distinct disease processes with different causes represented in the collective term *periodontal disease* and that it would be more realistic to classify the various types according to age of onset, severity of bone loss, and presence or absence of local and systemic factors.

There is an extensive literature dealing with the effects of local and systemic factors in the pathogenesis of periodontal disease; however, the identification of genetic factors has proved to be extremely complex and has met with little success. This complexity has made it difficult to design studies that are able to control for the numerous variables and multiple factors that contribute to cause periodontal disease. Nevertheless, studies show that the disease is similar to dental caries in that it is widespread, shows extensive variability in how it is expressed clinically, and is influenced by environmental conditions, such as diet, oral hygiene, and occlusion.

Although there are certain diseases and syndromes that occur due to single gene mutations or chromosomal abnormalities in which severe periodontal disease is a consistent clinical feature, the most common cause of periodontal disease or susceptibility to its process is certainly multifactorial with several genes playing a role in the pathogenic process. Table 4-1 lists many of these disorders with their apparent or known mode of inheritance. Detailed descriptions of many of these disorders appear in other chapters in this book (for example, cementum, hematologic disorders, mucous membrane disorders).

Another disorder that deserves mention is called *juvenile periodontosis* and has received much attention in the dental literature. It is characterized by destruction of the periodontal structures and early loss of permanent teeth. The alveolar bone loss observed in this disorder is vertical and occurs primarily around the first permanent molars and central and lateral incisors. Loss of these teeth occurs during adolescence or early adulthood.

Table 4-1. Diseases commonly accompanied by periodontal pathology

Disease	Mode of inheritance*
Inherited systemic or metabolic disorders	
Acatalasemia	AR
Hypophosphatasia	AR
Agammaglobulinemia	XL and AR
Connective tissue diseases	
Ehlers-Danlos syndrome	AD
Mucopolysaccharide disorders	
Hurler's syndrome	AR
Hunter's syndrome	XL
Scleroderma	?
Hereditary amyloidosis	AD
Hereditary gingival fibromatosis	AD
Chromosomal disorder	
Trisomy 21	
Hematologic or vascular diseases	
Cyclic neutropenia	?AD
Thalassemia	AR
Sickle cell disease	AR
Hereditary telangiectasia	AR
Sturge-Weber syndrome	?AD
Angio-osteohypertrophy	?AD
Diffuse angiokeratosis (Fabry's disease)	XL
Dermatological diseases	
White sponge nevus	AD
Pachyonychia congenita	AD
Hereditary benign intraepithelial dyskeratosis	
Darier's disease	AD
Epidermolysis bullosa	
Dystrophica	AD and AR
Letalis	AR

*AR, autosomal recessive; AD, autosomal dominant; XL, X-linked.

This disease has most frequently been observed in single, isolated instances; however, recent reports by Benjamin and Baer[52] and Bixler[54] demonstrate a strong familial tendency with good evidence for an autosomal dominant pattern of inheritance (Fig. 4-4).

Standard genetic tools are most useful in identifying disorders that result from a clear-cut single abnormal gene. Common periodontal disease is not a single gene defect as shown by population studies. Many genes with additive effects concerned with production of characters or properties such as periodontal disease are continuously variable and present a normal distribution in the population.

The complex nature of genetic factors in periodontal disease makes their isolation extremely difficult in a human population.

The human family studies that have been done to determine the role of heredity in periodontal disease suggest that genetic factors are present, although the exact nature of this influence is not certain. The major problem encountered in any attempt to compare studies is that few have used standardized methods of diagnosis or classification of the clinical pathological conditions that were observed.

A few family pedigree studies on periodontal disease allow for some generalizations concerning the role of genetics as a cause.

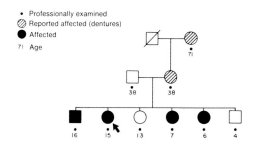

Fig. 4-4. Pedigree of family exhibiting autosomal dominant pattern of inheritance for juvenile periodontosis. (Modified from Bixler, D.: Genetic aspects of dental anomalies in children. In McDonald, R. E.: Dentistry for the child and adolescent, ed. 2, St. Louis, 1974, The C. V. Mosby Co.)

Dickmann,[57] in a study of forty-seven families with periodontal disease, reported that the disorder appeared to be transmitted as a dominant trait. Similarly, Rojahn[63] concluded that a dominant mode of inheritance with variable penetrance was responsible for the periodontal conditions in the families he studied. He observed that if a child exhibited periodontal disease, 87% of the time one parent was similarly involved.

More recently studies have been done on the periodontal status of Japanese and Hawaiian families.[55, 64] In both of these studies, schoolchildren were examined and evaluated by means of a standardized periodontal index. Schull and Neel[64] showed a significant increase in the frequency of gingivitis among Japanese children of consanguineous marriages. They noted an increase in the frequency of gingivitis of between 6% and 13% in children of first-cousin marriages as compared to unrelated controls. This increase in the incidence of periodontal disease in inbred populations was also observed by Witkop and associates[66] in the Brandywine triracial isolate of southern Maryland.

Chung and co-workers[55] reported a highly significant correlation between periodontal disease (gingivitis) and racial intermixture in 9912 Hawaiian schoolchildren. Russell's method of scoring periodontal disease using the Periodontal Index (PI) on twelve anterior teeth was used. Greene and Vermillion's OHI-S technique was used to assess the children's oral hygiene. The authors took differences in oral hygiene into consideration in evaluating their data. Their results showed that children of Hawaiian ancestry had a distinctly higher prevalence of periodontal disease than other racial groups. They also found that there was a significant effect of the hybridity of the children when major racial crosses were involved. The effect was that the hybrid children had an average periodontal score closer to the parental race with the lower mean.

These family studies as a group tend to support a polygenic influence, although the influence of recessive gene or genes in the cause of periodontal disease cannot be ruled out.

Twin studies

Few reports have been published describing studies of periodontal disease in twins, which one might expect to be a rewarding endeavor as in the case of dental caries, since complex multifactorial traits in humans are amenable to twin analysis. Reiser and Vogel[62] were primarily concerned with the occurrence of subgingival calculus in a population of twins who were divided into groups of monozygotic and dizygotic twins. They found that the intrapair variability of calculus formation among fraternal twins was about fifteen times as great as that noted in identical twins. In the twin pairs they studied, of which at least one member had a particular type of defect, monozygotic pairs were more concordant than dizygotic pairs. These results seem to indicate that there is a correlation between genetic factors and calculus formation.

Gorlin and associates[59] recently reviewed the literature on genetic aspects of periodontal disease and concluded that it is an extremely complex problem in which the isolation of such factors is difficult due to the joint action of many genes (polygenetic) with limited effects and considerable effect due to environmental factors. Future investigations in this area should consider the approach to the problem of heterogeneity by breaking the broad subject of periodontal disease down into specific subclassifications, such as calculus, induced periodontal pathologic conditions, or juvenile periodontosis, so that one would be more likely to discover a simple hereditary mechanism if one exists.

MALOCCLUSION

Before engaging in a detailed discussion on the genetic aspects of malocclusion, an attempt should be made to define certain frequently used terminology. The concept of *occlusion* pertains to the dynamic relationship between the teeth in the same dental arch as well as between the arches when the teeth are brought together. The term *normal occlusion* is arbitrary but is taken by most investigators to be a class I molar relationship with ideal alignment of all teeth and represents a situation that occurs in approximately 35% of the population. In a study[94] of Finnish children, frequencies of Angle malocclusions in mixed and permanent dentitions were found to be as follows:

Class I (normal)		34.7%
Class I malocclusion		42.0%
Class II malocclusion		19.6%
Class III malocclusion		3.7%

Among the elements that must be considered when discussing occlusion are (1) size of the maxilla, (2) size of the mandible, (3) size of the teeth, (4) structure of the teeth, (5) presence of supernumerary or congenitally missing teeth, (6) arch form, and (7) soft tissue structure of the lips and perioral musculature. It is significant that many of these factors have individually been shown to be genetically determined and are discussed elsewhere in this book. To define the term *malocclusion* is somewhat easier, since we can say that it is a significant deviation from normal occlusion. The use of this term clinically is based primarily on its value as a treatment role, rather than its use as a system of classification. In these terms, malocclusion may be defined as a deviation from normal that is sufficient to warrant orthodontic intervention.

The absence of a clear definition of normal or ideal occlusion has made it difficult to measure the incidences of normal and abnormal occlusion and to make valid comparisons of data reported by different investigators. Most investigators have utilized the Angle classification and its modifications in describing malocclusion and reporting its incidence in various populations.

There is good evidence from data derived from population, family, and twin studies to support the generalization that genetics plays an important role in nearly every aspect of craniofacial development, including occlusion. These same studies have also revealed that occasionally remarkable differences occur in the facial patterns of parents and children, siblings, and even identical twins, which emphasizes the critical role the environment plays in their development.

The question of whether nature or nurture

has the greater influence in the cause of malocclusion has been a moot point since the early days of orthodontics. Kingsley,[84] in his 1891 treatise on oral anomalies, is definite in ascribing inheritance as a major factor in producing malocclusion. Angle[67] was equally as adamant in his belief that "malocclusions arise from local causes." This dichotomy, heredity versus environment, is a misleading framework in which to consider the phenomenon of malocclusion. Although there are a number of diseases or syndromes that have as one of their characteristics various types of malocclusions (Chapters 15 and 17), the majority of occlusal disharmonies are caused by a combination of genetic and environmental factors.

That there is a significant genetic component to the phenomenon of malocclusion in man is evident to an orthodontist from even a cursory examination of the relatives (parents and siblings) of patients who present for treatment. In support of this clinical impression there are numerous reports of kindreds in which the occurrence of specific types of malocclusion, such as mandibular prognathism and Class II malocclusion, recur with a high frequency.

Class II malocclusion

Harris and his colleagues at the University of Michigan have done extensive studies on Angle Class II, Division I, patients for whom they have been able to document that the patterns of craniofacial growth that lead to the malocclusion are inherited. Their investigations have shown that in the Class II patient, the mandible is significantly more retruded than in Class I patients; furthermore, the body of the mandible is slightly smaller, and the overall length is slightly shorter than in Class I patients. Robert[102] examined severe skeletal Class II malocclusions, which revealed that the differences between moderate and severe Class II malocclusions are a matter of degree and do not represent two heterogeneous skeletal patterns.

Much of the early literature concerning the inheritance of Class II malocclusion attributed the disorder to simple Mendelian genetics and made efforts to explain the familial occurrence of the disorder to autosomal or sex-linked genes with incomplete penetrance or variable expressivity. More recently, however, the concept of polygenic inheritance has generally come to be recognized as the genetic mechanism by which Class II malocclusion segregates within families.

Harris[77] used the polygenic model and a multivariate statistical approach to analyze the large number of measurable variables represented in the craniofacial complex. The data for these studies have been derived from extensive orthodontic records consisting of cephalometric head films and dental casts from entire families.

If the assumption that various characteristics of the craniofacial complex are under the control of more than one gene (are polygenic) has validity, these studies should show a higher correlation between the patient and his immediate family than data from random pairings of unrelated siblings. This assumption was borne out, and the average correlation coefficient for the craniofacial measurements was approximately $r = 0.5$, which would be expected in individuals sharing approximately half their genes. Tooth size measurements also reportedly approach a correlation of $r = 0.5$, which would support the contention that teeth are also under polygenic control. The most important observation derived from these studies is the fact that dental occlusion is highly dependent on the craniofacial skeleton.

Mandibular prognathism

One of the best known examples of a genetic trait in humans passing through several generations is the pedigree of the so-called Hapsburg lip, which consisted of a prominent lower lip accentuated by a prognathic mandible. Haecker[75] studied the portraits of royal personages over several generations and concluded that the trait originated with Princess Cimburga of Massovia, the wife of Ernst the Iron, and passed through Frederick III of Austria (1415-1493) and several succeeding generations to Maria Theresa (1717-1780)

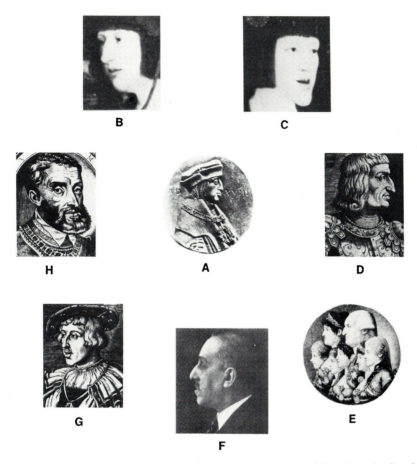

Fig. 4-5. Portraits of individuals from several generations of the royal Hapsburg family, demonstrating celebrated prominent lower lip accentuated by prognathic mandible. **A,** Maximilian I. **B,** Philip I. **C,** Charles V. **D,** Rudolph I. **E,** Maria Theresa and family. **F,** King Alfonso of Spain. **G,** Ferdinand I. **H,** Karl V.

(Fig. 4-5). The trait is interestingly enough observed in King Alfonso of Spain as late as the twentieth century (Fig. 4-5). Strohmayer[111] concluded from his detailed pedigree analysis of the Hapsburg family that the trait for mandibular prognathism was transmitted through several generations as autosomal dominant.

Other investigators have reported simple Mendelian inheritance as the cause for mandibular prognathism. McKusick[91] reported dominant inheritance in a black family. Involvement in four successive generations of a family was reported by Stiles and Luke.[109]

It should be noted that these are exceptions and do not provide sufficient information to make accurate predictions of mandibular growth and malocclusion in the vast majority of families in which class III occlusion and mandibular prognathism have been shown to be polygenic traits.

Suzuki[112] studied 1362 persons from 243 Japanese families. In the families in which the propositus demonstrated mandibular prognathism, there was a significantly higher incidence of this trait in other members of his family than was demonstrated in the families of propositi with normal occlusion. Of the family members of prognathic propositi, 34.3% demonstrated the trait, whereas in the families of individuals with normal occlusion, only 7.5% had the trait. In five families in which both parents were prognathic, 40% of the children were affected. If one parent was affected, 20.2% of the children were affected; if neither parent was affected, only 11.2% of the children were prognathic. Suzuki concluded that mandibular prognathism resulted from a "complicated hereditary mechanism."

Iwagaki[82] studied 2461 Japanese dental students in whom he recorded an incidence of 6% for mandibular prognathism. Through detailed family histories he determined that the occlusion of the parents and siblings of the students was markedly different in the families of those students who were prognathic. If the mother was affected, 18% of her offspring were similarly affected. If the father was prognathic, 31% of his offspring shared the trait. If neither parent had mandibular prognathism, only 4% of the children were affected. If there were no prognathic children in the family, only 2% of the parents were affected, and if the student demonstrated a normal occlusion, only 3% of his siblings were affected. Iwagaki suggested that, based on his data, mandibular prognathism was familial and perhaps transmitted as an autosomal recessive trait.

There are numerous other reports in the literature in which a small number of pedigree have been analyzed and the authors have concluded that prognathism is variously inherited as a dominant trait,[86] a dominant trait with incomplete penetrance,[109] and a simple recessive trait.[82] Schulze and Weise[106] and Schulze[105] examined sixteen families with 104 individuals demonstrating mandibular prognathism. They concluded from these studies that the inheritance was rather irregular and the penetrance was estimated at 70% with variable expressivity.

Kraus and co-workers[86] reported that class III malocclusion and mandibular prognathism is inherited as a simple recessive trait in Eastern Aleuts, but in Caucasian populations it was transmitted as a dominant trait.

Schulze[105] tabulated the degree of concordance for mandibular prognathism between monozygotic and dizygotic twins from several published reports. He found that concordance among monozygotic twins was six times higher than among dizygotic twins, which,

Table 4-2. Concordance for prognathism among twin pairs collected from published reports, 1924 to 1965*

	Concordance	Discordance
Monozygotic twins (21 pairs)	17 (81%)	4 (19%)
Dizygotic twins (15 pairs)	2 (13.3%)	13 (86.7%)

*Modified from Gorlin, R. R.: In Gorlin, R. J., and Goldman, H. M., editors: Thomas oral pathology, St. Louis, 1970, The C. V. Mosby Co.

according to Penrose,[100] supports a polygenic hypothesis as the primary cause for this trait (Table 4-2).

A variety of other abnormalities of tooth position and occlusion have been described in which both heredity and environment play important roles.

Diastema

Medial diastema refers to a condition characterized by a space of 1 mm or greater between the maxillary central incisors. It is important to distinguish between a *true diastema,* which is caused by a persistent tectolabial frenum, and *pseudodiastema,* which is caused by a divergent longitudinal axis of the incisors.

Hereditary factors as a cause of true medial diastema have been studied by numerous investigators who have published extensive pedigrees for the trait.[76, 113, 114] Trauner[114] reported that among twenty-one probands, 43% had similarly affected parents or siblings. Weninger[116] studied twenty-four families, observing as many as four generations in some, and suggested autosomal dominant inheritance. Tobias[113] reported concordance for the trait in monozygous twins. Korkhaus[85] studied seventeen pairs of dizygous twins in which only one pair was discordant for diastema yet found nine cases of discordance in twelve pairs of monozygous twins, casting some doubt on the single gene hypothesis.

Animal studies

Numerous studies using experimental animals have been designed to explore the effects of heredity on the craniofacial complex and the production of dental malocclusion.

Malocclusion resulting from some clearly apparent skeletal deformities has been demonstrated in the following animals:

1. Class II malocclusion in long-haired dachshunds[74]
2. Class III malocclusion in rabbits[70]
3. Retrognathia in sheep[98]
4. Class III malocclusion with achondroplasia in cattle[72]

In many cases this malocclusion has been attributed to classical Mendelian patterns of inheritance.

Of particular interest are the breeding experiments with dogs carried on by Stockard[110] and reported in the orthodontic literature by Johnson.[83] Various malocclusions were obtained when dogs with long, narrow skulls were crossed with dogs having short, broad skulls. The conclusions drawn from these observations were that individual features of the craniofacial complex (that is, mandibular length) were inherited according to Mendelian principles independently of other portions of the skull. It seems more likely, however, that this conclusion is a bit far reaching and that it is more realistic to think of the craniofacial complex as a closely knit complex of genetically and environmentally controlled interrelationships.

Population studies

Additional support for a genetic factor as a cause of malocclusion comes from anthropological studies of various populations and ethnic groups in which reported prevalences of malocclusion vary greatly from population to population (Table 4-3).

Although the basis for the observed differences in incidence of malocclusion is not clear, some of the variability could certainly be attributed to the methods used in classifying malocclusion and to the differences in age of the study populations.

Alternatively, there is some convincing evidence from population studies that indicates that genetic factors are also a cause of malocclusion. Schull and Neel[104] showed a consistent adverse effect of inbreeding on

Table 4-3. Frequency of normal occlusion in various populations

Population	Percent normal occlusion
Xavante Indian[97]	95
White children (Maryland)[92]	18
Eskimo children[95]	44
Japanese children[104]	41
Chippewa Indian children[73]	34
Black children (Chicago)[69]	57

malocclusion in Japanese children, which caused them to conclude that there was a strong possibility of recessive genes being involved in the production of malocclusion.

Among physical anthropologists, it is commonly believed that severe malocclusions are more prevalent in modern, civilized human groups than in most primitive populations. This difference would seem to be fertile ground for investigations toward the understanding of why malocclusion occurs and to what extent genetics and environment play a role as causes. One of the most common explanations given for this apparent increase is the increase in hybridization that has occurred as one of the side effects of civilization and is supported by the experiments of Stockard,[110] which produced a great diversity of occlusal anomalies in dogs by hybridizing breeds with dissimilar facial and cranial shapes. The large amounts of intermixture of different racial stocks is said to have disrupted the adaptation between tooth size and jaw size that has evolved in more primitive inbred societies through natural selection.

The possibility of detrimental effects of human hybridization was studied by Chung and Niswander,[18] who examined the offspring of matings between individuals of different races that represented the most diverse genetic crossing that can be found in human populations in sufficient numbers to study. The study was done on Hawaiian schoolchildren to detect and study racial variation in the prevalence of malocclusion and to investigate the possible effects on racial crossing as related to genetic heterozygosity. Hawaii is an ideal location for such a study because its population is composed of diverse racial groups with a high frequency of racial inter-marriage under relatively uniform environmental conditions. The data revealed that although there was ample evidence for differences in occlusion characteristics between races, there was no significant effect of hybridization through racial crossing that would indicate an increase in facial disharmonies. It was concluded that the children of inter-racial matings had no increased risk of malocclusion.

Family studies

In addition to the family studies cited in the discussion of the genetic aspects of mandibular prognathism, several other investigations have attempted to identify the genetic factors that predispose to malocclusion in man. Hughes and Moore[80] were among the earliest investigators to hypothesize a polygenic concept on inheritance in the craniofacial complex. They observed that craniofacial growth and structure is under strong hereditary control and expressed this concept in percentages of inheritability between parents and siblings. They concluded that the mandible and maxilla were under separate genetic control and that certain portions of individual bones, such as the mandible, were inherited independently.

Stein and associates[108] limited their cephalometric study of several families to angular measurements only. The resulting correlation coefficients, although somewhat equivocal, showed greater significance between sibling pairs than between parent and sibling combinations.

Morrees[93] subdivided cephalometric tracings into a series of horizontal and vertical planes, which he superimposed to note familial patterns for various facial proportions. Margolis[90] studied sixty-eight families using cephalometric radiographs. He divided the mandible and maxilla, as seen on lateral head films, into segments, noted concordance and discordance of each segment, and analyzed these results using a chi-square test. He concluded that certain aspects of mandibular

and maxillary structure appeared to be greatly influenced by heredity.

More recently, similarities between siblings with respect to facial structure and types of malocclusion have been studied by Niswander.[96] Several characteristics of the occlusion in 578 pairs of siblings in junior and senior high school children in Utah were recorded. Correlation coefficients within sibling pairs were all low but nonetheless positive for individual characters.

Anterior crowding, malalignment and rotation of lower teeth, and overjet all had correlations in the range of 0.20 to 0.25, whereas crossbite, overbite, and upper rotations and malalignment gave correlations between 0.10 and 0.19. Great similarities were noted between siblings where the frequency of malocclusion is significantly decreased among brothers and sisters of index cases with normal occlusion, whereas the siblings of index cases with malocclusion tended to have the same type of malocclusion much more frequently than would be expected from the dental population.

The results from this study are similar to the data collected on 1613 sibling pairs whose occlusions were examined by Chung and Niswander[18] in Hawaii. In that study, sibling correlation for incisor width was 0.421. For malalignment, overjet, overbite, crowding, and spacing, correlations ranged between 0.214 and 0.282 and were highly significant. Buccal and lingual crossbites had correlations of 0.101 and 0.124, respectively.

Twin studies

The study of craniofacial relationships in twins has provided much useful information concerning the role of heredity in malocclusion. As with any research involving twins, this literature is fraught with problems due to the methods employed for determining zygosity in the study populations, making the validity of many of the conclusions questionable.

Goldberg[71] studied fifteen pairs of identical twins and concluded that arch form was determined largely by heritable factors and that environmental influences were minimal.

Wylie[117] was among the first investigators to attempt to quantify specific craniofacial features derived from cephalometric head films. He studied fifteen families, of which thirteen had like-sexed twins of undetermined zygosity. His findings showed no significant correlations or relationships.

Snodgrasse[107] studied a kindred that contained a pair of twins in which he demonstrated a lower variability in occlusion between the twins than among other siblings and concluded that genetics must be responsible for the similarities.

Brodie and Newman[68] studied a set of adult male triplets and concluded that two of the members were monozygotic based on dermatoglyphics, anthropometrics, and cephalometric findings. They superimposed lateral head tracings and posterior-anterior tracings of skull films from these individuals and compared these data with those obtained from other siblings. The conclusions were that superimposition of total head outlined tracings provided little information as to the role of heredity in craniofacial growth or the establishment of genetic factors in occlusion.

Lundstrom[89] studied a sample of 100 monozygotic and 102 dizygotic twins in which little attempt was made to ascertain or confirm zygosity. In a later work in which fifty pairs of identical twins and fifty pairs of fraternal twins were studied, this time with comparisons of red cell antigens on the twins only, the conclusions were similar to the first study and are of a general nature. Lundstrom presented his results on histograms, which illustrate that genetic factors have a greater influence than nongenetic factors for most craniofacial distances and angles studied.

Leech[87] reported a pair of twins who were proved by rigorous dizygosity determinations to be monovular or identical, one of whom exhibited a class II, division I malocclusion and the other of whom had a class II, division II malocclusion. Analysis of muscle behavior using electron myography caused Leech to conclude that the differential muscle behavior patterns observed in these two twins were responsible for the different types of malocclusion.

Horowitz and co-workers[79] studied adult monozygotic and dizygotic twins using lateral head cephalograms. The statistics derived from their data indicated that there was a highly significant hereditary variation in the anterior cranial base, mandibular body length, and total and lower face height.

In a similar study, Hunter[81] used cephalometric analyses on seventy-two like-sexed twins and concluded that the strongest genetic component of variability was for facial height measurements rather than for measurements of facial depth.

Kraus and associates[86] studied six sets of like-sexed triplets to quantitate the effects of genetic factors in the determination of craniofacial structure. They studied seventeen skeletal traits from lateral and frontal head film tracings and concluded that the structure of all the bones of the craniofacial complex was under rather rigid control of hereditary factors. To explain the variability they did observe in craniofacial outline in monovular twins, they surmised that although heredity governs structure, environmental factors in their multitudinous facets have much influence on the bony elements, which combine to achieve the harmonious or unharmonious head and face.

Watnick[115] recently studied thirty-five pairs of monozygotic and thirty-five pairs of dizygotic like-sexed twins. He used multivariant and univariant statistical analyses of variance of vector and area differences that were obtained from cephalometric tracings of the mandible in this population. He concluded that the analysis of small unit areas within the craniofacial complex that represent local growth sites revealed that there are different modes of control within the same bone. Certain of these "unit areas," such as the lingual symphysis, lateral surface of the ramus, and frontal curvature of the mandible are predominantly under genetic control. Other unit areas such as the antegonial notch are predominantly affected by environmental factors. Other areas, such as the posterior border of the ramus and the labial symphysis, appear to be controlled equally by genetic and environmental factors.

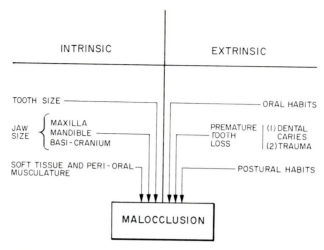

Fig. 4-6. Diagrammatic representation of multifactorial aspects of malocclusion.

The use of twin studies in the analysis of craniofacial structure has provided us with a better understanding of the relative roles of genetic and environmental factors in the determination of these characteristics. Comparisons of intrapair variances for monozygotic and dizygotic twins by univariate statistical methods demonstrates significant hereditary influences studied. It is probably safe to assume that heredity is at least as important as environment in determining the relationship between various craniofacial elements and that occlusion, be it normal or abnormal, is a polygenic trait. As such, it is subject to considerable environmental modifications as are all polygenic traits (Fig. 4-6).

REFERENCES

1. Bonaiti-Pellie, C., and Smith, C.: Risk tables for genetic counselling in some common congenital malformations, J. Med. Genet. **11**: 374-377, 1974.
2. Carter, C. O.: Multifactorial genetic disease. In McKusick, V. A., and Claiborne, R., editors: Medical genetics, New York, 1973, H. P. Publishing Co., Inc.
3. Carter, C. O., and Evans, K. A.: Inheritance of congenital pyloric stenosis, J. Med. Genet. **6**:233-254, 1969.
4. Falconer, D. S.: The inheritance of liability to certain diseases, estimated from the incidence among relatives, Ann. Hum. Genet. **29**:51-76, 1965.
5. Fraser Roberts, J. A.: An introduction to medical genetics, London, 1973, Oxford University Press.
6. Gottesman, I., and Shields, J.: A polygenic theory of schizophrenia, Proc. Natl. Acad. Sci. U.S.A. **58**:199-205, 1967.
7. Gruneberg, H.: Genetic studies on the skeleton of the mouse. IV. Quasicontinuous variation, J. Genet. **51**:95, 1952.
8. James, J. W.: Frequency in relatives for an all or none trait, Ann. Hum. Genet. **35**:47-50, 1971.
9. Kidd, K. K., and Spence, M. A.: Genetic analysis of pyloric stenosis suggesting a specific maternal effect. (In press.)
10. Reich, T., James, J. W., and Morris, C. A.: The use of multiple thresholds in determining the mode of transmission of semi-continuous traits, Ann. Hum. Genet. **36**:163-184, 1972.
11. Simpson, N. E.: Multifactorial inheritance, a possible hypothesis for diabetes, Diabetes **13**: 462-471, 1964.
12. Stewart, R. E.: Histopathology of cranial growth centers in achondroplasia, J. Dent. Res. **54**:163, Feb., 1975.
13. Suarez, B., and Spence, M. A.: The genetics of hypodontia, J. Dent. Res. **53**:781-785, 1974.

Dental caries

14. Bachrach, F. H., and Young, M.: A comparison of the degree of resemblance in dental characters shown in pairs of twins of identical and fraternal types, Br. Dent. J. **21**:1293-1304, 1927.
15. Böök, J. A., and Grahnén, H.: Clinical and genetical studies of dental caries. II. Parents

and sibs of adult highly resistant (caries-free) propositi, Odontol. Revy **4**:1-53, 1953.

16. Bossert, W. A.: The relation between the shape of the occlusal surfaces of molars and the prevalence of decay, J. Dent. Res. **13**: 125, 1933.

17. Caldwell, R. C., and Finn, S. B.: Comparisons of the caries experience between identical and fraternal twins and unrelated children, J. Dent. Res. **39**:693-694, 1960.

18. Chung, C. S., and Niswander, J. D.: Genetic and epidemiologic studies of oral characteristics in Hawaii's schoolchildren. V. Sibling correlations in occlusion traits, J. Dent. Res. **54**:324-329, 1975.

19. Chung, C. S., Niswander, J. D., Runck, D. W., Bilben, S. E., and Kau, M. C. W.: Genetic and epidemiologic studies of oral characteristics in Hawaii's schoolchildren. II. Malocclusion, Am. J. Hum. Genet. **23**:471-495, 1971.

20. Chung, C. S., Runck, D. W., Niswander, J. D., Bilben, S. E., and Kau, M. C. W.: Genetic and epidemiologic studies of oral characteristics in Hawaii's schoolchildren. I. Caries and periodontal disease, J. Dent. Res. **49**:1374-1375, 1970.

21. Chung, C. S., Witkop, C. J., and Henry, J. L. A.: A genetic study of dental caries with special reference to PTC taste sensitivity, Am. J. Hum. Genet. **12**:231-245, 1964.

22. Dahlberg, G., and Dahlberg, B.: Über Karies und andere Zahnveränderungen bei Zwillingen, Uppsala Läkerf. Forh. **47**:395-416, 1942.

23. Finn, S. B.: Heredity in relation to caries resistance. In Wolstenhome, G. E. W., editor: Caries resistant teeth, Boston, 1965, Little, Brown & Co.

24. Finn, S. B., and Caldwell, R. C.: Heredity and dental caries, Arch. Oral Biol. **8**:571, 1963.

25. Goodman, H. O., Luke, J. E., Rosen, S., and Hackel, E.: Heritability in dental caries, certain oral microflora and salivary components, Am. J. Hum. Genet. **11**:263-273, 1959.

26. Grainger, R. M., Paynter, K. J., and Shaw, J. H.: J. Dent. Res. **38**:105, 1959.

27. Green, G. E.: A bacteriolytic agent in salivary globulin of caries-immune human beings, J. Dent. Res. **38**:262-275, 1959.

28. Green, G. E., Wilson, R. M., Via, W. F., and Bixler, D.: A study of the genetics of immunity to human dental caries, 41st General Meeting of International Association for Dental Research, Pittsburgh, 1963.

29. Gustafsson, B. E., Quensel, C. E., Lanke, L. S., Lundquist, C., Grahnem, H., Bonow, B. E., and Krasse, B.: Vipeholm dental caries study: the effect of different levels of carbohydrate intake on caries activity in 436 individuals observed for 5 years, Acta Odontol. Scand. **11**:232, 1954.

30. Hatton, M. E.: Measure of the effects of heredity and environment on eruption of the deciduous teeth, J. Dent. Res. **34**:397-401, 1955.

31. Horowitz, S. L., Osborne, R. H., and DeGeorge, F. V.: Caries experience in twins, Science **128**:300-301, 1958.

32. Hunt, H. R., and Hoppert, C. A.: Inheritance of susceptibility to caries in albino rats, J. Am. Coll. Dent. **11**:33-37, 1944.

33. Hunt, H. R., Hoppert, C. A., and Rosen, S.: Genetic factors in experimental rat caries. In Sognnaes, R. F., editor: Advances in experimental caries research, Washington, D.C., 1955, American Association for the Advancement of Science.

34. Kifer, P. E., Hunt, H. R., Hoppert, C. A., and Witkop, C. J.: Comparison between widths of fissures of lower molars of caries-resistant and caries-susceptible albino rats, J. Dent. Res. **35**:620-629, 1956.

35. Klein, H.: The family and dental disease. IV. Dental disease (DMF) experience in parents and offspring, J.A.D.A. **33**:735, 1946.

36. Klein, H., and Palmer, C. E.: Studies on dental caries. V. Familial resemblance in caries experience in siblings, Public Health Rep. **53**:1353-1364, 1938.

37. König, K. G.: Dental morphology in relation to caries resistance with special reference to fissures as susceptible areas, J. Dent. Res. **42** (pt. 2):461-476, 1963.

38. Larson, R., and Simms, M.: Double mating: Its use to study heritable factors in dental caries, Science **149**:982, 1965.

39. Lehner, T., Cardwell, J. and Clarry, E.: Immunoglobulins in saliva and serum in dental caries, Lancet **1**:1294-1297, 1967.

40. Mandel, I. D., and Zengo, A. N.: Genetic and chemical aspects in caries resistance. In Mergenhagen, S. E., and Scherp, I. W., editors: Comparative immunology of the oral cavity, NIH 73-438, Washington, D.C., 1973, U.S. Department of Health, Education, and Welfare.

41. Mansbridge, J. N.: Heredity and dental caries, J. Dent. Res. **38**:337-347, 1959.

42. Niswander, J. D.: Genetics of common dental disorders, Dent. Clin. North Am. **19**:197, Jan., 1975.

43. O'Roark, W. L., and Leyschon, C.: Dental-caries prevalence as related to blood groups, J. Dent. Res. **42**:1530, 1963.

44. Schull, W. J., and Neel, J. V.: The effects

of inbreeding on Japanese children, New York, 1965, Harper & Row, Publishers.

45. Shaw, J. H., and Griffiths, D.: Arch. Oral Biol. 3:247, 1961.

46. Sims, W.: The concept of immunity in dental caries. II. Specific immune responses, Oral Surg. 34:69-86, 1972.

47. Turner, N. C., Bell, J. T., Scribner, J. H., and Meyer, J. Z.: Concordance of identical twins in salivary acidity-alkalinity: monozygotic twins and siblings compared in respect to salivary tests for titratable alkalinity and titratable acidity, J. Hered. 86:44-45, 1954.

48. Warren, L. A.: A family study of exceptional resistance to dental caries, Master's thesis, Bloomington, Ind., 1968, Indiana University.

49. Weisenstein, P. R., and Green, G. E.: Clinical and bacteriological studies of caries-immune human beings, J. Dent. Res. 36: 390-694, 1957.

50. Witkop, C. J., Jr., Barros, L., and Hamilton, P. A.: Public Health Rep. 77:928, 1962.

51. Witkop, C. J., Jr.: Genes, chromosomes and dentistry, J. Am. Dent. Assoc. 68:845-858, 1964.

Periodontal disease

52. Benjamin, S. D., and Baer, P. N.: Familial patterns of advanced alveolar bone loss in adolescence (periodontosis), Periodontics 5: 82-88, 1967.

53. Benjamin, S. D., and Baer, P. N.: Familial patterns of advanced alveolar bone loss in adolescence (periodontosis), J. Am. Soc. Psychosom. Dent. Med. 5:82-88, 1967.

54. Bixler, D.: Genetic aspects of dental anomalies in children. In McDonald, R. E.: Dentistry for the child and adolescent, ed. 2, St. Louis, 1974, The C. V. Mosby Co.

55. Chung, C. S., Runck, D. W., Niswander, J. D., Bilben, S. F., and Kau, M. D. W.: Genetic and epidemiologic studies of oral characteristics in Hawaii's schoolchildren. I. Caries and periodontal disease, J. Dent. Res. 49: 1374-1375, 1970.

56. Coccia, C. T., McDonald, R. E., and Mitchell, D. F.: Papillon-Lefèvre syndrome; precocious periodontosis with palmar-plantar hyperkeratosis, J. Periodontol. 37:404-414, 1966.

57. Dickmann, A.: Die Verebung der Paradentose (dissertation), München, 1935.

58. Gorlin, R. J., Stallard, R. E., and Shapiro, B. L.: Genetics and periodontal disease, J. Periodontol. 38:5-10, 1967.

59. Gorlin, R. J., Sedano, H., and Anderson, V. E.: The syndrome of palmar-plantar hyperkeratosis and premature periodontal destruction of the teeth—a clinical and genetic

analysis of Papillon-Lefèvre syndrome, J. Pediatr. 65:895-908, 1964.

60. McKusick, V. A.: Heritable disorders of connective tissue, ed. 4, St. Louis, 1972, The C. V. Mosby Co.

61. Nishimura, E. T., Hamilton, H. B., Kobara, T. Y., Takahara, S., Oxura, Y., and Foi, K.: Carrier state in human acatalasemia, Science 130:333-334, 1959.

62. Reiser, H. E., and Vogel, F.: Über die Erblichkeit der Zahnsteinbildung beim Menschen, Dtsch. Zahnaertzl. Z. 13:1355-1358, 1958.

63. Rojahn, H.: Familienuntersuchungen bei Paradentose (dissertation), Heidelberg, 1952.

64. Schull, W. J., and Neel, J. V.: The effects of inbreeding on Japanese children, New York, 1965, Harper & Row, Publishers.

65. Takahara, S.: Progressive oral gangrene, probably due to lack of catalase in the blood (acatalasemia); report of nine cases, Lancet 2:1101-1104, 1952.

66. Witkop, C. J., et al.: Medical and dental findings in the Brandywine isolate, Ala. J. Med. Sci. 3:382-403, 1966.

Malocclusion

67. Angle, E. H.: Treatment of malocclusion of the teeth, ed. 7, Philadelphia, 1907, S. S. White Manufacturing Co., pp. 52-54, 58, 559-553.

68. Brodie, A., and Newman, H.: In Petersen, W. F.: Man—weather—sun, Springfield, Ill., 1947, Charles C Thomas, Publisher, pp. 3-11.

69. Emrich, R. E., Brodie, A. G., and Blayney, J. R.: Prevalence of class I, class II, and class III malocclusions (Angle) in an urban population: an epidemiological study, J. Dent. Res. 44:947-953, 1965.

70. Fox, R., and Crary, D.: Mandibular prognathism in the rabbit, J. Hered. 62:23-27, 1971.

71. Goldberg, S.: Biometrics of identical twins from the dental viewpoint, J. Dent. Res. 9: 363-409, 1929.

72. Gregory, K. E., Koch, R. M., and Swiger, L. A.: Malocclusion—a hereditary defect in cattle, J. Hered. 53:168, 1962.

73. Grewe, J. M., Cervenka, J., Shapiro, B. L., et al.: Prevalence of malocclusion in Chippewa Indian children, J. Dent. Res. 47: 302-305, 1963.

74. Gruneberg, H., and Lea, A. J.: An inherited Jaw anomaly in long-haired dachshunds, J. Genet. 39:285, 1940.

75. Haecker, V.: Der Familientypus der Hapsburger, Z. Abst. Verenb. 6:61-89, 1911.

76. Harnisch, H.: Zur Vererbung des Diastema

mediale, Zahnaerztl. Rundschr. **49:**913-920, 1940.

77. Harris, J. E.: A multivariate analysis of the craniofacial complex, Ann Arbor, Mich., 1963, University of Michigan School of Dentistry.

78. Harris, J. E.: Genetic factors in the growth of the head: inheritance of the craniofacial complex and malocclusion, Dent. Clin. North Am. **19:**151-160, 1975.

79. Horowitz, S. L., Osborne, R. H., and DeGeorge, F. V.: A cephalometric study of craniofacial variation in adult twins, Angle Orthod. **30:**1-5, 1960.

80. Hughes, B. O., and Moore, G. R.: Heredity, growth, and the dento-facial complex, Angle Orthod. **11:**127-222, 1941.

81. Hunter, W. S.: A study of the inheritance of craniofacial characteristics as seen in lateral cephalograms of 72 like sexed twins, Europ. Orthod. Soc. Rep. Congr. **41:**59-70, 1965.

82. Iwagaki, H.: Hereditary influence of malocclusion, Am. J. Orthod. Oral Surg. **24:**328-336, 1938.

83. Johnson, A. L.: The constitutional factor in skull form and dental occlusion, Am. J. Orthod. Oral Surg. **26:**627-63, 1940.

84. Kingsley, N. W.: Die Anomalien der Zahnstellung und die Defekte des Gaumens (translated by L. H. von Hollaender), Leipzig, Germany, 1881, A. Felix.

85. Korkhaus, G.: In Handbuch der Zahnheilkunde, vol. 4, Munchen, 1939, I. F. Bergmann.

86. Kraus, B. S., Wise, W. J., and Frie, R. A.: Heredity and the craniofacial complex, Am. J. Orthod. **45:**172-217, 1959.

87. Leech, H. L.: Angle's class II, division 1, and class II, division 2, in identical twins, D. Pract. **5:**341-345, 1955.

88. Litton, S. F., Ackerman, L. N., Isaacson, R. J., and Shapiro, B. L.: A genetic study of class III malocclusion, Am. J. Orthod. **58:**565-577, 1970.

89. Lundstrom, A.: Tooth size and occlusion in twins, ed. 2, Basel, Switzerland, 1948, S. Karger, A. G.

90. Margolis, H. L., Hodge, T. A., and Tanner, J. M.: Familial similarities in the craniofacial complex, Personal communication, 1968.

91. McKusick, V. A.: Heritable disorders of connective tissue, ed. 4, St. Louis, 1972, The C. V. Mosby Co.

92. Mills, L. F.: Epidemiologic studies of occlusion. IV. The prevalence of malocclusion in a population of 1,455 school children, J. Dent. Res. **45:**332-336, 1966.

93. Moorrees, C. F. A.: Genetic considerations in dental anthropology. In Witkop, C. J.,

editor: Genetics and dental health, New York, 1962, McGraw-Hill Book Co., pp. 101-110.

94. Myllärniemi, S.: Malocclusion in Finnish rural children: an epidemiological study of different stages of dental development (doctoral thesis), Helsinki, 1970, University of Helsinki.

95. Newman, G. V.: The Eskimo's dentofacial complex, U.S. Armed Forces Med. J. **3:**1653-1662, 1952.

96. Niswander, J. D.: Genetics of common dental disorders, Dent. Clin. North Am. **19:**197-206, 1975.

97. Niswander, J. D.: Further studies on the Xavante Indians. VII. The oral status of the Xavante of Simoes Lopes, Am. J. Hum. Genet. **19:**543-553, 1967.

98. Nordby, J. E., Terrill, C. E., Hazel, L. N., and Stoehr, J. A.: The etiology and inheritance of inequalites in the jaws of sheep, Anat. Rec. **92:**235-254, 1945.

99. Noyes, H. J.: A review of the genetic influence on malocclusion, Am. J. Orthod. **44:**81-98, 1958.

100. Penrose, L. S.: Cited by Vogel, F.: Lehrbuch der allgemeinen Humangenetik, Heidelberg, Germany, 1961, Springer Verlag.

101. Platt, H.: Beitrag zur Frage der Vereblichkeit von Zahn- und Kieferanonmalien (medical dissertation), Wurzburg, Germany, 1938.

102. Robert, J. C.: A cephalometric study of class II division I malocclusion, Thesis, Ann Arbor, Mich., 1967, University of Michigan.

103. Rubbrect, O.: A study of the heredity of the anomalies of the jaws, Am. J. Orthod. Oral Surg. **25:**751-79, 1939.

104. Schull, W. J., and Neel, J. V.: The effects of inbreeding on Japanese children, New York, 1965, Harper & Row, Publishers.

105. Schulze, C.: Über Zwillinge mit Progenie, Stoma **18:**250-266, 1965.

106. Schulze, C., and Wiese, W.: Zur Vererbung der Progenie, Fortschr. Kieferorthop. **26:**213-229, 1965.

107. Snodgrasse, R. M.: A family line study of cephalofacial growth, Am. J. Orthod. **34:**714-24, 1948.

108. Stein, K. F., Kelly, T. J., and Wood, E.: Influence of heredity in the etiology of malocclusion, Am. J. Orthod. **42:**125-41, 1956.

109. Stiles, K. A., and Luke, J. E.: The inheritance of malocclusion due to mandibular prognathism, J. Hered. **44:**241-245, 1953.

110. Stockard, C. H.: The genetic and endocrinic basis for differences in form and behavior, Philadelphia, 1941, Wistar Institute of Anatomy and Biology.

111. Strohmayer, W.: Die Vererburg des Haps-

burger Familientypus, Nova Acta Leopoldina 5:219-296, 1937.

112. Suzuki, S.: Studies on the so-called reverse occlusion, J. Nihon Univ. Sch. Dent. 5:51-58, 1961.

113. Tobias, P. V.: Teeth, jaws and genes, J. Dent. Assoc. S. Afr. 10:88-104, March, 1955.

114. Trauner, R., et al.: Die Verebung und Entwicklung der Zahn- und Kieferstellungsanomalien, Fortschr. Kieferorthop. 23:1-71, 1961.

115. Watnick, S. S.: Inheritance of craniofacial morphology, Angle Orthod. 42:339-351, 1972.

116. Weninger, M.: Zur Verebung des medianen Oberkiefertremas, Z. Morphol. Anthropol. 32:367-393, 1933.

117. Wylie, W. L.: A quantitative method for comparison of craniofacial patterns in different individuals, Am. J. Anat. 74:39-45, 1944.

5

The genetics of tooth size

ROSARIO H. YAP POTTER

Genetic variation in man may be observed at two levels. When the differences between individuals are qualitative or discrete, as in the blood antigens, genotypes may be identified and gene frequencies estimated. The other type of genetic variation affects continuous traits, such as height, weight, or tooth size, in which the differences between individuals are of degree rather than kind. Biometrical or quantitative genetics is concerned with the study of the latter type of variation.

Evidence that the continuous variation in a trait is genetic in origin comes from two sources, the similarity between relatives in human studies and the response to selection in experiments on laboratory organisms.

The genetics of quantitative traits in man has not been as extensively studied as qualitative traits for several reasons. These traits are usually determined by the alleles of many loci so that the Mendelian type of analysis is not appropriate. They are further modified by environmental conditions, which obscure the genetic picture. Finally, the necessary statistical methods are involved and, in the case of human studies, not fully developed.

Dental geneticists and clinicians are usually more familiar with the inheritance pattern of qualitative traits and genetic methods such as pedigree analysis than with the fundamental laws of quantitative genetics and the methods of analysis for continuous variables. In this chapter, the genetic basis of quantitative traits, the properties of these traits, and

the methods for their analysis will be briefly discussed along with the genetics of tooth size.

Until recently, the main contributions in the literature toward understanding the genetics of tooth dimension in man consisted of demonstrations of a highly significant genetic control of unitary tooth dimensions inferred from twin studies. On this basis, the clinical literature implies that the size of teeth is mainly an inherited trait and that the environment has little or no effect, leading orthodontists and pedodontists to attempt to predict a patient's tooth mass from those of the parents or of the siblings. As a rule, failures were encountered in such attempts. We now know that both genetic and environmental factors determine the variability of dental dimensions. It is hoped that the investigations cited in this chapter serve to illustrate the multifactorial nature of the determinants of tooth size: first, differential and interacting genetic components, then differential and interacting environmental components, and finally, interaction between genetic and environmental factors.

TOOTH SIZE AND CRANIOFACIAL EVOLUTION

Because of their high inorganic content, teeth are often the most identifiable and permanent of all paleontological materials. Skeletons, even skulls, are less permanent, and in many cases teeth and jaws are the only fossil remains available to anthropologists to provide a reliable basis for the identification, classification, and discussion of evolutionary relationships. Careful study of these specimens has demonstrated that a major morphological trend in evolution has been a reduction in the jaw elements from ancestral to modern hominid dentition with a simultaneous reduction in the size of the teeth and a simplification in their form and pattern.

Anthropological data indicate that the enlargement of the size of the brain was a major factor in the chain of evolutionary events from the lower primates to man. The expansion of the neurocranium occurred concomitantly with a reduction of the muzzle area of the lower primates, resulting in a significant change in the jaws of the hominids. During the reduction process, the craniofacial axis (a line from the anterior border of the foramen magnum through the sella turcica to the nasion), which was originally a straight line directed upward and forward in the lower primates, became bent at the sella in the anthropoid apes to assume an obtuse angle. In man, the anterior leg of this axis became more nearly horizontal, thereby depressing the face and diminishing the projection of the jaws. As a result, the dental elements were reduced in an anteroposterior direction, shortening the dental arches, which became wider posteriorly. Accompanying changes in the mandible included a shortening of the body and heightening of the ascending ramus, which resulted in a decrease in the gonial angle formed by these two components. The entire head was then balanced on the erect spine in an upright position.

The size and shape of the teeth are closely correlated with craniofacial evolution. It would also seem reasonable to expect an alteration in tooth size to occur with changes in tooth shape, form, and pattern. Profound size changes found in fossil teeth of varying age as well as in the dentitions of living populations are of concern in evolutionary studies. The trends of such changes have led anthropologists to conclude an adaptive significance of tooth size that has arisen chiefly through selection forces such as alterations in

diet and in the use of teeth in mastication or as tools.[14] Dental dimensions are also important in microevolutionary studies of groups within species such as the racial groups in man. The goal of microevolutionary studies is to explain within- and between-group differences that are due to accumulation of minute variations. Here the possible dental adaptations are much less obvious, and evolutionary processes other than selection must be considered, such as drift and admixture,[30] to account for genetic variability.

The variation of tooth size among racial groups has been widely recognized. In addition to differences in absolute size, differences in relative size of certain teeth have been demonstrated. For example, the largeness of upper lateral incisors relative to the central incisors in the Mongoloid peoples is not seen in other racial groups. Within racial groups, sex variations are also recognized in that males exhibit larger teeth than females to different extents for different teeth, with the largest sex difference occurring in the canines.

The assumption that evolutionary change is always toward reduction and that the trend is irreversible must be treated with caution. An example of reduction is that occurring in the mesiodistal dimension of the mandibular molars in accordance with an evolutionary change from the five-cusped Y occlusal groove pattern to the four-cusped + groove pattern.[13] Other examples are reduction in cusp number not only in the molars but also in the lower second premolars and reduction in tooth number in the case of missing teeth. Examples of intensification of morphological features in evolution are shovel-shaped incisors and Carabelli's cusps. In certain racial groups these features seem to compensate to a limited extent for the loss in total size. For example, the eastern Mediterraneans and Europeans have generally small teeth, but more than 40% of them have developed Carabelli's cusp on the upper molars. On the other hand, Melanesians have a large Carabelli cusp, and the Mongoloid peoples have the shovel-shaped incisors, although both groups still maintain relatively large teeth.

The genetics of dental variation based on descriptive information between and within racial groups can be better understood through Butler's "field" hypothesis,[10] which was adapted for the human dentition by Dahlberg.[12] This theory postulates that the dentition can be divided into several fields corresponding to the morphological tooth groups. Within each field, the "key" tooth is the genetically stable tooth. It is proposed that a "distance gradient" exists, so that the more distant a tooth is from the key tooth, the more variable it becomes. The key teeth are the central incisors, canines, first premolars, and first molars. The variable teeth are the lateral incisors, second premolars, and second and third molars. An exception is the incisor group in the mandible in which the centrals are more variable than the laterals. With this scheme, it is expected that in the course of evolution, the most distant teeth within the fields are those that are most likely to change in size and shape or to be lost.

GENETIC BASIS OF QUANTITATIVE TRAITS

The most tenable explanation for the continuous variability in a phenotypic trait is that the genetic variation depends on the simultaneous segregation of many genes affecting the trait, together with the superimposition of environmental effects. This type of genetic variability is also referred to as *multifactorial inheritance*. The genes concerned are subject to the same laws of transmission and have the same general properties as the single genes involved in the qualitative differences of Mendelian genetics. Genetic difference caused by the segregation of many genes is referred to as *polygenic variation,* and the genes concerned are referred to as *polygenes*. Fig. 5-1 illustrates the manner in which Mendelian segregation of genes is translated into genetic variation of continuous traits through polygenes.

Measurable traits observed in a population may be expressed in terms of means, variances, and covariances, the study of which is analogous to studying the genotype frequen-

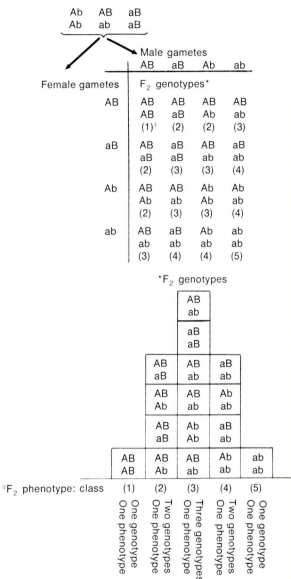

Fig. 5-1. Polygenic theory of continuous traits. F_2 genotypes are obtained with two genes, A and B, of equal and additive effect, ignoring dominance, epistasis, and environmental variation. Capital and small letters indicate the two alleles of a gene locus. Genotypes with same number of capital letters are expressed in same phenotypic class with no visible variation. Number of phenotypic classes is proportional to number of genes involved in trait: with three genes there are seven classes, with four genes there are nine classes, and with k genes there are $2k + 1$ classes.

cies and ratios of qualitative traits. The values for means, variances, and covariances are based on measurements of phenotypic traits from a group of individuals. The phenotypic value of a single individual from the group is any measured trait, such as the size of a tooth, and represents the combined effects of genotype and environment. The genotype refers to the particular array of genes possessed by the individual, and the environment consists of all nongenetic factors that influence the phenotypic measurement.

Components of genotypic variance

Parents transmit genes and not genotypes to their offspring. New genotypes are created in each generation as a consequence of the independent assortment and recombination of genes. When the transmission of a trait from parent to offspring is under consideration, it is apparent that the component of interest should focus on genes, not genotype. The portion of an individual's phenotypic variance that is due to his genotype is his genotypic or genetic variance, which is composed of additive effects, dominance, and epistatic effects of genes. The additive effects refer to the sum total of the unit effects of the genes carried by the individual that are involved in the trait, the summation being made over the pair of alleles at each locus and over all loci. Additive effects are therefore manifested when the gene is taken singly. When allelic genes are put together in pairs and a locus is considered, a nonadditive effect caused by dominance among the paired alleles at this locus will be manifested together with the additive effects. Dominance is therefore the interaction between alleles at one locus or the *within-locus* interaction, which, if present, will cause a more profound deviation of the genotype than when only additive effects are involved. When only one locus is considered, the genotypic variance of an individual is caused by the additive and the dominance effects. But in a polygenic trait the genotype refers to more than one locus, so that the genotypic variance may contain yet another nonadditive component. Epistasis is thus the effect of putting together two or more gene

loci, or the *between-loci* interaction. For a detailed account of these three components of genetic variance, the reader is referred to Falconer's *Quantitative Genetics*[15] or Mather and Jinks' *Biometrical Genetics*.[27]

Heritability

The proportion of the phenotypic variance that is attributable to the genotype is referred to as *heritability in the broad sense*. This ratio of genotype to phenotype variance measures the extent of genetic determination in the variability of a trait, but it does not tell us to what extent the trait is inherited. A perusal of genetic studies of tooth size indicates that the term *hereditary control* has been used interchangeably with the term *genetic control*. For polygenic characters, heritability differs from genetic control of variation; the former indicates the transmission of parental traits to offspring through the genes, and the latter indicates variation of an individual due to his genotype.

The additive component of genetic variance is that particular portion of the genotype which is associated with genes carried by the individual and transmitted to his offspring. The nonadditive components of genetic variance are due to dominance and epistasis. These sources constitute the total genetic variance of a polygenic trait. The proportion of the total genetic variance that is attributable to the additive effects of genes is an estimate of *heritability in the narrow sense*. This ratio, additive to total genetic variance, determines the extent to which a trait is inherited and thus the degree of resemblance between relatives. *Heritability in the narrow sense* is important for predictive purposes, since it estimates the reliability of an individual's phenotype as a predictor for the additive effects of genes that will exert an influence on the next generation.

In studies of prediction and of microevolutionary changes, the component of genetic variance that is of interest is the additive component, and the *heritability in the narrow sense* is the estimate used. It is important, therefore, to specify which type of heritability is being estimated. Since the experimental procedures of controlled breeding used to estimate additive genetic variance in animal and plant genetics are not applicable to humans, the heritability that is estimated from whatever type of human data is of limited value for practical purposes. Perhaps the only reasonable use of such estimates in man is to detect the presence of genetic variability. Even then, it must be remembered that these estimates necessarily assume complete independence of the genetic and environmental influences on the trait.

Properties of polygenic systems

The additive genetic variance is usually expressed as mean deviations from the population mean. Fig. 5-1 shows that the additive effects of the genes in an individual determine the mean genotype of the offspring generation, and, therefore, this individual's additive genotype is estimated from the mean value of the offspring. Since two parents contribute to the genotype of the offspring, one often reads in the literature that for a biometrical trait, the mean value of the offspring tend to be about halfway between the mean value of the parents and the population mean. In other words, the offspring tend to return to the mean value of the population regardless of the phenotypic extremes of the parents. To the uninitiated reader, an erroneous interpretation often arises that from generation to generation, the amount of variation around the population mean would thus be reduced, insofar as variability of the trait is attributed to genetic sources. A discussion of the properties of polygenic systems will explain the practically inexhaustible source of genetic variation.

With respect to continuous traits, the observed variation in the population is but a small fraction of the total genetic variability within the population. Polygenic systems possess two remarkable properties. First, the degree to which the trait is expressed depends more on the number of genes affecting the trait than on the particular genes present, so that similar phenotypes may actually be different in their genotypes. Fig. 5-1 shows that genotypes AaBb and aaBB will display a

phenotype (class 3) that is not distinguishable from the AAbb genotype. In other words, these three genotypes have the same phenotype with the similarity in phenotypic expression being due to balancing between A and a, B and b in the AaBb genotype, between AA and bb in the AAbb genotype, and between aa and BB in the aaBB genotype. The balancing leads to the second property of polygenes to conceal or store variability. This property is readily observed in the case of recessive traits, in which the recessive homozygotes will display the trait, whereas the heterozygotes will be the same as the normals, as in chondroectodermal dysplasia (Ellis–van Creveld disease) or acatalasia. The potential genetic variability is revealed only by the mating of two heterozygotes. The same type of concealment is displayed by heterozygotes in polygenic systems. For example, mating of two AaBb individuals will give offspring of the five phenotypes shown in Fig. 5-1, including those with extreme expressions of the trait, thereby revealing the variability hidden by the balancing effects of allelic genes in the heterozygote AaBb. In polygenic systems, however, the potential variation is not limited to heterozygotes. The mating of AAbb and aaBB individuals who are phenotypically indistinguishable from each other will likewise reproduce all the expressions of the trait in the third generation. The concealed variation has thus been revealed by recombination.

The proportion of concealed genetic variability depends on the number of genes in the polygenic system. The more genes involved in the trait, the greater is this proportion. Only a small fraction of the total genetic variability of a population is observed as differences between the individuals of a population, while the greater part is concealed in the form of genetic differences between individuals who do not display the full effects of their genes because of the way genes balance one another's effect.

Selection, the chief cause of evolutionary changes in a trait, can act on the trait only if individuals differ phenotypically. Therefore, to the extent that genetic variation is not phenotypically expressed, it is not acted on by selection. A large reserve of concealed polygenic variation is then expected to accumulate that is immune to the action of selection. Although mutation may account for some gene differences in a polygenic system, the increment added to the genetic variation due to mutation is negligible compared to the amount of accumulated genetic variation as just described.

OBJECTIVES IN GENETIC STUDIES OF TOOTH SIZE

Three major problems are posed in studying the genetics of tooth size. In the past, the question was often raised as to whether the portion of total variability of a trait in the population that is genetic in origin is detectable or not. Earlier literature on genetic control of tooth size consisted of studies directed mainly toward resolving this question and toward estimating the genetic fraction through a heritability estimate. An advantage of these studies is that the methods of analysis and the underlying statistical concepts were easily understood by dental geneticists. Unfortunately, evidences of significant genetic control of variability derived from these studies are inadequate to delineate satisfactorily the inheritance of tooth size for understanding genetic-environment interaction, for microevolutionary studies, or for clinical predictive purposes. Furthermore, the geneticist today is satisfied that phenotypic expressions are conditioned by the individual's genotype to various degrees. Although demonstration of a measurable genetic component is the first objective of biometrical studies, it is not by any means the final goal.

Beyond the question of relative magnitude of genetic effects is the question of gene action. In Mendelian or discrete inheritance, the mode of gene action is well understood. The gene or genes that affect a trait or cause a pathological entity are identified along with a description of the effects. In Mendelian inheritance, the pattern of inheritance of a trait is demonstrated according to dominance or recessivity. If the gene action is recognized, it follows that the products of inheritance

themselves become predictable. In the case of polygenic traits, it is impossible to analyze the genetic mechanism of transmission in these terms. For polygenic traits, the alternative is to enquire whether observed variation and covariation may be explained in terms following some known genetic concepts such as additive effects, dominance, epistasis, pleiotropy, and linkage. Recent studies of the genetics of tooth size have been directed toward partitioning the total genetic variance into its components as a basis for phenotype prediction. They have also been directed toward explaining phenotypic manifestations in terms of autosomal linkage or sex linkage. Linkage refers to the association in inheritance of polygenes and, in turn, of the phenotypic traits they control, due to their being located in the same autosome or sex chromosome. More recently, proposed multivariate analytic techniques have made it possible to study phenotypic correlations of multiple traits in terms of pleiotropy. Pleiotropy is the property of a gene or a polygene system whereby it affects two or more traits so that if the genes are segregating, they cause simultaneous variation in these traits to appear as phenotypic correlations. Human studies of twin and family data and animal studies were used in an effort to provide a more basic understanding of the genetic mode of transmission of these complex biometrical traits. The prevalence of symmetrical normal distributions in most anthropological traits has been interpreted to mean a greater importance of additive gene effects over dominance and epistasis. High correlations among anthropometric traits raise the question as to whether pleiotropy or linkage is the underlying genetic mechanism involved. Only when these genetic concepts are established for tooth size can a basis for phenotype prediction be identified.

A final and most important objective in studying multifactorial inheritance in man is to understand the effect of genotype-environment interaction. The application of human genetics differs from nonhuman genetics in which the goal is to change the genetic constitution to produce a desired phenotype, as in agricultural genetics and animal breeding programs. In man, a more realistic objective is to modify the environment either to prevent undesired phenotypes or to produce desired phenotypes. It must be remembered that a quantitative trait, such as tooth size, is measured from the phenotype and that the genetic constitution of an individual does not produce the trait by itself. Genes initiate growth and differentiation and then determine the individual's norm of reaction to the existing environment. Quantitative traits, therefore, are manifestations of an individual's developmental pattern that results from genetic-environment interactions.

In man, the question of genotype-environment interaction can best be approached by twin studies. Geneticists, however, have not optimally explored the potentials of twin research methods. This is primarily due to preoccupation with the problem of demonstrating the relative importance of genetics versus environment rather than with attention toward understanding their interaction. An example of this interaction is present as phenotypic correlations in antimeric tooth size, a phenomenon that is generally recognized among tooth morphologists. Interrelationships among multiple measured traits are results of both genetic and environmental factors, which may become complex. It is necessary to delineate these genetic and environmental causes of correlation to determine how genetic associations among multiple traits come about and whether environmental influences are the results of a single or of differential environmental factors. The "cross-twin" method[31] represents an effort in this direction. Recently, the development of multivariate techniques for analysis on twins has made it possible to explore this question in greater detail, as shown in the current twin studies[34] conducted at the Departments of Medical Genetics and Oral-Facial Genetics at the Indiana University Schools of Medicine and Dentistry.

HUMAN STUDIES ON TOOTH SIZE

The analytic methods in quantitative genetics, originally presented by Fisher,[16] depend principally on correlations between relatives and on the statistical procedure of *analysis of variance*. These methods were developed mainly for applying genetic principles to animal and plant breeding purposes, in which breed control is possible. In human studies, where planned experimental conditions are impossible, the limited efficiency of these statistical methods must be recognized. As an alternative, biometrical geneticists have devised and are continuing to devise different and appropriate methods of analysis for applications on commonly existing situations in man such as the occurrence of twins, consanguineous matings, population isolates, and population migration. Quantitative genetic analyses of tooth size in man are based on two genetic phenomena: resemblance between relatives, of which twins are a special kind, and inbreeding depression.

Twin studies

The twin method, when appropriately applied, provides geneticists with one of the most incisive and informative techniques available in man for the analysis of complex genetic traits.

Investigations using the twin method to interpret genetic control of tooth size generally aim at demonstrating a larger within-pair difference in dizygotic twins than in monozygotic twins. This procedure is based on the underlying principle that observed differences within a pair of monozygotic twins are due to environment and that differences within a pair of dizygotic twins are due to both environment and genotype. A comparison of the observed within-pair differences for twins in the two categories should provide a measure of the degree to which monozygotic twins are more alike than dizygotic twins. The larger this difference between the two twin categories, the greater the genetic effect on variability of the trait. The implied assumption here is that environmental effects are equal in the two twin categories.

The determination of zygosity was a serious problem for early researchers when classification of twins was based only on morphological criteria, so that there were always possibilities of a systematic misclassification of the most similar dizygotic twins as well as the most dissimilar monozygotic twins. At the present time, accurate zygosity classification is seldom a problem due to the ability to ascertain the large number of available polymorphic blood group and enzyme markers.

It must be recognized that the genotypic variance obtained from the twin method includes additive, dominance, and epistatic genetic effects, of which only the additive effects are directly transmittable from parent to offspring, and any heritability estimate derived from the twin data refers to *heritability in the broad sense.*

Studies on tooth size generally calculate for the ratio of dizygotic to monozygotic within-pair variances, and the significance of this difference is statistically tested. If most of the variability in a trait is environment-caused, the within-pair variances will be comparable in the two twin categories so that the ratio will approximate 1. The greater the genetic component of variance, the greater the difference will be between the dizygotic within-pair variance and the monozygotic within-pair variance, which results in an upward deviation of the ratio from unity. The work of Osborne and associates[31] typically illustrates this method of analysis. Their results demonstrated detectable genetic components of variation for the mesiodistal dimension of the six permanent anterior teeth on the right side that were studied in Caucasian twins, which showed a significantly greater within-pair variance in the dizygotic than in the monozygotic twins. In another investigation Horowitz and co-workers[21] indicated similar findings for the twelve anterior teeth studied.

From a Swedish twin sample, Lundström[25] arrived at essentially the same conclusions for the mesiodistal dimension of the permanent teeth from central incisors to first molars in all four quadrants. Although Lundström and some earlier workers used various methods to calculate for within-pair differences, a similar basic idea of comparing dizygotic with monozygotic within-pair differences was followed. All these twin data suggested varying extents in the genetic component of variability for different teeth.

In the work of Osborne and co-workers,[31] the documentation of a genetic basis for correlated dimensions of different teeth was first attempted. That some common factors involved in the determination of tooth size of different teeth may be genetic in origin received considerable support from a "cross-twin" method of analysis developed by these workers. Their findings indicated that the association between the mesiodistal dimension of adjacent anterior teeth is genetic in origin and not merely a consequence of within-individual mechanical or physiological influences, thus supporting a hypothesis of a genetic control for general tooth size (for the six permanent anterior teeth on the right side that were studied). Their results further indicated that in addition to common size factors, some genetically conditioned independence may be present to affect the size variation of individual teeth.

Osborne's work on twins is based on the univariate analytic method, in which the multiple tooth size variables, taken one at a time in the analysis, are treated as independent of each other. Tooth measurements from a set of teeth are highly correlated, however, suggesting that there are underlying genetic factors fundamental to the structure of these teeth. These same studies[31] suggest that one of the reasons adjacent teeth in a quadrant are highly interrelated is that they share some genes in common. Therefore the recently developed multivariate method, which considers correlated variables jointly as a system in an analysis, is a more appropriate approach in tooth size studies. In multivariate analysis, linear functions are derived from the tooth measurements, which would seem to be more directly related to causative effects that are common to the variables and would thus be more efficient than the separate measurements themselves for investigating genetic variability of tooth size.

Correlated characters are also of interest to the geneticist and the evolutionist. First, the genetic cause of correlations is chiefly through the pleiotropic action of genes. If the genetic correlation is caused by linkage to any extent, it is likely to diminish in magnitude through recombination in future generations with a consequent diminution of the correlated response. Second, studies of genetic correlations are highly relevant to the changes that might be expected to result from selection, since it is well known that intense selection for one biometrical trait commonly alters other traits as well. The concept of pleiotropic action of genes is pertinent toward understanding the role of selection in bringing about evolutionary changes. Evolution does not consist of changes of independent traits; what

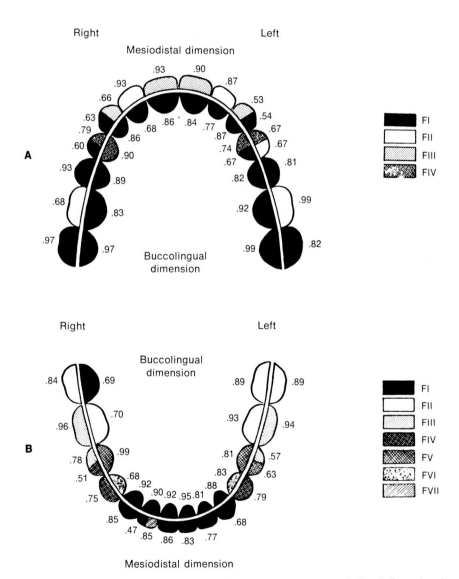

Fig. 5-2. Significant genetic factors. Outer half of teeth represents mesiodistal dimension; inner half represents buccolingual dimension. Largest loadings are shown, in some cases together with second largest loadings, to better depict genetic factors. Influence of identical genetic factors on antimeric tooth dimensions is striking. **A,** Four factors for maxillary teeth. Factor I appears to affect maxillary teeth in general, particularly buccolingual dimensions. **B,** Seven factors for mandibular teeth. Factor I appears to affect anterior teeth at both dimensions.

changes is the genetic system and the related developmental system as a whole.

In 1965 Vandenberg[7, 38] introduced his multivariate technique for the analysis of interrelated biometrical traits in twins and used it to characterize the independent genetic factors that were measured by a battery of psychological tests. This technique has the potential of revealing the pleiotropic actions of genes or of polygene systems. In addition, genetic correlations for multiple biometrical traits may readily be estimated. This analysis may be considered to be an extension of the univariate F test to the case of multiple correlated variables, which permits the identification of independent genetic factors that influence the traits in question. Utilizing this technique, we (Potter and co-workers[34]) presented the results of an analysis of mesiodistal and buccolingual dimensions of the permanent teeth from the central incisors to the second molars in Caucasian twins. Our results provide evidence that tooth dimension correlations are primarily genetic in origin, probably attributable to pleiotropic action of genes or, more likely, of groups of genes acting together as polygenic systems. We also demonstrated that this analytic method can lead to the identification of biologically meaningful genetic factors. Two such factors were consistently identified, as shown in Fig. 5-2. One genetic system appeared to affect the maxillary teeth in general, particularly their buccolingual dimensions. A second genetic system seemed to influence the mandibular anterior teeth at both their mesiodistal and labiolingual dimensions. The maxillary and mandibular dentitions were further demonstrated to be controlled by relatively independent genetic determinants, with the mandibular teeth being affected by a wider range of genetic factors, thus showing a greater genetic complexity than the maxillary teeth. These findings suggest a differential degree of evolutionary stability achieved in the teeth of the two jaws. Environmental effects seemed to be localized, that is, not common to a number of variables as the genetic effects, nor were they as interpretable. As a result, a greater number of environmental factors than genetic factors

were found to affect the same set of dental dimensions. More importantly, we observed overlapping genetic and environmental effects in that several measurements associated with one genetic factor were influenced in turn by a number of separate environmental factors, and a particular environmental factor influenced dimensions that were affected in turn by several independent genetic factors. Together with other genetic-environment interaction effects, this overlapping of common genetic and environmental determinants of tooth size may well be largely responsible for inconsistent or uninterpretable results of family data in the literature.

Family studies

It is generally recognized that man is a difficult subject for genetic studies based on family data, particularly in the case of complex polygenic inheritance. Despite certain methodological limitations, family studies potentially provide a means for quantifying genetic and environmental relationships in a way that twin studies cannot. The twin method has the advantage of determining the relative magnitudes of genetic versus environmental variance. However, genetic information given by such methods is that of total genotypic variance. The additive variance, which is the heritable component of the total genotypic variance, cannot be estimated from twin data alone. To delineate the inheritance of tooth size for predictive purposes in clinical practice or for microevolutionary analysis, it is necessary to demonstrate evidence for additive components of the genetic variance using family data.

To deduce the cause of resemblance in a family, the covariance between family members is the property of the population that we are seeking to measure. From observed covariances and correlations between family members, we can evaluate the relative magnitudes of the causal components of variance in terms of the additive effects of genes, dominance (within-locus interaction), or epistasis (between-loci interaction).

It must be pointed out once more that in human family studies, the methods depart considerably from the basic animal experimental procedures of controlled breeding, progeny test, and environment control for which Fisher[16] developed his original expected correlations between relatives. In dentofacial genetic studies, an interpretation of observed correlations between family members based directly on Fisher's theoretical correlations further assumes complete absence of environmental variation or complete similarity of environmental effects within families.

Early family studies on tooth size have reported parent-offspring correlations ranging from 0.31 to 0.51 for the mesiodistal dimension of the incisors and canines. Recent family investigations on tooth size tend to indicate that environmental factors cannot be ignored. Hanna and associates,[19] in a study on the mesiodistal widths of incisors of the permanent dentition, scored tooth size of family members as deviations from the midparental mean. Their findings showed a secular trend for greater tooth size in the offspring that the authors attributed to a difference in nutritional status between generations. After correcting the data for age and sex effects, they subjected the transformed scores to a multivariate analysis of statistical distance within families. From the results, these authors concluded that no significant within-family heterogeneity existed for the tooth dimensions studied and that the heterogeneity observed in the raw data before transformation resulted from environmental differences (such as age and sex) rather than from genetic differences within families.

In man, males are heterogametic (XY) and females homogametic (XX) with respect to the sex chromosomes. Sex-linked polygenes can thus affect the phenotypic expression of quantitative traits in the two sexes differentially if the X chromosome carries the major portion of the genes governing the trait. Garn and co-workers[17] have inferred sex-linked inheritance of tooth size from Pearson product moment correlations between siblings paired according to sex. Following the univariate method, sibling correlations were calculated for the mesiodistal dimension of all permanent teeth except third molars. The correla-

tions were then averaged over all the measurements studied. Their results showed that the mean of sister-sister correlations exceeded the mean of brother-brother correlations, which in turn exceeded the mean of brother-sister correlations. The rank order of these correlations follows that expected under the sex-linked model, assuming additive effects of genes with no environmental variation. The authors hypothesized a sex-linked inheritance of tooth size based on the magnitude of these mean correlations.

It must be pointed out that the Pearson product moment correlation is not appropriate for correlating brother-brother pairs or sister-sister pairs (and, for that matter, twin pairs) unless the two sets of data being correlated happen to have exactly the same mean and standard deviation. The usual Pearsonian r is referred to as the *interclass* correlation because it assumes that the two correlated variables can be separated and assigned to two distinct classes, X (the independent variable) and Y (the dependent variable). It is entirely arbitrary whether a given member of such pairs is X or Y, since there is no basis for assigning the member to one class or the other. Certainly, different assignments of each member of the pair to either class in computing the product moment correlations will result in different values of r. The *intraclass* correlation gives the coefficient of choice for this type of family member correlation, since statistically it is an unbiased estimate of the mean correlation coefficient in the population that is obtained from all possible assignments of each member of a pair to either one of the two classes being correlated. It is computed based on the *analysis of variance*.

The work of Garn and associates[17] has often been cited to favor the concept of sex linkage of genes controlling tooth size. Corroborating reports[2, 24] have been rather limited. As yet, available evidence is not entirely convincing due to the questionable statistical treatment of the data or basis of assigning sib pairs in the correlations. Contrasting evidence of no sex linkage has been shown by several workers through univariate analysis[9, 29, 36] and through multivariate analysis.[35] These inconsistent findings point out the difficulty in demonstrating sex linkage from family studies within the normal range of variation. Such a disparity might be attributable largely to environmental effects. For example, sex influence is another phenomenon that might be expected to affect within-family correlations to conflict statistically with sex linkage in the data. Sex influence may be considered as an outcome of interactions between the male or female phenotype with the genetic factors causing the trait. In other words, the same genes in different sexes have different manifestations because the sexes provide unequal conditions or environments for their manifestation. In the early days of Mendelism, many differences between the sexes were considered as the direct result of a sex-linked gene mechanism. We know now, however, that the male phenotype shows some variation from the female phenotype in nearly every trait studied. Most phenotypic traits are not directly sex linked, only indirectly sex influenced or sex controlled.

The most convincing demonstration of sex linkage in tooth size is through direct quantitative linkage studies with simple sex-linked traits. However, analytic methods available at present are not adequate for appropriate interpretations of linkage in man with respect to quantitative traits, and no such investigations have been conducted on tooth size.

In an attempt to approach the problem of genetic factors related to tooth size, some workers have resorted to an alternative approach through studying tooth shape and structure in abnormal individuals. For example, evidence accumulated in recent years has suggested a genetic basis for the clinical association between tooth size and hypodontia. Although the congenital absence of a tooth is a discrete (all-or-none) trait, it is postulated that the missing phenomenon occurs near the lower extreme of the distribution of tooth size, a continuous trait. The contention is that absence of a tooth and its size if present are both traits determined by the same polygenes, presumably through an underlying quasicontinuous distribution. Thus a reduction in size may reach the point where the threshold in the distribution is crossed and is manifest as a missing tooth.

If the polygenes governing tooth size and hypodontia were sex linked, we would expect a greater size reduction in females with hypodontia than in males. According to the Lyon[26] hypothesis, only one of the two X chromosomes in each cell in the female is genetically active. To the contrary, Baum and Cohen[6] have found greater mesiodistal size reduction in normal males with hypodontia than females with respect to the teeth adjacent to the one that was missing. This is contrary to the sex linkage hypothesis, and the authors suggested a more complicated mode of inheritance for these traits.

Another approach through a monogenic sex-linked trait was utilized by Nakata and associates.[28] They assessed the mesiodistal width of permanent teeth in female family members of male probands afflicted with anhidrotic ectodermal dysplasia, a known sex-linked recessive trait in which multiple missing teeth are syndromic. Mothers and some female siblings of affected males were shown to have relatively small teeth in the range of 0.11 to 1.82 standard deviations below the population mean for Japanese females. These data are supportive of both the sex-linked concept and Lyonization. No assessments of tooth size on the male probands (affected hemizygotes) together with the fathers and unaffected male sibs were reported in their preliminary study.

From these reports it appears that studies of abnormal individuals have not as yet yielded more definitive results. Conceivably, investigations of tooth size on patients with anomalies of X chromosome number would be profitable.

If appropriate quantitative linkage methods were available, such methods could also be used to test for autosomal linkage through genetic markers. Alternatively, tooth size has been studied in association with autosomal defects. Cohen and co-workers[11] found extensive mesiodistal size reduction in patients with Down's syndrome characterized by an extra chromosome in the G group. We may well expect investigations on other known autosomal chromosomal defects such as reduplications and translocations to reveal tooth size involvement. This line of evidence should suggest that the polygenes governing tooth size are located on the autosomes as well.

Kollar[23] has pointed out the complex integration of a large number of genes in coordinating tooth development to culminate in the final phenotype of tooth size and shape. Although it would seem that the size and shape of a tooth are both predetermined by its enamel organ, his experiments showed that it is the connective tissue of the papilla and not the epithelium that determines the development of the enamel organ and thus the future size and shape of the tooth. From reciprocal exchanges of enamel organs with the papillae between the incisor and the molar, he was able to demonstrate that an incisor enamel organ combined with molar papillae resulted in molar tooth buds. Apparently the enamel organ is induced by the connective tissue to reorganize the tooth bud according to the inherent genetic information of the papillae. Not only the genetic expression in the enamel organ and in the ameloblasts but also the genes in the dental pulp, odontoblasts, dental sac, and surrounding connective tissue are involved. Therefore it is doubtful that the complex genetic information determining the final tooth size is located largely on the X chromosome. Polygenes involved in tooth size are probably distributed throughout the autosomes as well. Furthermore, no mention of any particular evidence that specifies sex linkage could be found in the report of Grüneberg[18] on cross-mating experiments in the mouse, showing that molar size is conditioned by multiple genes of unknown number.

Fisher[16] originally estimated the causal components of genetic variance (additive effects, dominance, and epistasis) that were expected to contribute to covariances between relatives. These estimates were based on autosomal inheritance while omitting the effects of sex linkage. More recently, Kempthorne[22] and Bohidar[8] estimated these genetic components for autosomal and sex-linked inher-

Table 5-1. Coefficients of the variance components due to additive and dominance effects in sex-linked and autosomal inheritance of a quantitative trait*

Covariance of family members	Expected value of covariance
Father-son	$\frac{1}{2}\ \sigma_A^2$
Father-daughter	$\frac{1}{2}\ \sigma_A^2 + \frac{1}{2}\ \sigma_{As}^2$
Mother-son	$\frac{1}{2}\ \sigma_A^2 + \frac{1}{2}\ \sigma_{As}^2$
Mother-daughter	$\frac{1}{2}\ \sigma_A^2 + \frac{1}{2}\ \sigma_{As}^2$
Brother-sister	$\frac{1}{2}\ \sigma_A^2 + \frac{1}{4}\ \sigma_D^2 + \frac{1}{4}\ \sigma_{As}^2$
Full brothers	$\frac{1}{2}\ \sigma_A^2 + \frac{1}{4}\ \sigma_D^2 + \frac{1}{2}\ \sigma_{As}^2$
Full sisters	$\frac{1}{2}\ \sigma_A^2 + \frac{1}{4}\ \sigma_D^2 + \frac{3}{4}\ \sigma_{As}^2 + \frac{1}{2}\ \sigma_{Ds}^2$

*Modified from Potter, R. H., Yu, P. L., Dahlberg, A. A., Merritt, A. D., and Conneally, P. M.: Genetic studies of tooth size factors in Pima Indian families, Am. J. Hum. Genet. **20**:92, 1968.
$\sigma_A^2 =$ variance due to autosomal additive effect;
$\sigma_{As}^2 =$ variance due to sex-linked additive effect;
$\sigma_D^2 =$ variance due to autosomal dominance effect;
$\sigma_{Ds}^2 =$ variance due to sex-linked dominance effect.

itance jointly when they constructed the theoretical covariances between family members of the same or different sexes. Their model was modified and adopted by Potter and coworkers[35] when we analyzed covariances between family members on the size of the permanent dentition, as shown in Table 5-1.

In a family study of the Pima Indians in southern Arizona we made an effort to minimize environmental factors while evaluating autosomal or sex-linked additive effects and autosomal or sex-linked dominance effects. A multivariate approach through factor analysis was used to organize the original data of fifty-six tooth measurements (the mesiodistal and buccolingual dimensions of all permanent teeth, excluding the third molar) into three common factors on the basis of which each individual was given three factor scores. Covariances and correlations (interclass and intraclass) between family members were then calculated for all parent-offspring and sib-sib pairings based on these factor scores. Although total genetic variance was demonstrable in the data, we noted discrepancies between observed correlations and those expected on the basis of genetic relationships for conventional interpretation of any of the causal components in the model. The results led us to speculate that important environmental sources of variation exist that interact differentially with genotypes, particularly with those of different generations, and that the generally higher sib-sib correlations as compared to parent-offspring correlations further reflect environmental effects on tooth size, since sibs are more likely to share a common environment than are parents and offspring.

The studies that claim to show sex linkage in tooth size suggest that all teeth in the permanent dentition demonstrate such linkage. If this hypothesis is indeed tenable, it follows that the effect of sex linkage should be apparent when our tooth size factors are used in the analysis. On the contrary, our results failed to show any convincing evidence of sex-linked additive or dominance effects. Although parent-offspring correlations seem to suggest additive sex-linked effects for the mesiodistal dimension of the twelve anterior teeth, the observed sibling correlations contradict any such effects.

Bowden and Goose[9] have reported further evidence of no sex linkage from their observed parent-offspring, midparent-offspring, and sibling correlations for the mesiodistal dimension of the maxillary incisors and canines. Their data suggested that additive effects without dominance was the type of inheritance most likely for tooth size and confirmed the improved dietary hypothesis as an explanation for a secular trend in increased tooth size in the offspring.

Population study

A population method in quantitative genetics was utilized by Niswander and Chung[29] when they studied the effects of inbreeding on the mesiodistal dimension of the upper right central incisor in Japanese children. Their analysis on offspring of first, one and a half, and second cousin marriages compared to offspring of unrelated parents showed no effect of F (the coefficient of inbreeding) on the tooth dimension studied. The coefficient of inbreeding expresses the degree of relationship between an individual's parents, since it gives the probability that two alleles at a given gene locus in the individual are identical by descent, that is, derived from the same ancestor. They further observed a consistent increase of 15% to 20% in the variance of the tooth dimension as inbreeding increased from $F = 0$ (unrelated parents) to $F = \frac{1}{16}$ (parents are first cousins). The authors found that the added variability was not genetic in origin because, with further analysis, variance within sibships was the same for the offspring of unrelated parents as those observed in the offspring of first cousin marriages. In contrast, variance between sibships was increased almost 100% with inbreeding (from offspring of unrelated parents to offspring of first cousin marriages), which the authors attributed to the increased susceptibility of consanguineous children to environmental factors so that they reflect more easily the differences between families.

In the same study no evidence could be demonstrated to suggest sex linkage. Furthermore, data obtained from the offspring of first cousins and of unrelated parents showed that intraclass correlations for brother-sister pairs exceeded that of brother-brother pairs, which in turn exceeded that of sister-sister pairs. This relative rank ordering is inconsistent with the sex-linked hypothesis. Regression analysis of the tooth dimension on the coefficient of inbreeding for female first cousins also failed to demonstrate sex linkage.

Studies on asymmetry

Bilateral traits such as size of teeth on contralateral sides of the arch have been assumed to be under identical genetic control, that is, determined by the same genes. If this were true, then the phenotypic expression of the trait on the contralateral sides should be a function of identical developmental processes. Failure of the two sides to develop identically should reflect an underlying genetic instability suggesting that the study of asymmetry may afford a means of investigating the genetic stabilization of developmental processes. Asymmetry thus represents a measure of the developmental *noise* or interference encountered by the genes during ontogeny, which affects their attempts to render the same developmental message bilaterally. Asymmetry that favors the same side of the individual is called *directional,* and random or nondirectional difference between sides is designated as *fluctuating* asymmetry.

In a study of fluctuating asymmetry, Adams and Niswander[1] demonstrated a significant increase in dental (buccolingual dimension of the lower first molar) and dermatoglyphic (palm print) asymmetry within individuals who also manifested cleft lip with or without cleft palate. These authors postulated that polygenic systems normally buffer developmental processes against adverse environmental effects and that the substitution of deleterious genes causes the level of buffering to be lowered beyond the point where environmental disturbances may be compensated. Thus, in cleft lip with or without cleft palate for which a polygenic basis has been suggested, this developmental instability is manifested as increased dermatoglyphic and dental asymmetry.

Bailit and associates[5] provided further evidence to link fluctuating asymmetry in tooth size with genetic or environmental stress during development. These workers studied the mesiodistal dimension of all the permanent teeth except the third molars in four ethnic groups, the Tristanites, Nasioi, Kwaio, and Boston children. Intraclass correlations between right and left homologous teeth were calculated for each individual, which were then transformed into Fisher's *z* values. These scores were then averaged to obtain the mean tooth size asymmetry in each group. They were able to show significant differences in mean tooth size asymmetry among the ethnic groups. The order of these differences followed the predicted order of these groups ranked on ethnographic and medical bases as most to least stressed genetically and environmentally. They attributed this increase in fluctuating asymmetry to a general decrease in the coadaptation of different developmental systems in the presence of adverse genetic or environmental conditions.

Therefore asymmetry is a phenotypic manifestation of developmental *noise.*

When asymmetry was examined in relation to the coefficient of inbreeding F in the Tristanites, no significant linear relationship was found. That is, an effect of inbreeding (where genetic homozygosity is increased) on dental asymmetry could not be demonstrated. In this regard, Niswander and Chung[29] were also unable to show a clear effect of inbreeding on asymmetry of the maxillary central incisor in Japanese children, although they could not completely rule out such an effect.

According to C. W. Cotterman's unpublished lectures, the classical twin model may be used to assess the genetic and environmental bases of asymmetry and mirror imagery of bilateral traits. The following three statistically independent within-pair contrasts may be derived from the right and left measurements of twins to estimate three parameters: discordance, asymmetry, and mirror imagery.

Twin 1   Twin 2
$$R_1 + L_1 - R_2 - L_2 = \text{Discordance}$$
$$R_1 - L_1 + R_2 - L_2 = \text{Asymmetry}$$
$$R_1 - L_1 - R_2 + L_2 = \text{Mirror imagery}$$

With this scheme, discordance represents homolateral comparison that contrasts between co-twins on the same side, asymmetry refers to heterolateral comparison that contrasts between the two sides within individual co-twins, and mirror imagery (another aspect of asymmetry) is the co-twin–side interaction in the *analysis of variance.* Potter and Nance[33] utilized this method of constructing within-pair contrasts in documenting genetic and environmental effects on tooth size discordance, asymmetry, and mirror imagery. From within-pair contrasts, the within-pair variances were calculated for both the monozygotic and dizygotic twin types. The probability levels of the F ratio were used to test for significance of the variance estimates for the three parameters. We performed a univariate analysis for each of the mesiodistal and buccolingual dimensions of all permanent teeth excluding the third molars, using the same twin sample as a previously cited study.[34] Our results provided strong evidences for the existence of significant genetic determinants of almost all the individual tooth dimensions studied, but they provided little or no evidence for a genetic basis of asymmetry (and of mirror imagery as another aspect of asymmetry). The analysis gave no indication that monozygotic twinning was associated with an increased degree of either fluctuating asymmetry or mirror imagery when compared to dizygotic twins. In monozygotic twins, common environmental effects were observed to affect antimeric tooth dimensions in isolated instances. This is perhaps not surprising in view of the similarity in ontogeny and eruption pattern of the antimeres. The data on monozygotic twins further suggested that the increment of environmental discordance resulting from the twinning phenomenon was detectable over and above the developmental *noise* that caused asymmetry within individual co-twins.

The univariate study just mentioned failed to demonstrate a genetic basis for tooth size asymmetry. It would therefore seem reasonable to assume that the same genes control tooth size bilaterally. The previously described multivariate twin method proposed by Vandenberg[7, 38] is potentially useful to test this hypothesis further by seeking whether common genetic determinants influence antimeric dental dimensions. We reported results of applying this technique in the same twin study[34] as cited earlier in this chapter. The genetic factor patterns that emerged from the multivariate analysis are striking, as shown in Fig. 5-2, *A,* for the maxillary dentition and Fig. 5-2, *B,* for the mandibular dentition. Whenever a genetic factor is found to influence a dimension on the right side, it also appears to influence the corresponding dimension on the left side. We regard the extent to which antimeric tooth measurements are grouped together in the genetic analysis as a confirmation of the rather remarkable ability of this multivariate technique to extract biologically meaningful relationships between multiple biometrical traits such as tooth size. In monozygotic twins, common environmental effects were also found for a few sets

of antimeric teeth. This is perhaps not surprising in view of the similarity in ontogeny and eruption pattern of the antimeres.

ANIMAL STUDIES ON TOOTH SIZE

Human genetic studies through relatives and through populations suggest that although genetic variability is detectable, the environment clearly influences tooth size. Evidence on the specific environmental conditions associated with the size of teeth in man such as socioeconomic status, nutrition, climate, and systemic disease is not convincing. Since tooth size is largely determined during the prenatal period, maternal environment is expected to be a critical factor in the development of the trait.

Although there is little direct evidence of maternal effects on human tooth size, a few studies have reported that children premature by birth weight are retarded in dental eruption and have smaller teeth with more morphological defects.

Far beyond what is practicable in humans, close inbreeding and cross fostering methods as well as rigid control of the environment in animal studies allow for more definitive interpretations of genetic and environmental effects on tooth size, which may have important implications for man.

Specific maternal effects on tooth size in experimental animals have been the focus of several enquiries since Grüneberg[18] noted that independent of fetal genotype, third molar size in inbred strains of mice was smaller than in hybrids, and that the size of this tooth varies with certain unidentified maternal effects. Paynter and Grainger[32] showed evidence that measurable size differences of teeth in that rat could be produced by an alteration of the maternal diet. In their study, the offspring of rats fed with a diet either abnormally high in phosphate content or deficient in vitamin A had significantly smaller upper first molars than controls.

Holloway and co-workers[20] observed that in the offspring of rats fed a low-protein–high-sucrose diet, the molar teeth erupted later and were smaller in size than in the offspring of rats fed a normal diet. These authors noted that the smaller tooth size was due to a decrease in the distance between the outer borders of the dentin of the tooth rather than to a reduction in enamel thickness. Similar incidences of reduced molar size and delayed eruption in the offspring when pregnant female rats were fed a low-protein diet have been reported.

Bader[4] determined heritability (in the narrow sense) for the buccolingual width measured at right angles to an anteroposterior axis of three lower molars in the house mouse. That is, he estimated the proportion of the total phenotypic variance due to additive genetic effects. Based on specific mating schemes, the phenotypic variance was partitioned into additive genetic, maternal, and other environmental components. The results showed an abundance of additive genetic variance (66%) for the first and second molars and somewhat less (47%) for the third molar. Most importantly, maternal effects were estimated to be the largest single source of environmental variation of the tooth dimensions studied, with over half of the environmental variance and over a fourth of the total phenotypic variance contributed by this source. Maternal effects estimated from the environmental variance common to litters in the random-bred strain in this study are expected to constitute a considerably larger proportion of the variance in an isogenic strain.

It must be pointed out that any possible cytoplasmic inheritance cannot be separated from the effects of maternal environment according to present methods.

Other than cytoplasmic factors, maternal effects could be due to prenatal uterine environment or postnatal maternal effects such as lactation. A cross-fostering experiment on the house mouse was performed by Tenczar and Bader[37] to estimate the relative contributions of prenatal and postnatal maternal components to the variation of tooth size. Half of each litter of mice was reciprocally cross fostered, and the buccolingual widths of the second and third molars were studied. The results showed that 21% to 29% of the total variance in the width of the

second molar, which initiates differentiation in utero, could be attributed to prenatal factors, and only 7% to 11% could be attributed to postnatal factors. In contrast, the third molar, which initiates differentiation postnatally, did not exhibit significant prenatal effects on its size variation.

Fluctuating asymmetry on the buccolingual diameter of the three mandibular molars of the house mouse was investigated by Bader[3] among the wild, random-bred, inbred, and hybrid groups. Correlations between antimeric measurements in the genetically variable (wild and randombred) groups was found to be significantly higher than that in the isogenic (inbred and hybrid) groups. Furthermore, the hybrid group was reported to be considerably more symmetrical with respect to the third molar than the inbred group, and the difference was significant. These results supported the human studies conducted by Adams and Niswander[1] and by Bailit and associates,[5] which suggested that increased asymmetry is an indication of the inability of the genetic information to control development effectively in the presence of genetic or environmental stress. No indication of a general component of resistance to developmental *noise* in terms of asymmetry was found in Bader's study.

Evidence derived from animal studies has pointed to considerable environmental effects on tooth size variability that are seemingly exerted during ontogeny of the tooth, particularly near the onset of dentinogenesis and amelogenesis. These developmental processes occur during the prenatal and early postnatal period so that maternal effects are probably the most important source of environmental influence. Individual teeth vary in their susceptibility to these influences depending on the developmental timing and the extent of genetic determination of the particular tooth.

SUMMARY

The size of teeth is only one variable in a complex system of craniofacial development in man, the components of which generally show continuous variation. These variable traits are also the raw material for selection to act on to account for small cumulative changes in microevolution. The interest in tooth size among the dental geneticists, dental evolutionists, and dental clinicians is primarily in terms of phenotype prediction. Unfortunately, our present understanding of the genetics of tooth size falls short of allowing us to accurately predict tooth size. Within the last few years, however, computer usage has resulted in great strides in analytic techniques that have permitted tooth morphologists to bridge the gap toward understanding tooth size variation.

Univariate twin studies have established a detectable genetic component in tooth size variability. Family studies have demonstrated consistently that important environmental effects are superimposed on genetic effects to determine tooth size. From animal experimentation, these environmental influences were shown to be largely attributable to maternal effects, which consist of cytoplasmic inheritance, prenatal uterine environment (such as influenced by maternal diet), and postnatal maternal effects.

The additive and dominance components of genetic variance have not been clearly demonstrated from family data, nor has sex linkage in tooth size, probably because of superimposed environmental effects. Multivariate analysis has shown that correlated dental dimensions in an individual are influenced by common genetic factors that may or may not be identifiable. This common factor concept is in accord with the pleiotropic action of a gene or of a single gene set.

From twins, genetic-environment interactions have been illustrated in the form of estimated genetic and environmental correlations among tooth dimensions. An overlapping of genetic and environmental factors common to several measurements was shown. This type of interaction may be expected to cause difficulties in interpreting data obtained for genetic studies.

No genetic basis of tooth size asymmetry has been detected, and bilateral teeth may be assumed to be under identical genetic control with respect to their size. Asymmetry is thus a phenotypic manifestation of developmental *noise* attributable to environmental disturbances during tooth development.

This discourse should illustrate that quantitative genetics in man deals with the study of interactions of which the additive genetic effect is the simplest form and genetic-environment interaction the most complex. In dentistry, traits caused by discrete gene substitution have received a disproportionate amount of attention, even though these effects account for relatively few dramatic clinical entities. Such an entity may be better regarded as a special and rather rare case in the broad area of gene interactions, that is, it may be regarded as a special case of quantitative genetics with only one pair (or a few pairs) of genes involved in the causation of a trait.

REFERENCES

1. Adams, M. S., and Niswander, J. D.: Developmental "noise" and a congenital malformation, Genet. Res. **10:**313, 1967.
2. Alvesalo, L.: The influence of sex chromosome genes on tooth size in man: a genetic and quantitative study, Suom. Hammaslääk. Toim. **67:**3, 1971.
3. Bader, R. S.: Fluctuating asymmetry in the dentition of the house mouse, Growth **29:**291, 1965.
4. Bader, R. S.: Heritability of dental characters in the house mouse, Evolution **19:**378, 1965.
5. Bailit, H. L., Workman, P. L., Niswander, J. D., and MacLean, C. J.: Dental asymmetry as an indicator of genetic and environmental conditions in human populations, Hum. Biol. **42:**626, 1970.
6. Baum, B. J., and Cohen, M. M.: Patterns of size reduction in hypodontia, J. Dent. Res. **50:**779, 1971.
7. Bock, R. D., and Vandenberg, S. G.: Components of heritable variation in mental test scores. In Vandenberg, S. G., editor: Progress in human behavior genetics, Baltimore, 1968, The Johns Hopkins University Press.
8. Bohidar, N. R.: Role of sex-linked genes in quantitative inheritance, Fifth International Biometric Conference of the Biometric Society, Cambridge, 1963, E. & E. Plumridge.
9. Bowden, D. E., and Goose, D. H.: Inheritance of tooth size in Liverpool families, J. Med. Genet. **6:**55, 1969.
10. Butler, P. M.: Studies of the mammalian dentition: differentiation of the post-canine

dentition, Proc. Zool. Soc. Lond. B **109**:1, 1939.

11. Cohen, M. M., Garn, S. M., and Geciauskas, M. A.: Crown-size profile pattern in trisomy G, J. Dent. Res. **49**:460, 1970.

12. Dahlberg, A. A.: The changing dentition of man, J. Am. Dent. Assoc. **32**:676, 1945.

13. Dahlberg, A. A.: Relationship of tooth size to cusp number and groove conformation of occlusal surface patterns of lower molar teeth, J. Dent. Res. **40**:34, 1961.

14. Dahlberg, A. A.: Dental evolution and culture, Hum. Biol. **35**:237, 1963.

15. Falconer, D. S.: Introduction to quantitative genetics, New York, 1960, The Ronald Press Co.

16. Fisher, R. A.: The correlation between relatives on the supposition of Mendelian inheritance, Trans. R. Soc. Edin. **52**:399, 1918.

17. Garn, S. M., Lewis, A. B., and Kerewsky, R. S.: X-linked inheritance of tooth size, J. Dent. Res. **44**:439, 1965.

18. Grüneberg, H.: The genetics of a tooth defect in the mouse, Proc. R. Soc. Lond. (Biol.) **138**:437, 1951.

19. Hanna, B. L., Turner, M. E., and Hughes, R. D.: Family studies of the facial complex, J. Dent. Res. **42**:1322, 1963.

20. Holloway, P. J., Shaw, J. H., and Sweeney, E. A.: Effects of various sucrose:casein ratios in purified diets on the teeth and supporting structures of rats, Arch. Oral Biol. **3**:185. 1961.

21. Horowitz, S. L., Osborne, R. H., and De-George, F. V.: Hereditary factors in tooth dimensions; a study of the anterior teeth of twins, Angle Orthod. **28**:87, 1958.

22. Kempthorne, O.: An introduction to genetic statistics, New York, 1957, John Wiley & Sons, Inc., p. 339.

23. Kollar, E. J.: Histogenetic aspects of dermal-epidermal interactions. In Slavkin, H. C., and Bavetta, L. A., editors: Developmental aspects of oral biology, New York, 1972, Academic Press, Inc.

24. Lewis, D. W., and Grainger, R. M.: Sex-linked inheritance of tooth size—a family study, Arch. Oral Biol. **12**:539, 1967.

25. Lundström, A.: Tooth size and occlusion in twins, New York, 1948, S. Karger.

26. Lyon, M. F.: Gene action in the X-chromosome of the mouse, Nature **190**:372, 1961.

27. Mather, K., and Jinks, J. L.: Biometrical genetics, ed. 2, New York, 1971, Cornell University Press.

28. Nakata, M., Koshiba, H., Kindaichi, J., and Hamano, Y.: A genetic consideration on partial anodontia with ectodermal dysplasia, The 22nd annual meeting of the Japanese Division of the International Association for Dental Research program, Osaka, Japan, 1974.

29. Niswander, J. D., and Chung, C. S.: The effect of inbreeding on tooth size in Japanese children, Am. J. Hum. Genet. **17**:391, 1965.

30. Osborne, R. H.: Some genetic problems in interpreting the evolution of the human dentition, J. Dent. Res. **46**(supp.):945, 1967.

31. Osborne, R. H., Horowitz, S. L., and De-George, F. V.: Genetic variation in tooth dimensions: a twin study of the permanent anterior teeth, Am. J. Hum. Genet. **10**:350, 1958.

32. Paynter, K. J., and Grainger, R. M.: The relation of nutrition to the morphology and size of rat molar teeth, J. Can. Dent. Assoc. **22**:519, 1956.

33. Potter, R. H., and Nance, W. E.: A twin study on dental dimension. I. Discordance, asymmetry and mirror imagery, Am. J. Phys. Anthropol. **44**:391, 1976.

34. Potter, R. H., Nance, W. E., Yu, P. L., and Davis, W. B.: A twin study on dental dimension. II. Independent genetic determinants, Am. J. Phys. Anthropol. **44**:397, 1976.

35. Potter, R. H. Y., Yu, P. L., Dahlberg, A. A., Merritt, A. D., and Conneally, P. M.: Genetic studies of tooth size factors in Pima Indian families, Am. J. Hum. Genet. **20**:89, 1968.

36. Suarez, B. K.: The genetics of tooth size in man (thesis), Los Angeles, 1974, University of California at Los Angeles.

37. Tenczar, P., and Bader, R. S.: Maternal effect in dental traits of the house mouse, Science **152**:1398, 1966.

38. Vandenberg, S. G.: Multivariate analysis of twin differences. In Vandenberg, S. G., editor: Methods and goals in human behavior genetics, New York, 1965, Academic Press, Inc.

6

Genetic aspects of anomalous tooth development

GORDON H. DIXON
RAY E. STEWART

During early development of the human embryo, there is a migration of neural crest cells into the developing oral and facial region. As was pointed out in Chapter 1, these neural crest cells play a critical role in the development of tissues and organs in the areas of their destination. One of these roles is apparently to stimulate certain cells of the oral ectoderm to undergo differentiation into cells with odontogenic, or tooth-forming, potential.

At the beginning of the sixth week, there is a discrete proliferation of ectodermal cells along the margins of the developing jaws, which form two horseshoe-shaped plates known as the dental laminae.

At approximately 6½ weeks' gestation, localized proliferations of the lateral surface of the dental lamina result in primordial knoblike invaginations, which are destined to become the deciduous tooth buds. The succedaneous lamina develops from additional proliferation of the terminal portion of the lateral lamina of the developing primary tooth predecessors and eventuates in the permanent tooth buds.

The cells that constitute the enamel organ proper are all of ectodermal origin; however, the rate of cell division is not uniform throughout the bud. This disproportionate proliferation produces a bell-shaped structure that continues to increase in size and morphological complexity until the basic crown form of the future tooth is completed. A complex interaction between the ectodermally derived enamel organ and the underlying mesenchyme or dental papilla initiates the apposition of enamel and dentin matrix described in detail in Chapters 1, 7, and 8.

Anatomists and histologists have, for descriptive purposes, divided the various stages of development through which the tooth passes into several categories: (1) initiation (bud stage), (2) proliferation (cap stage), (3) histodifferentiation (bell stage), (4) morphodifferentiation, (5) apposition, (6) calcification, and (7) eruption.

Abnormalities can and do occur at any of these stages, resulting in a variety of clinical entities. The abnormalities may result from genetic or environmental factors or a combination of both. Fig. 6-1 lists the various stages and some of the clinical conditions that may result from excessive or deficient development at those stages.

An accurate estimate of the extent to which heredity influences the final size, form, and number of teeth (the number of loci contributing to various dental traits and the mode of genetic transmission of dental elements) has been of serious interest to dentists, geneticists, and anthropologists alike.

It is clear that the tooth, as it develops, is a hereditary unit in dynamic interplay with its environment, both affecting and being affected by its adjacent surroundings. These surroundings, also genetically determined, influence their environment and the tooth primordia therein. Thus identical tooth germs are influenced by various morphogenic areas to assume their normal shapes in their accustomed places within the dental arches. This is the basis by which Butler, an English paleontologist, developed the "field theory" for the mammalian dentition. He established three fields of influence within the dental

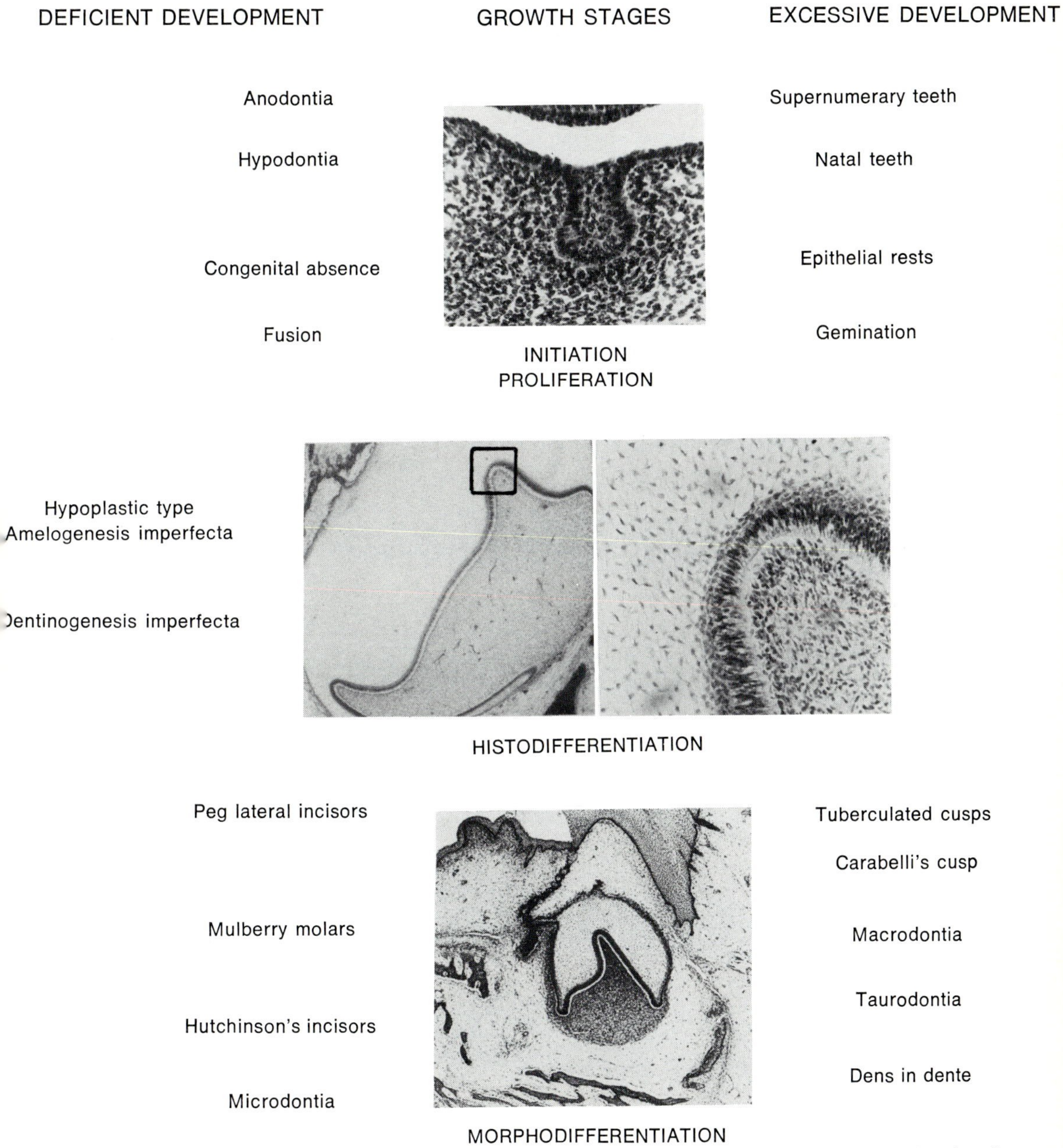

DEFICIENT DEVELOPMENT	GROWTH STAGES	EXCESSIVE DEVELOPMENT
Anodontia		Supernumerary teeth
Hypodontia		Natal teeth
Congenital absence		Epithelial rests
Fusion		Gemination

INITIATION
PROLIFERATION

Hypoplastic type
Amelogenesis imperfecta

Dentinogenesis imperfecta

HISTODIFFERENTIATION

Peg lateral incisors		Tuberculated cusps
		Carabelli's cusp
Mulberry molars		Macrodontia
		Taurodontia
Hutchinson's incisors		
		Dens in dente
Microdontia		

MORPHODIFFERENTIATION

Continued.

Fig. 6-1. Clinical conditions resulting from deficient or excessive development at various stages.

DEFICIENT DEVELOPMENT   GROWTH STAGES   EXCESSIVE DEVELOPMENT

Enamel hypoplasia
  Systemic
  Local
  Congenital

Enamel pearls

Hypercementosis

Dentinodysplasias

Odontoma

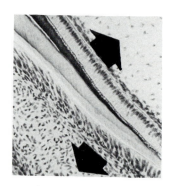

APPOSITION

Hypocalcified type
Amelogenesis imperfecta

Mottled enamel

Sclerotic dentin

Interglobular dentin

CALCIFICATION

Ankylosis

Impaction

Transposition

Neonatal teeth

Delayed eruption

Precocious eruption

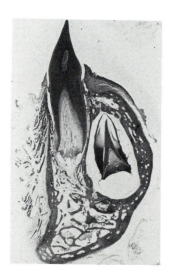

ERUPTION

Fig. 6-1, cont'd. Clinical conditions resulting from deficient or excessive development at various stages.

arch. The incisor, canine, and premolar/ molar fields were "anchored" by the central incisor, canine, and first molar, respectively. As the regions varied in size, so did the number of tooth primordia under their direct influence. According to this theory, the field of influence wanes as one progresses from the center of the region, and with distance each tooth becomes more variable and less like the dominant "anchor" tooth.

This theory was modified by Dahlberg[4] to account for the irregularities seen in the human dentition, that is, that the second premolar is more variable than the first premolar, and the mandibular central incisors are more variable than their lateral counterparts. Dahlberg's modifications do make it easy to visualize which teeth in the human dentition will vary the most in size and number; however, with these modifications goes much of the validity for a regional field theory.

Even with Dahlberg's modifications, a generalized morphogenic field of variable intensity is still a credible concept, which prompted Garn and associates[6] to hypothesize that the agenesis of third molars is an example of a field in which the most distal components are the most "unstable" teeth. Suarez[8] has suggested that a "variable" field influences the dentition and that in its weakest form the field may affect the development of only the late-forming third molars. In a stronger form both the incisor and premolar teeth may be affected.

More recently, Melnick and Shields[7] have proposed a model for the classification of various forms of structural anomalies, which they call "odonto-dysmorphogenesis." This model is based on the fact that the developmental steps leading to the formation of any organ, including teeth, involve a sequence of events that can generally be thought of as induction of cell groups, cellular migration, cellular interaction with a new "environment," and differentiation into specific tissue types. They cite Wasserman, who has proposed that the differential migration that leads to a precisely ordered characteristic pattern and arrangement is carried out by

cell-cell recognition or the "testing" of positional information. This is accomplished when the protein chains, composed of unique monomers protruding from the surface of one cell, interact with the matching protruding chains (PPC) of other cells. Thus the moving neural crest cells test the positional information of the cells over which they are moving and stop at that site for which they are programmed, resulting in an organization of mesenchymal fields. The cells of each field (incisiform, caniniform, molariform, glandular, and surface epithelium) possess positional information (unique protein chains) that are specific for each individual field.

According to Wasserman,[9] the PPC is responsible for the characterization of the mesoderm as either dental or nondental mesoderm encoded with specific pattern information. Each type of mesoderm will then direct and model the overlying oral epithelium to become either dental or nondental oral epithelium.

The model proposed by Melnick and Shields provides a coherent and unified classification of the various forms of odonto-dysmorphogenesis. The model includes two major causes, the first being mutational dysmorphogenesis. The first subclassification in this group would be mutant mesodermal organizer genes leading to aberrant cell surface proteins and thus to abnormal migration; the second subclassification would be mutant interpretational genes leading to an abnormal oral mesodermal type and thus to incorrect induction of the oral epithelium.

EVOLUTIONARY CONSIDERATIONS

Gabriel[5] has observed that there is a genetic pattern for tooth shape, whether it be in the shape of the crowns, the root form, or the most minute detail in cuspal anatomy. This genetic basis has evolved through the ancestry of mankind, and the morphological nature, eruption pattern, and number of teeth in the dentition of *Homo sapiens* and his lineage are the results of the ever-changing environment in which they existed.

That change is constant within our ecosystem is an axiom of life. Either an organism successfully adapts to this change, or it will succumb to the effects of its new environment. The phenotypic characteristics of the survivors will then be present in the genotype of future generations.

If the change is radical, the requirements for survival in the new system will be strict, and the range of variability in the structures and organs that lend fitness to those who survive will be small. Conversely, when the requirements for survival of the species are relaxed, increased variability and simplicity of these elements evolve. New gene mutations and formerly suppressed allelic patterns will find phenotypic expression in the new order.

Evidence for hereditary factors as determinants of tooth size, form, and number was recognized by physical anthropologists who had at their disposal the structural remains of skulls ranging over hundreds of thousands of years. From these materials it was evident that man adapted to fluctuations in environmental stress, both natural and those caused by the manipulation of his own surroundings. These changes in stress are reflected in the teeth of hominids to modern man. Basically, there has been an increase in the complexity of tooth form in response to natural selection followed by a relaxation that was accompanied by more variable and simpler dental forms. Variations in tooth shape and size have arisen in spatial and temporally segregated groups in a response to a multitude of environmental pressures.

Variations in the size and form of the anterior teeth have followed a rather complex evolutionary course. Incisors and canine tooth volume of early hominids diminished after the successful adoption of hand-held defensive weapons. This is apparent in the skulls of some Australopithecine hominids. As man became a successful hunter, the trend toward reduced tooth mass in the anterior region was reversed, and there was a substantial increase in the size and volume of the anterior segment, greater in the incisors than in the canines.

Dentofacial structures continued to evolve as man further learned to manipulate his environment. The teeth and supporting structures became a preferred tool. They were used as a vise, to grip, grasp, pull, and exert torsion.[10] Increased wear of the anteriors resulted in a selective advantage for increased volume of these teeth.

As man developed tools more sophisticated than his teeth in response to his growing cultural needs, a simplification of pattern and a reduction in tooth volume ensued. This relaxation probably occurred between the Neanderthal and Upper Paleolithic periods.[2]

The structure and form of the posterior dentition has followed a less involved course than the anterior complement. Extensive wear of the teeth of fossil hominids suggests a selective advantage for large occlusal surfaces of posterior teeth for mastication of a primarily vegetarian diet. A reduction in selection for this characteristic began when man added significant amounts of meat to his diet. This dietary shift to less abrasive foodstuffs occurred during the Australopithecine and *Homo erectus* phases.[1]

The beginning of man's use of fire in the temperate zone, approximately 400,000 years ago, resulted in the suspension of much of the remaining selective advantage for large posterior tooth mass,[3] since cooking of food further reduced the abrasive quality of the diet.

Further-evolution from a hunter-gatherer existence to a society oriented toward one of food cultivation and processing has occurred in all but the most primitive populations today. This alteration in dietary habits has greatly diminished the need for large premolar and molar volume and has made the posterior tooth volume that man maintains today superfluous for his present needs. This phenomenon has caused many anthropologists to conclude that the increased variability of the dentition seen in modern populations reflects the relaxation of selective stress for large tooth volume rather than a substitution of smaller teeth, as has been previously hypothesized.[10]

TOOTH FORM AND STRUCTURE

The genetics of tooth size are discussed in detail in Chapter 5; however, dental anomalies that are reflected in alterations of tooth size will be discussed concurrently in this section. Tooth size has been shown to have a genetic component.[35] It is probable that a number of loci are involved.[44] The genetic aspects of aberrations in tooth form, however, are poorly understood and have not been widely studied.

Peg-shaped lateral incisors

The maxillary lateral incisor is the most variable tooth in the anterior complement.[24] It is clear that reduced or hypoplastic maxillary laterals are a variable expression of the gene for congenitally missing lateral incisors and will therefore be discussed in the section on anomalies of tooth number.

Shovel-shaped incisors

Incisors with prominent lateral margins creating a hollowed lingual surface are called *shovel-shaped*. The trait is most commonly seen on maxillary lateral and central incisors, less frequently on mandibular incisors, and is rarely observed on canines[37] (Fig. 6-2). There is a continuous distribution of the trait from slight marginal proliferation to double-shoveled teeth, with proliferation affecting both palatal and facial marginal surfaces.[31]

Interpopulation variations are extreme, suggesting a genetic factor as a cause of shovel-shaped incisors. The trait is so common in the Mongoloid race that Moorrees[33] considers the trait to be a racial characteristic. Moderate to heavy shoveling is seen in 9% of American Caucasians, 17% of Africans, 73% of Japanese, and 96% to 100% of American Indians and Eskimos.[12, 25, 37, 46] Nonshoveled incisors were found in the majority of offspring born of Japanese mothers and Caucasian fathers, suggesting a recessive mode of inheritance.[23]

Turner[51] concluded that the inheritance of shovel-shaped incisors followed a simple Mendelian pattern; however, a study of 100 Chinese[31] has shown this to be improbable and suggests a polygenic model as the mode of transmission for shovel-shaped teeth.

Dens invaginatus

Dens invaginatus or dens in dente is most frequently seen in maxillary lateral incisors but has been reported in other teeth (Fig. 6-3). The defect may not be obvious clinically; however, radiographs show a continuum of this pathologic condition from a slight invagination to defects that extend into the radicular portion of the affected tooth.[34] The trait presumably results from an early invagination of the enamel epithelium.

Kong[27] reported a 2.5% incidence among Mongoloid peoples. He found the prevalence in Chinese to be 3.6%. A 1.4% prevalence was noted for Malay and Indians.

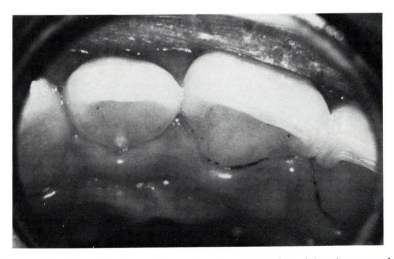

Fig. 6-2. Central and lateral incisors with prominent marginal ridges giving rise to morphological characteristic called shovel-shaped incisors.

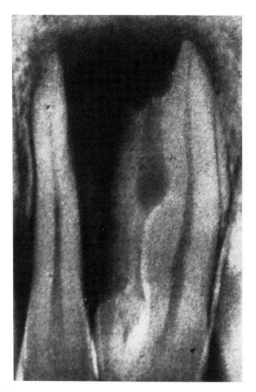

Fig. 6-3. Intraoral radiograph of permanent anterior tooth showing dens invaginatus. Note periapical radiolucency, which has resulted from periapical pathological condition secondary to carious involvement of dental pulp.

Grahnen and Lindahl[21] found a frequency of 3% in Swedes. A familial study of Swedish children indicated a high incidence of dens invaginatus in relatives of probands, in whom 43% of the parents and 32% of the siblings were affected. There was no sex difference noted in either group. They concluded that either a recessive or dominant model could fit their data. Shafer[40] and Amos[11] observed the traits in 1.8% and 5.1% of American Caucasians, respectively. The condition is rare in Negroes. Conclusive evidence for a single gene hypothesis is lacking; however, an autosomal dominant or possible polygenic model must be considered as the probable genetic mechanism of dens invaginatus. See p. 254 for additional discussion of dens invaginatus.

Dens evaginatus

Dens evaginatus describes a cone-shaped elevation of enamel situated in the central groove or lingual ridge of the buccal cusp of permanent premolar and molar teeth. This anomalous condition has been referred to in the literature as tuberculated teeth and accessory cusps.[15a]

The causative event leading to dens evaginatus occurs early in odontogenesis. Either an outfolding of the enamel epithelium or a

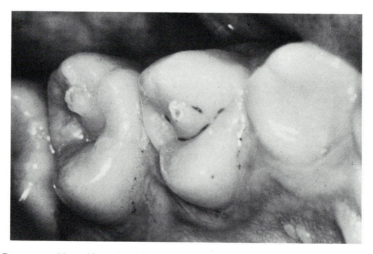

Fig. 6-4. Permanent bicuspid teeth with accessory central cusps commonly referred to as tuberculated teeth. Note polyplike cusps emanating from occlusal surface of both first and second bicuspids.

transient focal hyperplasia of the primitive pulpal mesenchyme gives rise to an evaginated area on the occlusal portion of affected teeth.

The tubercle can and usually does consist of all three dental tissues, enamel, dentin, and pulp.[34a]

As an isolated trait, dens evaginatus was thought to be restricted to the Mongoloid racial group until a recent report of the anomaly in a Caucasian-Greek girl.[47a]

The incidence among Mongoloid peoples ranges from 1.0 to 4.3%. However, in an ethnically pure Eskimo village, Hoffman[23a] observed the aberrant structure in 15% of the inhabitants. The variability in incidence among Mongoloids suggests the presence of genetic factors with differences in gene frequencies (Table 6-1).

Reports of familial occurrences have been few.[23a, 30a, 32, 54a] Recently we have observed the trait in a father and two daughters of a Guatemalan Indian family. Concordance was noted in twins from a Thai study.[37a]

Curzon[16a] hypothesized an X-linked factor involved in the expression of the characteristic. However, wide variabilities in male-to-female ratios from 1:0.76 to 1:3.0 have made it difficult to substantiate his supposition.

Autosomal dominance with decreased penetrance is the most likely inheritance.

Dens evaginatus has also been noted as a component in the syndrome of lobodontia, which was reported in a Caucasian family.[37b] (See Chapter 8 for additional discussion of this trait.)

Carabelli's trait

Carabelli's trait describes a morphological alteration that is normally located on the palatal surface of the mesiolingual cusp of maxillary permanent and deciduous molars. Morphological variations range from a definite cusp or tubercle to a small indented pit or fissure[19] (Fig. 6-5). Carabelli's cusp may be related to an evolutionary trait that developed in response to attrition on the occlusal surfaces of the molar teeth to the level of the cusp, in which case this fifth cusp added to the tooth volume and chewing surface.

Population studies show striking differences between Mongoloid and Caucasian races; the trait is present in as high as 90% of Caucasians[39] and is reportedly rare in Mongoloid peoples.

Table 6-1. Prevalence of dens evaginatus by population groups

Author	Year	Nationality	Incidence (%)
Kato[25a]	1937	Japanese	1.09
Sumiya[45]	1959	Japanese	1.88
Lau[30a]	1955	Chinese	1.29
Wu[53a]	1955	Chinese	1.44
Yip[54a]	1974	Chinese	3.62
		Malays	1.07
		East Indians	0.00
Reichart[37a]	1975	Thai	1.01
Merrill[32]	1964	North American Indians and Eskimos	4.30
Curzon[16a]	1970	Keewatin Eskimos	3.00

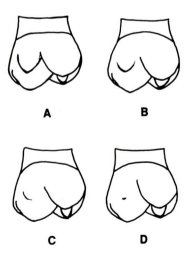

A   B

C   D

Fig. 6-5. Diagrammatic representation of morphological variations associated with Carabelli's trait, which describes mesiolingual cusp frequently found on maxillary molars, which ranges from definite accessory cusp or tubercle, **A,** to small pit or fissure on mesiolingual surface, **D.**

Pedersen[36] found Carabelli's trait practically absent in East Greenland Eskimos but frequent in Eskimo-Caucasian hybrids. The trait was observed in only 5.7% of Arizona Indians.[28] The trait occurred infrequently in Bantus.[42]

Dietz[20] concluded that Carabelli's trait has an autosomal dominant mode of inheritance. From studies of eight extensive pedigrees, Kraus[28] suggested a model of "two allelic autosomal genes without dominance." Lee and Goose[31] demonstrated that neither of these models was satisfactory to explain their data and that a multifactorial mode of transmission was more tenable.

Recent evidence in twins[13] has indicated that Carabelli's trait may not have a strong genetic component. The concordance rate for this trait in monozygotic males and females is 56.5% and 47.0%, respectively, whereas that of dizygotic males and females is 48.3% and 43.1%, respectively suggesting significant influence by environmental factors.

Paramolar tubercles

The paramolar tubercle, or Bolk's cusp, is seen most frequently on the buccal surface of the mesiobuccal cusp in permanent and deciduous molars[29] (Fig. 6-6). Exaggerated paramolars may result in a supernumerary structure called a *paramolar tooth* in the interproximal space of the molar teeth.[14]

The occurrence of paramolar tubercles varies among populations. The structure is almost never seen in Caucasians or Negroes[17]; however, Kustaloglu[29] found the trait in 2% to 3% of Malaysians and American Indians. Dahlberg[17] observed paramolar tubercules in 31% of a group of Pima Indians, indicating a genetic basis for paramolar tubercles and paramolar teeth.

Concordance for the structure in a pair of monozygotic twins was reported by Saheki.[38]

Occlusal patterns

Fissures and grooves in the molar teeth of Mongoloid individuals tend to be deeper and extend closer to the tooth borders when compared with those in Negroes and Caucasians.[50] Another molar characteristic that shows a racial preference is wrinkling of the enamel surface, which is common in Bantu[15] and Mongoloid[50] populations.

There is little racial difference in the number of cusps exhibited on maxillary molars, but this feature shows a wide degree of variance in the mandibular molar teeth. The frequency of a sixth cusp on the mandibular first molar was reported to be 0 to 1.9% in Caucasians, 2% in American Negroes, approximately 3% in African Negroes, from 5.2% to 31.6% in Japanese, and 54.4% in Polynesians.[47]

There are three major mandibular molar

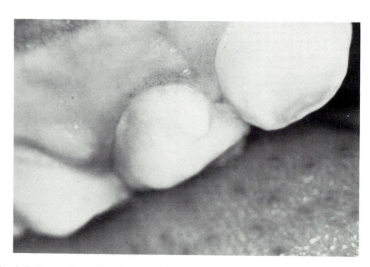

Fig. 6-6. Paramolar tubercle or Bolk's cusp on buccal surface of deciduous molar.

occlusal patterns: a primitive Y fissure configuration, a + type, and an X pattern, which is considered to be the most advanced anthropologically[47] (Fig. 6-7). Population data from Table 6-2 indicate a definite genetic basis for occlusal patterns of the mandibular molars.

Excessive enamel

Enamel extension onto the root surface and even into the furcation areas of molars is a more prevalent finding in the extracted teeth of Mongoloid populations as opposed to other racial groups.[50]

Enamel pearls are nodular excrescences usually located at the bifurcation of multi-rooted teeth. They may consist of only enamel, enamel and dentin, or enamel, dentin, and pulp tissues. These structures arise from local activity of the remnants of Hertwig's epithelial root sheath before it is reduced to rests of Malassez.

The hereditary nature of these structures is hypothesized from variable population frequencies. Enamel pearls were seen in 30% of Ainu and 3% of Japanese peoples.[15] Pedersen,[36] in a comparative study of Danes

and Greenland Eskimos, found a much higher incidence in the latter.

Pindborg[37] has suggested that enamel pearls and enamel extensions onto root surfaces may be a variable expression of the same phenomenon.

Root morphology

Mongoloid roots are simpler in form than those of Caucasians or Negroes,[37] and a genetic determination of some radicular traits can be postulated from interracial variations in root structure. Premolar teeth are more commonly single rooted in Mongoloids as opposed to other races.[36, 50] Division of premolar roots into multiple structures is most common among the Bantus.[42] Double-rooted mandibular premolars occur with an increased frequency in Turner's (XO) syndrome, in which 20% of a group of affected patients were observed to have the trait (Fig. 6-8). There is little racial variation in the number of maxillary molar roots[30]; however, the root form is shorter and less divergent in the maxillary molars of Mongoloid peoples when compared to those of Caucasians.[36, 50]

The most racially distinct trait observed in mandibular molar root is an extra distolingual root frequently seen in Mongoloid groups. The characteristic was noted ten times as frequently in Eskimos than in Caucasians[36] and was not seen by Shaw[42] in Bantus. Tratman[49] found none in European Caucasians, 0.2% in Asiatic Indians, 8% in Chinese, and 11% in Malaysian peoples.

The term *taurodontism* describes another aberation in root structure and was proposed by Sir Arthur Keith[26] in 1913. The phenome-

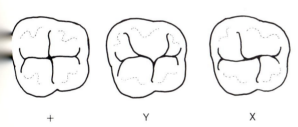

+   Y   X

Fig. 6-7. Three major mandibular molar occlusal patterns, which consist of +, Y, and X configuration.

Table 6-2. Mandibular molar groove patterns in various populations*

	Permanent first molars (%)				Permanent second molars (%)			
	Number of teeth	Y	+	X	Number of teeth	Y	+	X
Caucasians	878	66.6	19.8	13.6	950	15.2	27.8	57.0
Japanese	6375	64.9	33.0	2.1	5630	3.8	71.6	24.6
Polynesians	170	82.4	12.3	5.3	79	10.1	38.0	51.9

*Modified from Suzuki, M., and Sakai, T.: Occlusal surface patterns of lower molars and second deciduous molars among the living Polynesians, Am. J. Phys. Anthropol. **39**:305-315, 1973.

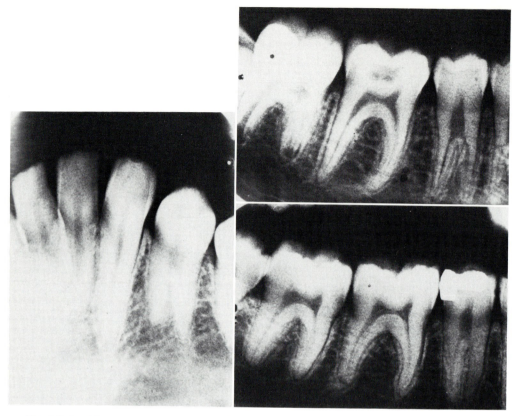

Fig. 6-8. Double-rooted mandibular premolars are visible on intraoral radiographs from patients with (XO) Turner's syndrome.

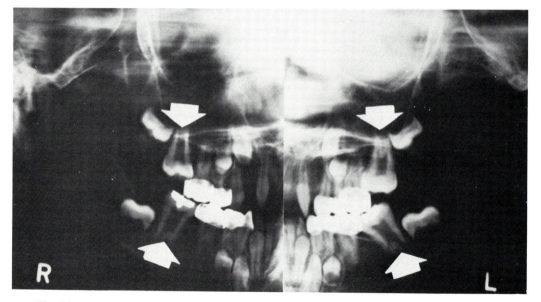

Fig. 6-9. Apicoocclusal enlargement of pulp chambers of mandibular and maxillary first permanent molars, commonly called taurodontism.

non is characterized by an apical-occlusal enlargement of the pulp chamber accompanied by a striking alteration in external root configuration (Fig. 6-9). The trait is thought to arise when Hertwig's epithelial root sheath fails to invaginate at the proper time.

The role that genetics plays in the cause of taurodontism is not clear. The fact that the relative frequency with which the trait occurs in various human populations is variable suggests that a genetic component may be at work. Taurodontism is found rarely in modern Caucasians[22] but is seen with higher frequency among certain modern populations that have lived under relatively primitive conditions in the recent past such as Aleuts,[33] Eskimos,[30] Bantus of South Africa, and Australoid people.[41] Witkop[23] reports of ongoing studies among Guatemalan Indians in which taurodontism is found in as much as 20% of the population.

A family in which this autosomal dominant trait was transmitted to five males and seven females over three generations has been reported.[43]

Coon[15] postulates that taurodontism is a genetically determined trait that offers a selective advantage in populations that use their teeth as tools. Further evidence for a genetic component to the taurodont phenomenon in association with a particular type of dental enamel defect is reported by Winter and associates,[52] who presented a family in which taurodontism and amelogenesis imperfecta are inherited together as an autosomal dominant trait. Crawford[16] reports another family in which a similar association between amelogenesis imperfecta and taurodontism exists.

There is some evidence that indicates that certain forms of taurodontism are not inherited as a simple genetic trait. The trait has been observed in a number of patients with various types of chromosome abnormalities, including a patient with a G-E translocation who also had dyschondrosteosis[54] and has been reported in several patients with abnormal numbers of X chromosomes. The actual frequency with which taurodon-

tism occurs in X-aneuploid patients is not known. Witkop reports that taurodontism occurs with high frequency in XXXXY patients and presented a single extracted hypertaurodont molar said to be from such a patient.[53]

Stewart[43] reported two cases of patients with X chromosome aneuploidy, XXY and XXXXY, both of whom had taurodontism. He speculated that the degree of taurodontism may be related to the number of X chromosomes present.

Thuline[48] has observed taurodontism in two patients with an XXYY chromosomal constitution and in one with XXXY syndrome.

TOOTH NUMBER

A number of terms have been used to describe the congenital absence of teeth in the primary and/or the permanent dentition. *Hypodontia* connotes the absence of only one or a few teeth. The term *oligodontia* implies agenesis of numerous teeth and is commonly associated with systemic abnormalities. *Anodontia* is the extreme expression of oligodontia and indicates the total absence of dental complement. This rare condition has been reported in the most severe forms of ectodermal dysplasia.

Congenital absence of teeth may arise from a variety of pathogenetic mechanisms. One cause is physical obstruction or disruption of the dental lamina, as seen in orofaciodigital (OFD) syndrome, in which hyperplastic connective tissue frenulae cover the dental lamina in the mandibular incisor area. Space limitation is a possible factor in the failure of third molar development; competition for minimum nutritional requirement in a spatially constricted area could cause tooth germ regression and agenesis. Functional abnormalities of the dental epithelium or its underlying mesenchyme could also produce hypodontia.

Hypodontia

Hypodontia is rarely seen in other mammalian species, including nonhuman primates.[115] The condition has not been reported in hominid dentitions before the Upper

Paleolithic period[115]; however, it is a frequent finding in *Homo sapiens* today.

Agenesis in the primary dentition is uncommon and is extremely rare in areas other than the incisor region; it has been reported more often in the maxilla than in the mandible.[103]

Variation in racial incidence is substantial and suggests a genetic component for hypodontia of the deciduous dentition. One study reported a frequency of 0.5% for Swedish children with a range of 0.1% to 0.7% for Caucasians.[66] Saito[106] estimated hypodontia at 5% in the primary dentition of Japanese children. Familial reports are sparse, but concordance in monozygotic twins has been reported.[102]

Hypodontia of permanent teeth is so common that it is considered by many to be a variant of normal. In fact, it has been postulated that man is now in an intermediate stage of tooth development. A dental formula of one incisor, one canine, one premolar, and two molars per quadrant has been proposed for future man.[66, 103]

Some studies have suggested a higher incidence of missing teeth in females[59, 91, 94, 100, 102] yet others were unable to substantiate this finding.[64, 118]

The prevalence of hypodontia of permanent teeth among races differs. In Caucasians, agenesis of teeth other than the third molar ranges between 2.3% and 9.6%.[103] Niswander and Sujaku[100] indicated a prevalence of 6.6% in Japanese, and Terasaki and Shiota[117] found a similar frequency in Japan. A study of Israelites found hypodontia highest among Orientals in that country.[105]

A familial tendency was noted by Grahnen[73] where agenesis was found in a greater proportion of proband relatives than in a random population. He conducted an extensive review of the literature on the heredity of congenitally missing teeth and quoted several workers who have reported concordance for hypodontia in monozygotic twins. Gravely and Johnson[77] reported the variation in expression of hypodontia in three pairs of monozygotic twins, supporting the view that this phenomenon is genetically determined

but that its expression is affected by nongenetic factors.

Grahnen[73] concluded that the genetic cause of hypodontia in the permanent dentition was one of "autosomal dominance showing incomplete penetrance and variable expression." Gorlin and Pindborg[72] also postulated a single gene locus.

Suarez,[115] in a study of data collected by Grahnen,[73] determined that hypodontia in the permanent dentition best fits a polygenic model. He has assumed that a morphogenic field of variable intensity affects teeth and that the most unstable structures, that is, third molars, second premolars, and maxillary lateral incisors, are under the greatest environmental influence. Woolf[118] also postulated that multiple genes and genotypes control the development of the permanent dentition, and a recent study in Israel[64] supports the multifactorial hypothesis.

Congenital absence of teeth and reduction in tooth size have been associated by clinicians for over a century. In 1870 McQuillan[93] published a pedigree in which hypodontia and hypopalsia of the maxillary lateral incisors were found concurrently and in successive generations. Since then, numerous pedigrees have been published linking the two characteristics as being an expression of the same disorder (Fig. 6-10).

Hypodontia of third molars has been associated with absence, hypoplasia, and reduced size of the remaining teeth.[59, 100, 115, 118] A correlation between hypoplasia and hypodontia of teeth other than the third molar has been reported.[100, 115] In experimental animals, Grüneberg[79] has shown a relationship between agenesis and reduction. He reported that a tooth germ must reach a critical size during a particular stage of development, or the structure will regress. Suarez[115] has statistically shown that hypodontia and reduction in the tooth size are controlled by the same or related gene loci and that continuous distribution of tooth size is another indication that hypodontia is transmitted polygenically.

In the permanent dentition, hypodontia is most commonly seen in third molar teeth. The prevalence of individuals lacking one or

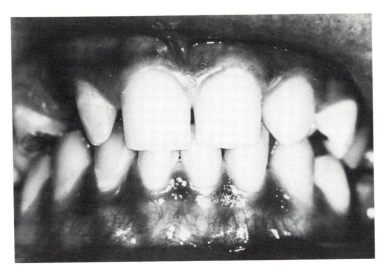

Fig. 6-10. Simultaneous occurrence of peg-shaped permanent lateral incisor on right and congenitally missing permanent lateral incisor on left, which demonstrates frequent relationship of these two phenomena, which are an expression of same gene defect.

more third molars varies from approximately 1% in some African Negroes and Australian Aboriginal samples to an estimated 30% in Japanese populations.[112] Incidence in Caucasian populations varies from 10% to 25%. Pedersen[102] noted a significant difference between East Greenland Eskimos (37%) and mixed natives from Southwest Greenland (30%). He concluded that these population frequencies reflect a genetic basis for third molar agenesis.

Family studies in Sweden reported that agenesis of third molars is more frequent among relatives of the propositi (30%) than among the general population (22%).[73] A polygenic inheritance is the most probable model for third-molar agenesis in man.

Laboratory studies of inbred mouse strains that normally have three molars have shown significant population differences.[112] Frequencies of 17.9%, 2.3%, and 0.1% were reported for the three different strains, suggesting a genetic component.

Excluding the third molars, second premolars are the most frequently absent teeth in studies involving Caucasian populations, with a range of 0.8% to 6.4%.[103] A Japanese study cited a prevalence of 1.8%.[100]

Grüneberg[78] reported a pedigree in which a mother and two of her children were missing second premolars. Concordance in monozygotic twins is not uncommon.[71, 108] Discordance is rare[108] but indicates exogenous factor influence.

An autosomal dominant syndrome featuring premolar agenesis, hyperhidrosis, and cavities prematura (PHC syndrome) was reported in twenty-five affected people in four generations of a Swedish pedigree.[58] Inheritance is either by a polygenic mode or an autosomal dominant mode with incomplete penetrance and variable expression.

The maxillary lateral incisor is the most studied tooth in the human dentition. Hypodontia and hypoplasia occur frequently, and often both traits are present in the same individual.

Since McQuillan[93] published the first pedigree genetically linking the two characteristics, many pedigree reviews have indicated complete dominance with variable expression as the mode of genetic transmission for the trait.[92, 97, 98, 107] However, the same authors have documented pedigrees with dominance showing incomplete penetrance and families that would best fit a recessive model.

An interesting family was reported by

Table 6-3. Frequency of absent and reduced maxillary lateral incisors among various populations*

Population	Reduced (%)	Absent (%)	Approximate ratio (reduced: absent)
Caucasians	3.1	3.2	1:1
Hawaiians	1.7	1.7	1:1
American Negroes	3.7	2.0	2:1
Japanese	4.7	1.1	5:1
Chinese	7.7	0.15	50:1

*Modified from Montagu, M. F. A.: The significance of the variability of the upper lateral incisor teeth in man, Hum. Biol. 12:328-358, 1940.

Sergi.[110] All affected members of the pedigree of three generations showed identical expressions of reduced lateral incisors on the left maxillary quadrant and absent lateral incisors on the right.

Intrapopulation differences are sizable[97] (Table 6-3). The trait has not been observed in Australian Aborigines[61] or Bantus.[111]

A group of inbred Swiss villagers illustrates the genetic control of the maxillary lateral incisor trait.[85] Fully one third of the individuals possessed the trait, and 20% of the population had congenitally missing lateral incisors.

Familial data gathered by Woolf[118] in Utah have produced a wealth of data concerning reduced and absent maxillary lateral incisors. Of the proband's first-degree relatives, 17.7% possessed the trait, whereas only 2.8% of the controls were positive. The fact that values were similar in siblings and parents (15.7% and 20%, respectively) and that fathers transmitted the trait equally to their sons and daughters prompted Woolf to hypothesize that the characteristic was transmitted as an autosomal dominant trait with reduced penetrance and variable expression. A polygenic model for this single tooth trait, however, could not be ruled out.

Hypodontia of the maxillary lateral incisor is significantly higher in patients with endocrinopathies[108] and is seen in 15% of Down's

syndrome (trisomy 21) cases and 11% of retarded individuals in general.[103] Agenesis is also common in cleft lip and palate patients.

Familial studies have suggested different modes of inheritance. Miller[95] and Castro[63] have both reported a dominant characteristic in three generations. Incomplete dominance was possible in a large pedigree recorded by Huskins,[83] and an X-linked mode has been suggested by Dahlberg.[67]

Review of pedigrees would indicate a multifactorial mode of inheritance.

Racial variations in Caucasian and Mongoloid populations are significantly different for agenesis of the mandibular lateral incisors. In Japanese, the prevalence is as high as 4.8%, and frequencies of less than 1% in Caucasians[108] suggest a hereditary background.

Concordance in monozygotic twins for agenesis was observed in three cases by Goldberg[71] and is not an uncommon finding.[103]

Agenesis of the maxillary canine is rare, the highest frequency being 0.15% in Caucasians.[103] A dominant mode of transmission was described by Grüneberg,[78] who observed a family with absence of the maxillary canines and retention of deciduous cuspids in seven members of three generations. Dolamore[69] described the trait in a father and son. Concordance in twin brothers has also been reported.[80]

Hypodontia is a characteristic of anhidrotic ectodermal dysplasia, an X-linked recessive syndrome, incontinentia pigmenti, an X-linked dominant trait, and Rieger's syndrome, an autosomal dominant condition.

Hypodontia is also seen in orofaciodigital (OFD) syndrome, an X-linked dominant trait, Hallermann-Streiff syndrome, and premolar aplasia–hyperhidrosis–canities prematura (PHC) syndrome, an autosomal dominant syndrome.

Hyperodontia

As in the case of hypodontia, hyperodontia of the primary dentition is rare. The condition is seen in approximately 0.5% of children.[75] Supernumerary deciduous teeth are more prevalent in males and are most frequently located in the maxillary anterior region. Extra permanent teeth were reported in 30% of Swedes who had a history of hyperodontia in the primary dentition.[76]

Although hyperodontia has been observed in all tooth-bearing areas of the permanent dentition, it is seen most frequently in the maxilla by a ratio of 9:1.[57] The trait shows a sex predilection in a ratio of 2:1 for males.[99, 101] Supernumerary teeth are commonly

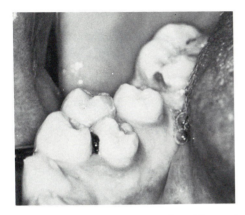

Fig. 6-11. Hyperodontia, illustrated in this case by occurrence of two supernumerary mandibular premolars. This phenomenon occurred bilaterally in case illustrated.

hypoplastic and often erupt ectopically (Fig. 6-11).

Several reports indicate that there is a difference in the incidence of hyperodontia between the Mongoloid and Caucasian races. Niswander and Sujaku[100] and others[106, 117] have cited frequencies greater than 3% in Japanese populations. An incidence of between 1% and 3% has been observed in Caucasians.[62, 76, 101, 107, 114]

The rarity of supernumerary teeth in regions other than the maxillary incisor and molar areas has made studies of the genetics of the condition difficult.

Mesiodens are conical in shape and located at or near the midline in the incisal region of the maxilla (Fig. 6-12). When mesiodens erupt, they are normally found either palatal to or between the central incisors and frequently cause an improper alignment of the central incisors. The sex ratio is 2:1 favoring the males.[57] There is a dearth of information concerning populations other than Caucasians. A study of Eskimos estimated the prevalence of mesiodens at 0.77%, which falls within the range for Caucasians (0.15% to 1.4%).[103, 109]

Familial incidences of multiple affected

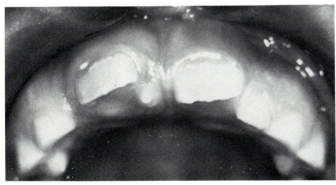
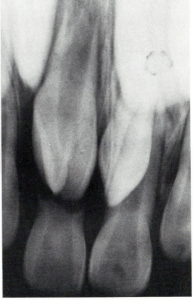

B

Fig. 6-12. Median diastema between maxillary permanent central incisors, which resulted from the presence of, **A,** midline supernumerary tooth or mesiodens. **B,** Intraoral radiograph demonstrating presence of supernumerary structures near midline between erupting permanent central incisors.

siblings[56, 81, 109] and the occurrence of mesiodens in successive generations[81, 87, 109] have
been cited. Hammond-Williams[81] reported a
female proband whose grandfather was also
affected; however, neither parent had the
trait. Another case of skipping a generation
was reported by Sedano and Gorlin.[109]
Keeler[87] reported a pedigree involving four
generations. Some individuals presented with
a supernumerary tooth, and others had
"twisted teeth." Sedano and Gorlin[109] believe
mesiodens to be governed by an autosomal
dominant trait with lack of penetrance. A
multifactorial mode must be considered.

Paramolar teeth may be located in the
interproximal spaces on the buccal aspect of
molar teeth. The hereditary nature of this
trait is discussed in the portion of this chapter
dealing with paramolar tubercles (p.
132).

Multiple supernumerary teeth are seen
with increased frequency in cases of cleidocranial dysplasia (Fig. 6-13), an autosomal
dominant syndrome, and Gardner's syndrome, which is also inherited as an autosomal dominant. Hyperodontia has been
reportedly associated with Hallermann-Streiff
and orofaciodigital syndrome. Supernumerary
teeth in the maxillary lateral incisor area are
a frequent finding in cleft lip and palate patients.

When considering specific teeth, a review
of pedigrees reveals that a single gene substitution may be responsible for the occurrence
of supernumerary teeth in individuals and in
families. However, Niswander and Sujaku[100]
have analyzed the data from family studies
and have demonstrated that of the Mendelian
models only an autosomal recessive mode of
inheritance could possibly fit the data for
hyperodontia of the permanent dentition.
They suggest a multifactorial mode of inheritance. Thus it is most likely that hyperodontia is under the control of a number of
different loci and that the genetics are similar
to the polygenic scheme of hypodontia.

Gemination, twinning, and fusion

Gemination is an abortive attempt by a
single tooth bud to divide and occurs due to
the invagination of the developing dental
organ. The extent of invagination in the
crown and/or root would determine the degree of cleavage (Fig. 6-14).

The term *twinning* indicates that the cleavage is complete, resulting in the formation of
a supernumerary tooth that is usually a mirror image of its adjacent partner (Fig. 6-15).

The hereditary factors of tooth gemination
are probably similar to those affecting the
dental lamina and resulting in hyperodontia.

Fusion is the embryological union of nor-

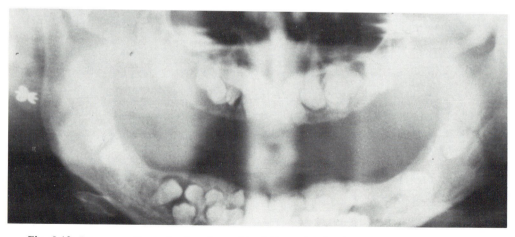

Fig. 6-13. Panorex radiograph of patient with cleidocranial dysplasia demonstrating numerous
unerupted permanent teeth with multiple supernumerary structures. This patient had worn
denture for 17 years supported by these unerupted teeth.

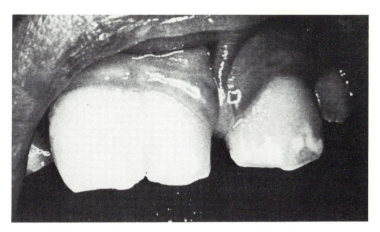

Fig. 6-14. Gemination of primary central incisors.

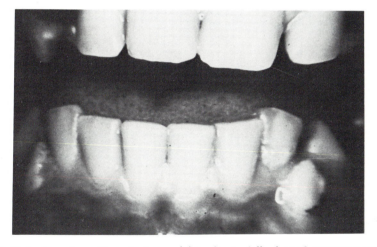

Fig. 6-15. Twinning of maxillary incisors, giving rise to fully formed supernumerary, which resembles its adjacent partner.

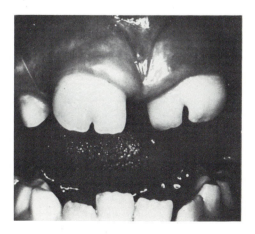

Fig. 6-16. Fusion between central and lateral incisors, which, in this case, probably occurred late in development, giving rise to bifid crowns with almost twice normal mesiodistal dimensions of single tooth and nearly equaling combined dimensions of normal central and lateral incisors.

mally discrete dental organs (Fig. 6-16). If fusion occurs early, the two developing teeth will unite to form a single tooth of almost normal size. However, if fusion occurs late in development, one tooth almost twice the normal size or a tooth with a bifid crown will result.[113]

A persistence of the interdental lamina has been demonstrated in fused incisors in dogs[82] and is a probable factor in the fusion of human teeth.

Racial variations have been noted in populations. Saito[106] observed a 5% incidence of fusion in Japanese, whereas studies of Caucasian populations found a prevalence of the trait to be less than 0.5%.[108]

Moody and Montgomery[98] reported three large pedigrees for fused teeth in which the affected individuals are all males. Although no mention is made of this striking phenomenon, these pedigrees are highly suggestive of Y-linked or holandric transmission for this trait.

Bilateral fusion in mandibular incisors was observed in sisters.[75] Concordance was reported in monozygotic twin girls and a brother.[108]

Fusion has been observed in a strain of Lakeland terriers,[82] demonstrating a pattern of inheritance. Fusion of the first and second molars has been noted in rice rats by Sofaer,[112] who postulated a single gene control of the trait.

Based on available reports, the genetic cause of fusion is probably autosomal dominant with reduced penetrance.

ERUPTION

The normal eruption sequence of the primary dentition is similar in all populations. The central incisors are the first teeth to erupt in children. They are followed by the lateral incisors, first molars, canines, and second molars, in that order.[144] Various factors have been implicated in the control of eruption; those most commonly cited are genetic, environmental, and systemic.

The genetic control of deciduous tooth eruption has been estimated at 78%.[133] Population studies show no significant intraracial

variation in emergence of primary teeth in American, Swiss, French, English, or Swedish Caucasians,[144] although several investigators have observed interracial variations. Tanner[149] found no advancement in Africans who had early skeletal maturation; however, MacKay and Martin[140] reported that Bantus had earlier eruption than Caucasians. Meredith[143] observed no significant difference between American Caucasians or Negroes, yet one report[128] places Negroes significantly ahead. Koreans[126] have been reported slightly advanced, and Australian Aborigines[122] have somewhat retarded tooth emergence when compared to Caucasians.

Familial data are scant, but twin studies have shown intraclass correlations for monozygotic twins to be 0.91% as opposed to 0.56% for dizygotic twins.[133]

If deciduous teeth emerge before the first 3 months of life, they are classified as premature (Fig. 6-17). Of these teeth, ones that are present at birth are called *natal teeth*, and those which erupt during the neonatal period, from birth to 30 days, are designated *neonatal teeth*.[141] Of the total, 90% are primary teeth (85% of which are mandibular incisors), and 10% are supernumerary calcified structures frequently referred to as *predeciduous teeth*[22] (Fig. 6-18). There is no apparent sex predilection. Natal teeth appear

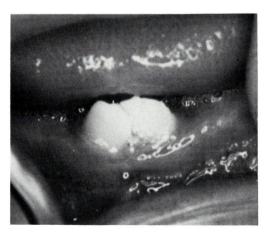

Fig. 6-17. Natal teeth in newborn infant, which, on radiographic examination, were determined to be prematurely erupted primary central incisors.

more frequently than neonatal teeth in a ratio of 3:1, although they are an expression of the same characteristic.[132]

Familial occurrences have been reported frequently in the literature. Natal and neonatal teeth were seen in three generations of a single family.[123, 132, 141] Natal teeth have been reported in two children born of the same mother but different fathers[134] and in two half-siblings with the same father.[120]

Concordance for natal teeth has been reported in twins.[121, 151] Capon[124] observed natal teeth in twin girls whose father had the trait. Neonatal teeth have been observed in twin girls.[119]

The hereditary transmission has been most characteristic of an autosomal dominant trait.[123]

Natal and neonatal teeth are reportedly associated with three syndromes: chondroectodermal dysplasia or Ellis–van Creveld syndrome (autosomal recessive), Hallermann-Streiff syndrome (autosomal dominant), and pachyonychia congenita (autosomal dominant).[123]

The eruption sequence of permanent teeth is more variable than that of the deciduous dentition and is illustrated in Table 6-4.[144]

Genetic factors in tooth eruption are clearly present. Monozygotic twins have been shown to have a concordance rate as high as 0.9

Table 6-4. Eruption standards for northern temperate zone Caucasian children*

Eruption sequence†	Tooth	Mean age of eruption in years	
		Males	Females
1	$\overline{6\,|\,6}$	6.2	5.9
2	6 | 6	6.4	6.2
3	$\overline{1\,|\,1}$	6.5	6.3
4	1 | 1	7.5	7.2
5	$\overline{2\,|\,2}$	7.7	7.3
6	2 | 2	8.7	8.2
7 Males (8) (Females)	4 | 4	10.4	10.0
8 Males (7) (Females)	$\overline{3\,|\,3}$	10.8	9.9
9	$\overline{4\,|\,4}$	10.8	10.2
10	5 | 5	11.2	10.9
11	$\overline{5\,|\,5}$	11.5	10.9
12	3 | 3	11.7	11.0
13	$\overline{7\,|\,7}$	12.1	11.7
14	$\overline{7\,|\,7}$	12.7	12.3

*Modified from Pindborg, J. J.: Pathology of the dental hard tissues, Philadelphia, 1970, W. B. Saunders Co.
†Eruption measured at time of tooth emergence.

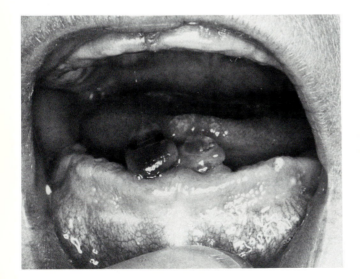

Fig. 6-18. Predeciduous teeth in newborn infant, which, by radiographic examination, were determined to be supernumerary calcified structures with primary incisors being in normal position and unerupted.

for dental development and eruption,[129, 137, 138] and dizygotic twins and siblings show a significantly lower concordance, although development in siblings is much closer than in unrelated individuals.[129, 131, 135]

An X-linked component has been hypothesized for tooth development and eruption[131]; however, this conclusion based on sib-sib correlations has met with much criticism.[142, 148] Evidence for X-linkage is meager at best,[148] and it can be argued that early eruption in females is hormonally mediated.

Racial differences have been reported with respect to tooth eruption times.[125, 130, 135, 139, 140] However, apparent population variations must be viewed with considerable caution due to the many exogenous influences on development of the permanent dentition.

Garn and associates,[130] controlling satisfactorily for variables such as sex, birth order, and nutrition, has shown rather convincingly that American Negroes have substantially advanced eruption times when compared to American Caucasians. Most studies indicate that eruption patterns are significantly affected by environmental as well as genetic factors.[144]

Socioeconomic levels are known to affect nutrition, personal hygiene, and related factors. Retarded eruption of anterior teeth and accelerated emergence of the posterior dentition has been linked to low socioeconomic status in all racial groups.[130, 139] Lee[139] suggests that anterior teeth reflect the general status of the child, and the posterior dentition is a mirror of the oral hygiene as a factor in the preservation of primary teeth.

Low birth weight but not birth order has been associated with delayed emergence of permanent teeth.[148] Conversely, early eruption has been associated with increased birth weight.[144] In monozygotic twins the child with the higher recorded birth weight has shown an advance in eruption time.[144]

Although nutrition has been implicated as a factor in dental development, teeth are at a substantially lower risk than are skeletal and other somatic structures for detrimental environmental influences. One study of nutrition was shown to correlate only slightly with dental development,[129] with nutritional factors contributing less than 1%.[148]

Precocious eruption is observed less commonly than retarded eruption in primary teeth. Delayed eruption may be due to systemic disorders and has been reported as associated with several syndromes.

Delay in permanent tooth eruption is associated with Down's syndrome, cleidocranial dysostosis, hypothyroidism, hypopituitarism, several types of craniofacial synostosis, and hemifacial atrophy.[144]

Precocious eruption is rare but seen in cases of precocious puberty, hyperthyroidism, hemifacial hypertrophy, and in affected areas of the dental arch in Sturge-Weber syndrome.

Premature loss of primary teeth can also affect eruption time and sequence of the permanent dentition. The condition has been observed in acrodynia, Hand-Schüller-Christian disease, hypophosphatasia, and Papillon-Lefèvre syndrome.

Ankylosis is defined as an aberration of tooth eruption in which the continuity of the periodontal ligament has been compromised. This results in a progressive loss of occlusal contact when a tooth becomes stabilized in the arch and the adjacent teeth continue to move in an occlusal direction (Fig. 6-19). The term *submergence* has been used to describe the same phenomenon, but since it does not accurately describe the loss of occlusal height, most investigators have preferred the term *ankylosis*.[147] The incidence of ankylosis has been determined to be approximately 1.3% in two large population studies.[147]

The precise biological mechanism by which a tooth becomes ankylosed has yet to be described. Via,[150] in a study of 2342 patients, found the frequency of ankylosis among siblings to be 44%, as compared to a frequency of 1.3% in the general population. He concluded that the occurrence of ankylosed deciduous teeth has a definite familial tendency and is probably an inherited trait.

Stewart and Hansen[147] reported the presence of concordant patterns of ankylosis in monozygotic twins who had ankylosis of six deciduous molars in identical locations, which, they believed, indicated a significant

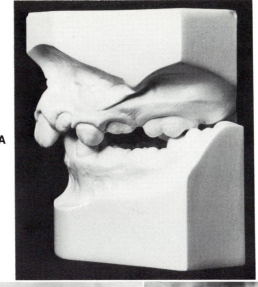

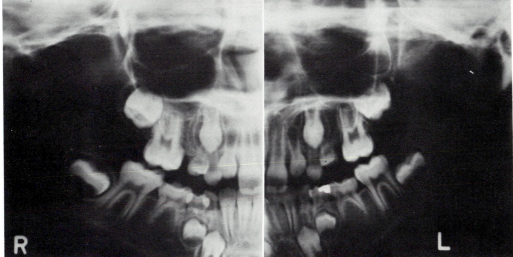

Fig. 6-19. A, Study models of patient in mixed dentition who demonstrates ankylosis of maxillary and mandibular primary molars. **B,** Panorex radiograph demonstrating bilateral occurrence of ankylosis of primary molars. Also note congenital absence of both first and second maxillary premolars and mandibular second premolars, which is phenomenon frequently observed in association with ankylosis of primary teeth.

genetic component to the cause of this anomaly.

The association between ankylosed primary teeth and multiple enamel defects has been reported by Rule.[146] A review of the reported cases of ankylosed primary teeth reveals a frequent association of these two phenomena and leads to speculation regarding the role of the enamel epithelium in the development of these anomalies and the possibility of a single gene or closely linked genes giving rise to both.

REFERENCES

1. Brace, C. C.: In Montagu, A., editor: Culture and the evolution of man, New York, 1962, Oxford University Press.
2. Brace, C. C.: In Montagu, A., editor: The concept of race, London, 1964, Collier-Macmillan Publishers.

3. Coon, C. S.: The origin of the races, ed. 1, New York, 1962, Alfred A. Knopf, Inc.
4. Dahlberg, A. A.: The changing dentition in man, J. Am. Dent. Assoc. 32:676, 1945.
5. Gabriel, A. C.: Genetic types in teeth, Sydney, Australia, 1948, Australian Medical Publishing Co.
6. Garn, S. M., Lewis, A. B., and Vicinus, J. H.: Third molar agenesis and reduction in the number of other teeth, J. Dent. Res. 41: 717, 1962.
7. Melnick, M., and Shields, E.: Personal communication, 1975.
8. Suarez, B. K.: The genetics of tooth size in man, Ph.D. dissertation, Los Angeles, 1974, University of California at Los Angeles.
9. Wasserman, G. D.: Molecular control of cell differentiation and morphogenesis—a systemic theory, New York, 1972, Marcel Dekker, Inc.
10. Wolpoff, M. H.: Metric trends in hominid dental evolution, Cleveland, 1972, The Press of Case Western Reserve University.

Tooth form and structure

11. Amos, E. R.: Incidence of small dens in dente, J. Am. Dent. Assoc. 51:31-33, 1955.
12. Bailit, H. C.: Dental variations among populations: an anthropologic view, Dent. Clin. North Am. 19:125-139, 1975.
13. Biggerstaff, R. H.: Heritability of the Carabelli cusp in twins, J. Dent. Res. 52:40-44, 1973.
14. Bolk, L.: Problems of human dentition, Am. J. Anat. 19:91, 1916.
15. Coon, C. S.: The origin of the races, ed. 1, New York, 1962, Alfred A. Knopf, Inc.
15a. Coon, C. S.: An introduction to fossil man. In Coon, C. S.: The origin of the races, ed. 1, New York, 1962, Alfred A. Knopf, pp. 356-357.
16. Crawford, J. L.: Concomitant taurodontism and amelogenesis imperfecta in the American Caucasian, J. Dent. Child. 37:83-87, 1970.
16a. Curzon, M. E., Curzon, J. A., and Poyton, H. G.: Evaginated odontomes in the Keewatin Eskimo, Br. Dent. J. 129:324-328, 1970.
17. Dahlberg, A. A.: The evolutionary significance of the prorostylid, Am. J. Phys. Anthropol. 8:15-25, 1950.
18. Dahlberg, A. A. (1956). Cited by Lasker, G. W., and Lee, M. M. C.: Racial traits in the human teeth, J. Forensic Sci. 2:401-419, 1957.
19. Dahlberg, A. A.: Analysis of the American Indian dentition. In Brothwell, D. R., editor: Dental anthropology, ed. 5, Oxford, England, 1963, Pergamon Press, Ltd.
20. Dietz, V.: A common dental morphotropic factor, the Carabelli cusp, J. Am. Dent. Assoc. 31:784-789, 1944.
21. Grahnen, H., and Lindahl, B.: Supernumerary teeth in the permanent dentition, a frequency study, Odontol. Revy 12:290-294, 1961.
22. Hammer, J. E., Witkop, C. J., and Metro, P. S.: Taurodontism, Oral Surg. 18:409-418, 1964.
23. Hanihara, K.: Studies on the deciduous dentition of the Japanese and the Japanese-American hybrids, J. Anthropol. Soc. Nippon 64:95-116, 1956.
23a. Hoffman, B.: Cited by Merrill, R. G.: Occlusal anomalous tubercles on premolars of Alaskan Eskimos and Indians, Oral Surg. 17:484-406, 1964.
24. Horowitz, S. L.: Clinical aspects of general research in dentistry, J. Dent. Res. (Suppl.) 42:1330-1343, 1963.
25. Hrdlicka, A.: Shovel-shaped teeth, Am. J. Phys. Anthropol. 3:429-465, 1920.
25a. Kato, K.: Contribution to the knowledge concerning the cone-shaped supernumerary cusp in the center of the occlusal surface on premolars of Japanese, Nehon Shika Gakukai Zasshi 30:28-49, 1937.
26. Keith, A.: The antiquity of man, London, 1925, Williams & Norgate, Ltd.
27. Kong, Y. W.: The prevalence of dens invaginatus in maxillary incisors, Dent. J. Malaysia Singapore 12:9-14, 1972.
28. Kraus, B. S.: Carabelli's anomaly of the maxillary molar teeth, Am. J. Hum. Genet. 3:348-355, 1951.
29. Kustaloglu, O. A.: Paramolar structures of the upper dentition, J. Dent. Res. 41:75-83, 1962.
30. Lasker, G. W., Lee, M. M. C.: Racial traits in the human teeth, J. Forensic Sci. 2:401-419, 1957.
30a. Lau, T. C.: Odontomes of the axial core type, Br. Dent. J. 99:219-225, 1955.
31. Lee, G. T. R., and Goose, D. H.: The inheritance of dental traits in a Chinese population in the United Kingdom, J. Med. Genet. 9:336-339, 1972.
32. Merrill, R. G.: Occlusal anomalous tubercles on premolars of Alaskan Eskimos and Indians, Oral Surg. 17:484-496, 1964.
33. Moorrees, C. F. A.: The Aleur dentition: a correlative study of dental characteristics in an Eskimoid people, ed. 1, Cambridge, Mass., 1957, Harvard University Press.
34. Oehlers, F. A.: Dens invaginatus, Oral Surg. 10:1204-1218, 1302-1316, 1957.
34a. Oehlers, F. A. C., Lee, K. W., and Lee,

E. C.: Dens evaginatus (evaginated odontome), Dent. Pract. **17**:239-244, 1967.

35. Osborn, R. H., Horowitz, S. L., and De-George, F. V.: Genetic variation in tooth dimensions: a twin study of the permanent anterior teeth, Am. J. Hum. Genet. **10**:350-356, 1958.

36. Pedersen, P. O.: The East Greenland Eskimo dentition, Copenhagen, 1949, C. A. Reizel.

37. Pindborg, J. J.: Pathology of the dental hard tissues, Philadelphia, 1970, W. B. Saunders Co.

37a. Reichart, P., and Tantiniran, D.: Dens evaginatus in the Thai, Oral Surg. **39**:615-621, 1975.

37b. Robbins, I. M., and Keene, H. J.: Multiple morphologic dental anomalies: report of a case, Oral Surg. **17**:683, 1964.

38. Saheki, M.: On the heredity of the tooth crown configurations studied in twins, Acta Anat. Nippon **33**:456-470, 1958.

39. Schulze, C.: Developmental abnormalities of the teeth and jaws. In Gorlin, R. J., and Goldman, H. M., editors: Thoma's oral pathology, ed. 6, St. Louis, 1970, The C. V. Mosby Co.

40. Shafer, W. G.: Dens in dente, N. Y. State Dent. J. **19**:220-225, 1953.

41. Shaw, J. C. M.: Taurodont teeth in the South African races, J. Anat. **62**:476-498, 1928.

42. Shaw, J. C. M.: The teeth, the bony palate, and the mandible in Bantu races of South Africa, London, 1931, John Bale Sons & Danielsson.

43. Stewart, R. E.: Taurodontism in X-chromosome aneuploid syndromes, Clin. Genet. **6**: 341-344, 1974.

44. Suarez, B. K.: The genetics of tooth size in man, Ph.D. dissertation, Los Angeles, 1974, University of California at Los Angeles.

45. Sumiya, Y.: Statistic study on dental anomalies in the Japanese, J. Anthropol. Soc. Nippon **67**:171-173, 1959.

46. Suzuki, M., and Sakai, T.: Shovel-shape incisors among the living Polynesians, Am. J. Phys. Anthropol. **22**:65-72, 1964.

47. Suzuki, M., and Sakai, T.: Occlusal surface patterns of lower molars and second deciduous molars among the living Polynesians, Am. J. Phys. Anthropol. **39**:305-315, 1973.

47a. Sykaras, S. N.: Occlusal anomalous tubercle on premolars of a Greek girl, Oral Surg. **38**: 88-91, 1974.

48. Thuline, H.: Rainier School, Buckley, Washington, personal communication, 1970.

49. Tratman, E. K.: Three-rooted lower molars in man and their racial distribution, Br. Dent. J. **64**:264-274, 1938.

50. Tratman, E. K.: A comparison of the teeth of peoples, Indo-European racial stock with the Mongoloid racial stock, Yearbook Phys. Anthropol. **6**:272-314, 1950.

51. Turner, C. G.: Microevolutionary interpretations from the dentition, Am. J. Phys. Anthropol. **30**:421-426, 1969.

52. Winter, G. B., Lee, K. W., and Johnson, N. W.: Hereditary amelogenesis imperfecta: a rare autosomal dominant type, Br. Dent. J. **127**:137-164, 1969.

53. Witkop, C. J.: Manifestations of genetic diseases in the human pulp, Oral Surg. **32**:278-316, 1971.

53a. Wu, K. L.: Survey on mid-occlusal tubercles in bicuspids, China Stomatol. Mag. **3**:294, 1955.

54. Wyandt, H. E., Hecht, F., Lovrien, E. W., and Stewart, R. E.: Study of a patient with apparent monosomy 21 owing to translocation: 45, xx, 21-, +(18S⁺), Cytogenetics **10**: 413-426, 1971.

54a. Yip, W. K.: The prevalence of dens evaginatus, Oral Surg. **38**:80-87, 1974.

Tooth number

55. Bailit, H. L.: Dental variations among populations: an anthropologic view, Dent. Clin. North Am. **19**:125-139, 1975.

56. Baker, C. R.: Similarity of malocclusion in families, Int. J. Orthod. **10**:459-462, 1924.

57. Bhaskar, S. N.: Synopsis of oral biology, ed. 4, St. Louis, 1973, The C. V. Mosby Co.

58. Böök, J. A.: Clinical and genetic studies of hypodontia, Am. J. Hum. Genet. **2**:240-263, 1950.

59. Brekhus, P. G., Oliver, C., and Montelius, G.: A study of the pattern and combination of congenitally missing teeth in man, J. Dent. Res. **23**:117-131, 1944.

60. Burman, L.: Dentition of identical twins, J. Am. Dent. Assoc. **31**:705-706, 1944.

61. Campbell, T. D.: Cited by Schultz, A. H.: The hereditary tendency to eliminate the upper lateral incisors, Hum. Biol. **4**:34-40, 1932.

62. Castaldi, C. R., et al.: The incidence of congenital dental anomalies in the age group 6-9, J. Dent. Res. **43**:802, 1964.

63. Castro, F. M.: Inherited and congenital causative factors in malocclusion, J. Am. Dent. Assoc. **15**:1206, 1928.

64. Chosach, A., Eidelman, E., and Cohen, T.: Hypodontia: a polygenic trait—a family study among Israeli Jews, J. Dent. Res. **54**: 16-19, 1975.

65. Clayton, J. M.: Congenital dental anomalies occurring in 3,557 children, J. Dent. Child. **23**:206-208, 1956.

66. Coon, C. S.: The origins of the races, ed. 1, New York, 1962, Alfred A. Knopf, Inc.

67. Dahlberg, A. A.: Inherited congenital absence of six incisors, deciduous and permanent, J. Dent. Res. **16**:59-62, 1937.

68. Dependorf (1912). Cited by Grahnen, H., and Granath, L.: Numerical variations in primary dentition and their correlations with the permanent dentition, Odontol. Rev. **12**: 348-351.

69. Dolamore, W. H.: Absent canines, Br. Dent. J. **68**:5-8, 1925.

70. Douglas, B. L., and Kresberg, H.: Mesiodens, Dent. Radiogr. Photogr. **30**:70-73, 1957.

71. Goldberg, S.: The dental arches of identical twins, Dent. Cosmos **72**:869-881, 1930.

72. Gorlin, R. J., and Pindborg, J. J.: Syndromes of the head and neck, New York, 1964, McGraw-Hill Book Co.

73. Grahnen, H.: Hypodontia in the permanent dentition: a clinical and genetical study, Odontol. Rev. **7**:1-100, 1956.

74. Grahnen, H.: Hereditary factors in relation to dental caries and congenitally missing teeth. In Witkop, C. J., editor: Genetics and dental health, New York, 1962, McGraw-Hill Book Co.

75. Grahnen, H., and Granath, L.-E.: Numerical variations in primary dentition and their correlation with the permanent dentition, Odontol. Revy **12**:348-357, 1961.

76. Grahnen, H., and Lindahl, B.: Supernumerary teeth in the permanent dentition, Odontol. Revy **12**:290-294, 1961.

77. Gravely, J. F., and Johnson, D. D.: Variation in expression of hypodontia in monozygotic twins, Dent. Pract. **21**:212, 1971.

78. Grüneberg, H.: Two independent inherited tooth anomalies in one family, J. Hered. **27**: 225-228, 1936.

79. Grüneberg, H.: The pathology of development: a study of inherited skeletal disorders in animals, Oxford, England, 1963, Blackwell Scientific Publications, Ltd.

80. Hallett, G. E. M.: Fourteen cases of congenital absence of canines, Br. Dent. J. **97**: 228-230, 1954.

81. Hammond-Williams, C.: Supernumerary teeth heredity, Br. Dent. J. **56**:500, 1934.

82. Hitchin, A. D., and Morris, I.: Geminated odontome, J. Dent. Res. **45**:575-583, 1966.

83. Huskins, L. L.: On the inheritance of any anomaly of human dentition, J. Hered. **21**: 279-282, 1930.

84. Ivy, R. H.: A case of non-eruption of entire permanent denture, Dent. Cosmos **75**:689-690, 1933.

85. Joehr, A. C.: Reduktionserscheinungen an den oberen seitlichen schneidezaehnen, Arch. Klaus Stifr. Vererbungstorsch **9**:73-133, 1934.

86. Keeler, C. E., and Short, R.: Hereditary absence of upper lateral incisors, J. Hered. **25**:391-392, 1934.

87. Keeler, C. E.: Heredity in dentistry, Dent. Cosmos **77**:1147-1163, 1935.

88. Korkhaus, G.: Die Vererbung der Anomalien der Zahnzahl, Korrespbl. Zahnaertze. **53**:435, 1929.

89. Korkhaus, G.: Stroungen des Zahnwechsels und die Retention der Zuhne, Vjschr. Zahnheilkd. **46**:55-68, 1930.

90. Korkhaus, G.: Uber den Einfluss der Eerbmasse auf das Gebiss: Befunde an Drillingen unde Vierluingen, Dentsch. Zahn Mund Kieferheilkd. **8**:247-270, 1941.

91. Lasker, G. W.: Genetic analysis of racial traits of the teeth: Cold Spring Harbor Symposia on Quantitative Biology **15**:191-203, 1950.

92. Mandeville, L. C.: Congenital absence of permanent maxillary lateral incisor teeth: a preliminary investigation, Ann. Eugenics **15**:1-10, 1949.

93. McQuillan, J. H.: Hereditary transmission of dental irregularities, Dent. Cosmos 12, 1870.

94. Meskin, L. H., and Gorlin, R. J.: Agenesis and peg-shaped permanent maxillary lateral incisors, J. Dent. Res. **42**:1476-1479, 1963.

95. Miller, M. A.: An inherited dental anomaly in a Japanese family, J. Hered. **32**:313-314, 1941.

96. Milles, L.: Inheritance of skeletal anomalies, J. Hered. **19**:28-46, 1928.

97. Montagu, M. F. A.: The significance of the variability of the upper lateral incisor teeth in man, Hum. Biol. **12**:328-358, 1940.

98. Moody, E., and Montgomery, L. B.: Hereditary tendencies in tooth formation **21**:1174-1176, 1934.

99. Niswander, J. D.: Effects of heredity and environment on development of dentition, J. Dent. Res. **42**:1288-1296, 1963.

100. Niswander, J. D., and Sujaku, C.: Congenital anomalies in Japanese children, Am. J. Phys. Anthropol. **21**:569-574, 1963.

101. Parry, R. R., and Iyer, V. S.: Supernumerary teeth amongst orthodontic patients in India, Br. Dent. J. **111**:257-258, 1961.

102. Pedersen, P. O.: The East Greenland Eskimo dentition, Copenhagen, 1949, C. A. Reizel.

103. Pindborg, J. J.: Pathology of the dental hard tissues, Philadelphia, 1970, W. B. Saunders Co.

104. Rantanen, A. V.: On the frequency of the missing and peg-shaped maxillary lateral incisor among Finnish students, Am. J. Phys. Anthropol. **14**:491-496, 1956.

105. Rosenzweig, K., and Gabarski, D.: Numerical aberrations in the permanent teeth of grade

school children in Jerusalem, Am. J. Phys. Anthropol. **23**:277-284, 1965.

106. Saito, T.: A genetic study on the degenerative anomalies of deciduous teeth, Jap. J. Hum. Genet. **4**:27-53, 1959.

107. Schultz, A. H.: The hereditary tendency to eliminate the upper lateral incisor, Hum. Biol. **4**:34-40, 1932.

108. Schulze, C.: Developmental abnormalities of the teeth and jaws. In Gorlin, R. J., and Goldman, H. M., editors: Thoma's oral pathology, ed. 6, St. Louis, 1970, The C. V. Mosby Co.

109. Sedano, H. O., and Gorlin, R. J.: Familial occurrence of mesiodens, Oral Surg. **27**:360-362, 1969.

110. Sergi, S.: Cited by Schultz, A. H.: The hereditary tendency to eliminate the upper lateral incisors, Hum. Biol. **4**:34-40, 1932.

111. Shaw. Cited by Schultz, A. H.: The hereditary tendency to eliminate the upper lateral incisors, Hum. Biol. **4**:34-40, 1932.

112. Sofaer, J. A.: Genetic variation and tooth development, Br. Med. Bull. **31**:107-110, 1975.

113. Sperber, G. H.: Genetic mechanisms and anomalies in odontogenesis, J. Canad. Dent. Assoc. **33**:433-442, 1967.

114. Stafne, C. E.: Supernumerary teeth, Dent. Cosmos **74**:653-659, 1932.

115. Suarez, B. K.: The genetics of tooth size in man, Ph.D. dissertation, Los Angeles, 1974, University of California at Los Angeles.

116. Sumiya, Y.: Statistic study on dental anomalies in the Japanese, J. Anthropol. Soc. Nippon **67**:171-172, 1959.

117. Terasaki, T., and Shiota, K.: Roentgenological study of supernumerary teeth in the incisal region of the upper jaw, J. Jap. Stom. Soc. **2**:231, 1953.

118. Woolf, C. M.: Missing maxillary lateral incisors: a genetic study, Am. J. Hum. Genet. **23**:280-296, 1971.

Eruption

119. Allwright, W. C.: Natal and neonatal teeth, Br. Dent. J. **105**:163-172, 1958.

120. Asana, D. J.: A male infant born with two lower central incisor teeth, Indian Med. Gaz. **56**:16, 1921.

121. Balard, B.: A case of twins with teeth present at birth, Dent. Sci. J. Aust. **4**:44, 1924.

122. Barrett, M. J., and Brown, T.: Eruption of deciduous teeth in Australian Aborigines, Aust. Dent. J. **11**:43-50, 1966.

123. Bodenhoff, J., and Gorlin, R. J.: Natal and neonatal teeth, Pediatrics **32**:1087-1093, 1963.

124. Capon, P. G.: A case of the presence of teeth in twins at birth, Br. Dent. J. **44**:1106, 1923.

125. Dahlberg, A. A., and Menegaz-Bock, R. M.: Emergence of the permanent teeth in Pima Indian children, J. Dent. Res. **37**:1123-1140, 1958.

126. Duk Jin Yun: Eruption of primary teeth in Korean rural children, Am. J. Phys. Anthropol. **15**:261-268, 1957.

127. Eveleth, P. B.: Eruption of permanent dentition and menarche of American children living in the tropics, Hum. Biol. **38**:60-70, 1966.

128. Furguson, A. D., Scott, R. B., and Bakwin, H.: Growth and development of Negro infants, J. Pediat. **50**:327-331, 1957.

129. Garn, S. M., Lewis, A. B., and Kerewsky, R. S.: Genetic, nutritional and maturational correlates of dental development, J. Dent. Res. **44**:228-242, 1965.

130. Garn, S. M., Nagy, J. M., Sandusky, S. T., and Throwbridge, F.: Economic impact on tooth emergence, Am. J. Phys. Anthropol. **39**:233-238, 1973.

131. Garn, S. M., and Rohmann, C. G.: X-linked inheritance of developmental timing in man, Nature **196**:695-696, 1962.

132. Hals, E.: Natal and neonatal teeth, Oral Surg. **10**:509-521, 1957.

133. Hatton, M. G.: A measure of the effect of heredity and environment on eruption of the deciduous teeth, J. Dent. Res. **34**:397-401, 1955.

134. Herpin, A.: Les dents à la naissance (abstr.), Dent. Cosmos **54**:121, 1912.

135. Hiernaux, J.: Ethnic differences in growth and development, Eugen. Quart. **15**:12-21, 1968.

136. Hurme, V. O.: Ranges of normalcy in eruption of permanent teeth, J. Dent. Child. **16**:11-15, 1949.

137. Korkhaus, G.: Die erste Dentition und der Zahnwechsel im Licht der Zwillingsforschung, Vjschr. Zahnheilkd. **45**:414-430, 1929.

138. Korkhaus, G.: Stroungen des Zahnwechsels und die Retention der Zahne, Vjschr. Zahnheilkd. **46**:55-68, 1930.

139. Lee, M. M. D., Low, W. D., and Chang, K. S. F.: Eruption of the permanent dentition of southern Chinese children in Hong Kong, Arch. Oral Biol. **10**:849-861, 1965.

140. MacKay, D. H., and Martin, W. J.: Dentition and physique of Bantu children, J. Trop. Med. Hyg. **55**:265-275, 1952.

141. Massler, M., and Savara, B. S.: Natal and neonatal teeth, J. Pediatrics **36**:349-359, 1950.

142. Mather, K., and Jinks, J. K.: Correlation between relatives arising from sex-linked genes, Nature **198**:314-315, 1963.

143. Meredith, H. V.: Order and age of eruption

for the deciduous dentition, J. Dent. Res. 25:43-66, 1946.

144. Pindborg, J. J.: Pathology of the dental hard tissues, Philadelphia, 1970, W. B. Saunders Co.

145. Rantanen, A. V.: The age of eruption of the third molar teeth, Acta Odontol. Scand. (Suppl.) 25:48, 1967.

146. Rule, J. T.: The relationship between ankylosed primary molars and multiple enamel defects, J. Dent. Child. 39:29-35, 1972.

147. Stewart, R. E., and Hansen, R. H.: Ankylosis and partial anodontia in twins: a case report, J. Calif. Dent. Assoc. 2:50, 1974.

148. Suarez, B. K.: The genetics of tooth size in man, Ph.D. dissertation, Los Angeles, 1974, University of California at Los Angeles.

149. Tanner, J. M.: Growth at adolescence, ed. 2, Oxford, England, 1962, Blackwell Scientific Publications, Ltd.

150. Via, M.: Submerged deciduous molars: familial tendencies, J. Am. Dent. Assoc. 69: 127-129, 1964.

151. Waiss, A. S.: Congenital teeth, Med. Rec. 50:803, 896.

7

Heritable defects of enamel

CARL J. WITKOP, Jr.
JOHN J. SAUK, Jr.

FORMATION OF NORMAL ENAMEL

Mammalian enamel occurs as the product of a group of highly differentiated ectodermal cells, the enamel organ. In the development of the enamel organ, a series of cellular changes occurs, resulting in the formation of four distinct layers: (1) the outer dental epithelium, (2) the stellate reticulum, (3) the stratum intermedium, and (4) the inner enamel epithelium. These four layers develop before any enamel formation. During those periods when enamel is not yet formed, the enamel organ exerts an influence that results in differentiation of odontoblasts. Thus the ultimate shape of the enamel-dentin junction is determined. Subsequent to the initiation of dentin production by odontoblasts, the cells of the inner dental epithelium (ameloblasts) begin to form enamel. The initial formation of enamel occurs at the occlusal or incisal surface of the developing tooth, and as enamel formation continues in these regions, additional ameloblasts form enamel proximally until the process terminates at the cervical regions of the developing crown. Thus the primordial cells of the dental lamina are the ancestors for subsequent generations of daughter cells of the inner enamel epithelium. In addition, the primordial cells contain the genetic information necessary for enamel formation, which will be transmitted to subsequent generations of daughter cells, resulting in a uniform expression from the incisal or occlusal surfaces to cervical portions of a tooth.

As the enamel organ prepares for the process of amelogenesis, the character of its four layers changes. The inner dental epithelium, or ameloblasts, become tall columnar cells with hyperchromatic nuclei that are polarized away from the developing enamel front. The stratum intermedium changes, and the area occupied by the stellate reticulum is reduced. The stellate reticulum and the external dental epithelium are condensed and form a layer of cells between the stratum intermedium and the connective tissue. Just before enamel formation, the enamel organ is invaded by vascular elements that penetrate the outer portion of the enamel organ and become proximate to the ameloblasts (Fig. 7-92). The initiation of enamel formation and its final form and character are dependent on a number of processes that are mediated by the ameloblasts. Enamel formation may be divided into three processes: (1) formation and secretion of an organic matrix, (2) mineralization of the matrix, and (3) maturation of enamel.

This work was supported in part by National Institutes of Health grant DE AM 03686.

151

Production of organic matrix

The elaboration of enamel matrix requires a specific intracellular arrangement of cellular organelles. During early differentiation, the ameloblasts become tall columnar cells.[56, 129] The internal organization of the secretory ameloblasts, beginning adjacent to the stratum intermedium, consists of a region of basal terminal bars, followed by a zone of mitochondria, a nucleus, a zone of endoplasmic reticulum, a Golgi system, another zone of endoplasmic reticulum, a distal terminal bar, and a Tomes' process, which is located proximal to the organic matrix elaborated. The mitochondria, which provide the energy for the cellular processes, are most proximate to vascular elements, which invade the stellate reticulum before enamel formation. The nucleus contains the genetic code for matrix formation and transcribes its code to messenger RNA, which translates this message to the ribosomes. Matrix is synthesized in endoplasmic reticulum and assembled in a system of Golgi and endoplasmic reticulum, resulting in membrane-bound granules and vacuoles, the secretion granules. The secretion granules approach the periphery of the Tomes' process and fuse with the plasma membrane. At the point of union, an opening occurs, and the contents of the granule are released into the extracellular space.[130]

Mineralization of the matrix

From the onset of amelogenesis, the secretion of organic matrix is a steady, regular process. The mineralization of enamel matrix occurs through apatite crystal nucleation and begins either immediately after matrix production or concomitantly with matrix secretion. The nucleation process is rapid, and the full c-axis length of the crystals is attained during the time of the secretion of a few microns of matrix.[3, 151] The growth of enamel in outer axial dimensions is slower and is not yet completely understood. Scott and associates[152] have summarized the mineralization process as occurring in three general phases. The first phase is the rapid deposition of the long, slender crystals. The second phase involves growth in width and thickness.

At this stage, matrix production is essentially complete. The remainder of crystal growth is a slow process; this is the process at which enamel reaches its final high level of mineral content and, as such, is defined as maturation.[151, 152]

Maturation of enamel

The process of maturation occurs periodically during stages of amelogenesis. During these periods, enamel crystallites become larger, and matrix is returned to the ameloblasts. Concurrent with these periods, the ameloblasts are modified from secretory cells to transporting cells.[130]

Shape of mineralizing front and formation of enamel prisms

The shape of the mineralizing front determines the shape and form of enamel prisms. Utilizing transmission and scanning electron microscopy, Boyde[13] was able to describe the shape of the mineralizing front in two patterns of dental enamel prisms. The mineralizing front was found to have three profiles according to the plane of section. Tangential sections revealed a honeycomb appearance. The individual spaces or cells of this pattern filled in progressively from one side as the plane entered deeper into the enamel. Longitudinal sections revealed a sawtooth profile, and transverse sections showed a repetitive, boxlike profile. At the mineralization front, crystallites grew perpendicular to the front of the cervical floors of the depression. However, at the lateral walls and cuspal walls, the orientation was more nearly parallel. Thus the abrupt concavities in the shape of the mineralizing front cause abrupt changes in the orientation of the developing crystallites. Boyde[13-15] and Boyde and Lester[16] suggest that the plane at which crystallite orientation changes is the plane of the classical prism sheaths of enamel prisms. The latter is based on observations that the prism boundaries in developing enamel do not contain material different from the surrounding enamel. The higher concentration of organic material at the prism sheaths in adult enamel is, then, presumably acquired during enamel maturation through the mobilization of matrix back to the ameloblasts. Enamel matrix possessing qualities of a thixotropic gel is forced parallel with crystallite direction back toward the ameloblasts. Matrix accumulates at the prism boundaries because in these regions the crystallites end and there is imperfect packing of crystallites,[13] and matrix becomes trapped and cannot be returned.

At the termination of enamel formation, ameloblasts lose their Tomes' process projections, and the mineralizing front becomes flat. The crystallites are then aligned parallel and perpendicular to the surface, and, since there are no changes in orientation, there are no prisms formed; hence the final prismless zone.[13]

Thus in the enamel defects that result in pitted hypoplastic surfaces[142] or disturbances that result in brown striae of Retzius or incremental lines, there is an early demise of ameloblasts or cessation of their secretory activity. The surface of the completed tissue will then contain depressions (pits) originally occupied by Tomes' processes of ameloblasts.[15]

Nature of enamel matrix

The proteins constituting the organic matrix of developing dental enamel in a number of animal species have been found to possess certain unique and similar features so that they may be considered as a separate class of extracellular proteins that are referred to as *enamelins* or *amelogens*.[64]

The amino acid composition of the organic matrix of developing enamel is characterized by a high proline content and elevated concentrations of glutamic acid, histidine, and leucine.[21, 23, 49, 66, 68] These matrices also contain peptide-bound o-phosphoserine.[67]

Glimcher[64] has noted that in enamelins 3- and 4-hydroxyproline are present as well as hydroxylysine. Hexose and hexosamine were found in equal amounts, and galactose and galactosamine were the principal sugars.[22, 44, 64] Acid mucopolysaccharides and glycopeptides have been isolated and identified. The acid mucopolysaccharide content has been estimated to be 0.2%. Glycopeptides were noted to contain quantities of carbo-

hydrate ranging up to 20%. The oligosaccharide moiety of these matrices contained galactosamine, galactose, and mannose in a ratio of 4:3:1.[64]

According to Glimcher, at high molarity EDTA and alkaline pH, the organic matrix of enamel is almost completely insoluble. However, at a low ionic strength, low temperatures, and a neutral pH, almost 90% of the enamel proteins may be extracted (neutral soluble enamel proteins, NSEP). The remaining proteins are soluble in dilute acid.[64] Electron-microscopic observations and amino acid analysis have revealed that the NSEP are morphologically identical to the enamel tubules within the rods or prisms, and the acid-soluble proteins are associated with the prism sheaths.[64, 69]

Twenty-six components of NSEP have been identified by disc electrophoresis. Glimcher states that this large number of compounds may represent a large series of distinct peptides or degradation products of a select number of high-molecular-weight proteins that are hydrolyzed during maturation.[64]

Physical chemical characterization of NSEP has revealed that as a group they exist as a large number of aggregate complexes of similar size.[64] Monomeric units have been noted to possess molecular weights from 6000 to 18,000, and the aggregates were noted to have molecular weights of up to 1 and 2 million.[49, 64, 68]

Some of the most homogeneous peptides are copolymers of a limited number of amino acids, that is, proline, glutamic acid, leucine, and tyrosine.[64]

Many of the proteins have been studied in both the solid state and after precipitation from solution and are noted to exist in a cross-beta configuration.[64] In solution, a small percentage of the peptides of the NSEP remained in their beta conformation, and most were noted to exist as random coils.[64, 65]

An interesting biological finding is that during calcification and maturation, 90% of the proteins originally in the developing enamel are lost. The matrix that remains after these processes has a composition different from that of developing enamel by consisting of low-molecular-weight peptides. Glimcher believes that this indicates that there has been hydrolysis of peptide bonds and removal of the organic matrix. In addition, this process has been selective in that the overall amino acid composition of embryonic enamel matrix is markedly changed from that in mature enamel matrix.[64] Thus mature enamel contains glycine and glutamic and aspartic acids, in addition to serine phosphate as the most prominent amino acids.[64]

Recently, Glimcher has isolated two homogeneous phosphorylated polypeptides from NSEP. The molecular weights of these polypeptides are both approximately 6000. In addition, all the serine residue in each of the peptides was phosphorylated, and the sequence of the serine phosphate residue in one of the peptides was suggested by Glimcher to be glut-o-phospho-leucine and in the other glut-o-phospho-serine-tyrosine.[64]

FORMATION OF ABNORMAL ENAMEL

Some gene mutations affecting the structure or composition of enamel usually result in alterations detectable only in the enamel; others may also involve alterations in other tissues or metabolic processes.[181, 185] In general, these mutations result in one of the following: insufficient enamel being formed (hypoplasia); a marked deficit of initial calcification of the organic matrix (hypocalcification); a defect in the formation of crystalline apatite in various components of the enamel rods or enamel sheaths (hypomaturation); a deposition of exogenous material frequently of a pigmented nature; or a combination of these processes. Currently we have insufficient knowledge concerning the exact structural or enzymatic protein alteration involved in these defects to make a precise chemically based classification of these disorders. The classification developed here will be based on the local or general effects of the mutation, the predominant type of deficit seen clinically and histologically, and the mode of inheritance. The rationale for developing a classification based on these three criteria is that each of them contributes both practical and theoretical points of differentiation for conditions that may closely resemble one another.

The conceptual value of separating those traits which affect only the specialized enamel organ from those conditions which involve other tissues or generalized metabolic processes as well is that this division suggests that those conditions with only dental involvement are determined by genes that regulate functions unique to the highly differentiated and specialized odontogenic cells, whereas those with general effects result from genes that regulate less differentiated cells or general metabolic or regulatory systems. One problem inherent in such a division is that it depends on our ability to detect abnormalities in other tissues or systems. The absence of striking lesions in other tissues may lull one into assuming that there are none. An excellent example is the otodental syndrome. This disorder has striking, gigantic globe-shaped posterior teeth apparent even to lay persons (Fig. 7-1).[75] What is less striking is the high-frequency hearing loss in affected individuals. Generally the audiogram is normal up to

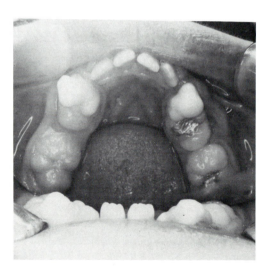

Fig. 7-1. Globodontia in patient with otodental syndrome. Condition spares incisor teeth in both dentitions and usually involves cuspids and teeth posterior to cuspids. Patient has erupted permanent incisor teeth. Primary cuspids have exfoliated. Note massive globe-shaped primary molar teeth. (Courtesy Dr. W. J. Streed, St. Cloud, Minn.)

6000 cycles but with a sharp reduction in the higher frequencies. In small kindreds this feature is easily overlooked because high-frequency hearing damage is a common sequela of high-intensity environmental noise. The association of the tooth anomaly and the hearing loss became apparent only after careful investigation of large kindreds by Levin and Jorgenson.[96] There is also the reverse set of circumstances to consider. Generalized disorders may affect the dental tissues, but because they are silent and cause no changes detectable by the usual methods employed in oral examination, it is assumed that the dental tissues are uninvolved. Fabry's disease is an excellent example. The deficiency of the enzyme ceramide trihexosidase permits the accumulation of a large amount of trihexosyl ceramide in the dental pulp, which is detectable by special histological methods or chemical extraction but rarely causes clinical dental features of diagnostic value.[40] A third pitfall in assuming that if the defect involves only dental tissues, it reflects genes controlling processes unique to dental development, comes from evidence that certain dominant mutations in the heterozygous state have detectable effects only in teeth but in the homozygous state have marked alterations in other systems. Dominant mutations that probably affect structural protein synthesis may possibly show a threshold effect in the heterozygous state in such tissues as enamel, which normally has less than 2% organic material. A reduction of about half of a particular protein in the heterozygote may cause an easily detectable alteration but would not become clinically significant in tissues containing larger amounts of the protein until the material was even further reduced as in the homozygous state. Such an example may be the xeroderma, talipes, and enamel defect (XTE syndrome) reported by Moynahan.[118] In the kindred reported, an enamel defect segregated as an autosomal dominant trait. Two children were the offspring of consanguineous affected parents. These children showed, in addition to a severe enamel defect, xeroderma, skin blisters, photophobia, oligophrenia, and clubfoot.

The general clinical features of an enamel defect provide the initial step in diagnosis of the condition by the clinician. Simply by noting whether the enamel has formed to full normal thickness on newly erupted or developing teeth, one may differentiate the hypoplastic conditions from the hypocalcified and hypomaturation forms of enamel defects. Generally the hardness of the enamel differentiates the hypocalcified from the hypomaturation forms. Hypocalcified enamel is so soft that it can be removed by a prophylaxis instrument, whereas hypomaturation forms admit the tip of an explorer under firm pressure, and enamel is lost by chipping from the underlying normal-appearing dentin. Not all conditions in which enamel is lost from teeth are intrinsic enamel defects. It is surprising how many referrals from dentists of patients with "defective enamel" are actually patients with hereditary opalescent dentin or dentinogenesis imperfecta, conditions primarily with defective dentin and with relatively minor or no changes in the histological features of enamel. The histological features of the enamel structure give a general clue to the steps in enamel formation that are under genetic control. In general, the hypoplastic forms reflect defects in differentiation or viability of ameloblasts and defects of matrix formation. The hypocalcified forms reflect defects of matrix structure and calcium-phosphate deposition. The hypomaturation forms reflect alterations in rod and rod sheath structure. As will be seen, the genetic control of enamel formation is probably exceedingly complex if the number of different mutations affecting enamel formation is any indication of the number of genes involved in normal formation. We do not know how many loci are involved, but present evidence suggests that a minimum of one X-chromosomal and three autosomal loci are involved in nonsyndromal defects of enamel. Linkage studies offer an introductory step in determining the genetic control map of enamel formation.

There are several theoretical and practical reasons for separating what appear to be similar clinical conditions when the modes of inheritance of these traits are different in different families.

The mode of inheritance gives a clue to the type of protein that is altered by the gene mutation. Proteins may be divided into enzymatic and structural or specialized protein. Enzymatic proteins are synthesized in relatively minute amounts, but their effect in regulation of biochemical pathways is disproportionately greater than their amount. Structural proteins are synthesized in relatively large quantities. In the diploid cell, each autosomal locus is represented twice, once on each homologous chromosome. A mutant gene on one chromosome paired with a normal gene on the other (heterozygous) would code for mutant protein or no protein, whereas the normal gene would produce about half of the normal amount of protein as produced by the homozygous normal. If only half of the normal enzymatic protein is made, then relatively minor changes result, since in most biochemical systems this is sufficient enzymatic activity to provide a nearly normal enzymatic function. On the other hand, if only half of a structural protein is normal, the effect is more readily detectable. Thus as a general rule it appears that most recessive traits are defects in enzymatic proteins, and most dominant traits are defects in structural proteins. In most instances, a search for enzymatic defects in dominantly inherited defects would be a less likely research hypothesis than a search for a defective structural protein.

Heterogeneity among enamel defects is common.[180] The mode of inheritance is useful in the detection of genetic heterogeneity. Many defects appear clinically and histologically similar but differ in the manner in which they are inherited. Does a patient with what appears to be disease *A* but without some of the usually encountered features of disease *A* have a variant of the condition, or does he have a different disease, *B?* If it can be shown that the patient inherited his disease in a manner different from the inheritance of disease *A*, then we can be confident that he has a disease based on a different mutation and must have a different disease. Each specific mutation is the specific etiological

mechanism for one specific disease. Autosomal dominant hypomaturation amelogenesis imperfecta and X-linked hypomaturation amelogenesis imperfecta may appear so similar in affected males as to be indistinguishable clinically. Yet we know by the mode of inheritance in families that they are controlled by genes on different chromosomes, and therefore, in the absence of a possible presently undetectable chromosomal translocation, they are probably caused by different genes.

The mode of inheritance is also important in counseling the patient. Because the clinical appearances of the various defects of enamel are frequently similar, it is better to construct a detailed family pedigree and to determine how the trait is inherited in that particular family than to rely on published modes of inheritance.

INHERITED DEFECTS PRIMARILY INVOLVING ENAMEL— AMELOGENESIS IMPERFECTA

Hereditary defects of enamel unassociated with generalized defects are considered types of amelogenesis imperfecta.[171, 185, 186] Amelogenesis imperfecta of all types occurs in the general population in a ratio of about 1:14,000. The most common type of amelogenesis imperfecta is the autosomal dominantly inherited hypocalcification of enamel, which occurs in a ratio of about 1:20,000.[173-176]

Attempts to classify the various forms of amelogenesis imperfecta began with Weinmann and co-workers[162] by distinguishing hypoplastic and hypocalcified forms on clinical criteria. Darling[35] demonstrated that clinical criteria alone were insufficient to distinguish some forms that showed clinical similarities but had radiographic and histological differences. Hals[79, 80] demonstrated that histological criteria alone may show both hypoplasia and hypocalcification at the microscopic level in teeth that grossly may show only one or the other of these features. A series of publications by Winter and co-workers[168, 171, 172] in England and by Witkop and associates* in the United States demon-

---

*See references 173-176, 179, 180, 183, 185.

strated that clinical, histological, and genetic criteria must all be used to classify these defects. Essentially, the basic classification presented here is a modified compilation of those presented by Winter's and Witkop's groups.

Many patients with the hypoplastic and hypocalcified forms of enamel defects have anterior open bite. Schulze[145-148] has classified cases with anterior open bite separately from those lacking this characteristic. We believe that anterior open bite is a secondary effect rather than a direct pleiotropic effect of the gene mutation. Although it occurs in high frequency of up to 60% in some types of hypoplastic and hypocalcified defects, many individuals within kindreds having the enamel defect do not have anterior malocclusion. Furthermore, over 30% of 164 persons examined with dentinogenesis imperfecta in the Brandywine isolate had anterior open bite.[184, 185] Thus the presence or absence of anterior open bite does not distinguish between specific genetic mutations. Many patients with anterior open bite are those who complain of sensitivity to hot and cold and who have teeth with rough surfaces. Perhaps this leads to a tongue thrust habit, which could account for the prevalence of open bite in these conditions.

Generally, patients with all forms of amelo-genesis imperfecta are good candidates for full-crown restorations. Dentin and root form are usually within normal variation. Pulp chamber size frequently may be prematurely reduced from secondary dentin, which allows placement of anterior restorations at an earlier age than in normal teeth. The high incidence of malocclusion in these defects complicates full-mouth restoration, but in general these patients respond well to orthodontic procedures. Posterior stabilization with full crowns should precede anterior restoration.

Hypoplastic amelogenesis imperfecta

The hypoplastic forms of amelogenesis imperfecta include those disorders in which all or a localized portion of the enamel does not reach normal thickness during development. In general, these conditions appear clinically as thin enamel on teeth that do not contact each other mesiodistally, as pits in the enamel, or as vertical or horizontal fissures in the enamel.

Autosomal dominant pitted hypoplastic amelogenesis imperfecta. In autosomal dominant pitted hypoplastic amelogenesis imperfecta, the enamel of both the primary and secondary dentitions usually approaches normal thickness, but with pinpoint- to pinhead-sized pits randomly distributed over the sur-

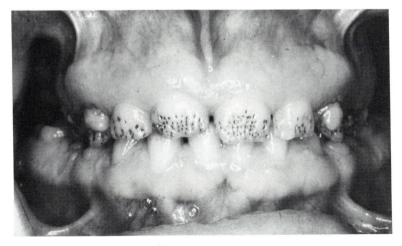

Fig. 7-2. Pitted hypoplastic amelogenesis imperfecta in moderately severely affected patient. Staining in bottom of pits gives impression of black dots on enamel. Note tendency of pits to have both vertical and horizontal arrangement in rows and columns. (Courtesy Dr. Joseph Giansanti, Lexington, Ky.)

face (Fig. 7-2). The enamel on newly erupted teeth is hard with a normal yellow-white color. Staining of the pits frequently occurs after exposure to the oral environment, giving the teeth a black, pockmarked appearance. Usually both dentitions are affected, but in some cases the primary teeth may have smooth but thin enamel. The pits involve the labial surfaces to a greater degree than the lingual surfaces but with some incisors having thin enamel on the labial surface. Winter[168] notes that in some families the pits tend to be arranged in vertical columns. Some of our patients have the pits oriented in both rows and columns (Fig. 7-2). Variation in the number of teeth involved and the number of pits in the enamel is seen in families. This type of amelogenesis imperfecta may resemble the enamel defect seen in some forms of rickets, fever hypoplasia, pseudohypoparathyroidism, and epidermolysis bullosa. The first two conditions usually show horizontal arrangement of the defect, and the other general symptoms distinguish the latter conditions.

Histological sections show that the incremental lines of Retzius bend down under the bottom of the pits, which may have an area of hypocalcified enamel at this point.[80]

Pitted hypoplastic amelogenesis imperfecta is inherited as an autosomal dominant trait. Male-to-male transmission has been observed in kindreds. This is a moderately well-defined entity with sporadic cases occurring. Cases and families that represent this condition are those of Darling (group 1, Fig. 5 1a, 1b),[35] Hals, 1958, same cases 1962 (family 1),[79, 80] Rushton (Fig. 3),[138] Winter (Figs. 5 and 6),[168] and Schulze[148] (type IIf). Possible cases are those of Weyman[165] (sporadic, no history in family) and Toller[160] (case 1).

Autosomal dominant local hypoplastic amelogenesis imperfecta. In autosomal dominant local hypoplastic amelogenesis imperfecta, the hypoplastic defect is a horizontal row of pits, linear depressions, or one large hypoplastic area in the enamel with hypocalcification of the enamel adjacent to and below the hypoplastic area (Fig. 7-3). These defects appear most prominent on the buccal

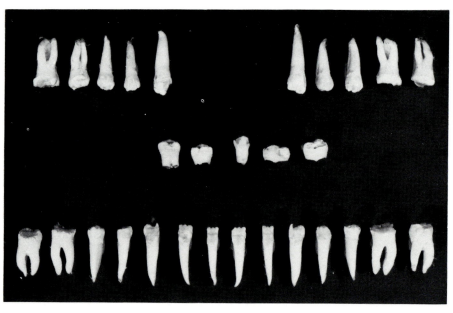

Fig. 7-3. Teeth extracted from patient with autosomal dominant local hypoplastic amelogenesis imperfecta illustrating horizontal nature of lesion affecting primarily middle third of buccal surface of both primary and secondary teeth. (Courtesy Dr. R. A. Vickers, Minneapolis, Minn.; from Witkop, C. J., Jr., and Rao, S.: Birth Defects **7**[7]:153-184, 1971.)

surfaces of the teeth involving the middle third of the enamel, although in some the lesion is placed more incisally or occlusally and the lingual aspect may be involved (Fig. 7-4). The incisal edge or occlusal surface is usually not involved. Only primary teeth or teeth in both dentitions may be involved. All teeth may be affected, but individuals within affected kindreds usually show a variation in the number of teeth affected and in the severity of the lesion. The pattern does not correspond with specific time in development of the teeth as seen in tetracycline or other environmental insults. Changes are most consistently found on the buccal surfaces of primary molars and bicuspids. In mildly affected adults, the lesion may be represented only by minor defects and hypocalcified areas in the middle third of the buccal and to a lesser extent lingual enamel (Fig. 7-4).

Histologically, the enamel shows defects in the buccal and lingual enamel (Fig. 7-5). The defective enamel shows a combination of hypoplastic and hypomaturation alterations. The enamel rods are disoriented, course in twisted patterns, show a bending of incremental lines toward the dentinoenamel junction, and show void defects in the prism sheath area and occasionally within the enamel rods. This latter feature resembles the defect in the hypomaturation forms of amelogenesis imperfecta. Figs. 7-6 and 7-7 are SEM photomicrographs through the defective area. The surface of the enamel has small pits that are similar to those seen in developing normal enamel and represent the impressions of

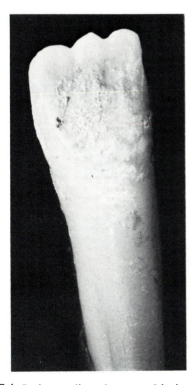

Fig. 7-4. Lesion on lingual aspect of incisor tooth affects enamel on middle third of crown. This tooth also illustrates that this disorder may have hypomature enamel as well as hypoplastic features. (Courtesy Dr. R. A. Vickers, Minneapolis, Minn.)

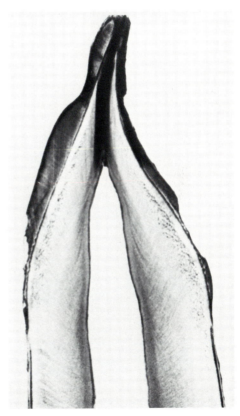

Fig. 7-5. Ground section of incisor tooth from patient with local hypoplastic amelogenesis imperfecta demonstrates localization of lesion to buccal and lingual aspects of middle portion of crown. (×10.) (From Sauk, J. J., Vickers, R. A., Copeland, J. S., and Lyon, H. W.: Oral Surg. **34**:60, 1972.)

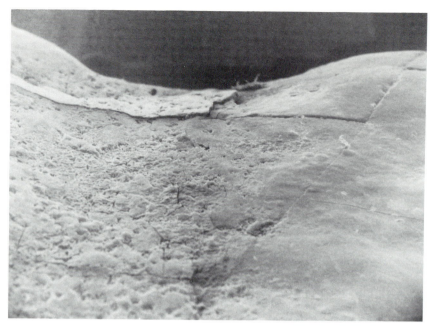

Fig. 7-6. Low magnification of hypoplastic area on surface of enamel. Pits and craters vary in size from size of small pits seen in developing enamel to deep craters and are dispersed throughout areas of more normal-appearing enamel. Peripheral to central area are smooth, unaffected zones of normal enamel. (×55; tilt angle 45 degrees.) (From Sauk, J. J., Vickers, R. A., Copeland, J. S., and Lyon, H. W.: Oral Surg. **34:**60, 1972.)

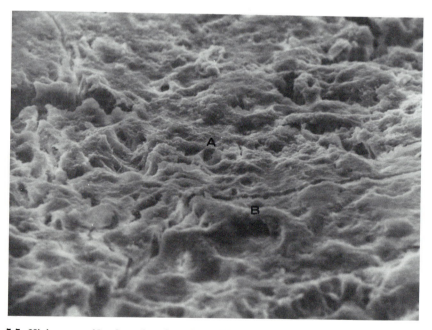

Fig. 7-7. Higher magnification of surface defect illustrated in Fig. 7-6 demonstrates two types of depressions. At *A,* small pit is seen similar in size and shape to that seen on surface of developing normal enamel, and at *B,* crater possibly represents local failure of group of ameloblasts or vascular defect. (×550; tilt angle 45 degrees.) (From Sauk, J. J., Vickers, R. A., Copeland, J. S., and Lyon, H. W.: Oral Surg. **34:**60, 1972.)

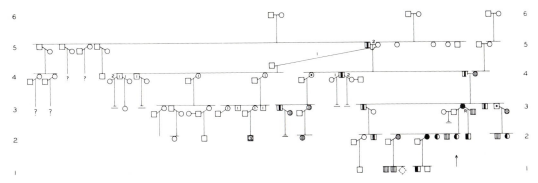

Fig. 7-8. Kindred of local hypoplastic amelogenesis imperfecta. Half-shaded symbols indicate primary dentition affected and secondary dentition unerupted. Vertical-lined symbols are persons personally examined without trait. (From Witkop, C. J., Jr.: Genetic diseases of the oral cavity. In Tiecke, R. W.: Oral pathology, New York, 1965, McGraw-Hill Book Co. Copyright 1965; used with permission of McGraw-Hill Book Co.)

Tomes' processes. In addition, there are larger pits and deep craters throughout the area (Fig. 7-7). There is also a disorder in the enamel prisms similar to that seen in the hypomaturation forms of amelogenesis imperfecta. Electron probe data indicate that the enamel below the hypoplastic defect has two distinct layers of enamel that differ in their mineralization. Enamel adjacent to the dentinoenamel junction has a mineral content more closely approximating normal enamel, whereas that in the outer segment approaches the mineral content of hypomature enamel. The mineral content in weight percent of normal enamel averaged over a 10 nm zone was found by Sauk and associates[144] to be 31.13 ± 0.91 calcium, 17.15 ± 0.67 phosphorus, and a Ca:P ratio of 2.04 ± 0.45; outer zone enamel had 29.71 ± 1.11 calcium, 13.01 ± 0.91 phosphorus, and a Ca:P ratio of 1.89 ± 0.67.

Examples of this condition have been reported by Witkop[173, 176] (Fig. 7-8), Sauk and associates,[144] and probably some cases of Darling.[35]

Autosomal dominant smooth hypoplastic amelogenesis imperfecta. In autosomal dominant smooth hypoplastic amelogenesis imperfecta, the enamel is thin, hard, and glossy with a smooth surface (Fig. 7-9). The enamel of newly erupted teeth is yellow. The color of erupted teeth may vary from an opaque

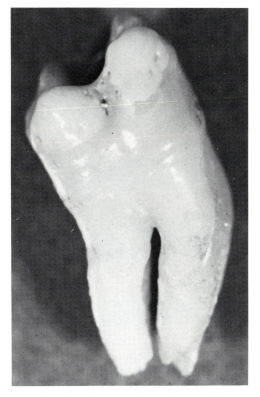

Fig. 7-9. Tooth from patient with smooth hypoplastic amelogenesis imperfecta showing thin, shiny, smooth, clinically hard enamel.

white to a translucent brown hue. The enamel is approximately a fourth to an eighth of the normal thickness, giving the appearance of teeth prepared for jacket crowns. The teeth do not meet at the contact points. Some of the enamel may be missing on newly erupted teeth, especially on the incisal or occlusal third, and it may be chalky in the interproximal areas (Fig. 7-10). Some of these are due to resorption of the enamel before eruption, since in this condition delay and failure of eruption of teeth occur with resorption of the teeth in the alveolus. Some teeth may be congenitally absent.

On radiographs (Fig. 7-11), the enamel appears missing or is represented by a faint, narrow, radiodense outline of the crown. Pulpal calcifications may be present in both erupted and unerupted teeth. Multiple teeth may undergo resorption within the alveolus.

Sections of the impacted teeth undergoing resorption within the alveolus show areas of resorption of the tooth structure and deposition of osteodentin and osteoid. Remnants of enamel organ are present over the partially resorbed teeth and may undergo cystic degeneration in some cases. Unerupted teeth may have deposition of cementum over the enamel (Fig. 7-12). In some impacted teeth, cementum may cover the enamel entirely. Adjacent to unerupted teeth are found remnants of odontogenic epithelium with small round calcified bodies, which Weinmann and associates[162] called *enameloid conglomerates* but which may include cementoid bodies. These are seen in many other types of tooth defects associated with disturbances in tooth development. They are most frequently seen in several types of amelogenesis imperfecta, odontodysplasia, congenitally missing teeth in which there is some attempt at tooth formation with odontogenic remnants, and impacted dens in dente. Histological sections show three major features. Most consistently found are short enamel rods. Ground sections show that the enamel rods have thick prominent enamel rod sheaths, seen best in polarized light.[47] Some areas of enamel are covered with a structureless horizontally oriented laminated calcified layer up to 1 mm in thickness. This layer may be covered by a prominent hyalinized enamel cuticle containing cell remnants. Microradiographs show normal contrast between enamel and dentin, suggesting that the calcification of the enamel approaches normal (Fig. 7-13). Although the

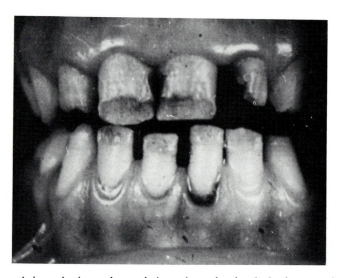

Fig. 7-10. Smooth hypoplastic amelogenesis imperfecta showing lack of contact between teeth. Gross pitting seen on incisal areas is from resorption of enamel before eruption. (From Weinmann, J. P., Svoboda, J. F., and Woods, R. W.: J. Am. Dent. Assoc. **32:**397, 1945. Copyright by the American Dental Association. Reprinted by permission.)

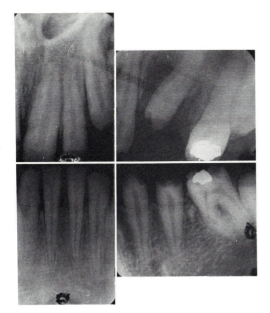

Fig. 7-11. Radiographs of patient with autosomal dominant smooth type of amelogenesis imperfecta showing thin enamel on all teeth and unerupted teeth. In many areas enamel layer cannot be distinguished on radiograph. (Courtesy Dr. Joseph P. Weinmann.)

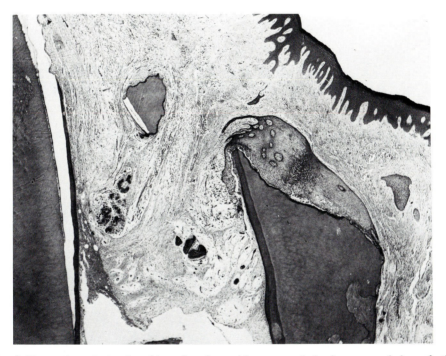

Fig. 7-12. Section of alveolar ridge of patient with autosomal dominant smooth hypoplastic amelogenesis imperfecta demonstrating remnants of two unerupted teeth. Note layer of cementum covering space occupied by thin layer of enamel on tooth at left. Small foci of odontogenic elements in center of photomicrograph contain small calcified bodies. Tooth on right is covered with remnants of odontogenic epithelium, and crown has been nearly completely resorbed. (From Weinmann, J. P., Svoboda, J. F., and Woods, R. W.: J. Am. Dent. Assoc. **32:**397, 1945. Copyright by the American Dental Association. Reprinted by permission.)

histological sections show a laminated structureless enamel surface in many areas, some areas are not covered with this layer. SEM photomicrographs may show both perikymata and imbrication lines usually associated with normally formed enamel (Fig. 7-14).

The condition is inherited as an autosomal dominant trait with high penetrance and has been reported in large well-documented kindreds. Similar reported cases are those of Weinmann and associates[162] (family D), Darling[35] (group 3), Erpenstein and Wannen-

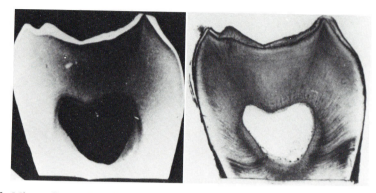

Fig. 7-13. Microradiograph on left shows normal contrast between enamel and dentin. Compare with ground section photographed with transmitted light on right. (×10.) (From Weinmann, J. P., Svoboda, J. F., and Woods, R. W.: J. Am. Dent. Assoc. **32:**397, 1945. Copyright by the American Dental Association. Reprinted by permission.)

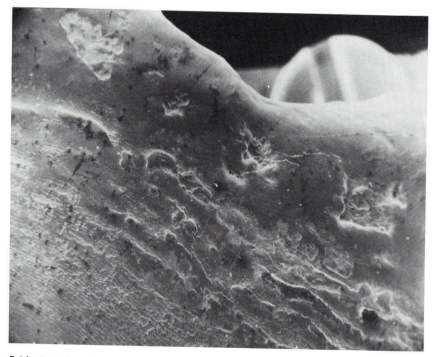

Fig. 7-14. Scanning electron photomicrograph of surface of enamel on cusp of tooth from patient with smooth hypoplastic amelogenesis imperfecta showing perikymata similar to those seen on normal enamel. (×24.)

macher,[47] Prince and Lilly,[124] Witkop and Sauk,[186] Burzynski and co-workers,[24] and possibly that of Wennstrom.[163]

Autosomal dominant rough hypoplastic amelogenesis imperfecta. In autosomal dominant rough hypoplastic amelogenesis imperfecta, the enamel is hard with a rough, granular surface. It may chip from the underlying dentin rather than abrade away as seen in the smooth type. The teeth are white to yellow-white in color when newly erupted and are not as subject to attrition as those with the smooth form (Fig. 7-15). The enamel is a fourth to an eighth normal thickness, resulting in teeth that appear to have been prepared for jacket crowns. An occasional tooth may have thicker enamel at the cervical aspect. The teeth do not meet at the contact points but retain more of the normal outline of a tooth in contrast to the smooth form, in which the teeth have more nearly paralleled sides without the normal mesial and distal bulges. Both primary and secondary teeth are affected in this condition.

Radiographically, there is a thin but distinct line of enamel covering the teeth, which contrasts well from the dentin (Fig. 7-16). In contrast to the smooth form, impacted and partly resorbed teeth are less frequently seen in this type of defect but do occur.

Histological sections show two main types of defects. Most prominent and frequently seen is a complete absence of enamel with definite rod structure, most of the enamel consisting of a horizontal, laminated, highly calcified structure in which only a few faint, vertically arranged structures are seen, which may be attempts at rod formation. The dentinoenamel junction below this type of enamel is flat without scallops. Where the enamel is thicker, there are prominent large peaks in the dentinoenamel junction. The overlying enamel consists of rods running in various directions as seen in gnarled enamel (Fig. 7-17). The lines of Retzius are markedly distorted. The Hunter-Schreger bands are accentuated (Fig. 7-18). This type of enamel may be covered with a lamellar type of structure in which only faint impressions of rods are discernible or distorted rods extend to the surface, which shows minute depressions.

This condition is inherited as an autosomal dominant trait. Similar cases are those of Rushton,[134, 138] Darling[35] (one case from Rushton in group 3), Witkop[173, 176] (Fig. 32-23), Hals[79, 80] (family 2), Finn,[50] and prob-

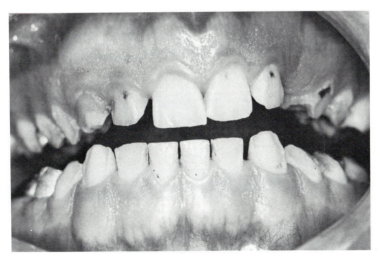

Fig. 7-15. Rough hypoplastic amelogenesis imperfecta showing lack of contact between teeth having granular vitreous enamel surface. Hypocalcified areas seen in smooth hypoplastic type are not seen. (From Witkop, C. J., Jr.: Genetic diseases of the oral cavity. In Tiecke, R. W.: Oral pathology, New York, 1965, McGraw-Hill Book Co. Copyright 1965; used with permission of McGraw-Hill Book Co.)

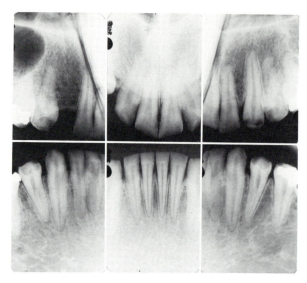

Fig. 7-16. Radiographs of patient in Fig. 7-15 with rough hypoplastic amelogenesis imperfecta. Only a thin layer of radiodense enamel can be seen outlining crowns. (From Witkop, C. J., Jr.: Genetic diseases of the oral cavity. In Tiecke, R. W.: Oral pathology, New York, 1965, McGraw-Hill Book Co. Copyright 1965; used with permission of McGraw-Hill Book Co.)

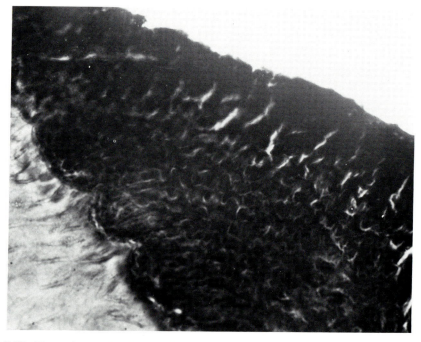

Fig. 7-17. Photomicrograph of ground section through gnarled enamel area adjacent to prominent peaks in dentinoenamel junction. Note disorientation and short atypical enamel rods. (×20; ground section, trichrome stain.)

ably those of Kinase[89] and Fischman and Fischman.[51] Previous classification of the case of Prince and Lilly[124] as rough type is an error (Witkop and Sauk).[186]

Autosomal recessive rough amelogenesis

imperfecta (**enamel agenesis**). In enamel agenesis, the teeth, when newly erupted, have a distinct yellow color like that of normal dentin. The surface is rough and granular, resembling ground glass (Fig. 7-19). There

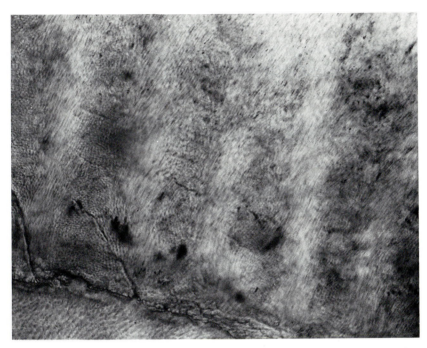

Fig. 7-18. Photomicrograph of ground section through more normal-appearing area of enamel over flat dentinoenamel junction. Note prominent Hunter-Schreger bands, which are not usually seen under transmitted light by which specimen was photographed. (×100; ground section, unstained.)

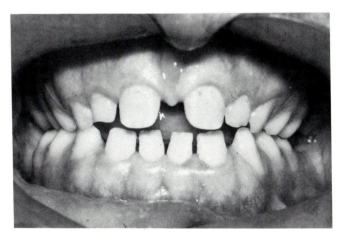

Fig. 7-19. Autosomal recessive hypoplastic amelogenesis imperfecta (enamel agenesis). Teeth do not meet at contact points, are yellowish brown in color, and have little clinical evidence of enamel formation.

is nearly complete lack of any enamel formation detectable clinically or on radiographs. The teeth are widely spaced and do not meet at the contact points. All patients seen with this form of enamel defect have had anterior open bite. Numerous teeth are missing in the erupted dentition and are represented in the radiographs as unerupted teeth undergoing resorption. Both dentitions are affected.

Radiographs show no evidence of enamel (Fig. 7-20). Many permanent teeth remain impacted and undergo partial resorption within the alveolus. The teeth have normal-appearing roots and pulp chambers. Serial ground sections of both erupted and unerupted teeth show a flat dentinoenamel junction and normal dentin except in resorbed teeth, in which masses of tertiary dentin form apically from the resorption processes in the crown. The surface of the dentin in many areas of both erupted and unerupted teeth has no enamel (Fig. 7-21). Other areas of the impacted teeth are covered by a layer of calcified cuticle with fragments of atypical enamel organ remnants arranged in a cystic pattern around the crown. Small, round calci-fied bodies may be present in the enamel epithelium. In other areas on erupted teeth, the dentin is covered by a hard, granular, vitreous lamellar layer of calcified globular material (Fig. 7-22) or lamellar vitreous material resembling the lamellar layers seen in sections of agates (Fig. 7-23). This layer is about 7 μm thick at the thickest point (Figs. 7-22 and 7-23). The lamellar enamel layer is covered by remnants of cuticular material, which stain red in Masson's trichrome stain.

This is a rare form of amelogenesis imperfecta. Only two families with this condition have been observed by the authors. In one family, the affected individuals were identical twin boys who had four normal sibs and normal parents. No consanguinity was known within two generations. Ancestors of both parents came from the same village in Yugoslavia, however. The other family had one affected girl and a normal brother. There were no other affected relatives in the kindred and no known consanguinity. The patient described by Frank and Bolender[55] possibly represents another example of this condition. The patient of Catena and associates[27] had a

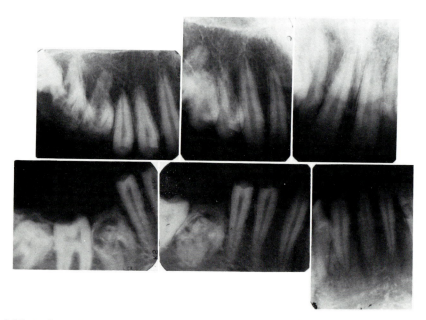

Fig. 7-20. Radiographs of patient with autosomal recessive hypoplastic amelogenesis imperfecta show no discernible enamel on erupted and unerupted teeth. Crowns of many unerupted teeth are being resorbed within alveolus.

similar enamel defect but also dry, wrinkled skin and an inability to close her eyelids.

X-linked (dominant) smooth hypoplastic amelogenesis imperfecta. The clinical appearance of the enamel in males hemizygous for the trait is different from the appearance of the enamel in females heterozygous for the defect. Primary and secondary teeth are affected in both sexes. In males, the enamel is smooth, shiny, thin, and yellow-brown (Fig. 7-24). Teeth do not meet at the contact points. Occlusal and incisal abrasion is

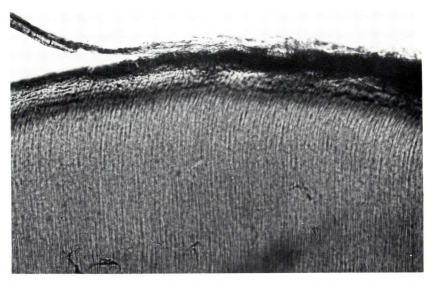

Fig. 7-21. Photomicrograph of ground section of unerupted unresorbed tooth from patient with autosomal recessive hypoplastic amelogenesis imperfecta through area devoid of any structure resembling enamel. Only a thin layer of laminated material resembling calcified enamel cuticle covers dentin. Line of dentinoenamel junction lacks scallops. (×200; ground section.)

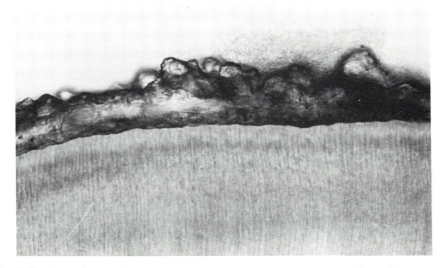

Fig. 7-22. Photomicrograph of ground section of erupted tooth from patient with autosomal recessive hypoplastic amelogenesis imperfecta through area covered by globular vitreous material having no structures resembling normal enamel rods. (×240; ground section, unstained.)

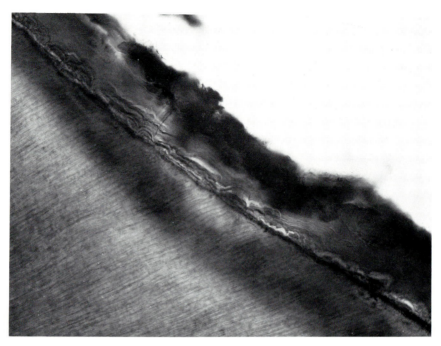

Fig. 7-23. Photomicrograph of dentin and enamel through area of erupted tooth from patient with autosomal recessive hypoplastic amelogenesis imperfecta. Dentinoenamel junction is flat, and enamel is represented by layers of calcified material resembling agate. (×240; ground section, Masson's trichrome stain.)

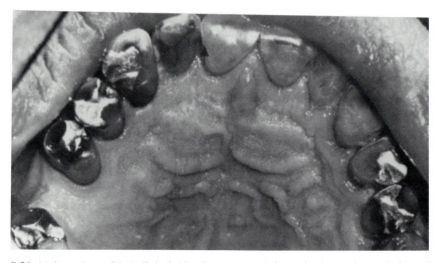

Fig. 7-24. Male patient with X-linked (dominant) smooth hypoplastic amelogenesis imperfecta has thin enamel that can be noted, *arrow,* in areas of attrition on anterior teeth. Surface of enamel is smooth and shiny. (From Berkman, M. D., and Singer, A.: Birth Defects 7[7]:204-209, 1971.)

marked in adults. On radiographs, males show a thin outline of enamel over the teeth that contrasts fairly well from the dentin (Fig. 7-25). Other structures appear normal. In females the trait is expressed as alternating vertical bands of enamel of nearly normal thickness interspersed with bands of hypoplastic enamel (Fig. 7-26). Occasionally, dentin may be visible in the bottoms of the hypoplastic grooves. The vertical bands are randomly distributed and are of varying widths. There is no symmetry in the patterns on homologous teeth from the right and left arches. Even in females, many teeth do not always meet at the contact points. These bands can be seen in radiographs and are especially prominent in anterior teeth (Fig. 7-27). An occasional af-

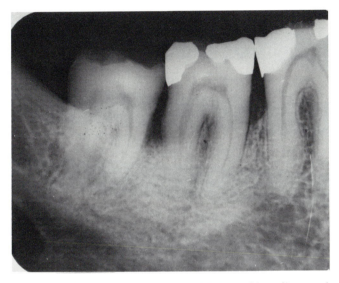

Fig. 7-25. Radiograph of male patient seen in Fig. 7-24 shows thin radiopaque layer of enamel of normal radiodensity. (From Berkman, M. D., and Singer, A.: Birth Defects **7**[7]:204-209, 1971.)

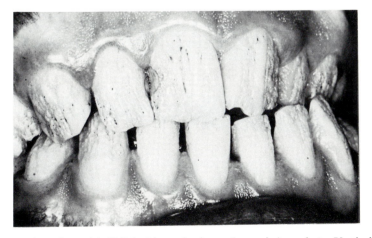

Fig. 7-26. Female patient with X-linked hypoplastic amelogenesis imperfecta. Vertical bands of hypoplastic enamel and enamel approaching normal thickness are seen arranged in random pattern over teeth. Note lack of symmetry of bands on homologous teeth in right and left arch. (From Rushton, M. A.: Proc. R. Soc. Med. **57**:53, 1964.)

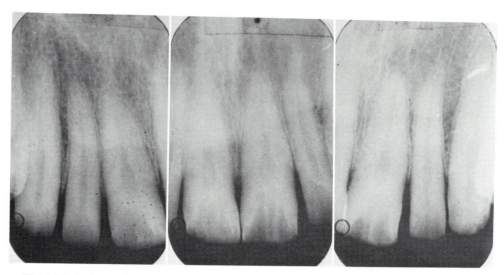

Fig. 7-27. Radiographs of female patient with X-linked smooth hypoplastic amelogenesis imperfecta demonstrating appearance of vertical bands of hypoplastic and more normal enamel. (From Berkman, M. D., and Singer, A.: Birth Defects **7**[7]:204-209, 1971.)

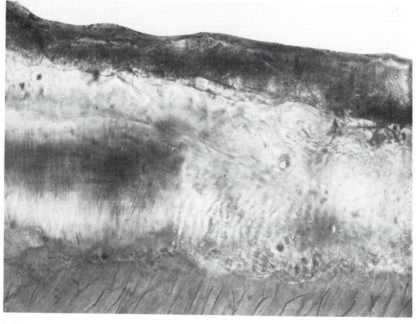

Fig. 7-28. Photomicrograph of ground section of male patient with X-linked hypoplastic amelogenesis imperfecta. Three areas of different appearance are seen. At left, enamel rods are indistinct and appear fused. At right, short enamel rods can be distinguished with incremental lines of decreased width. Glasslike structureless material covers surface. Reduced number of scallops but with accentuated peaks are seen at dentinoenamel junction. (From Schulze, C.: Dtsch. Zahn. Mund. Kieferheilkd. **16**:108, 1952.)

fected female may show a tooth or teeth that have nearly all hypoplastic enamel, but in other females a tooth or teeth may be nearly normal. As in many forms of amelogenesis imperfecta, anterior open bite is a frequent associated finding but varies within kindreds.

The histological appearance of the enamel in males shows a variable pattern from different areas. Overall, the enamel is reduced to from an eighth to a fourth normal thickness. The dentinoenamel junction is usually scalloped but with occasional exaggerated peaks. In some areas, the enamel has a homogeneous appearance in which the enamel rods are indistinct and appear fused (Fig. 7-28, *left*), and in other areas the rod structure can be discerned with reduction in the distance between enamel rod incremental lines (Fig. 7-28, *right*). A vitreous structureless layer covers the surface of these shortened rods.

This condition is inherited as an X-linked trait, with females showing vertical banding of hypoplastic and normal enamel consistent with the Lyonization effect of genes on the X chromosome in heterozygous females (see discussion of Lyonization under "X-linked hypomaturation amelogenesis imperfecta") (Fig. 7-29). Numerous examples of this condition have been reported by Zahn,[189] Fish,[52] Schulze[145-148] (types IIa, b, c), Darling[35] (group 2), Rushton,[138] Weyers[164] (same cases as Schulze), and Berkman and Singer.[12] Possible cases are those of Spokes[156] and Haldane.[77]

Hypomaturation amelogenesis imperfecta

The hypomaturation forms of amelogenesis imperfecta are characterized clinically by enamel that has a mottled brown-yellow-white appearance and is generally of normal thickness such that teeth meet at contact points. The enamel is softer than normal and tends to chip from the dentin. The enamel approaches the radiodensity of dentin.

Autosomal dominant hypomaturation-hypoplastic amelogenesis imperfecta with taurodontism. Winter and co-workers[172] described a large kindred in which hypomaturation-hypoplastic enamel and taurodontism was inherited as an autosomal dominant trait. They believed that the condition as seen in this family was a unique trait and was distinguishable from the trichodentoosseous syndrome in that none of the affected family members demonstrated nail defects, tightly curly hair or sclerosteosis, which are found in the syndrome in addition to the enamel and taurodontic defect.[169] Winter[169] has also encountered additional families who have the enamel and taurodontic defect but without the other features of the trichodentoosseous syndrome. Gulmen[74] has examined a family in which some members have all features of the trichodentoosseous syndrome and other affected members have only the enamel and taurodontic defects. Some affected individuals in the kindred had tightly curly hair in infancy and childhood but did not show this feature by early adulthood. The nail and bone defect in trichodentoosseous syndrome

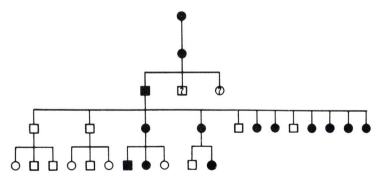

Fig. 7-29. Kindred of X-linked smooth hypoplastic amelogenesis imperfecta demonstrating that trait is passed from affected men to all of their daughters but none of their sons. (Modified from Haldane, J. B. S.: J. Hered. **28**:58, 1937.)

is not a consistent finding, probably affecting from 30% to 50% of affected patients.[99]

There is possibly a separate autosomal dominantly inherited defect consisting of hypomaturation-hypoplastic enamel defect and taurodontism. However, in light of the kindreds of Lichtenstein and co-workers[99] and Gulmen,[74] the cases may represent variations in expressivity of the trichodentoosseous syndrome. The findings will be described in detail in the section on that syndrome.

X-linked (recessive) hypomaturation amelogenesis imperfecta. In X-linked hypomaturation amelogenesis imperfecta, both the primary and secondary teeth are affected, but with a different clinical appearance of the primary and secondary teeth in males and a difference in the appearance of the teeth in males and females.

The most striking defect is found in affected males. The permanent teeth are a mottled yellow-white color but may darken with adsorption of stains with age (Fig. 7-30). The enamel approaches normal thickness, but occasionally in severely affected males there is a slightly reduced thickness to the enamel. However, in most cases the teeth meet at the contact points and have a normal contour. The enamel at the cervical aspect of tooth crowns tends to be better formed. The enamel is softer than normal, and the point of an explorer can be forced into the surface. Although these teeth chip and abrade more easily than normal teeth, the loss of enamel does not proceed as rapidly as that seen in the hypocalcified forms. The primary teeth of affected males have a ground glass opaque white appearance. An occasional patient shows a slight yellow cast to the enamel of primary teeth. The color of enamel in primary teeth can best be described as an opaque white with translucent white mottling. The surface is moderately smooth. It is not shiny smooth as seen in the smooth hypoplastic forms or rough and granular as seen in the rough hypoplastic forms but approaches that of normal teeth.

In females, both the primary and permanent teeth show alternating vertical bands of white opaque enamel and normal translucent enamel (Fig. 7-31). These bands vary in width and are randomly distributed over the crown. There is no symmetry in homologous teeth from the right and left sides of the arch. Transillumination may aid in demonstrating these bands in the enamel. They may

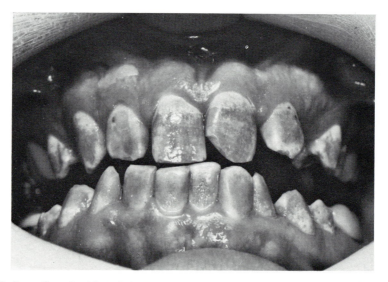

Fig. 7-30. Boy affected with X-linked hypomaturation amelogenesis imperfecta shows mottled yellowish white appearance to enamel that tends to chip from crowns. (From Witkop, C. J., Jr.: Oral Surg. **23:**174, 1967.)

be difficult to photograph, being essentially a contrast of opaque white with translucent white. Fig. 7-32 is a camera lucida projection of the teeth of an affected female with an overlay tracing of the defective enamel bands.

Radiographs of the teeth of affected males show approximately the same radiodensity of enamel and dentin. We have been unable to demonstrate a banding appearance in the radiographs of teeth from affected females.

Histologically, the ground sections of teeth from affected males show a striking defect occupying primarily the outer half of the enamel (Fig. 7-33). The enamel adjacent to the normally scalloped dentinoenamel junction may closely approximate the structure of

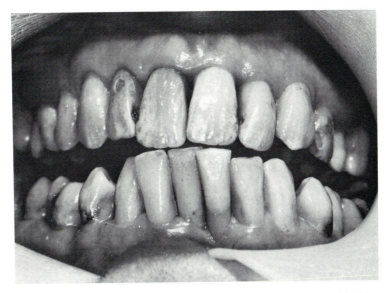

Fig. 7-31. Mother of boy illustrated in Fig. 7-30. Women heterozygous for X-linked hypomaturation amelogenesis imperfecta show vertical bands of opaque white and translucent normal-appearing enamel as best seen on patient's right maxillary central incisor. (From Witkop, C. J., Jr.: Oral Surg. **23**:174, 1967.)

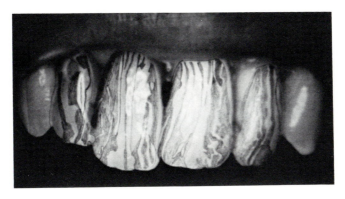

Fig. 7-32. Camera lucida tracing of hypomature enamel bands (dark) and normal translucent enamel (light) of woman heterozygous for X-linked hypomaturation amelogenesis imperfecta. Note lack of symmetry of vertical bands on homologous teeth from right and left sides of arch as expected of Lyonizing defect on X chromosome. (From Witkop, C. J., Jr.: Oral Surg. **23**: 174, 1967.)

normal enamel. The midportion or outer portion of the enamel shows a striking defect in nearly all enamel rod sheaths in this area. The enamel rod sheaths may be entirely lacking, filled with pigmented derbris or with an eosinophilic staining (hemotoxylin and eosin or Masson's trichrome) material.

In the ground sections, these prismatic sheath defects may enlarge and cross the rod itself, forming structures resembling an exclamation mark (Fig. 7-34). Some of these spaces fuse with spaces from adjacent rod sheath areas, obliterating several rods. These structures appear to be spaces in the prism sheath area. Toward the outer midhalf of the enamel, they obliterate the rod structure. A reversion to more nearly normal conditions

prevails at the surface, with fewer of the rods showing interprismatic defects. The Hunter-Schreger band effect is disrupted. In carefully decalcified sections, the rod sheath area may be observed filled with an eosinophilic material on Masson's trichrome stain, resembling the thixotropic gel found in the ends of developing ameloblasts in normal amelogenesis.

Scanning electron micrographs of this type of enamel indicate that a fibrillar type of enamel is found. The interprismatic area is reduced or absent, and a fibrous-appearing enamel rod remains (Fig. 7-35). Scanning sections throughout the thickness of the enamel show that normal-appearing enamel prisms and interprismatic enamel are found primarily in the first 1 to 2 mm of enamel

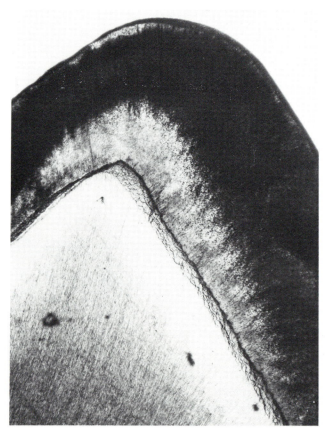

Fig. 7-33. Ground section of tooth from boy affected with X-linked hypomaturation amelogenesis imperfecta illustrating low-powered view of cusp with most severe defect involving outer portion of enamel. Dentinoenamel junction is normally scalloped. (×20; ground section, unstained.)

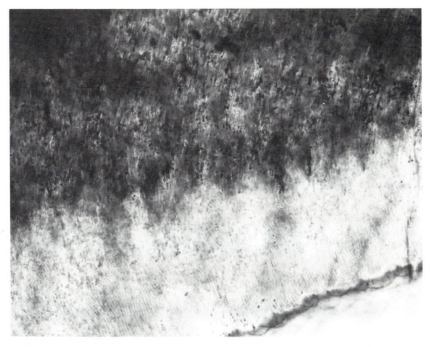

Fig. 7-34. Unstained ground section through enamel of boy with X-linked hypomaturation amelogenesis imperfecta. Rod sheath areas contain spaces filled with stained material. (×200.)

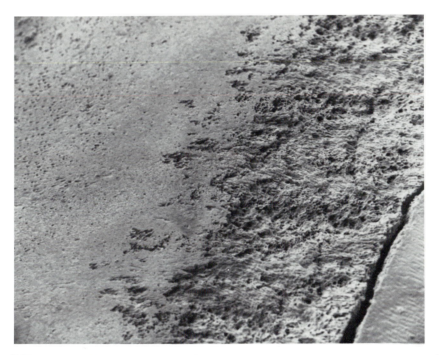

Fig. 7-35. Scanning electron-microscopic view of cut surface of enamel from tooth of boy with X-linked hypomaturation amelogenesis imperfecta. Specimen has been polished and etched. Area of low mineral content on left does not etch as rapidly as area of higher mineral content adjacent to dentinoenamel junction on right. Spaces and holes in left part of specimen occur primarily in rod sheath area. (×110; ground section, polished and etched.)

adjacent to the dentin. The surface of the enamel is porous, allowing entrance into the enamel of oral fluids and stains (Fig. 7-36), but the teeth are not prone to decay.

Histological and ultrastructural observations of the enamel from females heterozygous for this defect show that their teeth have two distinct forms of enamel occurring in vertically arranged bands. One type of band contains enamel rods structurally resembling those of normal enamel, and the other bands have enamel structurally resembling that seen in affected males. Enamel from heterozygous females appears marbled on scanning at low magnification, which correlates with the vertical stripes seen in the clinical photograph. The marbled areas clearly demonstrate two zones of different enamel (Fig. 7-37). These zones also differ in calcium and phosphorous content and suggest that enamel from heterozygous females is composed of two gene products, one similar to the mutant enamel of affected males and the other having the

same mineral content as enamel from normal males. Sauk and associates[143] used an electron probe scan to compare the area encompassing bands of normal and abnormal enamel in a heterozygous female's teeth with the enamel of her affected son and a normal male. As the probe moved across areas in the mother's enamel clinically resembling the enamel of normal males, the probe analysis of calcium and phosphorous content of this area was identical to that of the normal male control. When the probe approached those areas which in the SEM photographs resembled those of her affected son's enamel, the values of calcium and phosphorous dropped, approaching those obtained for the enamel of the son (Fig. 7-38). These results are interpreted to indicate that the mother has two types of genetically determined enamel, one type being normal and the other similar to the mutant enamel possessed by her son.

The basic biochemical defect is unknown in this disorder. The mineral content is less

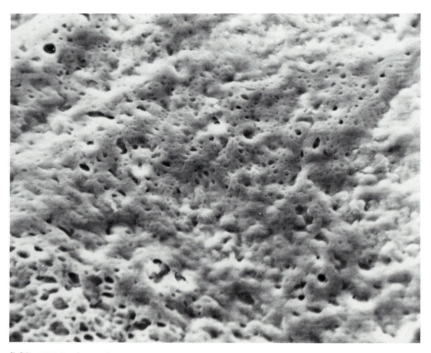

Fig. 7-36. SEM photomicrograph of surface of enamel of tooth from boy with X-linked amelogenesis imperfecta shows porous nature of enamel. This probably explains why these teeth darken with age, since this enamel could be penetrated by oral stains. Despite this porosity, which is also seen in autosomal recessive form, these teeth are not prone to decay. (×2200.)

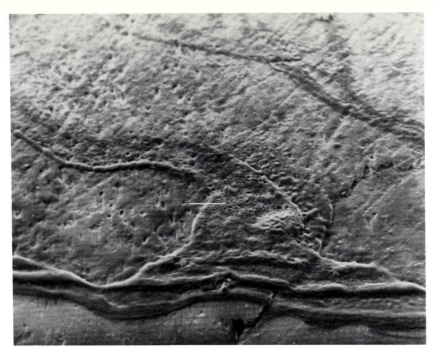

Fig. 7-37. SEM photomicrograph of surface enamel of tooth from woman heterozygous for X-linked hypomaturation amelogenesis. Band of hypomature enamel courses left to center, through surrounding more normal-appearing enamel. Note porous nature of enamel in band similar to that seen in all of enamel of her son in Fig. 7-36. Line on photograph represents approximate tract in comparable polished sections of electron probe used to analyze mineral content of normal and hypomature enamel as seen in Fig. 7-38.

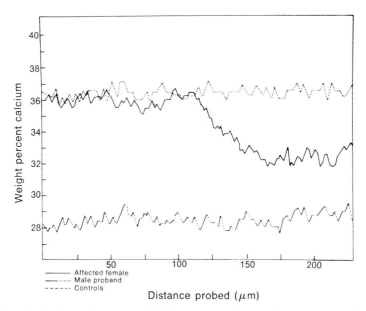

Fig. 7-38. Levels of calcium in comparable 225 μm scan of enamel from normal male (control), affected male, and across two zones (Fig. 7-37) of differing enamel in affected female. Scan across enamel of heterozygous female is like that of normal male until area of enamel resembling that of her affected son is approached, where it then drops toward levels seen in her son's enamel. (From Sauk, J. J., Lyon, H. W., and Witkop, C. J., Jr.: Am. J. Hum. Genet. **24:** 267, 1972.)

Table 7-1. Electron-microprobe data for calcium and phosphorous*

	Weight percent		
	Calcium	*Phosphorus*	*Ca/P*
Affected male	29.74 ± 0.35	14.30 ± 0.10	2.08 ± 0.04
Control (naval recruits)	36.16 ± 0.55	17.33 ± 0.26	2.08 ± 0.01
Heterozygous female (normal area)	35.94 ± 0.35	16.08 ± 0.20	2.15 ± 0.05
Heterozygous female (mottled area)	32.96 ± 0.58	15.24 ± 0.23	2.09 ± 0.03

*From Sauk, J. J., Jr., Lyon, H. W., and Witkop, C. J., Jr.: Electron optic microanalysis of two gene products in enamel of females heterozygous for X-linked hypomaturation amelogenesis imperfecta, Am. J. Hum. Genet. **24:**267, 1972.
The ± values indicate standard deviation from the mean.

than that seen in normal teeth (Table 7-1). However, an analogy with the development of normal enamel leads to the speculation that the defect may involve the resorption of thixotropic gel from the periphery of the calcifying rod back into Tomes' process. Boyde,[13] in an ultrastructural study of enamel, demonstrated that the enamel rod sheaths are composed of the same materials as the prisms, the main difference being one of a different orientation of crystallites. Crystallites are laid down parallel to the end of Tomes' process. This arrangement of developing crystals is a partial sphere, the crystallites at the periphery constituting the enamel rod sheath having an orientation different from those in the prisms. The latter are parallel to long axis of the prism, and those at the periphery are short, comprising the enamel rod sheath in the fully formed enamel.

It is in the rod sheath area that most of the remobilization of the organic matrix gel back into Tomes' process of the ameloblast occurs. This sequence Boyde describes as "maturation."

The higher concentration of organic material at the prism sheaths of adult enamel is presumably acquired during "maturation," via the remobilization of the organic matrix gel. The pressure gradient causing this movement of thixotropic gel (Eastoe[43]) must force it parallel with the crystal direction and back toward the ameloblasts. The accumulation of more organic matrix at the prism boundaries is thus simply explained because this is the only region at which crystallites end and because the more imperfect packing of crystallites at this plane, where the orientation on either side is different (from adjacent sheaths), causes the existence of more spaces which are not filled with crystalline material.*

If one accepts this process as that of maturation, then the type of defect seen in the hypomaturation forms of amelogenesis imperfecta and in opaque white spots is compatible with a defect in this stage of calcification. The fact that there is a mutation causing accumulation of large amounts of organic material in spaces normally occupied by the rod sheath suggests that the mutation interferes with the remobilization of the gel and further suggests that maturation is under a genetic control mechanism that is distinct and separate from the process of calcification.

Genetic investigations of several families by Witkop[179] and by McLarty and co-workers[113] show that only males have the mottled yellow-brown teeth, whereas females have vertically striped teeth. If the trait in question is designated as mottled yellow teeth, then this inheritance pattern is compatible with an X-linked recessive mode of inheritance. However, heterozygous females show some aspects of the defect, having vertically striped teeth (Fig. 7-39). This feature is similar to that seen in obligate heterozygous females in the X-linked dominant hypoplastic amelogenesis imperfecta kindreds.

An explanation for this type of vertical banding of two distinct types of enamel in

*From Boyde, A.: The development of enamel structure, Proc. R. Soc. Med. (Odontol.) **60:**923, 1967.

females can be deduced from what is proposed as the mode of action of the X chromosomes in females. In 1961, Lyon[102] advanced the hypothesis that in females only one X chromosome per somatic cell is genetically active during interphase. The other X chromosome, represented by the Barr body (sex-chromatin body), retains its heterochromatic properties and hence is probably inactive. The hypothesis proposes that early in embryogenesis each somatic cell of the female reaches a "time of decision" regarding whether a paternal X (X^p) or a maternal X (X^m) shall be the active chromosome in that particular cell. The hypothesis suggests that either the X^p or the X^m chromosome is selected at random. Once the decision is made, all the descendants of this embryonic cell retain the activity of the selected chromosome. Thus females are a mosaic of cell clones as regards the activity of the X chromosome in somatic cells.

Up until the time the cells of the enamel organ establish the outline form of the tooth,

the cells containing either the X^m or X^p are free to migrate and, by differential proliferation, to change their relationship to each other. Once the outline form of the tooth begins, clone lines of inner enamel epithelial cells, which eventually develop into ameloblasts, become fixed. As daughter cells of any one inner enamel epithelial cell are added at the proliferating end of the dental organ, this clone line will have a vertical distribution in the completed enamel organ. The enamel then produced by this clone line will also have a vertical distribution. In essence, the type of alternating vertical banding of normal and abnormal enamel demonstrated in these females can be interpreted as a record in the enamel of the particular X chromosome governing different clone lines of ameloblasts. This type of X-linked hypomaturation defect has been described by Witkop[173, 176, 179] and by McLarty and associates.[113] Possibly this is also the same as Darling's[35] group 4a and the defect described by Cameron and Bradford.[25]

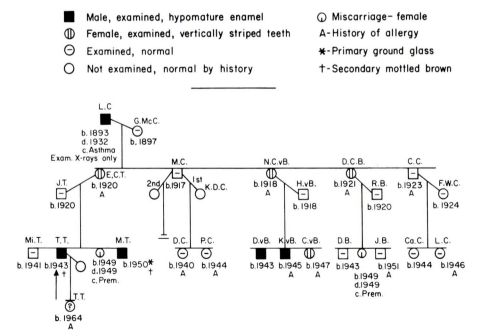

Fig. 7-39. Kindred of hypomaturation amelogenesis imperfecta compatible with X-chromosomal trait showing Lyonization in heterozygous females as vertically striped teeth. (From Witkop, C. J., Jr.: Oral Surg. **23**:174, 1967.)

Autosomal recessive pigmented hypomaturation amelogenesis. In autosomal recessive pigmented hypomaturation amelogenesis, primary and secondary dentitions are affected. The enamel has a milky to shiny agar-brown color on newly erupted teeth but may become more deeply stained on contact with exoge-

nous agents (Fig. 7-40). The enamel is of normal thickness and tends to chip from the dentin, especially around restorations. Resorption of the incisal or occlusal enamel may occur before eruption of teeth (Fig. 7-41). Some areas on the enamel are more severely involved, approaching the hypocalcified types.

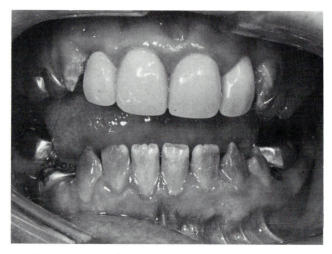

Fig. 7-40. Oral condition of girl with autosomal recessive pigmented hypomaturation amelogenesis imperfecta shows shiny mottled appearance of enamel, which is mottled yellow-brown color. Maxillary canine teeth erupted with defects seen and probably were places resorbed before eruption. (From Witkop, C. J., Jr., Kuhlmann, W., and Sauk, J.: Oral Surg. **36:**367, 1973.)

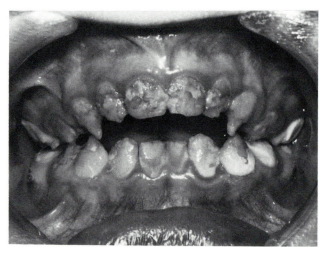

Fig. 7-41. Primary dentition of affected sister of girl in Fig. 7-40 shows that primary teeth are also partially resorbed before eruption. Note heavy deposits of calculus, which fluoresced reddish violet under ultraviolet light. Anterior open bite is feature often seen in many types of amelogenesis imperfecta. (From Witkop, C. J., Kuhlmann, W., and Sauk, J.: Oral Surg. **36:**367, 1973.)

Patients with this condition tend to form large amounts of calculus (Fig. 7-41), and many show a type of calculus that contains a pigment-forming organism. Calculus of this type fluoresces intense red-violet and may lead to the erroneous diagnosis of porphyria.

On radiographs the enamel is less radiodense than normal and does not contrast well with the dentin (Fig. 7-42). Root and pulp structure appear normal. Teeth may be seen undergoing resorption within the alveolus.

Ground sections of unerupted teeth show the presence of a brown pigment occupying a localized band of enamel midway between the dentinoenamel junction and the surface of the enamel (Fig. 7-43). In addition, there are spaces in the interrod areas forming exclamation point–shaped lacunae (Fig. 7-44). These spaces may extend across the rod, interrupting rod continuity. The incremental lines in the enamel rods in these areas are either absent, indistinct, or exaggerated, depending on the presence of gel inclusions within the rod as well as the prism sheath area (Fig. 7-45). The striae of Retzius are absent or indistinct. The pigment does not give the histochemical reaction expected for blood pigments. Carefully decalcified sections of enamel stained with Masson's trichrome stain show that the spaces in the enamel sheath areas are filled with a pink staining material resembling the thixotropic gel seen at the ends of developing ameloblasts in normal enamel (Fig. 7-46).

Longitudinal SEM sections of teeth with hypomaturation pigmented form of amelogenesis imperfecta show that the enamel is homogeneous and of low mineral content. The only portion of the enamel approaching normal calcification is adjacent to the dentinoenamel junction (Fig. 7-47). At higher magnification (Fig. 7-48), the affected enamel shows a homogenous structure with little or no classic prism formation. The surface of the enamel is porous, similar to that seen in the X-linked type (Fig. 7-36). Despite this feature, the teeth are not prone to decay, and several patients have been caries free.[183]

In affected males with the X-linked variety, the microscopic lesion primarily affects the

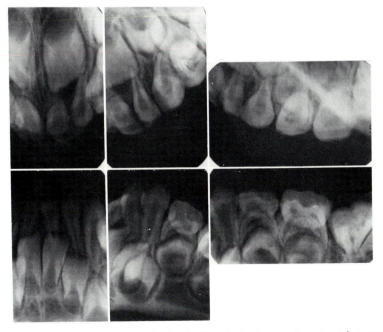

Fig. 7-42. Radiographs of patient in Fig. 7-41. Note lack of normal contrast between enamel and dentin in teeth of both dentitions. (From Witkop, C. J., Kuhlmann, W., and Sauk, J.: Oral Surg. **36:**367, 1973.)

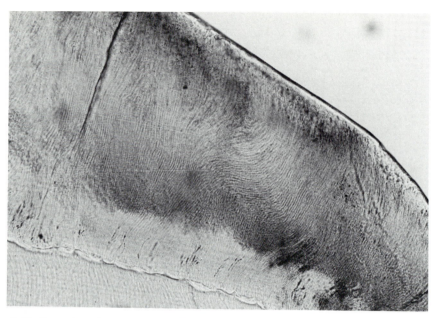

Fig. 7-43. Ground section of unerupted third molar from girl with autosomal recessive pigmented hypomaturation amelogenesis imperfecta showing that most marked changes are in outer three fourths of enamel. (×125; ground section, unstained.) (From Witkop, C. J., Kuhlmann, W., and Sauk, J.: Oral Surg. **36**:367, 1973.)

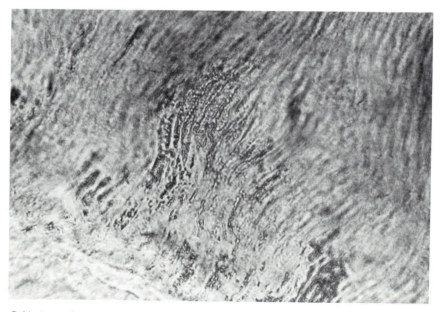

Fig. 7-44. Ground section of enamel from unerupted molar of girl with pigmented hypomaturation amelogenesis imperfecta demonstrates spaces in interprismatic areas of enamel rods in which incremental lines are indistinct or distorted. (×500; unstained.) (From Witkop, C. J., Kuhlmann, W., and Sauk, J.: Oral Surg. **36**:367, 1973.)

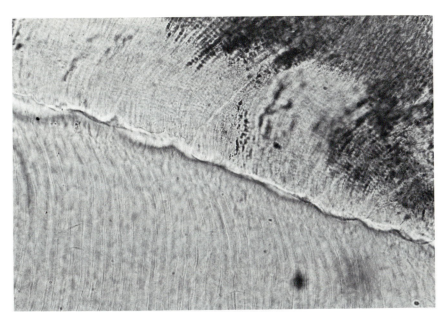

Fig. 7-45. Ground section of dentin and enamel from patient with pigmented hypomaturation shows scalloped dentinoenamel junction and enamel rods with accentuated pigment containing incremental striations, which become obliterated in enamel rods in upper right portion of photograph. (×312.) (From Witkop, C. J., Jr., Kuhlmann, W., and Sauk, J.: Oral Surg. **36:**367, 1973.)

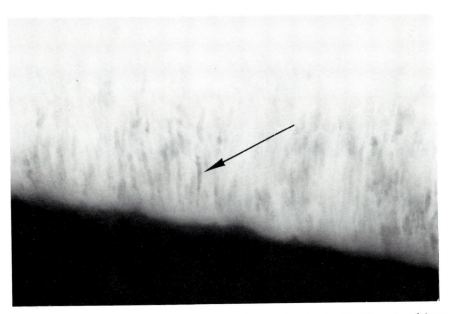

Fig. 7-46. Decalcified section through dentin and enamel stained with Masson's trichrome. Note interprismatic areas filled with material, *arrow,* that stained pink. (×500; decalcified, Masson's trichrome stain.) (From Witkop, C. J., Jr., Kuhlmann, W., and Sauk, J.: Oral Surg. **36:**367, 1973.)

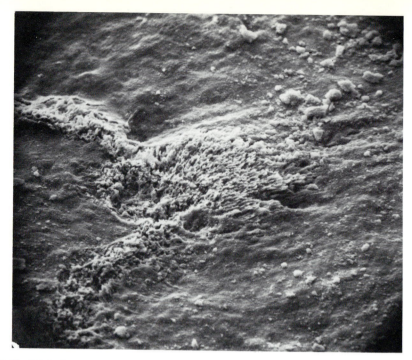

Fig. 7-47. SEM view of pigmented hypomaturation amelogenesis imperfecta at dentinoenamel junction shows that mature well-calcified prisms are found only in this region. Most enamel is homogeneous-appearing hypomature enamel. (×200.) (From Witkop, C. J., Jr., Kuhlmann, W., and Sauk, J.: Oral Surg. 36:367, 1973.)

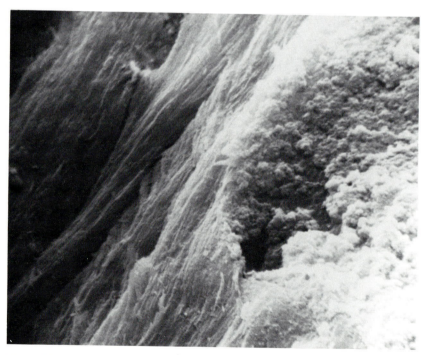

Fig. 7-48. SEM scan through section of enamel near surface reveals fibrous enamel associated with interprismatic void filled with material like thixotropic gel. (×5000.) (From Witkop, C. J., Kuhlmann, W., and Sauk, J.: Oral Surg. 36:367, 1973.)

prism sheath area, whereas in the autosomal recessive pigmented hypomaturation type the defect involves both the prism sheaths and the main body of the rod. Possibly the defect in this condition involves an enzyme depolymerizing the thixotropic gel. This system would envision that normal enamel formation involves first a depolymerization of the thixotropic gel (the enzyme possibly defective in this condition) and the enzymatic resorption of the depolymerized thixotropic material into the retreating ameloblast or Tomes' process (the enzyme possibly defective in the X-linked hypomaturation type).

This is a rare form of amelogenesis imperfecta, if reports in the literature are any indication of prevalence of the trait. In one family, the parents were first cousins once removed,[176] and in the other three families we have seen, no evidence of consanguinity could be found. A previously unreported kindred appears in Fig. 7-49.

Cases reported have been those of Witkop[173, 176, 179] and Witkop and co-workers.[183] Other possible examples of this defect are those of Rygge[139] and Gustafson and associates.[76]

Snow-capped teeth. Snow-capped teeth is a fairly common disorder in which varying proportions of the enamel on the incisal or occlusal aspects of the crowns of teeth have an opaque white appearance. The opaque whiteness of the enamel may be solid or flecked, appears clinically to involve only the surface of the enamel, and resembles the appearance of enamel seen in white spots. The junction line of opaque white enamel and translucent enamel is often sharp (Fig. 7-50). The pattern of affected teeth has a distinct anterior-posterior relationship and does not show a correlation with the chronological order of tooth development. Within families, the number of teeth affected varies among affected individuals. Maxillary teeth tend to be more severely involved than mandibular teeth. The pattern of the defect on teeth, anterior to posterior, resembles that which would be obtained if a denture were dipped into white paint. Some affected persons have incisors through second molars showing opaque enamel on the incisal or occlusal third to eighth of the crown. Others have only incisors through first molars or incisors through second bicuspids, and so forth, such that mildly affected persons show the defect only on central and lateral incisors. The opaque white enamel does not have the iridescent sheen seen in the white-frosted-ridge appearance of enamel with mild fluorosis. Both primary and secondary teeth are affected; however, it is not known whether a person with affected primary teeth will have succedaneous permanent teeth always affected.

Histologically, the defect involves the surface enamel or enamel lying below the first millimeter of normal-appearing surface enamel. The defect involves primarily enamel rod sheaths that contain disoriented enamel crystals. This suggests that the ameloblasts during the last stage of enamel rod formation lose the ball-shaped Tomes' processes, which may become somewhat flattened such that the peripheral crystallization in the enamel rod sheath is disturbed. The anatomical distribution of the defect is possibly caused by a loss of complete ameloblastic function in the last stages of amelogenesis in the ameloblasts forming incisal or coronal enamel. These areas are where enamel tends to be the thickest, and at this point they seem to become incapable of forming the last micromillimeters of normal enamel.

The condition has been observed to segre-

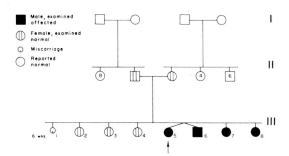

Fig. 7-49. Kindred of pigmented hypomaturation amelogenesis imperfecta. There was no known parental consanguinity within two generations before generation I.

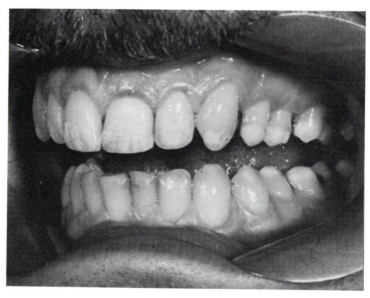

Fig. 7-50. Patient with snow-capped teeth shows white opaque hypomature enamel involving incisal and occlusal aspects of crowns. Note straight-line relationship of defect from anterior to posterior teeth in pattern inconsistent with chronological order of tooth development. (From Witkop, C. J., Jr.: Genetic diseases of the oral cavity. In Tiecke, R. W.: Oral pathology, New York, 1965, McGraw-Hill Book Co. Copyright 1965; used with permission of McGraw-Hill Book Co.)

gate as an autosomal dominant trait in several kindreds but with variable expressivity as to the number of teeth affected and with an occasional lack of penetrance, since individuals with affected parents but who do not themselves show the defect (at least in their permanent teeth) have had affected children. The prevalence is about one in 2000. The condition has been described by Witkop and co-workers[176, 185, 186] and by Winter and Brook.[171]

Hypocalcified amelogenesis imperfecta

Autosomal dominant hypocalcified amelogenesis imperfecta. In autosomal dominant hypocalcified amelogenesis imperfecta, the enamel on newly erupted teeth and unerupted and unresorbed teeth is of normal thickness, although occasional areas of hypoplasia are seen on the middle third of the labial surface (Fig. 7-51). The enamel is so soft, however, that it may be lost soon after eruption, leaving a crown composed only of dentin. The enamel has a cheesy consistency and can be scraped from the dentin with a prophylaxis instrument or penetrated easily with a dental explorer. The enamel at the cervical portion of the crown is often better calcified than that on the other portions of the crown. Newly erupted teeth are covered with a dull, lusterless, opaque white, honey colored, or yellow-orange-brown enamel. The enamel is lost rapidly in the softer supracervical areas, leaving areas of exposed dentin, which may be exquisitely sensitive. Numerous teeth may fail to erupt or have marked delay in eruption. Anterior open bite has been recorded in over 60% of the cases observed and is well demonstrated in published photographs of the condition* (Fig. 7-52).

Patients with this condition are exceedingly prone to form calculus rapidly, even to a greater degree than are patients with the autosomal recessive hypomaturation type of defect. We have seen patients develop calculus covering the entire tooth within 3 months

---

*See references 30, 35, 83, 140, 168, 176.

after a thorough prophylaxis. Many have acute and chronic periodontitis adjacent to these large masses of calculus. Fig. 7-52 shows a patient who actually developed intraoral stalactites of calcium salts.

Radiographically, the enamel fails to contrast with the dentin, and often the dentin is more radiodense than the enamel. As the enamel at the cervical aspect of the tooth is usually better calcified and the loss of enamel is uneven, the teeth have a distinct moth-eaten appearance on radiographs (Fig. 7-53). Occasionally unerupted teeth can be seen in radiographs undergoing resorption.[161]

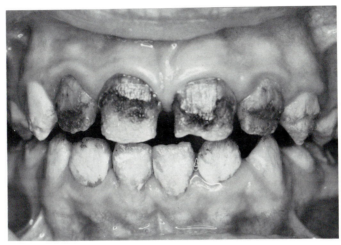

Fig. 7-51. Girl with hypocalcified amelogenesis imperfecta showing that enamel tends to be better formed near cervical aspect of crown. On newly erupted teeth (canines) enamel is usually of normal thickness but extremely soft.

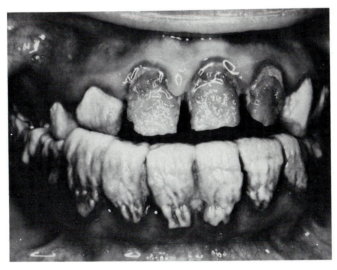

Fig. 7-52. Patient with hypocalcified amelogenesis imperfecta showing massive accumulation of calculus, particularly on mandibular teeth, a feature common to this type of enamel defect. In this patient accumulation was so massive that stalactites of calculus overhung vestibular gingivae. (From Giansanti, J. S.: J. Am. Dent. Assoc. **86:**675, 1973. Copyright by the American Dental Association. Reprinted by permission.)

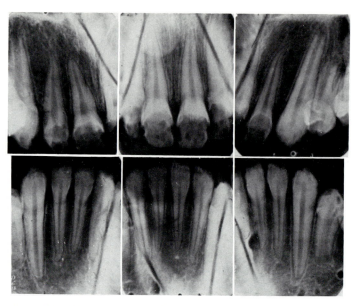

Fig. 7-53. Radiographs of boy with hypocalcified amelogenesis imperfecta illustrating moth-eaten appearance of crowns of teeth. Note lack of normal contrast between enamel and dentin.

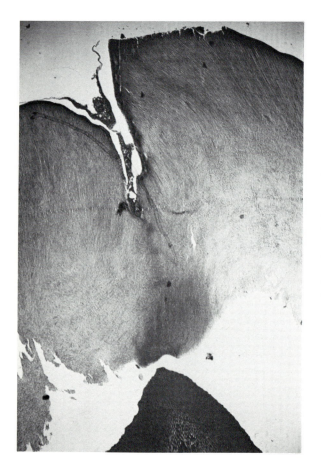

Fig. 7-54. Decalcified section of enamel from unerupted third molar tooth of boy with hypocalcified amelogenesis imperfecta. Enamel matrix has been maintained but shows artifactual separation from dentin. Dentino-enamel junction shows scalloping. Preserved enamel matrix resembles that in developing normal enamel. Remnants of enamel cuticle appear in fissure. (×20; decalcified, Masson's trichrome stain.)

Histologically the enamel of unerupted teeth is of normal thickness, and often enamel matrix of both erupted and unerupted teeth will be retained after decalcification. Chaudhry and associates[30] state that the organic content of the enamel is 9.66%, as compared with normal enamel, which has 4.88% organic material. In our series, the organic content of enamel from these teeth has ranged from 8.7% to 14.2%, with mean values of twelve teeth being 11.6%. The enamel matrix in ground and decalcified sections appears normal but hypocalcified (Fig. 7-54). In occasional spots on the surface, a pattern of fine

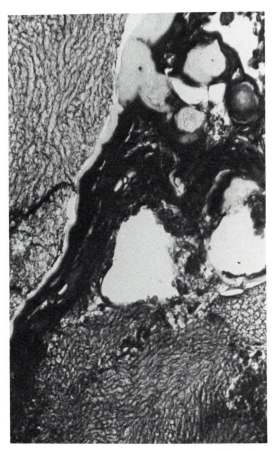

Fig. 7-55. Higher magnification of specimen in Fig. 7-54 demonstrates cuticular material extending into fissure. Globular and laminated calcified structures are found within cuticle. (×400; decalcified, Masson's trichrome stain.)

fibrils that deviate 30 to 40 degrees vertically from the prisms can be seen and have been described by Hals[79, 80] and discussed by Rushton[137] as being present in some normal teeth. Weinmann and associates[162] and Rushton[137] describe a cuticular layer overlying the surface of the enamel of unerupted teeth. Beginning from the enamel surface, there is first a multiple fine-layered cuticlelike substance, then a denser area that stains more deeply and more closely resembles classical enamel cuticle but appears to be only a more densely packed region of the finely laminated inner substance. Below this are cellular remnants of reduced enamel epithelium. Fig. 7-55 shows this cuticular material extends deeply into occlusal grooves of molars and contains globular and laminated calcified material. Listgarten[100] failed to find evidence of collagen fibrils in this cuticle from patients with amelogenesis imperfecta and believed it was associated with degeneration of reduced enamel epithelium. Study of the histological features of this defect by light microscopy gives the impression that the defect is more severely expressed as an intraprismatic calcification defect. If one compares this defect with that seen in the X-linked hypomaturation type of amelogenesis imperfecta, it seems that the latter condition has its main defect in the interprismatic zone or the rod sheaths.

SEM photographs of longitudinal sections of surface zones of enamel reveal large intraprismatic zones that do not contain any material and appear as voids (Fig. 7-56).[142] These zones may possibly result from localized aplasia of ameloblasts. The surface of the enamel shows the presence of voids and fibrous disoriented enamel prisms (Fig. 7-57). These prisms have a fibrillar character to them, suggesting hypomineralization of the prisms. Crypts on the surface of the enamel resemble those seen in the rough forms of hypoplastic amelogenesis imperfecta, thus suggesting a local hypoplastic component to the defect.[142] The enamel rods, where fully formed, have normal-appearing incremental cross striations (Fig. 7-58).

This defect may be due to an altered enamel matrix that structurally does not per-

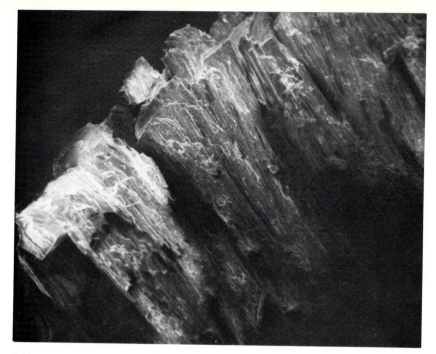

Fig. 7-56. Untreated fracture specimen of enamel from unerupted tooth of 20-year-old man with hypocalcified amelogenesis imperfecta. Longitudinal section shows numerous voids and disoriented enamel prisms extending below surface. (×500; untreated.) (From Sauk, J. J., Jr., Cotton, W. R., Lyon, H. W., and Witkop, C. J., Jr.: Arch. Oral Biol. **12:**771, 1972.)

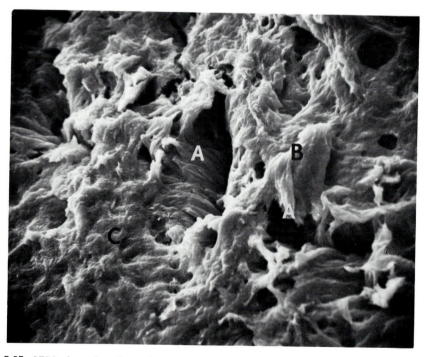

Fig. 7-57. SEM view of surface of enamel from patient with hypocalcified amelogenesis imperfecta. Untreated surface shows voids, *A,* fibrillar disoriented enamel prisms, *B,* and completely formed enamel prisms, *C.* (×750; untreated.) (From Sauk, J. J., Jr., Cotton, W. R., Lyon, H. W., and Witkop, C. J., Jr.: Arch. Oral Biol. **12:**771, 1972.)

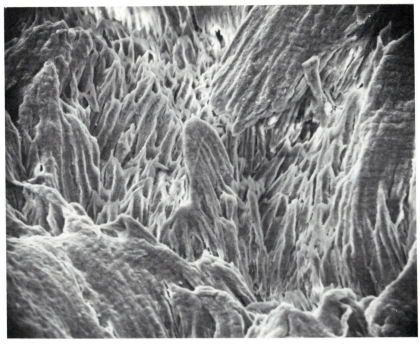

Fig. 7-58. SEM appearance of EDTA-treated surface enamel from a patient with hypocalcified amelogenesis. Enamel rods contain normal-appearing cross striations. (×500; EDTA etch.) (From Sauk, J. J., Jr., Cotton, W. R., Lyon, H. W., and Witkop, C. J., Jr.: Arch. Oral Biol. **12:**771, 1972.)

mit normal calcification to begin. The structural mutation may affect the keratin-like material of the enamel matrix.

This is the most common form of amelogenesis imperfecta. Similar cases showing autosomal dominant inheritance have been reported by Sato,[140] Euler,[48] Weinmann and associates[162] (families M and L), Darling[35] (group 4B), Witkop (Figs. 32-26 and 32-27),[173, 176] Chaudhry and co-workers[30] (families B, D, F, ?K), Toller[160] (cases 3 to 5), Laird,[94] Rushton,[137] Finn,[50] Winter (Fig. 4),[168] Pindborg (Figs. 84 to 87),[121] Schulze (Figs. 3-82 to 3-84),[147] Sauk and associates,[142] Winter and Brook,[171] and Giansanti.[62] Possible cases are some of those of Keeler[88] and those of Macklin[104] and Hiyama and Kanai.[83]

Autosomal recessive hypocalcified amelogenesis imperfecta. Autosomal recessive inheritance for a hypocalcified form of amelogenesis imperfecta is not well established. We have seen two affected girls with two normal

sisters from a family wherein the putative parents were unaffected. Clinically, radiographically, and histologically the findings were more severe than those seen in the autosomal dominant form.

Other possible cases wherein the parents were unaffected are those of Schulze,[146] Fluckinger[54] (cases 2 and 3), and questionable cases of Wittner[187] and Soifer.[155]

INHERITED DEFECTS OF ENAMEL ACCOMPANYING GENERALIZED DEFECTS

Hereditary defects, in which abnormal enamel is but one of several signs of these disorders, are numerous. All of these will not be described in detail, especially those in which defective enamel has been reported in relatively few instances. Enamel defects, as well as defects in tooth form, occur in high frequency in those disorders that have been generally classified as ectodermal dysplasias.[182] There are many disorders in which defective enamel has been reported, including those diseases in which the enamel defects may be only a chance association.[185] However, since many of these conditions are rare and have not been documented by a trained dental observer, they have not been included.

Only enamel has been observed defective in some of these conditions, and in others, both enamel and dentin and possibly cementum are known to be abnormal. In many instances teeth were not observed microscopically, so that it is not known with certainty whether structures other than enamel were involved. Thus this classification is tentatively based on these aspects as presently reported.

Inherited defects involving only enamel accompanying generalized defects

Amelo-onychohypohidrotic syndrome. A syndrome consisting of hypocalcified-hypoplastic enamel, onycholysis with subungual hyperkeratosis, seborrheic dermatitis of the scalp, and hypofunction of the sweat glands with rough, dry skin was first observed in a kindred of Caucasian ancestry to be inherited as an autosomal dominant trait by Witkop and associates.[182] Since the initial report, we have observed another kindred with this condition.

The enamel defect affects all teeth in both dentitions (Fig. 7-59). The teeth do not meet at the contact points. The general thickness of the enamel is less than normal but varies greatly in different areas of the crown. The enamel at the cervical portion of the teeth tends to approach normal thickness and is somewhat better calcified than that on other areas of the crown. The occlusal and incisal portions of the crowns may show evidence of partial resorption of enamel before eruption, giving these areas a rough, moth-eaten appearance. The middle third of the enamel is pitted on most teeth. The color of the enamel of newly erupted teeth varies from opaque white to a dark yellow-brown. Black-stained areas are found on teeth that have been in the oral cavity for a period of time. The hardness of the enamel varies considerably. Some areas, particularly on the deciduous incisors, are hard and smooth and approach the consistency of normal enamel. Other areas are covered with a soft, friable, chalky enamel that can be removed easily with a sharp

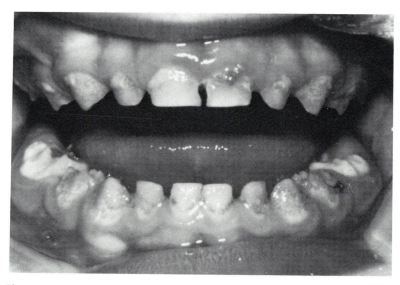

Fig. 7-59. Oral condition of 3-year-old boy with hypoplastic-hypocalcified enamel, onycholysis, and hypohidrosis. Enamel is rough and hypoplastic, with areas of soft hypomineralized enamel. Teeth were dark yellowish brown color. (From Witkop, C. J., Jr., Brearley, L. J., and Gentry, W. C., Jr.: Oral Surg. **39:**71, 1975.)

instrument. The deciduous teeth erupt at the expected time or are only slightly delayed. The eruption of the permanent dentition is markedly retarded, with some teeth never appearing in the oral cavity.

Radiographs show multiple unerupted teeth with resorption, beginning at the incisal or occlusal surface of the crowns (Fig. 7-60). Root formation and general outline of the teeth are not unusual. Patients have onycholysis of the distal quarter to half of all toenails and fingernails (Fig. 7-61). The nail plate is not elevated by the accumulation of keratinous debris under the nail.

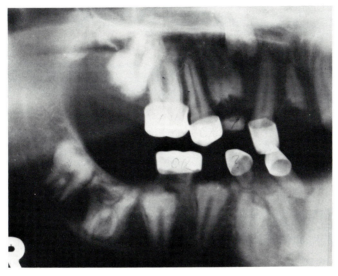

Fig. 7-60. Radiograph of 12-year-old boy with amelo-onychohypohidrotic syndrome shows delayed eruption of many teeth, which show radiographic evidence of destruction of crowns within alveoli. (From Witkop, C. J., Jr., Brearley, L. J., and Gentry, W. C., Jr.: Oral Surg. **39:**71, 1975.)

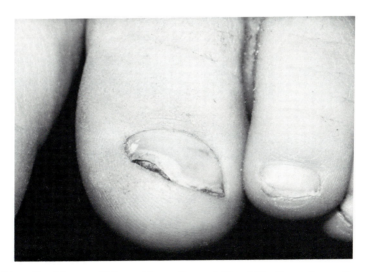

Fig. 7-61. Toenails of 3-year-old boy with amelo-onychohypohidrotic syndrome show subungual hyperkeratosis beneath nail plates of normal thickness and contour. (From Witkop, C. J., Jr., Brearley, L. J., and Gentry, W. C., Jr.: Oral Surg. **39:**71, 1975.)

Counts of sweat pores on finger-pad dermal ridges are within normal variation. Dermal printing of sweat glands under both stimulated and unstimulated conditions shows a marked decrease in the ability to produce sweat (Fig. 7-62).

All affected patients have had 2 to 4 mm waxy brown keratotic crusts with erythematous bases covered with dry scale throughout the scalp. In general, the skin is xerotic, with some demonstrating keratosis pilaris, particularly on the buttocks.

Histological sections of unerupted teeth show extensive resorptions of the crowns of many teeth (Fig. 7-63).

Two kindreds have been observed in which the condition segregates as an autosomal dominant trait (Fig. 7-64).

Oculodento-osseous dysplasia. Oculodento-osseous dysplasia, also described under the term *oculodentodigital dysplasia,*[72, 128] consists of (1) typical facies characterized by microphthalmus and microcornea with anomalies of the irides and a thin nose with ante-verted nostrils and hypoplasia of the area of the nose, (2) hypoplasia of enamel, (3) bony anomalies of the middle digits of the fifth finger, absence of the middle phalanx of second through fifth toes, and syndactyly and camptodactyly of the fourth and fifth fingers, and (4) thickened mandibular bone. Some patients have developed glaucoma and have had dry, lusterless hair that fails to grow to normal length. Blindness may result,[32] but longevity is not apparently reduced. Hypoplastic enamel is found on both primary and secondary teeth, which may not meet at contact points.[45, 125] Newly erupted teeth are yellow and have a grossly rough pitted surface (Fig. 7-65) with normal pulp chambers and root formation.

The enamel defect is apparent radiographically on unerupted teeth. The enamel contrasts normally from the dentin, but the gross rough enamel surface gives the teeth a moth-eaten appearance (Fig. 7-66).

The condition is inherited as an autosomal dominant trait. The condition is rare; less

Control   Patient

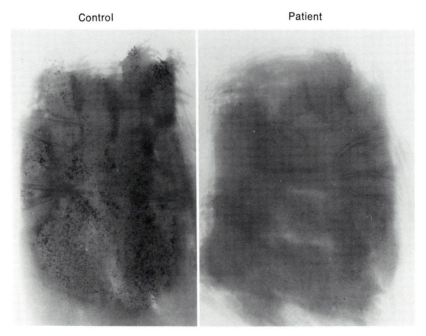

Fig. 7-62. Photographs of starch bond paper–iodine palm prints of normal control and patient with amelo-onychohypohidrotic syndrome at room temperature after a minute's contact with paper. Only a few scattered impressions of sweat glands are seen in subject's print. (From Witkop, C. J., Jr., Brearley, L. J., and Gentry, W. C., Jr.: Oral Surg. **39:**71, 1975.)

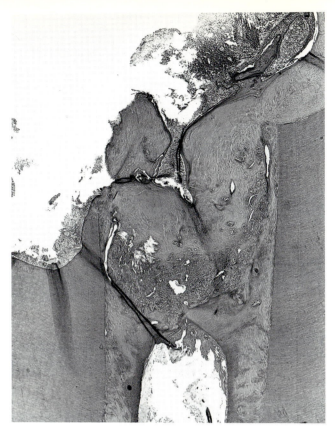

Fig. 7-63. Photomicrograph of decalcified section of unerupted tooth from patient with ameloonychohypohidrotic syndrome shows extensive resorption of crown by granulation tissue in which odontogenic elements persist at upper right. Note extensive secondary dentin and repeated attempts to form dentin bridges over pulp chamber. (×10; decalcified, hematoxylin and eosin.) (From Witkop, C. J., Jr., Brearley, L. J., and Gentry, W. C., Jr.: Oral Surg. **39:** 71, 1975.)

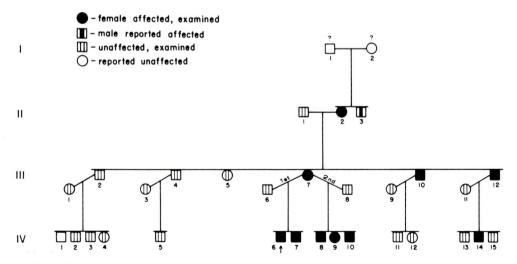

Fig. 7-64. Kindred chart of family with ameloonychohypohidrotic syndrome, which is compatible with autosomal dominant mode of transmission. (From Witkop, C. J., Jr., Brearley, L. J., and Gentry, W. C., Jr.: Oral Surg. **39:**71, 1975.)

than fifty families have been reported in the literature[63, 114, 116, 122, 159] since the description of Lohmann[101] in 1920. O'Rourk and Bravos[120] reported a similar condition that appears to be a unique example in a single patient. The patient differed from the classical syndrome in that the digital defect was different, and the patient had missing permanent teeth and conical lower incisors in addition to hypoplasia of enamel.

Tuberous sclerosis. Tuberous sclerosis may affect numerous body systems, but the most constant findings are the triad of adenoma sebaceum, epilepsy, and mental retardation, which characterize the disease. A variety of lesions arise in skin, nervous system, heart, kidney, and other organs due to a limited hyperplasia of ectodermal and mesodermal cells, resulting in mixed-cell tumors that rarely undergo malignant transformation and metastases.[93] A characteristic of the cells within these tumors is their giant size, so both hypertrophy and hyperplasia are found in these blastomatous lesions.[1]

The condition may be present at birth, but in most instances the infant has been judged normal at birth, with attention being drawn to the disease by the later appearance of seizures or retarded psychomotor development. One early sign present in about 85% of cases is the congenital white hypomelanotic ash–leaf-shaped macules.[53] These appear before any other skin lesion. They occur most frequently on the skin over the trunk and limbs, have a linear orientation, and can be demonstrated easily with a Wood's lamp at 360 nm.

Angiofibromas (adenoma sebaceum) develop on the face later, from 3 to 10 years of age, and are present in about 90% of patients

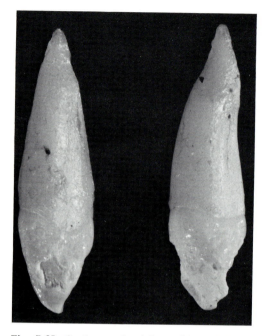

Fig. 7-65. Canine teeth of boy with oculodento-osseous dysplasia shows rough, pitted hypoplastic enamel most severely defective in midportion of crown, somewhat resembling that seen in local hypoplastic amelogenesis imperfecta. (From Gorlin, R. J., Meskin, L. H., and Geme, J. W.: J. Pediatr. **63:**69, 1963.)

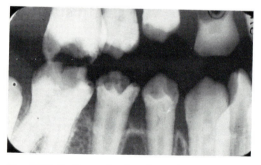

Fig. 7-66. Radiograph of patient with oculodento-osseous dysplasia shows moth-eaten appearance of crowns of teeth, normal contrast between enamel and dentin, and multiple denticles in pulp chambers and canals of many teeth. (From Gorlin, R. J., Meskin, L. H., and Geme, J. W.: J. Pediatr. **63:**69, 1963.)

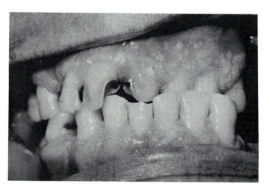

Fig. 7-67. Oral condition of woman with tuberous sclerosis. Note fibrous growths on gingivae.

over the age of 4 years.[126] These red to pink nodules with a smooth, glistening surface are most prominent on the nasolabial folds (Fig. 7-67), cheeks, skin, forehead, and scalp. Elephant hide or orange peel–like shagreen patches are areas of subepidermal fibrosis occurring in the trunk. Subungual fibromas commonly elevate the nail bed.

Oral lesions are present in about 11% of cases, according to Schürmann and co-workers.[150] These consist of fibrous growths and angiofibromas affecting the oral mucosa, primarily the mandibular anterior gingivae (Fig. 7-67). Fibrous growth of the lips, buccal mucosa, dorsum of the tongue, and palate has been described.[36, 71, 93, 103, 150] Hypertosis of the alveolar process has been noted.[136, 150]

Carol[26] noted gross linear enamel hypoplasia of the mesial edges of incisors and cuspids of one patient. Witkop and Rao[185] suggest that hypoplastic enamel may be associated with the condition, but details of the patients seen in Chile were not given. Hoff and associates[84] found small pit-shaped enamel defects on all tooth surfaces of all six patients described with the disorder. The number of pits ranged from one to eleven per tooth surface (Fig. 7-68). They occurred in no clear pattern, and the distribution on contralateral teeth was not symmetrical and did not follow a chronological pattern of development. Radiographically, the defects appeared as small, round, pin-sized radiolucencies in the enamel.[84]

These pits have a diameter of about 100 μm as seen by scanning electron microscopy (Fig. 7-69). They sometimes contain calcified material that appears to be calculus (Fig. 7-70). The craters, when viewed in section, penetrate from a third to nearly the full thickness of the enamel (Fig. 7-69). These tract defects in enamel appear to result from dysfunction of a small group of ameloblasts. Possibly small angioid lesions within the developing enamel are involved in the production of local ameloblast death.

The condition presents a variable but relatively poor prognosis because of the high frequency of tumors of the central nervous system, heart, and kidney. Mental retardation occurs in about 75% of the cases, and the majority of patients do not survive 25 years of age.

Tuberous sclerosis has been reported in all

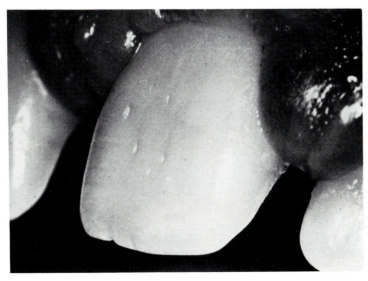

Fig. 7-68. Photograph of patient with tuberous sclerosis showing small pits on enamel of incisor tooth. (From Hoff, M., van Grunsven, M. F., and 's-Gravenmade, E. J.: Oral Surg. **40:**261, 1975.)

major races, and estimates of frequency vary from 1:14,000 to 1:100,000.[1, 82] From 0.1% to 0.5% of the population of mental institutions in the United States has been affected, and in Europe the condition has been found in 0.6% to 0.7% of the mentally institutionalized. The condition is inherited as an autosomal dominant trait with high lethality. About 85% of the cases appear to be new mutations.[20] The only adequate description of the enamel defect is that by Hoff and associates.[84]

Amelocerebrohypohidrotic syndrome. Amelocerebrohypohidrotic syndrome, described by Köhlschütter and co-workers,[90] consists of severe seizures, muscular spasticity and progressive mental retardation, hypoplasia of enamel, and hypohidrosis. The initial report of the disorder included four affected deceased and one living affected brother from a family living in a central valley of Switzerland. Since that time, two other families of Swiss origin, one with an affected boy and the other with two affected boys, have been seen by the original authors.

The affected children appear to develop normally during infancy until the onset of severe seizures from 11 months to 4 years of age. After the onset of seizures, there is a progressive mental retardation accompanied by muscular spasticity. Peripheral nerve conduction velocities and peripheral nerve histology are normal. The EEG is diffusely abnormal. Histological changes in the brain

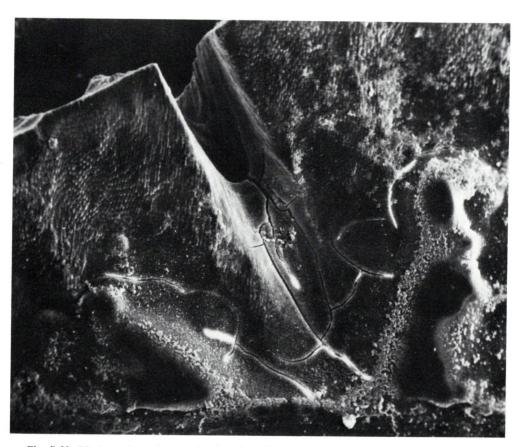

Fig. 7-69. Electron photomicrograph of section of enamel from tooth of patient with tuberous sclerosis. Pit seen courses through upper layers of enamel. (From Hoff, M., van Grunsven, M. F., and 's-Gravenmade, E. J.: Oral Surg. **40:**261, 1975.)

include diminished number of neurons, smaller glial cells, and ballooning of axons. Pericytes of vessels contain lipid droplets as seen by orthochromatic staining with acid cresyl violet. Similar degenerative changes are seen in electron microscopy.

Sweating is decreased spontaneously and when heat and pilocarpine are administered subcutaneously. Sodium and chloride levels in sweat are moderately elevated, and potassium is markedly elevated. Skin biopsies showed decreased numbers of sweat and sebaceous glands.

The enamel defect affects all teeth in both dentitions. Teeth do not meet at contact points. There is a nearly complete absence of enamel except for islands of thin enamel near the cervix of the crowns (Fig. 7-71). Radiographs of the teeth indicate that they have a normal pulp and root formation.

A large number of enzymatic determinations and other analyses ruled out a known mucopolysaccharidosis or glycolipidosis.

The specific inheritance of the disease has yet to be determined. The present kindreds are compatible with either an X-linked disorder, since all affected children have been boys, or an autosomal recessive trait.

The only families we know are those of Köhlschütter and associates.[90]

Epidermolysis bullosa. A number of vesicular disorders have been included under the term *epidermolysis bullosa.* Although these conditions can be distinguished generally by

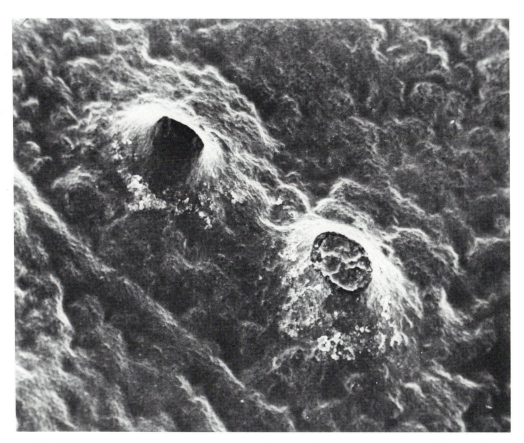

Fig. 7-70. Electron photomicrograph of enamel from patient with tuberous sclerosis. Two pits are seen in enamel. Pit on enamel surface at right is filled with calcified material, probably representing deposits of calculus. (From Hoff, M., van Grunsven, M. F., and 's-Gravenmade, E. J.: Oral Surg. **40:**261, 1975.)

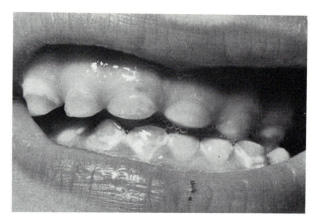

Fig. 7-71. Primary dentition of boy with amelocerebrohypohidrotic syndrome of Kohlschütter, showing hypoplastic enamel. Small islands of enamel appear on crowns in areas of exposed dentin. (From Kohlschütter, A., Chappuis, D., Meier, C., Tönz, O., Vassela, F., and Herschkowitz, N.: Helv. Paediatr. Acta **29:**283, 1974.)

their clinical and genetic features, there is no unanimously accepted classification of these diseases.[70] Most authors, however, recognize two autosomal dominant forms of the disease and two autosomal recessive types. These recognized types include the dominant simplex form, the dominant dystrophic (hypertrophic) form, the recessive dystrophic form, and epidermolysis bullosa letalis. General reviews are to be found in Bergenholtz and Olsson[11] and Gedde-Dahl.[61] (See also Chapter 12.)

Enamel defects have not been reported in the dominant simplex form, and oral mucosal involvement rarely occurs.[61] Furthermore, the occurrence of defective enamel and the type of enamel hypoplasia in the remaining three types is variable. In general, there is no correlation between the occurrence of defects of enamel and the severity of cutaneous involvement.[70, 132] There have been patients with the severely recessive dystrophic type without enamel involvement,[46] and patients with the dominant dystrophic form of the disease may rarely have hypoplastic enamel (Fig. 7-72).

In dominant dystrophic epidermolysis bullosa, onset of the first symptoms usually occurs late in infancy or in early childhood. Lesions are flat, pink bullae of the extremities, which heal with scarring. Thick, dystrophic nails accompany about 80% of patients who lack conjunctival and corneal lesions (Fig. 7-73). Oral mucosal lesions are found in fewer than 20% of cases. The condition improves with age. Gorlin[70] states that most authors agree that the teeth are uninvolved; however, the patient of Winter and Brook[171] shown in Fig. 7-22 is a rare exception and may indicate that genetically heterogeneous forms of the dominant type exist, as is indicated by the more severe cases described by Davidson[37] and Bart.[9]

Recessive dystrophic epidermolysis bullosa probably represents a genetically heterogeneous group of disorders. Bullae arise at pressure points and collapse, leaving large bleeding surfaces. Nikolsky's sign is frequently present. The hands may be enclosed in a glovelike epidermal sac, and subsequent scarring produces a claw deformity. Scars, milia, and pigment changes are frequent sequelae of the skin lesions. Mucosa is involved in infancy and affects more than a third of the patients. Esophageal lesions may scar, leading to stenosis and dysphagia. Vesicular separation occurs in the basal cell layer of skin and mucosa. The enamel defect varies in its clinical appearance, and there is no correlation between the enamel defect and the severity of the dermal disorder. Some patients have demonstrated random pitting of the enamel, with

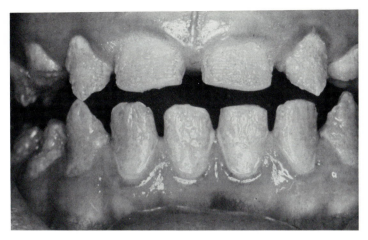

Fig. 7-72. Teeth seen in boy with autosomal dominant dystrophic epidermolysis bullosa show rough hypoplastic enamel involving entire dentition. This type of defective enamel is uncommonly seen in dominant dystrophic form of disease. (From Winter, G. B., and Brook, A. H.: Dent. Clin. North Am. **19:**3-24, 1975.)

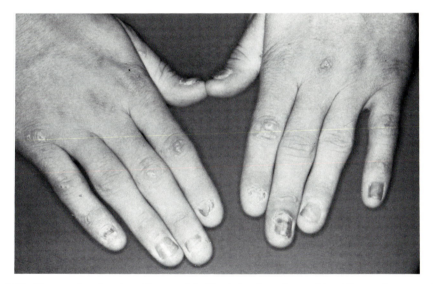

Fig. 7-73. Fingernails of patient illustrated in Fig. 7-72 show dystrophic nails seen in dystrophic forms of epidermolysis bullosa. (From Winter, G. B., and Brook, A. H.: Dent. Clin. North Am. **19:**3-24, 1975.)

the pits assuming a honeycomb pattern.[132, 135] Other patients who have died in infancy but after eruption of primary teeth have had brown, thin granular enamel.[6]

The histological changes when an enamel defect is present are probably similar in some cases to those seen in the lethal form. Epidermolysis bullosa letalis has its onset in the neonatal period, with death before 3 months of age. This form usually does not have milia, scarring, or pigment changes. Nails are involved early, with massive bullae, and are rapidly lost. Nearly all body surfaces seem to be involved in the process, but palms and soles are spared. Separation occurs at the intermembrane space between epidermis and dermis.[7]

Brain and Wigglesworth[19] and Arwill and

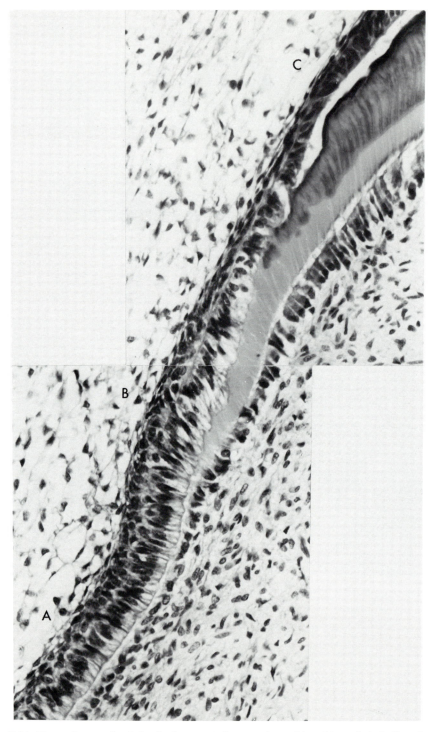

Fig. 7-74. Photomicrograph of developing tooth from patient with epidermolysis bullosa letalis shows that normal appearing ameloblasts at *A* become vacuolated after induction of dentin at *B* and at *C* show metaplastic characteristics, lose orientation, and lose Tomes' processes. Space represents enamel lost in decalcification. (From Gardner, D. G., and Hudson, C. D.: Oral Surg. **40:**483, 1975.)

co-workers[6] noted thin enamel, from 40 to 400 μm in thickness, on developing primary incisors. The prismless enamel was laminated with globular inclusions and had a granular surface and a lamellar appearance over most of the crown, the cervical enamel being better formed.[39] The enamel adjacent to the dentin and the surface of the enamel was better calcified than the intermediate layer. Along the surface and some distance from it were numerous calcified globules, which were also seen within the body of the enamel on the tooth. A moderate amount of interglobular dentin was scattered throughout the crown. In other areas, the enamel was folded in helical masses. The outer enamel epithelium

demonstrated metaplasia, and numerous microvacuoles containing keratin debris were distributed along the length of the partially reduced enamel epithelium. A hyalinized, structureless lamellar enamel from 50 to 200 μm thick was seen in decalcified sections.

Gardner and Hudson[59] made a detailed study of developing teeth in the lethal form of the disorder. The enamel epithelium initially differentiates into normal-appearing ameloblasts that induce differentiation of odontoblast from the cells of the dental papillae (Fig. 7-74, *A*). Simultaneously with the initial deposition of dentin, the dentino-enamel junction becomes highly irregular so that the subsequent intraface surface of the

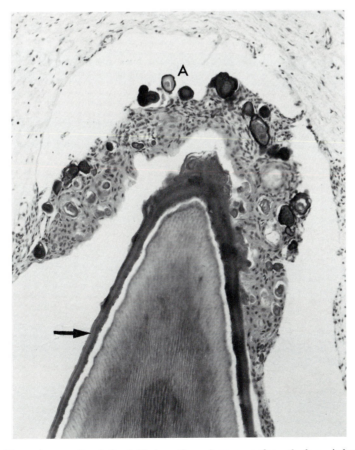

Fig. 7-75. Photomicrograph of decalcified section of unerupted tooth from infant who died with epidermolysis bullosa letalis. Tip of developing tooth is covered with laminated structureless material lacking normal enamel prisms, *arrow*. Odontogenic epithelium appears metaplastic and contains round calcified bodies with concentric laminations, *A*. (From Gardner, D. G., and Hudson, C. D.: Oral Surg. **40:**483, 1975.)

dentin becomes highly irregular. At this point, the ameloblasts abruptly appear abnormal, containing vacuoles and becoming disoriented (Fig. 7-74, *B*). There is a marked delay in the formation of enamel matrix. The ameloblasts lose their terminal processes and regress to metaplastic-appearing short cells with loss of nuclear polarization, terminal bars, and Tomes' processes (Fig. 7-74, *C*). The enamel matrix is scantily laminated and lacks prismatic form. The reduced enamel appears metaplastic with squamous characteristics and contains numerous irregularly concentric laminated calcified structures (Fig. 7-75).

Mucopolysaccharidoses. The mucopolysaccharidoses are storage diseases in which the progressive development of clinical signs parallels the accumulation of mucopolysaccharide in the tissues. In some of these disorders, mucopolysaccharides accumulate in the developing dental follicle, a feature that may be demonstrable on oral radiographs (Fig. 7-76). Small, widely spaced teeth may result, and these patients frequently have bruxism leading to attrition of occlusal and incisal enamel surfaces. These features have given the impression that the enamel is structurally defective. However, a structural defect in enamel has been demonstrated only in mucopolysaccharidosis IV (Morquio syndrome).[117] These syndromes have other orofacial features that vary with the age of onset and severity and are not all present in each specific syndrome. In general, these consist of coarse, thickened facial features, dwarfism, short neck, broad maxilla, widely spaced teeth, enlarged alveolar processes, flattening or concavity of the head of the condyle, and corneal opacities (see Stevenson[158] and McKusick[110] for details of each syndrome).

Seven general types of mucopolysaccharidoses have been distinguished by clinical, genetic, and biochemical criteria.[111] All are autosomal recessive traits except type II (Hunter's syndrome),[85] which is an X-linked trait. Three forms—type II (Hunter),[85] type III (Sanfilippo),[141] and type IV (Morquio)[117]—have two variants each, and other rare, unclassified types exist, which may represent allelic variants or allelic combinations of the major types.[110]

1. Type I (Hurler)[86]: excretes dermatan sulfate and heparan sulfate
2. Type II (Hunter)[85]: excretes dermatan sulfate and heparan sulfate
   a. Severe infantile form
   b. Mild adult form[41]
3. Type III (Sanfilippo)[141]
   a. Heparan sulfate sulfatase deficiency[92]
   b. N-Acetyl-α-D-glycosaminidase deficiency[119]
4. Type IV (Morquio)[18, 117]
   a. Possibly chondroitin sulfate N-acetylhexosamine sulfate sulfatase deficiency[109]; excretes keratin sulfate
   b. Non–keratin-sulfate excreting[110]
5. Type V (Scheie, late Hurler)[149]: excretes dermatan sulfate; most probably allelic with type I[112]; fibroblasts cross correct Sanfilippo A and Hunter, but not Hurler[166]
6. Type VI (Maroteaux-Lamy) [107]: excretes dermatan sulfate
7. Type VII (Sly)[154]: β-glucuronidase deficiency
8. Other mucopolysaccharidoses
   GM1 gangliosidoses
   I-cell disease
   Lipomucopolysaccharidosis

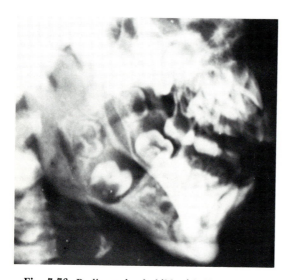

Fig. 7-76. Radiograph of child with Hurler's syndrome showing wide radiolucent area around crowns of developing first molar teeth. These pseudocystic areas are accumulations of mucopolysaccharides. (From Gardner, D. G.: Oral Surg. **32:**46, 1971.)

Mannosidosis
α-Fucosidosis
Metachromatic leukodystrophy variant
Farber's disease
Chondroitin sulfaturia

Mucopolysaccharidosis I (Hurler),[58] II (Hunter), and VI (Maroteaux-Lamy)[157] may show radiographic accumulation of mucopolysaccharides around developing teeth (Fig. 7-76).[28, 58, 127, 188] Histological evidence that these radiolucent areas represent accumulations of mucopolysaccharides was provided by Gardner.[57] Gardner[58] investigated the enamel by ground sections from patients with Hurler's and Hunter's syndromes and found the enamel to be structurally normal.

Mucopolysaccharidosis type IV (Morquio) is a dwarfing disorder with progressive spinal deformities, short neck, short, broad nose, and thick lips, giving a prominence to the lower face. Hearing loss is common, and aortic regurgitation occurs in a few patients. Diffuse corneal clouding is a frequent sign. Irregular cortical bone is found radiographically at the head of the condyle.[153]

The enamel of primary and secondary teeth is involved. The teeth do not usually meet at the contact points and are smaller than normal, with thin enamel of normal radiographic density.[60, 97, 153] Both primary and secondary dentitions are involved. The teeth are best described clinically as gray, dysplastic teeth with thin enamel and pointed cusps.[17, 95, 97, 108, 190] The enamel may be pitted, particularly on the buccal aspects, or it may have vertically arranged dimpling (Fig. 7-77). The enamel is of normal hardness. Half of the patients examined by Levin and associates[97] had anterior open bite.

Radiographs of patients show that all teeth of both dentitions are covered by a thin layer of enamel that contrasts well from dentin, suggesting that the enamel has a nearly normal mineral content (Fig. 7-78).

Patients with MPS III (Sanfilippo's disease) may show loss of enamel from bruxism, a common trait in this type of mucopolysaccharidosis. In addition, heavy deposits of tubular dentin and osteodentin may obliterate the pulp chambers, giving a radiographic ap-

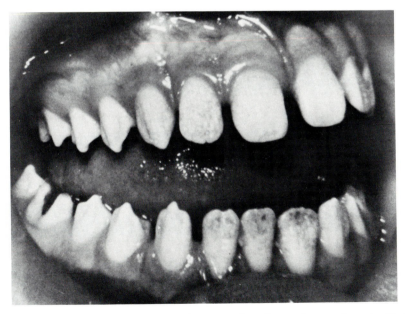

Fig. 7-77. Intraoral condition of patient with Morquio's disease (mucopolysaccharidosis type IV) shows widely spaced teeth covered with hypoplastic enamel with small dimples frequently arranged vertically on crown. Enamel of these teeth is often dirty gray. (From Levin, L. S., Jorgenson, R. J., and Salinas, C. F.: Oral Surg. **39**:390, 1975.)

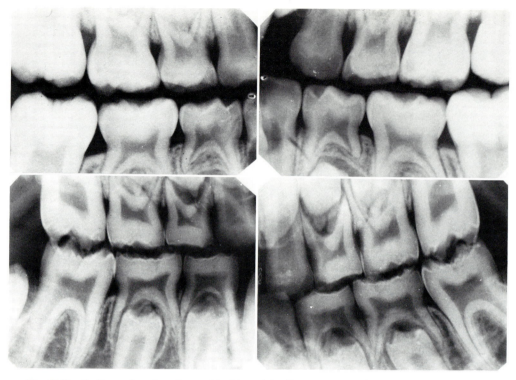

Fig. 7-78. Radiographs of patient with Morquio's disease (mucopolysaccharidosis type IV) demonstrate that enamel of both primary and secondary dentitions is thin but contrasts well from dentin. (From Levin, L. S., Jorgenson, R. J., and Salinas, C. F.: Oral Surg. 39:390, 1975.)

pearance not unlike that seen in opalescent dentin.

Inherited defects involving enamel and other tooth structures accompanying generalized defects

Trichodentoosseous syndrome. Trichodentoosseous syndrome consists of hypoplastic-hypocalcified enamel, taurodont teeth, tightly curly hair (Fig. 7-79), and cortical osteosclerosis. A family with affected members showing tightly curled hair, hypoplastic enamel, and laminated splitting of the superficial layers of nails or thick cornified nails was described by Robinson and co-workers.[131] The pulp chambers were described as small in anterior teeth, which had severe attrition, and in molars they "conformed to the flat configuration of the crown." However, a ground section illustrating the enamel defect also showed the enlarged pulp chambers and an apically placed bifurcation of an

obviously taurodont molar tooth (Fig. 7-80). Winter and associates[172] described an extensive kindred in which hypoplastic-hypocalcified enamel and taurodont teeth were inherited as an autosomal dominant trait, but they did not indicate that any of the affected members had unusual hair, nails, or bone. Crawford[33] described a patient with hypoplastic enamel and taurodont teeth, which also occurred in other family members, compatible with an autosomal dominant trait. The condition of the hair, nails, and bone was not described, but radiographs of the teeth illustrated dense bone in the maxilla and mandible. Subsequent investigation of the family indicated that those with the dental changes had tightly curly hair. Lichtenstein and Warson,[98] Lichtenstein and co-workers,[99] and Jorgenson and Warson[87] described an extensive kindred wherein affected members had, in addition to the hair and tooth defects, osteosclerosis of the bone cortex

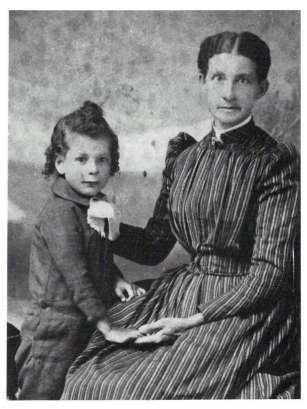

Fig. 7-79. Members of kindred with trichodentoosseous syndrome illustrating tightly curled hair exhibited by many affected persons. (From Robinson, G. C., Miller, J. R., and Worth, H. M.: Pediatrics **37**:498, 1966.)

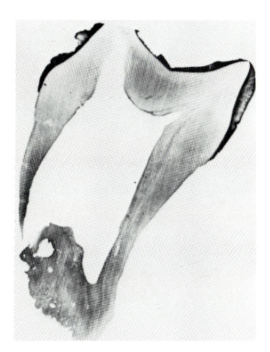

without increased cortical thickening. These examples probably represent the same defect,[185] since all features of the syndrome may not be present in all affected members of any one kindred. Tightly curled hair may be present at birth but may not be obvious when the same individual reaches adulthood.[74] Osteosclerosis is also variable and appears to be present in about 50% of the patients. The family described by Gulmen[74] has affected

Fig. 7-80. Ground sections of molar tooth from patient with the trichodentoosseous syndrome showing enlarged pulp chamber and apically placed bifurcation of taurodont-shaped tooth. Note thin layer of enamel. Pulp horns have been filled with secondary dentin. (From Robinson, G. C., Miller, J. R., and Worth, H. M.: Pediatrics **37**:498, 1966.)

individuals with taurodont teeth and enamel hypoplasia but without hair, nail, or bone defects at the time of examination, whereas others had various combinations of these defects. It appears that the enamel and taurodontic defects are the most constant features of the syndrome, followed by hair, bone, and nail defects.

Affected individuals usually first manifest the trait in infancy by developing a full head of tightly curled to kinky hair (Fig. 7-79). Some retain this hair feature into adulthood, but often the hair becomes straight.[74, 99] Affected family members have characteristic facies, being dolichocephalic with frontal bossing and square jaw. Psychosomatic milestones are normal. Radiographically, bone density of both flat and long bones may be from mildly to moderately increased, with osteosclerosis of skull base being the most consistently involved site. The trabecular architecture is usually fine without any alterations of general bone outline. Mandibular rami may be shortened with an obtuse inferior angle.[99]

The clinical appearance of the teeth is variable, presenting features of all of the various types of enamel defects, hypoplasia, hypomaturation, and hypocalcification of enamel.[33, 87, 115, 172] Primary as well as secondary teeth are involved in this syndrome, having both a taurodont configuration of molar teeth and a hypoplastic-hypomature enamel. The most frequently seen defect is hypoplasia of enamel, wherein the teeth appear small and do not meet at the contact points due to the thinness of the enamel (Fig. 7-81). Other patients have had enamel of full thickness that has a mottled yellow-white color resembling that seen in hypomaturation defects.[172] Some patients have mottled yellow-white enamel with pits distributed predominantly over the labial-buccal surfaces (Fig. 7-82). The teeth are susceptible to attrition and tend to wear down rapidly. This trait, combined with the histological finding of high pulp horns reaching the dentinoenamel junction similar to that seen in vitamin D–resistant rickets (hypophosphatemia), makes these patients susceptible to microexposure of the pulp horns with subsequent multiple abcesses, which have been reported in over 75% of affected patients.[87] Eruption of the primary dentition may be delayed, and many

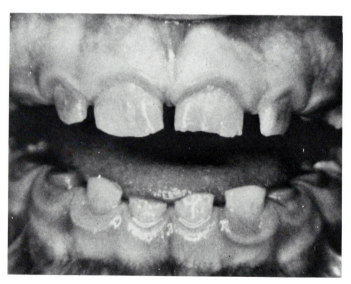

Fig. 7-81. Teeth of patient with trichodentoosseous syndrome show thin enamel such that teeth lack normal contour and do not meet at contact points. Note marked occlusal wear on teeth approaching that seen in hereditary opalescent dentin. (From Crawford, J. L.: J. Dent. Child. 37:83, 1970.)

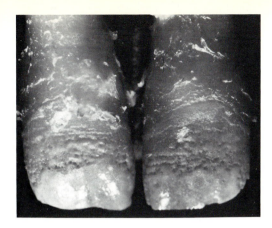

Fig. 7-82. Surface of enamel of patient with trichodentoosseous syndrome shows numerous pits in thin enamel. (Courtesy Dr. Ronald Jorgenson, Charleston, S.C.)

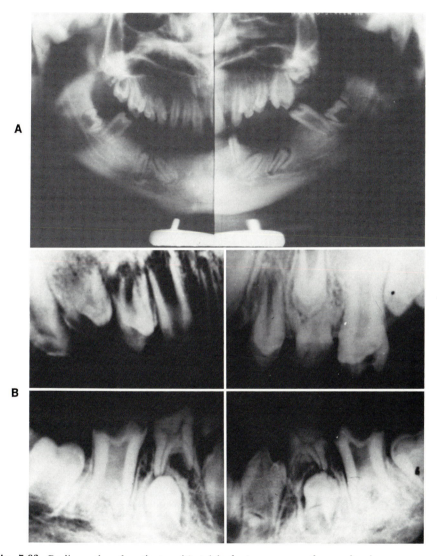

A

B

Fig. 7-83. Radiographs of patients with trichodentoosseous syndrome showing numerous unerupted teeth with large pulp chambers, A, and high pulp horns, B. Note thin layer of enamel, B, and taurodont molar teeth. (A from Jorgenson, R. J., and Warson, R. W.: Oral Surg. 36: 693, 1973; B from Crawford, J. L.: J. Dent. Child. 37:83, 1970.)

teeth of the secondary dentition may be un-erupted.

Radiographs of the teeth show thin enamel having normal contrast with the dentin or enamel of full thickness that has a radio-density similar to that of dentin. The molar teeth have a taurodontic form with delayed closure of the apices and frequently demonstrate periapical radiolucent areas subsequent to microexposure of the pulp.

Histological sections of teeth show enlarged pulp chambers, deposition of secondary dentin, and thin enamel with areas of hypoplasia or hypocalcification. Although taurodontism is difficult to demonstrate in anterior teeth, it is obvious that anterior as well as posterior teeth in this syndrome initially have large pulp cavities (Fig. 7-83), which may become reduced in size by secondary dentin. The enamel is thin on teeth of both dentitions. Local areas of enamel show features of calcification defects, having short hypomineralized enamel rods or having inclusions within the enamel. The defect described by Winter and associates[172] indicates that a band about 200 μm wide adjacent to the surface appears similar to normal enamel. Below this normal band, the enamel is hypomature with large prominent interprismatic spaces, prominent striae of Retzius, and prism cross striations. Near the dentinoenamel junction, the enamel has a band about 60 μm wide that contains large irregular opaque globules that distort the prism structure. These defects range up to 20 μm across and tend to lie at right angles to the enamel prisms. They resemble the vascular arcades seen in areas of inter-globular dentin of dentin dysplasia. The surface of the enamel is covered in part by a laminated homogeneous layer attached by processes that extend into the enamel surface. The dentin adjacent to the dentinoenamel junction shows some reduction in the number of dentinal tubules as a minor variation. Irregular secondary dentin may be deposited on the pulpal third of root dentin, tertiary dentin in the pulp horn areas, and amorphous denticles in the pulp tissue.[115]

The association of pitting hypoplasia, hypomature enamel, and taurodont teeth points

to a defect in the epithelial elements of the odontogenic organ, since the epithelial cells of the enamel organ establish the outline form of the tooth, induce odontoblastic differentiation, establish the area of bifurcation or trifurcation in multirooted teeth, and produce enamel. The presence of defective laminated nails and thick curly hair also supports an ectodermal defect. However, the sclerotic bone indicates that the defect involves mesenchymal as well as ectodermal structures. Possibly the defect involves a protein common to all of these structures.

All kindreds reported indicate an autosomal dominant mode of inheritance,* suggesting a defect in a structural protein common to the involved structures.

Pseudohypoparathyroidism (PHP).[2] Possibly two types of pseudohypoparathyroidism exist and are currently designated type I and type II. The basic chemical defect in PHP I is an unresponsiveness of target cells in bone and kidney to a parathyroid hormone.[8] The hormone is normal and is produced in adequate amounts but fails to stimulate adenyl cyclase to produce cyclic 3'-5' adenosine monophosphate, the cytoplasmic messenger, in adequate amounts to cause a phosphate diuresis in the kidney and resorption of calcium phosphate from bone.[29] PHP II has a normal rise in cyclic AMP after parathyroid hormone stimulation, so apparently it has an intact receptor hormone site on the target cells, but this is ineffective in causing a phosphate diuresis. Correction of this defect may ensue after calcium infusion.[133] The site of the chemical defect in type II is possibly an abnormality in cyclic adenosine monophosphate phosphodiesterase, the second step in the cytoplasmic cascade system. We are unaware of any differences in the teeth in the two types.

PHP is inherited as an X-linked trait[105, 177, 178] in which dental as well as biochemical manifestations vary according to the sex of the patient.[185] In general, males are more severely affected than females, although the latter are more commonly encountered. Sub-

---

*See references 33, 87, 98, 99, 115, 172.

jects with PHP have short neck, round facies (Fig. 7-84), thick, stocky body build, short digits (Fig. 7-85), most frequently the fourth metacarpal, extraosseous calcifications, most frequently lamellar calcifications of the falx cerebri and basal ganglia, thin, pitted enamel, hypocalcemia, and failure to respond to administered parathyroid extract with a normal phosphate diuresis and a rise in serum calcium.[123] Hypocalcemia leads to tetany, convulsions, and muscle cramps and may be mistaken for epilepsy, especially in infancy and childhood.

Within kindreds in which at least one individual has PHP, there are usually other individuals who have the morphological stigmata of PHP but who do not show the chemical abnormalities of PHP. These individuals, on testing their response to parathyroid extract, respond normally with a phosphate diuresis and a rise in serum calcium. These individuals are designated as having pseudopseudohypoparathyroidism (PPHP). Patients with PPHP have not been noted to have specific dental defects; the latter have been observed only in patients with PHP.[186]

Defective teeth have been found in from 37% to 50% of patients with PHP.[186]

The tooth defect is more severe in male than in female patients, as would be expected of an X-linked trait. The tooth defect affects teeth in the order of development. Thus, if first permanent molars are hypoplastic, teeth that develop subsequent to the first molars, such as bicuspids, cuspids, second and

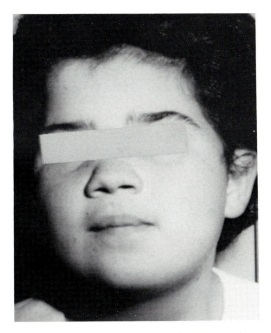

Fig. 7-84. Facies of patient with PHP tends to be round and full appearing. (From Croft, L. K., Witkop, C. J., Jr., and Glas, J.-E.: Oral Surg. **20:** 758, 1965.)

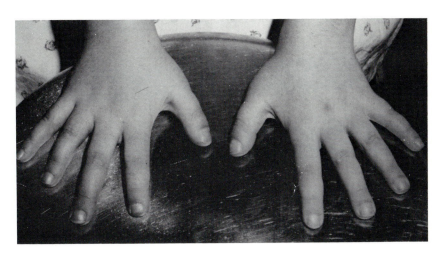

Fig. 7-85. Patients with PHP may have short digits, most frequently fourth finger due to short metacarpal bone. Note short finger on patient's right hand. (From Croft, L. K., Witkop, C. J., and Glas, J.-E.: Oral Surg. 20:758, 1965.)

third molars, are also defective. The most frequently affected group of teeth in female patients observed in our series were the bicuspid and second and third molar teeth. This pattern of tooth defects in PHP and the observation that some patients have been tested as PPHP at a young age who subsequently developed the chemical changes of PHP[10, 177, 178] suggest that the defect seen in teeth marks the chronological onset of the chemical changes of PHP. Primary teeth are rarely affected and have been observed to be involved in only one male patient in our series. Both male and female patients show delayed eruption of teeth of the secondary dentition, which also show defects of the enamel (Figs. 7-86 to 7-88). The involved teeth are grossly wedge shaped, having short roots and delayed closure of the root canal at the apices (Figs. 7-87 and 7-88). Male patients have thin enamel with small pits on the enamel surfaces

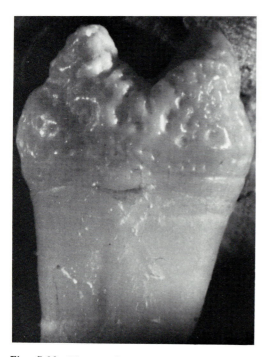

Fig. 7-86. Unerupted premolar tooth extracted from 12-year-old girl with PHP. Crown is covered with hypoplastic enamel characterized by random pitting. Enamel is hard and of normal color. (From Croft, L. K., Witkop, C. J., and Glas, J.-E.: Oral Surg. 20:758, 1965.)

(Fig. 7-88), whereas the affected teeth in female patients have enamel of essentially normal thickness with large pits randomly distributed over the crown (Fig. 7-86).[34]

Radiographic features found in any particular patient are variable depending on the sex and age of the patient at the time that the chemical changes of PHP appear in the patient. Male patients have small wedge-shaped teeth with short roots and delayed closure of apices (Fig. 7-88). Many teeth may still be within bony crypts beyond the age that the tooth is normally fully erupted (Fig. 7-88). Female patients show gross pitting of enamel, wedge-shaped teeth with short roots, delayed closure of apices, and most frequently involvement of bicuspid and second and third molar teeth only. This pattern of affected teeth in females is one which is most important for dentists to recognize. We have had a number of patients referred for Dilantin gingival hyperplasia with the question, "Why are the bicuspid and second and third molar teeth hypoplastic?" These patients have been children who have had unrecognized PHP, the hypocalcemic tetany being misdiagnosed as petit mal and treated with diphenylhydantoin (Dilantin).

Histological features of the enamel defect in female patients show that the enamel is grossly pitted with incremental lines of Retzius bending down under the individual pits, indicating a defect in development rather than a secondary defect produced by resorption of normally formed enamel wherein these lines would be interrupted (Fig. 7-89). There is normal contrast of enamel and dentin seen both on general radiographs and micrographs of tooth sections (Fig. 7-90), indicating that calcification of enamel is not grossly defective. The dentin contains numerous areas of interglobular calcification, which are most prominent near the root apices, which tend to be open beyond the age when normal apical closure occurs (Fig. 7-90). The dentin in affected teeth may show defects in calcification, particularly near the apices of the teeth, where areas of interglobular calcification are common (Fig. 7-91).

PHP is an X-linked trait with affected

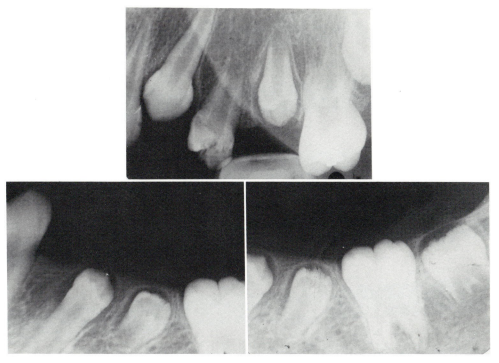

Fig. 7-87. Radiographs of 12-year-old girl with PHP show delayed eruption of teeth, pitted enamel on premolar and second molar teeth, and delayed closure of apices of teeth. (From Croft, L. K., Witkop, C. J., and Glas, J.-E.: Oral Surg. **20:**758, 1965.)

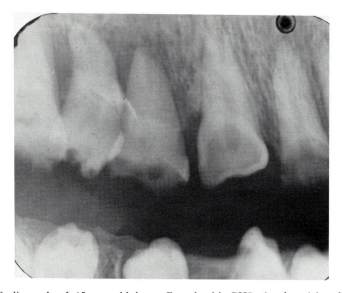

Fig. 7-88. Radiograph of 15-year-old boy affected with PHP showing delayed eruption of wedge-shaped teeth covered with layer of enamel that is thinner than that seen in affected females. Compare with Fig. 7-87. (From Witkop, C. J., Jr., and Rao, S.: Birth Defects **7**[7]: 153-184, 1971.)

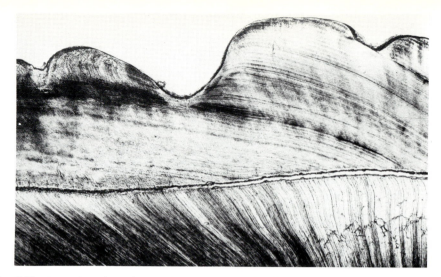

Fig. 7-89. Ground section of tooth from 12-year-old girl with PHP shows gross pitting of enamel. Developmental lines of Retzius bend beneath defect, indicating defect in development of enamel rather than resorption of fully formed enamel. (From Croft, L. K., Witkop, C. J., Jr., and Glas, J.-E.: Oral Surg. 20:758, 1965.)

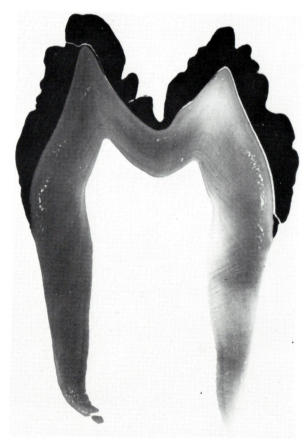

Fig. 7-90. Microradiograph of section of premolar tooth from 12-year-old girl with PHP shows normal contrast between enamel and dentin, indicating that there is no gross defect in mineralization of enamel. Apex of this tooth is still open at 12 years of age. (From Croft, L. K., Witkop, C. J., Jr., and Glas, J.-E.: Oral Surg. 20:758, 1965.)

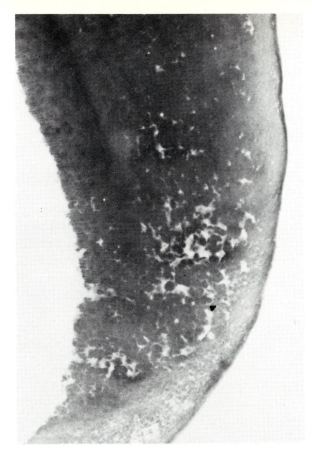

Fig. 7-91. Microradiograph of ground section of tooth from 12-year-old girl with PHP shows interglobular calcification of dentin adjacent to apex of root. (From Croft, L. K., Witkop, C. J., Jr., and Glas, J.-E.: Oral Surg. 20:758, 1965.)

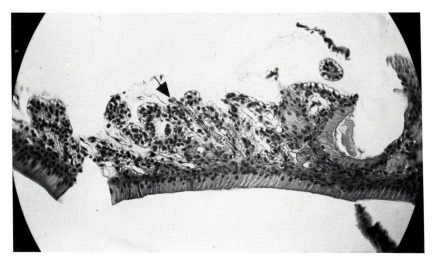

Fig. 7-92. Photomicrograph of enamel organ covering normal developing enamel shows penetration of stellate reticulum by blood vessels, *arrow,* which reach level of stratum intermedium. Defect in exchange of metabolites at these points could account for random pitting seen in teeth of females heterozygous for PHP. (From Ussing, M. N.: Acta Odontol. Scand. 13:123, 1955.)

males having thin enamel with small pits, whereas females have enamel of essentially normal thickness with large pits randomly distributed over the crown. The hypothesis proposed to explain this phenomenon[177] is that although the differences in males and females are due to a Lyonization effect, in contrast to the vertical distribution of normal and hypoplastic enamel bands seen in X-linked types of amelogenesis imperfecta in which the gene mutation most likely results in an abnormal function of individual ameloblasts, in PHP the mutation results in a defect in the vascular portion of the enamel organ.[177, 178] Normally, the outer enamel epithelium of the developing dental follicle is invaded at many points by capillary loops just before the elongation of the interenamel epithelial cells as they assume their mature configuration as functional ameloblasts. These loops penetrate the stellate reticulum and lie adjacent to the stratum intermedium (Fig. 7-92).

A random type pitting in females heterozygous for PHP and generalized thin enamel in hemizygous males could result if the gene action occurred at the anatomical site of the vascular loops. Females having both normal and abnormal clones of cells would have the random pitted pattern.

Kindreds wherein some patients have PHP and other relatives may have PHP or PPHP are compatible with an X-linked mode of inheritance.

Vitamin D–dependent rickets. In vitamin D–dependent rickets, the children are normal at birth, develop hypocalcemic, hypophosphatemic rickets in the latter half of the first year of life, and have generalized renal tubular dysfunction. This latter sign disappears on doses of vitamin D_2 or D_3 when given at about 100 times the usual daily allowance.

Two prominent features distinguishing vitamin D–dependent rickets[5] from vitamin D–resistant rickets (hypophosphatemia) are that the dependent form has hypoplasia of enamel and is inherited as an autosomal recessive trait, whereas hypoplastic enamel is an uncommon feature in hypophosphatemic vitamin D–resistant rickets, which is inherited as an X-linked disorder. Thus females may be as severely affected as males in vitamin D–dependent rickets.

Teeth that calcify postnatally are affected, the maternal normal chemistry apparently protecting the fetus. Typically, the permanent teeth show gross hypoplasia of incisal and occlusal enamel in the form of large pits (Fig. 7-93). The enamel may be mottled yellow-gray in color, resembling the enamel seen in

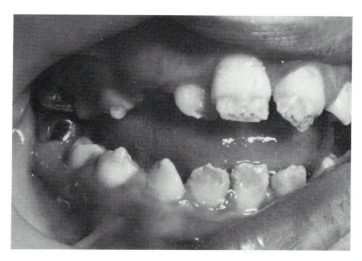

Fig. 7-93. Intraoral photograph of 15-year-old boy with vitamin D–dependent rickets showing characteristic hypoplastic enamel on incisal and occlusal aspects of secondary teeth. Enamel was opaque mottled yellow-gray in this patient.

hypomaturation defects. Primary teeth may be affected rarely. When enamel and dentin defects are present in the primary teeth, they usually spare the primary incisor teeth but affect the cuspid and molar teeth (Fig. 7-94).

In addition to hypoplasia of enamel, radiographic changes show large pulp chambers, high pulp horns, and delayed closure of root apices (Fig. 7-95). Children with de Toni-Debre-Fanconi syndrome have essentially the same dental changes.[186]

Microexposures of the pulp horns may occur, resulting in pulp death and periapical lesions. The response to vitamin D_2 or D_3 therapy is better than that seen in hypophosphatemic vitamin D–resistant rickets. Early treatment possibly would protect the child from having defects in teeth that develop subsequent to therapy.

The histological features of the teeth have been unreported to our knowledge, but they would be expected to show an enamel defect similar to that seen in PHP with the additional feature of areas of hypomaturation of enamel and large amounts of interglobular dentin throughout the crown and particularly near root apices.

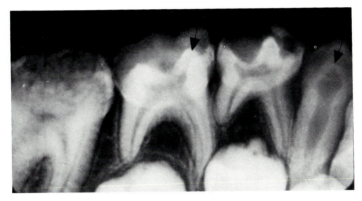

Fig. 7-94. Radiographs of patient with vitamin D–dependent rickets showing teeth with high pulp horns extending toward dentinoenamel junction, *arrows,* and hypoplastic enamel.

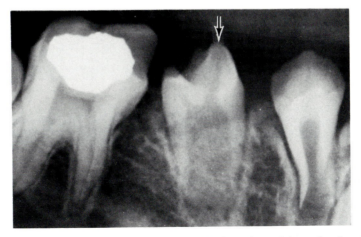

Fig. 7-95. Radiograph of patient with vitamin D–dependent rickets showing thin hypoplastic enamel covering crowns of teeth, high pulp horn in rotated second premolar reaching dentinoenamel junction, and delayed closure of root apices.

REFERENCES

1. Adams, R. D., and Reed, W. B.: Neuro-cutaneous diseases. In Fitzpatrick, T. B., et al.: Dermatology in general medicine, New York, 1971, McGraw-Hill Book Co., pp. 1386-1393.

2. Albright, F., Burnett, C. H., Smith, P. H., and Parson, W.: Pseudohypoparathyroidism—an example of Seabright-Bantam syndrome, Endocrinology 30:922, 1942.

3. Angmar-Mansson, B.: A quantitative microradiographic study on the organic matrix of developing human enamel in relation to the mineral content, Arch. Oral Biol. 16:135, 1971.

4. Archard, H. O., and Witkop, C. J., Jr.: Hereditary hypophosphatemia (vitamin D–resistant rickets) presenting primary dental manifestations, Oral Surg. 22:184, 1966.

5. Arnaud, C., Maijer, R., Reade, T., Scrivner, C. R., and Whelen, D. T.: Vitamin D dependency: an inherited postnatal syndrome with secondary hyperparathyroidism, Pediatrics 46:871, 1970.

6. Arwill, T., Bergenholtz, A., and Olsson, O.: Epidermolysis bullosa hereditaria. III. A histologic study of the teeth in the polydysplastic, dystrophic, and lethal forms, Oral Surg. 19:723, 1965.

7. Arwill, T., Bergenholtz, A., and Thilander, H.: Epidermolysis bullosa hereditaria. V. The ultrastructure of oral mucosa and skin in four cases of the letalis form, Acta Pathol. Microbiol. Scand. 74:311, 1968.

8. Aurbach, G. D., Patts, J. T., Jr., Chase, L. R., and Melson, G. L.: Polypeptide hormones and calcium metabolism, Ann. Intern. Med. 70:1243, 1969.

9. Bart, B.: Epidermolysis bullosa and congenital localized absence of skin, Arch. Dermatol. 101:78, 1970.

10. Bartter, F. C.: Hypophosphatasia. In Stanbury, J. B., Wyngaarden, J. B., and Fredrickson, D. S.: The metabolic basis of inherited disease, ed. 2, New York, 1966, McGraw-Hill Book Co., pp. 1015-1023.

11. Bergenholtz, A., and Olsson, O.: Epidermolysis bullosa hereditaria. I. Epidermolysis bullosa hereditaria letalis; a survey of the literature and report of 11 cases, Acta Derm. Venereol. (Stockh.) 48:220, 1968.

12. Berkman, M. D., and Singer, A.: Demonstration of the Lyon hypothesis in X-linked dominant hypoplastic amelogenesis imperfecta. In Bergsma, D.: Birth defects original article series, pt. 11, Orofacial structures, vol. 7, no. 7, Baltimore, 1971, The Williams & Wilkins Co., pp. 204-209.

13. Boyde, A.: The development of enamel structure, Proc. R. Soc. Med. (Odontol.) 60:923, 1967.

14. Boyde, A.: Electron microscopic observations relating to the nature and development of prism decussation in mammalian dental enamel, Bull. Group Int. Rech. Sci. Stomatol. 12:151, 1969.

15. Boyde, A.: The surface of the enamel in human hypoplastic teeth, Arch. Oral Biol. 15:897, 1970.

16. Boyde, A., and Lester, K. S.: The structure and development of marsupial enamel tubules, Z. Zellforsch. Mikrosk. Anat. 82:558, 1967.

17. Brabant, H., Werelds, R., and Klees, L.: Les altérations dentaires dans la maladie de Morquio, Rev. Stomatol. Chir. Maxillofac. 63:466, 1962.

18. Brailsford, J. R.: Chondro-osteo-dystrophy: roentgenographic and clinical features of child with dislocation of vertebrae, Am. J. Surg. 7:404, 1929.

19. Brain, E. B., and Wigglesworth, J. S.: Developing teeth in epidermolysis bullosa hereditaria letalis: a histologic study, Br. Dent. J. 124:255, 1968.

20. Bundey, S., and Evans, K.: Tuberous sclerosis: a genetic study, J. Neurol. Neurosurg. Psychiatry 32:591, 1969.

21. Burgess, R. C., and Maclaren, C.: Proteins in developing bovine enamel. In Stack, M. V., and Fearnhead, R. W.: Tooth enamel, its composition, properties, and fundamental structure, Bristol, England, 1965, John Wright & Sons, Ltd., pp. 74, 109.

22. Burgess, R. C., Nikiforuk, G., and Maclaren, C.: Chromatographic studies on carbohydrate components in enamel, Arch. Oral Biol. 3:8, 1960.

23. Burrows, L. R.: An investigation of proteins of human enamel matrix with special reference to the amino-acid hydroxyproline. In Stack, M. V., and Fearnhead, R. W.: Tooth enamel, its composition, properties, and fundamental structure, Bristol, England, 1965, John Wright & Sons, Ltd., pp. 59, 99.

24. Burzynski, N. J., Gonzalez, W. E., and Snawder, K. D.: Autosomal dominant smooth hypoplastic amelogenesis imperfecta, Oral Surg. 36:818, 1973.

25. Cameron, I. W., and Bradford, E. W.: Amelogenesis imperfecta: a case report of a family, Br. Dent. J. 102:129, 1957.

26. Carol, W. L. L.: Beitrag zur Kenntnis des Adenoma Sebaceum (Pringle) und sein Verhälthis zur Krankheit von Bourneville und von Recklinghausen, Acta Derm. Venereol. (Stockh.) 2:186, 1921-1922.

27. Catena, D. L., Miller, A. S., Leberman, O. F., Freeman, N. C., and Balick, N. L.: Consanguinity: report of a case, Oral Surg. **30:** 207, 1970.

28. Cawson, R. A.: The oral changes in gargoylism, Proc. R. Soc. Med. 55:1066, 1962.

29. Chase, L. F., Melson, G. L., and Aurbach, G. D.: Pseudohypoparathyroidism: defective excretion of 3′,5′-AMP in response to parathyroid hormone, J. Clin. Invest. 48:1832, 1969.

30. Chaudhry, A. P., Johnson, O. N., Mitchell, D. F., Gorlin, R. J., and Bartholdi, W. L.: Hereditary enamel dysplasia, J. Pediatr. **54:** 776, 1959.

31. Clark, R. D., Smith, J. D., Jr., and Davidson, E. A.: Hexosamine and acid glycosaminoglycans in human teeth, Biochim. Biophys. Acta 101:267, 1965.

32. Cowan, A.: Leontiasis ossea, Oral Surg. **12:** 983, 1959.

33. Crawford, J. L.: Concomitant taurodontism and amelogenesis imperfecta in the American Caucasian, J. Dent. Child. 37:83, 1970.

34. Croft, L. K., Witkop, C. J., Jr., and Glas, J.-E.: Pseudohypoparathyroidism, Oral Surg. **20:**758, 1965.

35. Darling, A. I.: Some observations on amelogenesis imperfecta and calcification of the dental enamel, Proc. R. Soc. Med. (Odontol.) **49:**759, 1956.

36. Davis, R. K., Bear, P. N., Archard, H. O., and Palmer, J. H.: Tuberous sclerosis with oral manifestations, Oral Surg. 17:395, 1964.

37. Davidson, B. C. C.: Epidermolysis bullosa, J. Med. Genet. 2:233, 1965.

38. Degering, C. I.: Amelogenesis imperfecta, a report of two cases, Oral Surg. 16:1051, 1963.

39. Delaire, J., Kerebal, B., and Billet, J.: Manifestation buccodentaires des epidermolysis bulleuses, Rev. Stomatol. Chir. Maxillofac. 61:189, 1960.

40. Desnick, S. J., Witkop, C. J., Jr., Krivit, W., Thies, J. K., and Desnick, R. J.: Fabry's disease: diagnostic confirmation by analysis of dental pulp, Arch. Oral Biol. 17:1473, 1972.

41. di Ferranti, N., and Nichols, B. L.: A case of Hunter syndrome with progeny, Johns Hopkins Med. J. 130:325, 1972.

42. Eastoe, J. E.: The amino acid composition of proteins from the oral tissues. II. The matrix proteins in dentine and enamel from developing human deciduous teeth, Arch. Oral Biol. 8:633, 1963.

43. Eastoe, J. E.: The chemical composition of bone and tooth, Adv. Fluorine Res. Dent. Caries Prevention 3:5, 1964.

44. Egyedi, H., and Stack, M. V.: The carbohydrate content of enamel, N.Y. State Dent. J. 22:486, 1956.

45. Eidelman, E., Chosack, A., and Wagner, M. L.: Orodigitofacial dysostosis and oculodentodigital dysplasia, Oral Surg. 23:311, 1967.

46. Endruschat, A. J., and Keenen, D. A.: Anesthetic and dental management of a child with epidermolysis bullosa dystrophica, Oral Surg. 36:667, 1973.

47. Erpenstein, H., and Wannenmacher, E.: Schmelzhypoplasie und offender Biss als autosomal dominant vererbtes Markmelspaar, Dtsch. Zahnaerztl. Z. 23:405, 1968.

48. Euler, H.: Über "angeborene Schmelzkypoplasien," Z. Stomatol. 42:337, 1944.

49. Fearnhead, R. W.: The insoluble organic component of human enamel. In Stack, M. V., and Fearnhead, R. W.: Tooth enamel, its composition, properties, and fundamental structure, Bristol, England, 1965, John Wright & Sons, Ltd., pp. 127-131.

50. Finn, S. B.: Dentin and enamel anomalies. In Witkop, C. J., Jr.: Genetics and dental health, New York, 1962, McGraw-Hill Book Co., pp. 219-245.

51. Fischman, S. L., and Fischman, I. C.: Hypoplastic amelogenesis imperfecta: report of a case, J. Am. Dent. Assoc. 75:929, 1967.

52. Fish, E. W.: Surgical pathology of the mouth, London, 1948, Sir Isaac Pitman & Sons, Ltd., pp. 359-383.

53. Fitzpatrick, T. B., Szabó, G., Hori, Y., Simone, A., Reed, W. B., and Greenberg, M. H.: White leaf-shaped macules, earliest visible sign of tuberous sclerosis, Arch. Dermatol. 98:1, 1968.

54. Fluckinger, G.: Drei falle von amelogenesis imperfecta hereditaria. Schweiz. Monatsschr. Zahnheilkd. 76:11, 1966.

55. Frank, R. M., and Bolender, C.: Amelogenesis imparfaite et retentions totales multiples des dents permanentes, Rev. Stomatol. Chir. Maxillofac. 63:23, 1962.

56. Frank, R. M., and Nalbandian, J.: Ultrastructure of amelogenesis. In Miles, A. E. W.: Structure and chemical organization of teeth, New York, 1967, Academic Press, Inc., pp. 399-446.

57. Gardner, D. G.: Metachromatic cells in gingiva in Hurler's syndrome, Oral Surg. 26: 782, 1968.

58. Gardner, D. G.: The oral manifestations of Hurler's syndrome, Oral Surg. 32:46, 1971.

59. Gardner, D. G., and Hudson, C. D.: The disturbance in odontogenesis in epidermolysis bullosa hereditaria letalis, Oral Surg. 40: 483, 1975.

60. Garn, S. M., and Hurme, V. O.: Dental defects in three siblings with Morquio's disease, Br. Dent. J. **93**:210, 1952.

61. Gedde-Dahl, T., Jr.: Epidermolysis bullosa: a clinical, genetic and epidemiologic study, Baltimore, 1971, The Johns Hopkins University Press.

62. Giansanti, J. S.: A kindred showing hypocalcified amelogenesis imperfecta: report of case, J. Am. Dent. Assoc. **86**:675, 1973.

63. Gillespie, F. D.: A hereditary syndrome: dysplasia oculodentodigitalis, Arch. Ophthalmol. **71**:187, 1964.

64. Glimcher, M. J.: Studies of embryonic and mature dental enamel; the "enamelins." In Chemistry and Physiology of Enamel, University of Michigan Symposium, Ann Arbor, Mich., 1971, University of Michigan Press, pp. 2-4.

65. Glimcher, M. J., Bonar, L. C., and Daniel, E. J.: Molecular structure of the protein matrix of bovine dental enamel, J. Mol. Biol. **3**:541, 1961.

66. Glimcher, M. J., Friberg, U. A., and Levine, P. T.: The isolation and amino acid composition of the enamel proteins of erupted bovine teeth, Biochem. J. **93**:202, 1964.

67. Glimcher, M. J., and Krane, S. M.: The identification of serine phosphate in enamel proteins, Biochim. Biophys. Acta **90**:477, 1964.

68. Glimcher, M. J., Mechanic, G. L., and Friberg, U. A.: The amino acid composition of the organic matrix and the neutral soluble and acid soluble components of embryonic bovine enamel, Biochem. J. **93**:198, 1964.

69. Glimcher, M. J., Travis, D. F., Friberg, U. A., and Mechanic, G. L.: The electron microscopic localization of the neutral soluble proteins of developing bovine enamel, J. Ultrastruct. Res. **10**:362, 1964.

70. Gorlin, R. J.: Epidermolysis bullosa, Oral Surg. **32**:760, 1971.

71. Gorlin, R. J., Chaudhry, A. P., and Kelln, E. E.: Oral manifestations of the Fitzgerald-Gardner, Pringle-Bourneville, Robin, adrenogenital, and Hurler-Pfaundler syndromes, Oral Surg. **13**:1233, 1960.

72. Gorlin, R. J., Meskin, L. H., and Geme, J. W.: Oculo-dento-digital dysplasia, J. Pediatr. **63**:69, 1963.

73. Gorlin, R. J., and Pindborg, J. J.: Syndromes of the head and neck, New York, 1964, McGraw-Hill Book Co., pp. 528-535.

74. Gulmen, S.: Personal communication, St. Louis, 1975, Washington University.

75. Witkop, C. J., Jr., Gundlach, K. K. H., Streed, W. J., and Sauk, J. J., Jr.: Globodontia in the otodental syndrome, Oral Surg. **41**:472, 1976.

76. Gustafson, G., Nystrom, P., and Stelling, E.: Five cases of pronounced enamel hypocalcification within the same family, Odontol. Tidskr. **55**:183, 1947, (abst.) Dent. Record **68**:75, 1948.

77. Haldane, J. B. S.: A probably new sex-linked dominant in man, J. Hered. **28**:58, 1937.

78. Hall, R. K.: Gross tooth hypocalcification in vitamin D resistant rickets, Aust. Dent. J. **4**:329, 1959.

79. Hals, E.: Hereditary enamel hypoplasia: investigations of two families, Odontol. Tidskr. **66**:562, 1958.

80. Hals, E.: Dentin and enamel anomalies: histologic observation. In Witkop, C. J., Jr.: Genetics and dental health, New York, 1962, McGraw-Hill Book Co., pp. 246-260.

81. Harris, R., and Sullivan, H. R.: Dental sequelae in deciduous dentition in vitamin D resistant rickets, Aust. Dent. J. **5**:200, 1960.

82. Haslam, R. H. A.: Tuberous sclerosis. In Bergsma, D.: Birth defects atlas and compendium, Baltimore, 1973, The Williams & Wilkins Co., p. 807.

83. Hiyama, K., and Kanai, T.: A clinical report of familial enamel hypoplasia, J. Stomatol. Soc. (Koku-Byo-Gakkai Zasshi) **17**:75, 1943.

84. Hoff, M., van Grunsven, M. F., Jongebloed, W. L., and 's-Gravenmade, E. J.: Enamel defects associated with tuberous sclerosis: a clinical and scanning-electron-microscope study, Oral Surg. **40**:261, 1975.

85. Hunter, C.: A rare disease in two brothers, Proc. R. Soc. Med. **10**:104, 1917.

86. Hurler, G.: Über einen Typ multipler Abartungen, vorwiegend am Skelettsystem. Z. Kinderheilkd. **24**:220, 1919.

87. Jorgenson, R. J., and Warson, R. W.: Dental abnormalities in the tricho-dento-osseous syndrome, Oral Surg. **36**:693, 1973.

88. Keeler, C. E.: Heredity in dentistry, Dent. Cosmos **77**:1147, 1935.

89. Kinase, H.: Regelung einer Klasse III nach Angle mit nachfolgendem Mantelkronenersatz bei "angeborener Schmelzhypoplasie" samtlicher Zahne, Z. Stomatol. **50**:543, 1953.

90. Köhlschütter, A., Chappuis, D., Meier, C., Tönz, O., Vassella, F., and Herschkowitz, N.: Familial epilepsy and yellow teeth—a disease of the CNS associated with enamel hypoplasia, Helv. Paediatr. Acta **29**:283, 1974.

91. Krane, S. M., Stone, M. J., and Glimcher, M. J.: The presence of protein phosphokinase in connective tissues and the phosphorylation of enamel proteins *in vitro,* Biochim. Biophys. Acta **97**:77, 1965.

92. Kresse, H., and Neufeld, E. F.: The Sanfilippo A corrective factor: purification and

mode of action, J. Biol. Chem. **247**:2164, 1972.

93. Lagos, J. E., and Gomez, M. R.: Tuberous sclerosis: reappraisal of a clinical entity, Mayo Clin. Proc. **42**:26, 1967.

94. Laird, W. R. E.: Hereditary amelogenesis imperfecta, Dent. Pract. **19**:90, 1968.

95. Langer, L. O., and Carey, L. S.: The roentgenographic features of the KS mucopolysaccharidosis of Morquio (Morquio-Brailsford's disease), Am. J. Roentgenol. **97**:1, 1966.

96. Levin, L. S., and Jorgenson, R. J.: Otodental dyplasia: a previously undescribed syndrome. In Bergsma, D.: Clinical delineation of birth defects. XVI. Urinary system and others, Baltimore, 1974, The Williams & Wilkins Co., pp. 310-312.

97. Levin, L. S., Jorgenson, R. J., and Salinas, C. F.: Oral findings in the Morquio syndrome (mucopolysaccharidosis IV), Oral Surg. **39**:390, 1975.

98. Lichtenstein, J. R., and Warson, R. W.: Syndrome of dental anomalies, curly hair and sclerotic bones. In Bergsma, D.: Birth defects original article series. XI. Orofacial structures, vol. 7, no. 7, Baltimore, 1971, The Williams & Wilkins Co., pp. 308-311.

99. Lichtenstein, J. R., Warson, R. W., Jorgenson, R. J., Dorst, J. P., and McKusick, V. A.: The tricho-dento-osseous (TDO) syndrome, Am. J. Hum. Genet. **24**:569, 1972.

100. Listgarten, M. A.: A mineralized cuticular structure with connective tissue characteristics on the crown of human unerupted teeth in amelogenesis imperfecta, a light and electron microscopic study, Arch. Oral Biol. **12**:877, 1967.

101. Lohmann, W.: Beitragzur Kenntnis des reinen Mikrophthalmus, Arch. Augenheilkd. **86**:136, 1920.

102. Lyon, M. F.: Gene action in the X-chromosome of the mouse *(Mus musculus L.)*, Nature **190**:372, 1961.

103. Mackler, S. B., Shoulars, H. W., and Burkes, E. J.: Tuberous sclerosis with gingival lesions, Oral Surg. **34**:619, 1972.

104. Macklin, M. T.: Absent tooth enamel, Eugenical News **23**:28, 1938.

105. Mann, J. B., Alterman, S., and Hills, A. G.: Albright's hereditary osteodystrophy comprising pseudohypoparathyroidism and pseudopseudohypoparathyroidism: with a report of two cases representing the complete syndrome occurring in successive generations, Ann. Intern. Med. **56**:315, 1962.

106. Marks, S. C., Lindahl, R. L., and Bawden, J. W.: Dental and cephalometric findings in vitamin D resistant rickets, J. Dent. Child. **32**:259, 1965.

107. Maroteaux, P., and Lamy, M.: Hurler's disease, Morquio's disease, and related mucopolysaccharidoses, J. Pediatr. **67**:312, 1965.

108. Maroteaux, P., Lamy, M., and Foucher, M.: La maladie de Morquio: étude clinique, radiologique et biologique, Presse Med. **71**:2091, 1963.

109. Matalon, R., Arbogast, B., and Dorfman, A.: Morquio's syndrome: a deficiency of chondroitin sulfate N-acetylhexosamine sulfate sulfatase (abst.), Pediatr. Res. **8**:436, 1974.

110. McKusick, V. A.: Heritable disorders of connective tissue, ed. 4, St. Louis, 1972, The C. V. Mosby Co., pp. 521-686.

111. McKusick, V. A.: Mendelian inheritance in man: catalogs of autosomal dominant, autosomal recessive, and X-linked phenotypes, ed. 4, Baltimore, 1975, The Johns Hopkins University Press, pp. 505-508, 643.

112. McKusick, V. A., Howell, R. R., Hussels, I. E., Neufeld, E. F., and Stevenson, R. E.: Allelism, nonallelism and genetic compounds among the mucopolysaccharidoses hypothesis, Lancet **1**:933, 1972.

113. McLarty, E. L., Giansanti, J. S., and Hibbard, E. D.: X-linked hypomaturation type of amelogenesis imperfecta exhibiting Lyonization in affected females, Oral Surg. **36**:678, 1973.

114. Meyer-Schwickerath, G.: Mikrophthalmussyndrome, Klin. Monatsbl. Augenheilkd. **131**:18, 1957.

115. Mjör, I. A.: The structure of taurodont teeth, J. Dent. Child. **39**:459, 1972.

116. Mohr, O. L.: Dominant acrocephalosyndactyly, Hereditas **25**:193, 1939.

117. Morquio, L.: Sur une forme de dystrophie osseuse familiale, Bull. Soc. Pediatr. Paris **27**:145, 1929.

118. Moynahan, E. J.: XTE syndrome (xeroderma, talipes and enamel defect): a new heredo-familial syndrome: two cases, homozygous inheritance of a dominant gene, Proc. R. Soc. Med. **63**:447, 1970.

119. O'Brien, J. S.: Sanfilippo syndrome: profound deficiency of alpha-acelyly-lucosaminidase activity in organs and skin fibroblasts from type-B patients, Proc. Natl. Acad. Sci. U.S.A. **69**:1720, 1972.

120. O'Rourk, T. R., Jr., and Bravos, A.: An oculo-dento-digital dysplasia. In Bergsma, D.: Birth defects original article series. II. Malformation syndromes, vol. 5, no. 2, New York, 1968, The National Foundation, pp. 226-237.

121. Pindborg, J. J.: Pathology of the dental hard tissue, Philadelphia, 1970, W. B. Saunders Co.

122. Pitter, J., and Svejda, J.: Über die Einfluss der Röntgenstrahlen auf die Entstchung von

Missbildungen der menschlichen Frucht, Ophthalmologica **123**:386, 1952.

123. Potts, J. T.: Pseudohypoparathyroidism. In Stanbury, J. B., Wyngaarden, J. B., and Frederickson, D. S.: The metabolic basis of inherited disease, ed. 3, New York, 1972, McGraw-Hill Book Co., pp. 1305-1319.

124. Prince, J., and Lilly, G.: Amelogenesis imperfecta: report of a case, Oral Surg. **25**: 134, 1968.

125. Rajic, D. S., and de Veber, L. L.: Hereditary oculodento osseous dysplasia, Ann. Radiol. **9**: 224, 1966.

126. Reed, W. B., Nickel, W. R., and Campion, G.: Internal manifestations of tuberous sclerosis, Arch. Dermatol. **87**:715, 1963.

127. Reilly, W. A., and Lindsay, S.: Gargoylism (lipochondrodystrophy), Am. J. Dis. Child. **75**:595, 1948.

128. Reisner, S. H., Kott, E., and Bornstein, B.: Oculodentodigital dysplasia, Am. J. Dis. Child. **118**:600, 1969.

129. Reith, E. J.: The ultrastructure of ameloblasts during matrix formation and maturation of enamel, J. Biophys. Biochem. Cytol. **9**: 825, 1961.

130. Reith, E. J., and Butcher, E. O.: Microanatomy and histochemistry of amelogenesis. In Miles, A. E. W.: Structure and chemical organization of teeth, New York, 1967, Academic Press, Inc., pp. 371-398.

131. Robinson, G. C., Miller, J. R., and Worth, H. M.: Hereditary enamel hypoplasia: its association with characteristic hair structure, Pediatrics **37**:498, 1966.

132. Rodermund, O. E.: Zahnveranderungen bei Epidermolysis bullosa, Dermatol. Wochenschr. **153**:350, 1967.

133. Rodriguez, H. V., Jr., Klahr, S., and Slatopolsky, E.: Pseudohypoparathyroidism type II: restoration of normal renal responsiveness to parathyroid hormone by calcium administration, J. Clin. Endocrinol. **39**:693, 1974.

134. Rushton, M. A.: A case of hereditary enamel hypoplasia, Br. Dent. J. **88**:300, 1950.

135. Rushton, M. A.: Teeth. In Sorsby, A.: Clinical genetics, St. Louis, 1953, The C. V. Mosby Co., pp. 382-397.

136. Rushton, M. A.: Some less common bone lesions affecting the jaws: tuberous sclerosis with jaw lesions, Oral Surg. **9**:298, 1956.

137. Rushton, M. A.: Surface of the enamel in hereditary enamel hypocalcification, Br. Dent. J. **112**:24, 1962.

138. Rushton, M. A.: Hereditary enamel defects, Proc. R. Soc. Med. **57**:53, 1964.

139. Rygge, J.: Trois cas de coloration brune de l'émail de toutes les dents chez trois enfants de même famille, Acta Odontol. Scand. **1**: 57, 1939.

140. Sato, M.: On a familial tooth hypocalcification, J. Jap. Dent. Acad. (Nikon-Shika-Gakkai-Zasshi) **32**:111, 1939.

141. Sanfilippo, S. J., Podosin, R., Langer, L. O., Jr., and Good, R. A.: Mental retardation associated with acid mucopolysacchariduria (heparitin sulfate type), J. Pediatr. **63**:837, 1963.

142. Sauk, J. J., Jr., Cotton, W. R., Lyon, H. W., and Witkop, C. J., Jr.: Electron optic analysis of hypomineralized amelogenesis imperfecta in man, Arch. Oral Biol. **12**:771, 1972.

143. Sauk, J. J., Jr., Lyon, H. W., and Witkop, C. J., Jr.: Electron optic microanalysis of two gene products in enamel of females heterozygous for X-linked hypomaturation amelogenesis imperfecta, Am. J. Hum. Genet. **24**:267, 1972.

144. Sauk, J. J., Jr., Vickers, R. A., Copeland, J. S., and Lyon, H. W.: The surface of genetically determined hypoplastic enamel in human teeth, Oral Surg. **34**:60, 1972.

145. Schulze, C.: Beitrag zur Frage der angeborenen Schmelzhypoplasie, Dtsch. Zahn. Mund. Kieferheilkd. **16**:108, 1952.

146. Schulze, C.: Über einen Fall von Hypoplasie du Hartsubstanzen bei Zahnen im Bereich des rechten Oberkiefers (Odontodysplia), Dtsch. Zahnaerztl Z. **11**:14-25, 1956.

147. Schulze, C.: Erbbedingte Strukturanomalien menschlicher Zahne, Acta Genet. Stat. Med. **7**:231, 1957.

148. Schulze, C.: Developmental abnormalities of the teeth and jaw. In Gorlin, R. J., and Goldman, H. M.: Thoma's oral pathology, ed. 6, vol. 1, St. Louis, 1970, The C. V. Mosby Co., pp. 96-183.

149. Scheie, H. G., Hambrick, G. W., Jr., and Barnes, L. A.: A newly recognized forme fruste of Hurler's disease (gargoylism), Am. J. Ophthalmol. **53**:753, 1962.

150. Schürmann, H., Greitehr, A., and Hornstein, O.: Krankheiten der Mundschleimhaut und der Lippen, ed. 3, Munich, Germany, 1966, Verlag Urban & Schwarzenberg, pp. 47-48.

151. Scott, D. B., Simmelink, J. W., and Nygaard, V.: Mineralization of dental enamel. In Avery, J. K.: Chemistry and physiology of enamel, Ann Arbor, Mich., 1971, University of Michigan Press, pp. 6-24.

152. Scott, D. B., Simmelink, J. W., Sevancar, J. R., and Smith, T. J.: Apatite crystal growth in biological systems. In Brown, W. E., and Young, R. A.: Structural properties of hydroxyapatite and related compounds, New York, 1972, Gordon & Breach, Science Publishers, Inc.

153. Sela, M., Eidelman, E., and Yatziv, S.: Oral manifestations of Morquio's syndrome, Oral Surg. **39**:583, 1975.

154. Sly, W. S., Quinton, B. A., McAlister, W. H., and Rimain, D. L.: Beta glucuronidase deficiency: report of clinical, radiologic and biochemical features of a new mucopolysaccharidosis, J. Pediatr. **82**:249, 1973.

155. Soifer, M. E.: Discolored hypoplastic teeth, Oral Surg. **6**:886, 1953.

156. Spokes, S.: Case of faulty development of enamel, Trans. Odontol. Soc. G. B. **22**:229, 1890.

157. Standish, M. L., and Gorlin, R.: Bone disorders affecting the jaws. In Gorlin, R. J., and Goldman, H. M.: Thoma's oral pathology, ed. 6, St. Louis, 1970, The C. V. Mosby Co., pp. 516-559.

158. Stevenson, R. E.: Mucopolysaccharidoses I, II, III, IV, V, VI. In Bergsma, D.: Birth defects atlas and compendium, Baltimore, 1973, The Williams & Wilkins Co., pp. 635-640.

159. Sugar, H. S., Thompson, J. P., and Davis, J. D.: The oculo-dento-digital dysplasia syndrome, Am. J. Ophthalmol. **61**:1448, 1966.

160. Toller, P. A.: A clinical report on six cases of amelogenesis imperfecta, Oral Surg. **12**:325, 1959.

161. Ussing, M. N.: The development of the epithelial attachment, Acta Odontol. Scand. **13**:123, 1955.

162. Weinmann, J. P., Svoboda, J. F., and Woods, R. W.: Hereditary disturbances of enamel formation and calcification, J. Am. Dent. Assoc. **32**:397, 1945.

163. Wennstrom, A.: Fall av amelogenesis imperfecta, Odontol. Foren. Tidskr. **27**:175, 1963.

164. Weyers, H.: Über eine regional auftretende Schmelzdysplasie (amelogenesis dysplastica) und ihre Beziehungen zu generalisierten Schmelzhypoplasien, Stoma **10**:177, 1957.

165. Weyman, J.: Two unusual cases of amelogenesis imperfecta, Br. Dent. J. **99**:228, 1955.

166. Wiesmann, U. N., and Neufeld, E. F.: Scheie und Hurler syndromes: apparent identity of the biochemical defect, Science **169**:72, 1970.

167. Wihr, N. L.: Abnormal dentition in vitamin D resistant rickets: a case report, J. Dent. Child. **37**:222, 1970.

168. Winter, G. B.: Hereditary and idiopathic anomalies of teeth number, structure and form, Dent. Clin. North Am. **13**:355, 1969.

169. Winter, G. B.: Personal communication, Guys Hospital, London, 1971.

170. Winter, G. B.: Personal communication, Eastman Dental Hospital, London, 1975.

171. Winter, G. B., and Brook, A. H.: Enamel hypoplasia and anomalies of the enamel. In Poole, A. E.: Symposium on genetics, Dent. Clin. North Am. **19**:3-24, 1975.

172. Winter, G. B., Lee, K. W., and Johnson, N. W.: Hereditary amelogenesis imperfecta: a rare autosomal dominant type, Br. Dent. J. **127**:157, 1969.

173. Witkop, C. J., Jr.: Hereditary defects in enamel and dentin, Acta Genet. Stat. Med. **7**:236, 1957.

174. Witkop, C. J., Jr.: Genetics and dentistry, Eugenics Quart. **5**:15, 1958.

175. Witkop, C. J., Jr.: Genetics and dentistry. In Hammons, H. G.: Hereditary counseling, New York, 1959, Hoeber, pp. 13-28.

176. Witkop, C. J., Jr.: Genetic diseases of the oral cavity. In Tiecke, R. W.: Oral pathology, New York, 1965, McGraw-Hill Book Co., pp. 786-843.

177. Witkop, C. J., Jr.: Inborn errors of metabolism with particular reference to pseudohypoparathyroidism, J. Dent. Res. **45**:568, 1966.

178. Witkop, C. J., Jr.: Genetic patterns in cutaneous neoplasms. In Berlin, N. I.: Basal cell nevus syndrome, Combined Clinical Staff Conference, National Institutes of Health, Ann. Intern. Med. **64**:403, 1966.

179. Witkop, C. J., Jr.: Partial expression of sex-linked recessive amelogenesis imperfecta in females compatible with the Lyon hypothesis, Oral Surg. **23**:174, 1967.

180. Witkop, C. J., Jr.: Heterogeneity in inherited dental traits, gingival fibromatosis and amelogenesis imperfecta, South. Med. J. **64**:16, 1971.

181. Witkop, C. J., Jr.: Genetics, Schweiz. Monatsschr. Zahnheilkd. **82**:917, 1972.

182. Witkop, C. J., Jr., Brearley, L. J., and Gentry, W. C., Jr.: Hypoplastic enamel, onycholysis, and hypohidrosis inherited as an autosomal dominant trait: a review of ectodermal dysplasia syndromes, Oral Surg. **39**:71, 1975.

183. Witkop, C. J., Jr., Kuhlmann, W., and Sauk, J. J., Jr.: Autosomal recessive pigmented hypomaturation amelogenesis imperfecta, Oral Surg. **36**:367, 1973.

184. Witkop, C. J., Jr., MacLean, C. J., Schmidt, P. J., and Henry, J. L.: Medical and dental findings in the Brandywine isolate, Ala. J. Med. Sci. **3**:382, 1966.

185. Witkop, C. J., Jr., and Rao, S.: Inherited defects in tooth structure. In Bergsma, D.: Birth defects original article series. XI. Orofacial structures, vol. 7, no. 7, Baltimore, 1971, The Williams & Wilkins Co., pp. 153-184.

186. Witkop, C. J., Jr., and Sauk, J. J., Jr.: Dental and oral manifestations of hereditary disease, Washington, D. C., 1971, American Academy of Oral Pathology.

187. Wittner, H. L.: Unusual case of hypocalcified enamel, J. Am. Dent. Assoc. **32**:210, 1945.

188. Worth, H. M.: Hurler's syndrome: a study of radiologic appearances in the jaws, Oral Surg. 22:21, 1966.

189. Zahn, H.: Über einen Fall bisher noch nicht beschriebenen Missbildung des Schmelzes der Milch-und der bleibenden Zähne, Medical dissertation, Wurzberg, Germany, 1935.

190. Zellweger, H., Ponseti, I. V., Pedrini, V., Stamler, F. S., and von Noorden, J. K.: Morquio-Ullrich's disease: report of two cases, J. Pediatr. 59:549, 1961.

8

Heritable disorders affecting dentin

DAVID BIXLER

In this chapter, heritable defects of dentin will be considered in two large groups: (1) those which are primary diseases of dentin itself and (2) those in which the dentin defect accompanies defects in other tissue systems. This latter category of secondary dentin defects contains both syndromes in which there is an obvious relationship between the dentin and other affected tissues (as in vitamin D–resistant rickets) and diseases that have no apparent relationship among the affected tissues (branchio-skeletal-genital syndrome).

A more detailed discussion of each of these groups of defects will be preceded by a section dealing with the embryology and biochemistry of dentin. This is an essential introduction for the reader to arrive at a basic understanding of dentin defects and to extend his thinking about etiology in each case. Wherever a heritable defect of dentin has been described and demonstrated, this approach should encourage the reader to hypothesize a fundamental biochemical or morphological defect that may be used to explain the disease spectrum.

EMBRYOLOGY OF DENTIN

The establishment of three primary germ layers in the embryo serves as the basis for differentiation of tissues and organs largely derived from each of the three layers. In regard to teeth, enamel and dentin develop from cells of ectodermal origin, whereas cementum has a mesodermal origin. The specific processes of cellular development, however, are much more complex and with regard to dentin involve the following sequential events:

1. Ectoderm divides into cutaneous and neural plate ectoderm, the latter giving rise to the neural tube.

2. Budding cells from the neural plate give rise to neural crest cells, which comprise a separate tissue akin to the three primary germ layers mentioned above.

3. Neural crest cells, although of ectodermal origin, give rise to tissues exhibiting properties of mesenchyme, which are thereby designated as ectomesenchyme in origin. (Mesenchyme is classified as tissue of mesodermal origin.)

4. Neural crest cells have migratory properties and move in the natural cleavage planes between ectoderm and mesoderm, giving rise to a myriad of structures of the head, face, and neck. Migration of neural crest cells in the trunk proceeds along two pathways, one alongside the neural tube and the other under the surface ectoderm. Essentially all of the neural crest cells giving rise to cranial structures follow the latter route.[5]

5. One of these neural crest derivatives appears to be the odontoblast cell, which ultimately gives rise to dentin.

Organogenesis

Potential odontogenic tissue can be identified as early as the twenty-eighth day of development in man and is characterized by ectodermal thickenings on the lateral margins of the stomodeum or primitive oral cavity. By the thirty-fifth day, four separate sites of odontogenic epithelium are recognizable, two in the maxilla and two in the mandible. These odontogenic epithelial islands coalesce on the thirty-seventh day to form the dental laminae, which are then two horseshoe-shaped plates, one in each jaw. Projections of the dental laminae into the subjacent mesenchyme at specific locations form the primordia of the primary *enamel* organs, ten in each jaw.

The enamel organ is a precursor of the tooth germ, which consists in toto of the enamel organ itself, a subjacent dental papilla, and a surrounding dental follicle. Thus the enamel organ is ectodermal in origin (inner enamel epithelium), whereas the dental papilla and dental follicle are ectomesenchymal in origin and are anlage of the dental pulp and peridontal apparatus. Recent evidence makes it probable that the neural crest cells that subsequently give rise to odontoblasts migrate into the dental papilla and differentiate there.[8]

Histogenesis

The initiation of enamel and dentin formation occurs when the preodontoblasts (neural crest cell derivatives) come into contact with the inner enamel epithelium destined to be ameloblasts. The remarkable sequence of events that follows has been described and experimentally manipulated.[3] They appear to consist of the following:

1. Preodontoblasts begin secretion of the predentin matrix between themselves and the preameloblasts. In this matrix are RNA-containing vesicles, which seem to be responsible for alterations in the basal lamina of the preameloblasts.

2. Matrix vesicles from these preodontoblasts come into close apposition with the preameloblast basement cell membrane and appear to alter it. This contact initiates the production of enamel matrix by preameloblasts.

3. Continued dentin matrix production by the cells now designated as odontoblasts occurs simultaneously with step 2.

The foregoing events clearly indicate that enamel and dentin are produced as the result of an inductive interaction between the two, with the ectomesenchymally derived odontoblast playing a critical role in initiation of tooth development. It is also now clear that the ectomesenchyme giving rise to the odontoblast is essential for determining tooth size and shape, since molar mesenchyme cultured with incisor epithelium gives rise to a molar tooth.[6, 7] Even lip epithelium may be induced to form enamel by odontoblastic mesenchyme. However, not all epithelia are competent to respond, so it appears that at least some general characteristics may be essential for an epithelium that is to be induced.[8]

The purpose of reviewing these events of morphogenesis is to emphasize the complex nature of odontogenesis, which is undoubtedly polygenically controlled. Therefore, it should not be surprising that the number of recognized, distinct heritable defects of teeth is growing every day.

THE BIOCHEMISTRY OF DENTIN

Dentin is composed principally of two tissues: (1) an organic matrix, which is the product of the odontoblast itself, and (2) an inorganic crystalline matrix, which is hydroxyapatite $[Ca_{10}(PO_4)_6(OH)_2]$ deposited within the organic matrix. A few brief comments about each of these matrices is appropriate.

Organic matrix

The primary product of the odontoblast is the organic matrix, which consists principally of the protein collagen, although a phosphoprotein necessary for mineralization is probably also an odontoblast product. From a conceptual standpoint, many authors have suggested that heritable diseases of dentin should ultimately be traceable to defects in a collagen protein, regardless of whether that defect lies in its primary, secondary, tertiary, or quaternary structure. As the following discussion will show, this concept is too simplistic and, in fact, inaccurate.

Primary protein structure is determined by

Table 8-1. Amino acid composition of normal human bone and dentin: number of residues per 1000 total residues recovered

	Bone	Dentin
Alanine	113.5	112.0
Glycine	319.0	319.0
Valine	23.6	25.0
Leucine	25.5	26.0
Isoleucine	13.3	10.0
Proline	123.4	115.0
Phenylalanine	13.9	14.0
Tyrosine	4.5	2.3
Serine	35.9	38.0
Threonine	18.4	19.0
Arginine	47.1	47.0
Methionine	5.3	5.2
Histidine	5.8	5.3
Lysine	28.0	23.0
Aspartic acid	47.0	55.0
Glutamic acid	72.2	73.0
Hydroxyproline	100.2	101.0
Hydroxylysine	3.5	8.4

Table 8-2. Collagen matrices of various cell types*

Cell type	Process	Collagen matrix type
Fibroblast	Fibrogenesis	Type I, $a_1(I)_2a_2$ Type III, $a_1(III)_3$
Odontoblast	Dentinogenesis	Type I
Ameloblast	Amelogenesis	Noncollagen matrix
Chondroblast	Chondrogenesis	Type II, $a_1(II)_3$
Osteoblast	Osteogenesis	Type I
Epithelia	Basal lamina formation	Type IV, $a_1(IV)_3$

*Modified from Slavkin, H. C., et al.: The role of extra-cellular matrix macromolecules upon cell differentiation. In Peeters, H., editor: Protides of the biological fluids, 22nd Colloquium, Oxford, England, 1975, Pergamon Press, Ltd.

which amino acids are placed in *what* order in the polypeptide chain. This process is under direct control of the genetic material (DNA) and is mediated by DNA-transcribed RNA. A considerable amount of evidence has accumulated regarding the amino acid composition of human collagen, both in bone and dentin. Table 8-1 shows data published by Eastoe and associates.[4]

Bearing in mind that the amino acid composition of bone collagen varies slightly, depending on the particular bone from which it was taken as well as the specific site in that bone, it can be seen that there is a high degree of similarity in amino acid composition between bone and dentin. This strongly suggests that there is little, if any, difference in the messenger RNA coding for bone or dentin collagen. The other essential feature of primary protein structure is identified in the specific sequence of amino acids in the primary polypeptide chain. As yet, sequencing of the amino acids in these collagen chains has not been accomplished, which leaves considerable doubt about the identity of the genetic loci specifying bone collagen and dentin collagen.

Secondary structure of collagen is typically alphahelical due to the nature of peptide linkage. Tertiary structure is much more complicated and is determined by the ability of the amino acids in the primary chain to form electrostatic and covalent bonds with reactive side groups, thereby producing a specific *intrachain* configuration. This intrachain bonding results in the production of a unique configuration for each polypeptide chain. The reader is referred to any contemporary text of biochemistry for more detailed discussion of the chemistry of these important concepts as they relate to molecular shape.

Quaternary structure results from the combination of two or more identical and/or different polypeptide chains to produce the functional protein molecule and thereby relates to the molecular interchain structure. The basic structural unit of collagen consists of three polypeptide chains, two of which are identical (designated a_1) and one of which is similar but different (designated a_2). Thus the simple collagen formula is $(a_1)_2a_2$. These chains combine in a spiral or twisting fashion to produce the basic unit designated as tropocollagen. The functional collagen matrix of either bone or dentin ultimately consists of multiple aggregations of tropocollagen called fibrils, which collectively make up the collagen fiber characteristic of the various connective tissues (Table 8-2).

Inorganic matrix and calcification

As mentioned above, the inorganic matrix of dentin is hydroxyapatite, which is the crystal structure characteristic of all mineralized tissues. Since this crystal structure is the end result of mineralization, when considering heritable defects of calcified tissue, it is often more useful to think of the calcification process rather than the end product itself.

Although collagen is the matrix of all calcified tissues, with notable exception of enamel (Table 8-2), and even though considerable evidence is available to indicate that only native collagen mineralizes whereas denatured collagen does not, it is not at all clear whether collagen should be considered the sole molecule responsible for initiating and completing the mineralization process. Carmichael and co-workers[2] have presented evidence for existence of a phosphoprotein in dentin that is covalently bound to collagen by an hydroxylysine-glycosidic linkage. This protein has an amino acid composition distinct from that of collagen. The significance of such a protein becomes apparent when one considers that the collagens of mineralized tissues are nearly identical to the collagens of soft, normally nonmineralized tissues such as skin and tendon (Table 8-2). If such a molecule is necessary for normal mineralization, the potential number of heritable dentin defects increases greatly, since one may now enumerate three classes of defects: (1) those involving the primary structure of collagen, (2) those involving the primary structure of the phosphoprotein, and (3) those interfering with the establishment of covalent linkages between the two. Preliminary evidence for the latter group is suggested by the paper of Eastoe and associates,[4] which compares the amino acid composition of collagen from os-

teogenesis imperfecta and dentinogenesis imperfecta, both heritable diseases of mineralized tissues. A detailed review of the calcification process itself has been published.[1]

PRIMARY DISEASES OF DENTIN

As the number of diseases that primarily involve dentin grows, the need for a classification has become apparent. In the following section, the classification proposed and published by Shields and co-workers[48] will be referred to. The nomenclature of this classification recognizes two basic groups, dentin dysplasias and the dentinogenesis imperfectas. Within each group, types are identified by Roman numerals. This system has the disadvantage of not supplying a readily recognizable, descriptive name (for example, opalescent dentin), but it has the advantage of not biasing the disease description with terminology that may subsequently prove to be inadequate, inappropriate, or even inaccurate. Within this classification the dentinogenesis imperfecta types are arranged in order of severity, with type I the least severe and type III the most severe. Hopefully the reader will use the system for reference purposes only and will not construe it to be the final work on etiologic classification of dentin diseases, about which little is known of the basic molecular defect.

Dentinogenesis imperfecta, Shields type I

Clinical features. Dentinogenesis imperfecta is only one of the several clinical manifestations of a generalized skeletal disease called osteogenesis imperfecta or OI.[21] These features may be listed as multiple bone fractures, hyperextensible joints, blue sclerae, progressive deafness, and dentinogenesis imperfecta. Two types of OI are recognized, depending on age of onset and severity, OI congenita and OI tarda. Both types may show teeth with the dentin defect. All of the observed abnormalities occur in tissues with major collagen components, and the fundamental defect has been suggested to reside in the collagen matrix. The presence of a dentin defect in this skeletal disorder is therefore not entirely unexpected. The dental features are unique, and even though they closely resemble the features of dentinogenesis imperfecta type II, they are described here as a separate entity. Although listed here in the category of a primary disease of dentin, it is probably more accurate to think of this disorder as a primary defect of the matrix that is common to both bones and teeth. It is not certain whether this type is actually a primary disease of dentin or of bone.

A striking amber translucency of both the primary and permanent dentitions may be seen. There is, however, considerable variation in expression, which ranges from all teeth affected to only a few showing a mild discoloration (Figs. 8-1 and 8-2). Those which are discolored often show enamel that chips and fractures away, which then permits more rapid attrition of the exposed, softer dentin.[53]

Radiographic features. Radiographs show that both dentitions may have teeth with accelerated pulpal obliteration (Fig. 8-3) with the obliteration occurring soon after eruption but sometimes even before eruption.[44, 57, 60] Short, constricted roots are observed in both dentitions.[28]

Histopathology. The dentinoenamel junc-

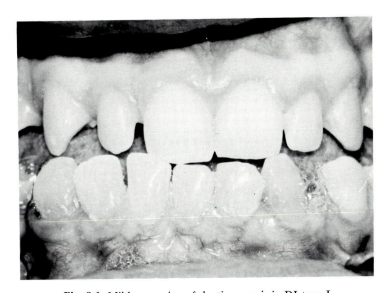

Fig. 8-1. Mild expression of dentinogenesis in DI type I.

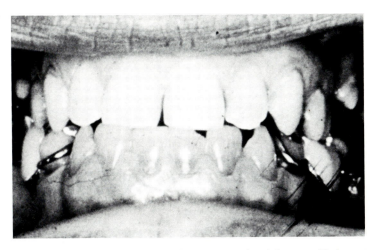

Fig. 8-2. Severe expression of dentinogenesis in DI type I involving mandibular anterior teeth.

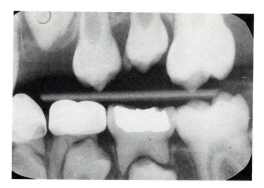

Fig. 8-3. DI type I. Partial obliteration of pulp chambers and root canals in deciduous dentition.

tion shows scalloping, but a normal layer of peripheral or mantle dentin can be seen.[22, 25, 28] Teeth have been noted in which no normal dentin is present.[9, 43] The normal-appearing mantle dentin, when present, merges with the dysplastic dentin, which often undergoes a proliferation sufficient to obliterate the pulp chamber and tooth canals.

Light microscopic examination of this abnormal dentin shows that it is often atubular or distinctly abnormal with considerable disorganization in tubule size and direction[33, 36] and an interglobular type of calcification.[16, 43]

Biochemical features. A comparison of collagen extracted from the bone of persons with osteogenesis imperfecta with bone collagen obtained from normal persons has failed to reveal any unusual amino acids present in OI.[4] Furthermore, the compositional differences were small, although collagen from the OI bone had a 7% to 9% deficiency in the more common amino acids (glycine, proline, and hydroxyproline) and 8% to 28% excess of amino acids with lipophilic side chains (leucine, isoleucine, valine, and phenylalanine). Interestingly, an excess of hydroxylysine was noted by Eastoe and associates[4]; others[2] have speculated on the importance of hydroxylation of lysine in various collagens. It is known that such hydroxylation residues are glycosidically linked to either galactose or the disaccharide glycosylgalactose.[51] The purpose of glycosylation is not clear, but it has been proposed to be important in the extrusion of collagen from

the cell,[13] collagen cross-linking,[51] fibrillogenesis[32] and even the calcification process itself.[52] Eastoe[8] has reported that amino acid analyses of OI suggest the presence of significant amounts of a noncollagen protein present, perhaps linked to these hydroxylysine groups. This might be a clue as to the molecular defect in OI, since Carmichael and co-workers[2] and others[18, 27, 50, 54] have shown that normal dentin has a phosphoprotein covalently linked to hydroxylysine, possibly related to normal mineralization. Thus an altered protein linked to the excess hydroxylysine groups present in bone from OI patients is conceivably responsible for the poor mineralization observed in the disorder.

Unfortunately, no comparable analytical data are available on collagen extracted from the dentin of patients with dentinogenesis imperfecta, type I. However, it is not unreasonable to presume similarity, if not identity, between bone and dentin collagen. Published data on amino acids from the normal tissues (Table 8-1) support this idea.

Inheritance. DI type I segregates as an autosomal dominant trait with variable expressivity in most families with osteogenesis imperfecta (Fig. 8-4). However, OI also has been documented to be an autosomal recessive trait with some families showing the most severe and even lethal form of this disorder, OI congenita. The inheritance of the dentin defect will follow that of the skeletal defect and may appear as either a dominant or a recessive trait. The clinical and radiographic features observed in the teeth are probably related to the degree of pulpal obliteration. This is observed to be highly variable ranging from normal dentin and pulp chamber to total chamber obliteration with the most minimal expression of affected dentin being the appearance of "vascular canals."[43, 60]

Dentinogenesis imperfecta, Shields type II (hereditary opalescent dentin)

Clinical, radiographic, and histopathological features (Figs. 8-5 and 8-6). Dentinogenesis imperfecta type II, also described in the literature as hereditary opalescent dentin,

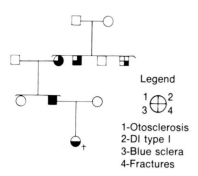

Legend

1 ⊕ 2
3 ⊕ 4

1-Otosclerosis
2-DI type I
3-Blue sclera
4-Fractures

Fig. 8-4. Pedigree of family with osteogenesis imperfecta. Three of the five affecteds have clinical evidence for DI type I as well.

has essentially the same clinical, radiographic, and histopathologic features as DI type I.*
The principal reasons for recognizing it as a separate entity are as follows:

1. Many families have been reported that demonstrate multiple members affected with DI type II who have none of the findings of osteogenesis imperfecta.[12, 38, 56, 60]

2. The within-family correlation of severity, coloration, and attrition is high in type II (low variability in gene expression), whereas there is considerable phenotypic variation in DI type I.[12]

---

*See references 10, 23, 26, 30, 55, 60.

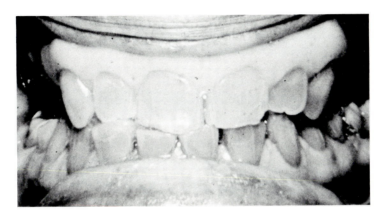

Fig. 8-5. Uniform expression of DI type II in all teeth.

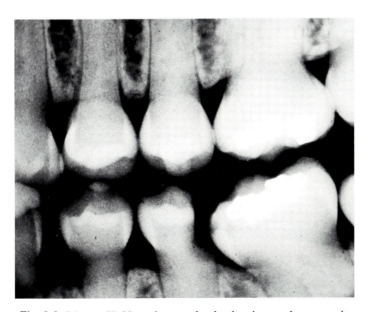

Fig. 8-6. DI type II. Note absence of pulp chambers and root canals.

3. In DI type II, both dentitions are equally affected employing both clinical and radiographic criteria,[47] and one never finds completely normal teeth.[12] By contrast, DI type I always shows the deciduous teeth to be more severely affected than the permanent teeth.[57]

Biochemical features. The specific biochemical defect in DI type II is not known. Many authors have suggested that the basic problem is a molecular collagen defect. Biochemical studies by Eastoe and associates[4] comparing collagen from normal dentin and DI type II dentin have shown only minor differences in amino acid content and amount with one exception. Hydroxylysine content of collagen from DI type II is elevated over that in normal dentin collagen. The significance of this finding is not known, but, as was speculated in the foregoing discussion of the molecular basis for DI type I, it may be related to the ability of such collagen to calcify. Several authors have suggested that phosphoproteins covalently linked to glycosylated hydroxylysine may be important in initiating the nucleation of apatite.[18, 27, 50, 54] Collagen is not the only potentially defective molecule. A wide variety of heritable defects of connective tissue have been described (including Marfan's syndrome, multiple types of Ehlers-Danlos syndrome, and many others), but it seems unlikely that all of these disorders should have a basic defect in the collagen molecule itself. Basic lesions will undoubtedly be found in other components of the extracellular matrix and at sites in the metabolic pathways where the reason for their effects on the structural integrity of connective tissue is not so apparent. Such reasoning also applies to heritable dentin defects, which may be etiologically classed in three groups: (1) primary defect in collagen, (2) primary defect in calcifying matrix (phosphoprotein defect?), and (3) primary defect in another metabolic pathway that results in production of mineralizing inhibitors. The latter system would be analogous to the detrimental effect of homocystine on collagen metabolism as seen in the disease homocystinuria. In this disease, the primary biochemical defect is not of collagen itself, but the phenotype produced by the inability of the person to metabolize homocysteine to cysteine closely resembles the phenotype of Marfan's syndrome, a disease thought to result from a primary collagen defect.

Epidemiology and inheritance. Dentinogenesis imperfecta type II represents one of the most common, dominantly inherited disorders in man and affects approximately one in every 8000 persons. Sporadic cases of the disorder are virtually unreported, which suggests that the mutation rate is low. It should be noted that DI type I, DD type II (p. 237), and tetracycline-stained teeth all may have the clinical appearance of DI type II opalescent dentin, and these other cases do occur in a sporadic fashion. Therefore any report of a sporadic case of DI type II or of an affected person with both parents normal that does not have clinical, radiographic, and histopathological data to confirm the diagnosis is open to serious doubt. Witkop and Rao[60] state that of 164 well-documented propositi, only five were reported to have neither parent affected. Three of these five cases have genotyping studies showing a paternal exclusion, and the other two had no such studies. One must conclude that the mutation rate for this dominant gene is indeed low.

It has also been demonstrated that penetrance for this trait is essentially complete (Fig. 8-7). Witkop and Rao[60] report only one instance in 362 possibilities in which a known gene carrier has failed to present any of the clinical stigmata of DI type II. However, even this person was subsequently shown to have at least the radiographic evidence for lack of pulp chambers and the positive histopathological findings of dentinogenesis imperfecta.

Not only is penetrance complete for this trait, but gene expression, at least within a sibship, is remarkably uniform. Bixler and associates[12] have reported that in sibships with multiple affecteds, the degree of discoloration was correlated with the severity of attrition. Furthermore, this correlation within a sibship was uniform even though there were differences between sibships. One important variable in gene expression is the age of the affected, since it has been clearly documented that this is a progressive disorder with older persons showing more pronounced clinical and radiographic changes.

Finally, DI type II is an autosomal trait (Fig. 8-7). Numerous instances of male-to-male transmission have been reported, and the sex ratio of affecteds, although varying somewhat from study to study, closely approximates the 1:1 expected for an autosomal trait.[12, 31, 49] Assuming that autosomal dominant inheritance is well established for DI type II, one wonders what the homozygous phenotype may be. Shokeir[49] has reported a family in which both parents had DI type II, who had four children: one normal male, two classically affected DI type II females, and one severely affected female

who was presumed to be homozygous for the DI type II gene. The radiographic appearance of her teeth at age 9 indicated marked thinning of dentin, which was reduced to a mere shell. The pulp chambers of these teeth were actually enlarged, raising the interesting question of a possible relationship between this presumed homozygous dentin malformation and what other authors have called "shell teeth."[42, 58]

The homozygous phenotype for almost all dominant genes is unknown. The reason is that such a homozygous genotype would result only when two affecteds marry. Assuming such marriages to occur only by chance, the probability of such a union of DI type II genes is $(8 \times 10^{-3})^2$, the product of the separate incidences of the defect. Even then, only a quarter of the offspring would by

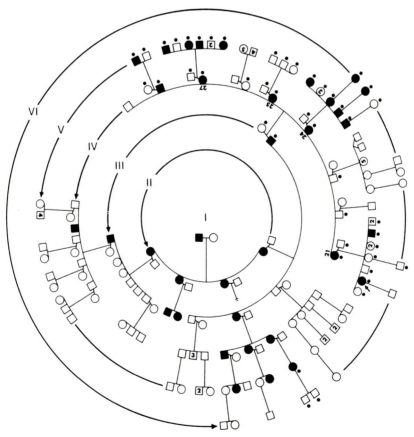

Fig. 8-7. Pedigree of DI type II. Male-to-male transmission confirms this as autosomal trait. (From Bixler, D., Conneally, P. M., and Christen, A. G.: J. Dent. Res. **48:**1196-1199, 1969.)

chance be homozygous affected, giving an overall probability of 1.6×10^{-5}, a rare event indeed.

Dentinogenesis imperfecta, Shields type III (Brandywine type)

Clinical features. Teeth with dentinogenesis imperfecta, Shields type III resemble those of DI types I and II in both coloration and shape. However, considerable phenotypic variability within this type is noted. The most commonly observed clinical characteristics are (1) opalescent color to the teeth, (2) both dentitions involved, and (3) bell-shaped appearance to the crowns.[58, 59]

Radiographic features. In the deciduous teeth there is a high degree of variability in radiographic appearance ranging from normal to that typically observed in DI type II. The unique feature seems to be the appearance of so-called shell teeth (Fig. 8-8). Witkop[58] has used this term to describe teeth in which dentin formation did not occur after the mantle layer of dentin was formed. He observed this unusual situation in eight of 252 affecteds in the Brandywine population, a triracial isolate in Maryland. Shell teeth have been described in two other instances, one by Rushton[42] as an isolated case and the other by Schimmelpfennig and McDonald[46] in a family with an enamel aplasia. The latter case was subsequently shown to be related to the Brandywine kindreds.[58] This condition seems unusual enough to justify a separate classification as DI type III, since

there have been *no* instances of shell teeth observed in all the cases of DI type II reported in the literature.

Further variation in radiographic appearance was noted by Witkop,[58] who reported three cases in which the primary teeth showed normal pulp chambers and canals but had the clinical and histopathological appearance of DI type II. These findings might be described as variability in gene expression and thereby represent the mildest manifestation of DI type III.

Finally, a third unique radiographic finding in this type of dentinogenesis is the occurrence of multiple pulp exposures in the deciduous dentition. Such a finding is essentially nonexistent in DI type II but perhaps not so remote for DI type I, in which some teeth may show relatively normal pulp chambers and canals.

Histopathology. Insufficient information is available on these teeth to adequately characterize their histopathology.

Biochemistry. No information is available on the biochemistry of DI type III.

Inheritance. The pedigree information provided by Hursey and co-workers[24] indicates an autosomal dominant trait. For the reasons stated previously, this appears to be a distinct type of dentinogenesis, although it is possible that the genes for DI types II and III are allelic. Linkage studies will be useful in resolving this question. As previously mentioned, shell teeth might be the expression of

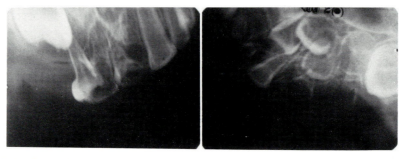

Fig. 8-8. Radiographic appearance of shell teeth, which has been observed in some cases of DI type III. (Courtesy Dr. Carl J. Witkop, Jr.; from Tiecke, R. W., editor: Oral pathology, New York, 1965, McGraw-Hill Book Co. Copyright 1965; used with permission of McGraw-Hill Book Co.)

the homozygous affected phenotype.[49] This idea is partially supported by finding eight such severely affected people in a total of 252 cases of DI in an inbred population.[58]

Dentin dysplasias

Shields type I

Clinical features. Shields type I dentin dysplasia, DD type I, has appeared in the literature under a variety of descriptive terms, including rootless teeth, nonopalescent and opalescent dentin, and radicular dentin dysplasia. Rootless teeth represent one of the significant, descriptive features of this disorder, but over the years *dentin dysplasia* has come to be the term of choice, and that preference will be continued here.

The permanent and deciduous teeth are of normal size, shape, and consistency,[17, 29, 34] although affected teeth occasionally show a slight amber translucency.[60] The most striking clinical feature is malalignment and malposition of teeth (Fig. 8-9). This problem is due to such extreme tooth mobility that even minor trauma may result in exfoliation. The reason lies in the failure to form normal root structure.

Radiographic features. Affected teeth have short roots with sharp, conical, apical constructions.[11] Associated with these short or blunted roots are multiple periapical radiolucencies, which, when seen in noncarious teeth, are of great value in making the diagnosis of dentin dysplasia type I.[41] Obliteration of the pulp is a significant feature of this disorder, which occurs preeruptively in the permanent dentition and produces a crescent-shaped, pulpal remnant that is visible radiographically but typically only in the permanent teeth, since total pulp chamber obliteration is a common feature of the deciduous dentition.[60] Root canals are absent. Occasionally, individual calcified masses can be observed in the pulp, but most often these are fused into a single mass that is continuous with root dentin.

Histopathology. In both dentitions the common finding is a layer of normal mantle dentin with most of the coronal dentin also unaffected.[14, 15, 41] However, areas of atubular dentin can be observed, most often in the deciduous teeth.[29] Below this normal dentin can be found the pulpal remnants, visible on radiographs as the crescent-shaped area. Apically from the pulpal tissue are large masses of calcified tubular dentin, atypical osteodentin, and even true denticles.[29, 48, 61] These mineralized structures appear to block the formation of a normal dentinal tubule pathway, and the tubules are shunted around

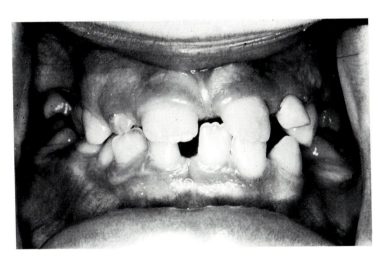

Fig. 8-9. DD type I. Clinical appearance of migrating teeth. (Courtesy Dr. Carl J. Witkop, Jr.; from Tiecke, R. W., editor: Oral pathology, New York, 1965, McGraw-Hill Book Co. Copyright 1965; used with permission of McGraw-Hill Book Co.)

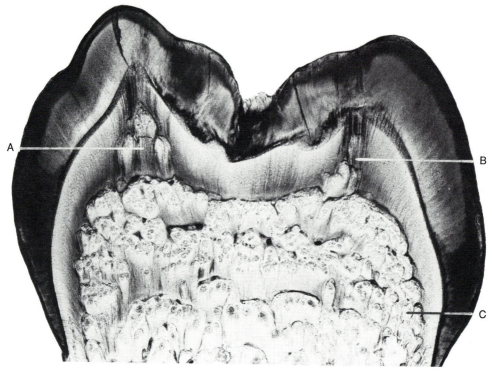

Fig. 8-10. DD type I. Ground section showing pulpal obliteration by abnormal dentin. Note variation in severity under cusp tips, *A* and *B,* and in pulp chamber, *C.*

them, thereby giving them the remarkable appearance of a stream of lava flowing around boulders (Figs. 8-10 and 8-11).

Although the primary defect in DD type I is unknown, Sauk and associates[45] have presented data from scanning electron microscope studies that indicate that the cascades of dentin observed as a typical feature of this disorder result from repetitive attempts to form root structure. The authors hypothesize that the primary defect, then, is in the epithelial component of the root sheath, which repetitively invaginates, first too soon and subsequently too often. The result would then be a series of abortive attempts to form root dentin. This suggestion does parallel the histopathological picture actually observed. Remarkably, that dentin which is formed is normal in architecture; it is abnormal principally in its anatomical orientation. The above explanation does not seem to consider the probable role of dentin as an inductive force in cementum formation. Since a pri-

mary dentin defect has already been demonstrated in DD type I, at this stage it seems unnecessary to postulate a primary defect in the root sheath epithelium.

The apical cysts that are noted on radiographic examination have a close histopathological resemblance to radicular cysts.[60]

Epidemiology and inheritance. Shields type I dentin dysplasia is a rare dentin condition estimated to have a population frequency of about one in 100,000 persons.[57] Only about thirty cases have been reported in the literature, and in many of these cases no family information is given.[29, 35] Several pedigrees show a dominant mode of inheritance with several examples of male-to-male transmission. No family studies are published that define the gene expression, but some variability exists. Several cases have been published that have shown no periapical cysts. Elzay and Robinson[17] have suggested that calcification of the dentinal papilla could be considered as a mild form of expression of dentin dysplasia

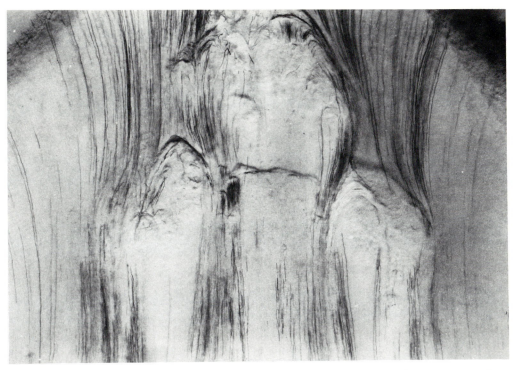

Fig. 8-11. DD type I. Higher magnification of Fig. 8-10 at *A* showing cascading appearance of dentinal tubule production. (From Logan, J., et al.: Oral Surg. **23:**338-342, 1967.)

type I. However, all gene carriers seem to be uniformly affected by obliteration of pulp chambers in both dentitions. Because of the lack of reported family information it is impossible to classify all published cases as sporadic or familial. Witkop[60] states that of six propositi known to him, only one had unaffected parents, and in this case there was no paternal exclusion by genotypic tests. This suggests that the majority of cases are familial and that the mutation rate for this gene is low. I am unaware of any cases occurring in non-Caucasian races that might be considered as negative evidence for multiple mutations contributing substantially to the present affected population. Another explanation for the presence of such rare traits occurring only in certain populations employs the founder principle. This states that when a natural population sends forth only a few founders to begin new populations, whatever genes these founders take with them, detrimental or beneficial, all stand a good chance of becoming stabilized in the new population because of a sampling accident. Thus a relatively rare trait such as dentin dysplasia could readily be confined to select groups by virtue of the founder effect.

Shields type II (anomalous dysplasia of dentin)

Clinical features. In dentin dysplasia, Shields type II, there is a significant color difference in the two dentitions. The primary teeth have an amber, translucent appearance closely resembling that of DI type II (Fig. 8-12). However, the permanent teeth are of normal color. There are no other distinctive clinical features that characterize this disorder, and in the cases studied at Indiana University we have specifically not observed an unusual attrition rate for these affected primary teeth.[17, 40, 48]

Radiographic features. Pulp chambers of the deciduous dentition eventually are completely obliterated (Fig. 8-13). Some pulp chamber may still be evident at 2 years of age,

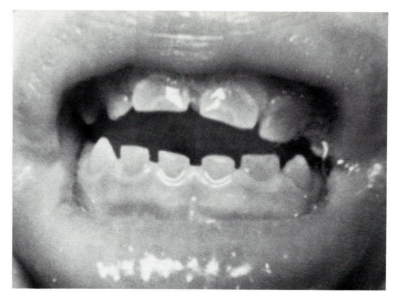

Fig. 8-12. DD type II. Uniform appearance of opalescent dentin to all teeth in only deciduous dentition. (Courtesy Dr. Edward Shields, Indianapolis, Ind.)

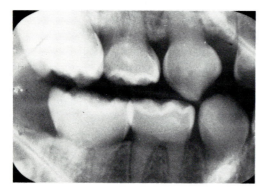

Fig. 8-13. DD type II. Absence of pulp chambers and root canals of deciduous teeth as seen in DI type II. (Courtesy Dr. Edward Shields, Indianapolis, Ind.)

but this is completely gone by 5 to 6 years of age. Obliteration never occurs before eruption. The radiographic appearance of the permanent dentition is different with pulp chambers evident in all teeth, although pulpal obliteration has been noted in incisors by 14 years of age. However, the anterior teeth and premolars typically have a pulp chamber and root canal that are thistle-tube in shape due to the radicular extension of the pulp cham-

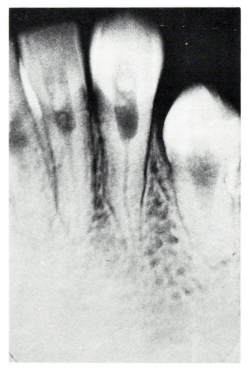

Fig. 8-14. DD type II. Permanent teeth showing peculiar thistle-tube shape to pulp chamber and multiple pulp stones. (Courtesy Dr. Edward Shields, Indianapolis, Ind.)

ber[19, 39, 40, 48] (Fig. 8-14). Almost all teeth show multiple accumulations of pulp stones in these unusually shaped pulp chambers.[39, 48] In contrast to DD type I, multiple periapical radiolucencies are not a feature of this disorder (Figs. 8-13 and 8-14).

Histopathological features. The deciduous teeth show a normal-appearing layer of coronal dentin with a sudden transition to amorphous and atubular dentin in the radicular portion.[48] Also noted are irregular arrangements of the dentinal tubules. Permanent teeth show essentially normal coronal dentin but with interglobular dentin appearing in the pulpal third.[40, 48] The radicular dentin, by contrast, is atubular, amorphous, and irregular in organization when tubules were present. Root canals are reduced in dimension. Also to be noted in the permanent teeth is the presence of multiple denticles, some false (concentric, lamellated) but mostly those of the true variety (unattached dentin) (Fig. 8-15). These histopathological findings are consistent with the radiographic and clinical findings, which suggest that a more complete and severe dysplasia of dentin is affecting the deciduous teeth, whereas the permanent teeth, although clearly affected, have a more normal and less severe picture.

Epidemiology and inheritance. There are four kindreds in the literature with sufficient documentation to be assigned the designation of DD type II.[19, 39, 40, 48] Another report by Ruston[43] probably represents the same entity. In addition, I have observed two other familial cases of DD type II, which have not been reported in the literature. In all these pedigrees an autosomal dominant mode of inheritance is clear. Furthermore, penetrance is high and may even be 100%. I have personally examined one family in which the disorder was originally classified in a 6 year old as DI type II. Both parents were said to be normal and, in fact, had normal-appearing teeth, which raised the question of a new mutation. However, radiographic examina-

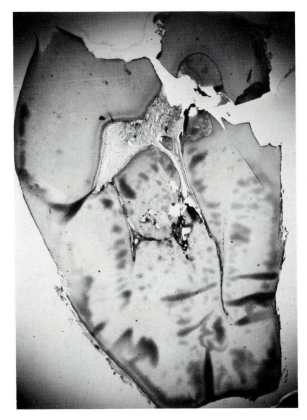

Fig. 8-15. DD type II. Affected maxillary second premolar showing true denticle surrounded by pulpal tissue. (From Shields, E. D., Bixler, D., and El-Kafrawy, A. M.: Arch. Oral Biol. **18:**543-553, 1973.)

tion of the father confirmed the diagnosis of DD type II, which emphasizes that this particular dentin disorder may be misdiagnosed and even missed entirely (nonpenetrance) if both clinical and radiographic evidence are not used for making the diagnosis.

No information is as yet available on gene expression or mutation rate. However, with only five kindreds reported, the trait would appear to be much rarer than DI type II and no more common than DD type I.

Numerous authors have described the presence of a normal-appearing mantle layer of dentin in their histological preparations of teeth with DI types I and II and DD types I and II. One might presume that the dentin matrix laid down for the mantle layer is somehow different, since it is so often described as normal even in the presence of the adjacent gross dentin matrix abnormality such as seen in DD type I. This presumption can even be extended to shell teeth (as seen in DI type III), since Rushton[42] has clearly demonstrated a relatively normal-appearing layer of mantle dentin about 1 mm thick in his shell teeth. Witkop[60] comments that mantle dentin is the most normal-appearing of all dentin in these teeth, but that it too shows areas that are not traversed by normal dentinal tubules. Herold[20] reported that the collagen fibril dimensions and its orientation within the entire dentin layer of teeth with dentinogenesis imperfecta (type II) closely resembles that of the mantle dentin layer in normal teeth. Thus the entire abnormal dentin layer of DI type II appears to be mantle dentin consisting of coarse fibrils (1000 Å) and thereby lacking the fine fibrils (500 Å) seen in normal circumpulpal dentin. He proposed that DI type II be considered a disease state resulting from a failure of the odontoblast to begin production of that dentin matrix consisting of the fine fibril. In light of the recent experiments of Croissant and co-workers[3] on epithelial-mesenchymal interactions in odontogenesis, one may presume that a normal mantle layer, essentially the predentin (or, as these workers call it, progenitor extracellular matrix), is a necessity

for normal enamel formation. In all of these heritable dentin defects the enamel is repeatedly described as normal in structure and amount. Therefore the odontoblastic agents employed for information transfer to ameloblasts, which in turn activate enamel protein synthesis, must be intact. From a developmental biology standpoint, these heritable dentin defects make it clear that at least two distinct programming mechanisms are at work in the odontoblast: (1) production of agent(s) for ameloblast induction and (2) production of a collagenous matrix representing the dentin.

Summary. It appears that these dentin defects have four salient features: (1) a monogenic mode of inheritance, (2) varying degrees of dentinal tubular disorganization, (3) essentially a normal layer of mantle dentin, and (4) true denticles. Regarding the latter, these are rare findings in normal teeth and must be distinguished from false denticles (pulp stones), which are relatively common. The presence of true denticles in these primary dentin diseases is difficult to explain but can be described as genetic pleiotropism. Apparently the abnormal dentin produced in these disorders is responsible for the production of abnormal epigenetic factors, which, in turn, induce the formation of true denticles. Under this concept, denticle formation is secondary to the primary dentin defect.

Table 8-3 summarizes the differential diagnostic findings in these three types of dentinogenesis imperfecta and the two types of dentin dysplasia.

Other disorders with primary defects of dentin

Odontodysplasia

Clinical and radiographic features. Odontodysplasia represents a localized arrest in tooth development. One may see a single tooth or even several teeth in the same quadrant with moderate to severe hypoplasia of the crowns. Chaudhry and co-workers[65] have reported a case in which three of the four quadrants of teeth were involved. Affected teeth are often discolored, depending on the severity of the enamel defect, and are espe-

Table 8-3. Diagnostic features of affected teeth in dentinogenesis imperfecta, types I, II, and III, and dentin dysplasia, types I and II

	DI-I	DI-II	DI-III	DD-I	DD-II
Clinical features					
Primary teeth amber, translucent	+	++	+	+	++
Secondary teeth discolored	+	++	++	–	–
Discoloration in both dentitions	+	++	++	–	–
Loose teeth	–	+	+	++	–
Rapid attrition of crowns	+	++	++	–	–
Fragile roots	+	+	+	+	–
Radiographic features					
Ovoid crowns	++	++	++	–	–
Short, tapering roots	+	+	+	++	–
Obliteration of pulp cavities					
Before eruption	+	+	+	++	–
After eruption	+	++	+	–	+
Horizontal line at DEJ (crescent-shaped pulp chamber)	–	–	–	++	–
Apical extension of pulp chamber	–	–	–	–	+
Multiple apical radiolucencies	+	+	+	++	–
Thistle-tube shape to pulp chamber	–	–	–	–	+
Reduced x-ray contrast of dentin	++	++	+	++	–
Pulp stones in pulp chamber	–	–	–	–	++
Histopathological features					
True denticles	+	+	+	++	++
False denticles	+	+	+	–	+
Features in common					
Primary teeth more severely affected	++	++	++	++	++
Normal mantle dentin	++	++	++	++	++
Abnormal radicular dentin	++	++	++	+	++
Normal enamel	+	+	+	++	++
Interglobular dentin	+	++	+	+	++
Scalloping of DEJ	+	+	+	++	++

Key: ++, typically evident in all teeth; +, variable in frequency or severity; – absent.

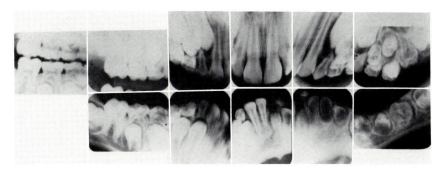

Fig. 8-16. Odontodysplasia affecting several teeth in right maxilla. (Courtesy Dr. Carl J. Witkop, Jr., Minneapolis, Minn.)

cially susceptible to dental caries with local infection a common complication. When deciduous teeth are affected, the permanent successors are also often involved.[63, 67] However, affected permanent teeth may be observed underlying normal deciduous predecessors.[67] Interestingly, defective teeth are often unerupted or delayed in their eruption.[62]

Radiographs show these teeth to have large pulps, little dentin, and only a thin layer of enamel (Fig. 8-16). A ghostlike appearance is often commented on.[63, 67] The roots are poorly outlined and typically shortened.

Histopathological features. Microscopic examination of the dentin shows atubular tracts, increased tubule size, and an irregular path for those tubules present. Large areas of interglobular dentin are often noted. Mantle dentin is less severely affected but still has significant abnormalities. Denticles are sometimes noted, but these are typically of the false type.[63] The cementum is normal in appearance.

Incomplete fusion of dentinal tracts at the incisal edge of anterior teeth has been observed, which means that the pulp chamber may be open to the oral cavity, a good explanation for the periapical infection that is so often observed.[62] Ground sections of affected teeth show both hypoplasia and hypocalcification of the enamel.

The cause of this disorder is unclear and no familial cases have been reported. This observation coupled with the localized nature of the defect makes an hereditary basis unlikely. Zegarelli and associates[68] have enumerated several possible explanations, including nutritional deficit, trauma, infection, and radiation. None of these can satisfactorily explain all reported cases. Rushton[67] has commented that the tooth or teeth involved give clues to the timing of the developmental defect, and even the latest dates of these are often so early in development as to clearly exclude such explanations as trauma and dental infection. Prenatal histories are not helpful in this regard. Bergman,[64] Abrams,[62] and Rushton[67] speculate that a somatic mutation might account for localized develop-

mental arrest in the enamel organ epithelium. One might expect that such a defect in the primary dental anlagen could be transmitted to the permanent anlagen, thereby resulting in both dentitions affected, a situation noted in several instances.[62, 63]

Melnick and Shields[66] have presented a model of odontomorphogenesis that can be used to explain various types of dental dysplasias, such as other anomalies that occur as single or multiple events in the same individual. The authors suggest that, regardless of the particular malformation, all represent aberrant odontogenesis during histodifferentiation and morphodifferentiation. In this model, mutation in a somatic cell may be critical, especially one occurring in a cell mass having an important role in initiating an inductive process or in providing essential cell positional information. Odontodysplasia is a defect of odontomorphogenesis occurring at an early stage (all three dental tissues are affected), probably involving the neural crest cells, which are thought to give rise to dentin (dentin is the inductive force behind enamel and cementum formation). Therefore a somatic mutation involving such a neural crest cell seems likely.

The following outline presents a possible classification of odontomorphogenetic defects as suggested by Melnick and Shields.[66]

A. Mutational dysmorphogenesis
  1. Mutant mesodermal organizer genes
    a. Anodontia
    b. Supernumerary teeth
    c. Predeciduous teeth
    d. Multiple odontomas
    e. Odontodysplasia
  2. Mutant mesodermal interpretational genes
    a. Anodontia, partial or complete
    b. Absence of single tooth or pair of homologous teeth
    c. Peg-shaped lateral incisors
    d. Microdontia
    e. Macrodontia
    f. Schizodontism (gemination)
    g. Dens invaginatus
    h. Dens evaginatus
    i. Single odontomas
B. Environmental dysmorphogenesis
  1. Syndontism (fusion)

Hereditary dysplasias of enamel and dentin. There are reports in the literature indicating the existence of an hereditary dysplastic defect involving both enamel and dentin. At this time it is impossible to say in which structure the primary defect resides. However, recalling the essential inductive role of odontoblasts in initiating enamel formation, I presume a primary dentin defect.

In 1953, Schimmelpfennig and McDonald[46] described a case of what they called "enamel and dentin aplasia." The primary teeth were of brownish color in this 4-year-old Negro boy. There was marked attrition of the crowns and several resultant pulp exposures. No enamel was clinically apparent on the primary teeth, and the remaining dentin was so translucent that the pulp chamber outline and the pulp tissue itself were visible on the occlusal surface. No dental caries was present. Several of the anterior teeth were slightly mobile due to advanced root resorption, conceivably a normal process at this age. Six-year molars erupted during the observation period and were noted to be partially covered with a thin, grayish coat of enamel. This enamel did not extend into the depth of the pits and fissures of the molars, and dentin was visible there.

Radiographs confirmed a generalized lack of enamel on the primary teeth, although some enamel with reduced density and thickness was noted on the permanent teeth (Fig. 8-17). Multiple periapical radiolucencies were observed at the apices of some of the teeth with exposed pulps. Pulp chambers and root canals appeared to be large. No teeth were missing, and the alveolar bone was normal in appearance.

Ground sections were made of several teeth, which showed the enamel to have an amorphous appearance and to be without the normal enamel structures. The dentinoenamel junction was atypical and showed a lack of scalloping. There appeared to be a relatively thin layer of normal mantle dentin, but since only ground sections were reported, more detailed comment is impossible. The remainder of the dentin was grossly abnormal with dentinal tubules reduced in number and irregular in their course with excessive branching.

The cementum was normal-appearing and cellular in type. The pulp chambers were again commented on as being large, and there was no evidence of secondary dentin formation in these severely abraded teeth.

From this description, the term *dysplasia of enamel and dentin* seems appropriately descriptive, since both a hypoplasia and dysplasia of the enamel and dentin are present. Schimmelpfennig and McDonald used the term *aplasia* to describe this case, which is erroneous since both enamel and dentin were actually formed, although imperfectly.

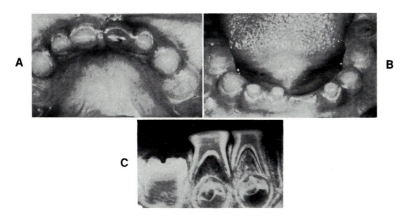

Fig. 8-17. Enamel and dentin dysplasia, dominant type. Note severe abrasion with near pulp exposure, **A** and **B**, and almost total absence of enamel, **C**. (From McDonald, R. E.: Dentistry for the child and adolescent, ed. 2, St. Louis, 1974, The C. V. Mosby Co.)

Heredity. Family history revealed that this child's father had the same clinical appearance for both sets of his teeth and had a full-mouth extraction at an early age. By history, six of the father's seven sibs were similarly affected, as was his mother. This history denotes an autosomal dominant trait, since there are at least three generations of affecteds (vertical transmission of the trait) and male-to-male transmission (X-linkage ruled out).

There are other reports in the literature suggesting that a combined hereditary enamel-dentin defect may exist. Olson[73] described a family in which dominant inheritance of a gross lack of enamel on teeth in both dentitions was noted. Tooth color resembled that seen in the family described above. However, the pulp chambers were of normal size, and no description of the dentin was offered, suggesting that this could be one of the dominant forms of amelogenesis imperfecta. Two other reports[70, 71] also describe this disorder, but again a failure to describe the dentin by the authors makes classification impossible. Siirila and Heikinheimo[75] reported a defect in the permanent teeth of a 15-year-old boy, which they called odontogenesis imperfecta. The enamel was markedly hypoplastic, and the dentin showed changes similar to those described for dentinal dysplasia type I. Such dentin proliferation, although abnormal, is not concordant with that seen in the family of Schimmelpfennig and McDonald.

Another possible example occurred in a family of affecteds reported by Helfer and Cuttita.[69] They described amber-colored deciduous teeth in an 8-year-old boy who had severe crown attrition. Radiographs showed severe pulpal recession with dentin filling most of the pulp chamber. This dentin phenotype appears to be the opposite of that observed by Schimmelpfennig and McDonald but does somewhat resemble the case of Siirila and Heikinheimo.[75] Again, no dentin studies were made by the authors. In this family, four generations of affecteds were identified, but no affected male had offspring, so X-linkage remains a possibility. Both tissues were affected in this case reported by Helfer and Cuttita, but the disorder cannot be placed in the separate categories of either amelogenesis or dentinogenesis. Neither does the trait as they describe it seem to resemble closely any of the previously described possible cases of enamel and dentin dysplasia.

From the foregoing reports at least one entity seems probable, an autosomal dominantly inherited dysplasia of both enamel and dentin. However, at least one other genetic type seems certain. Kimura and Nakata[72] have examined two Japanese girls with clinical features of (1) yellowed teeth with significant attrition and (2) delayed eruption of permanent teeth in the younger girl and failure of eruption (except for central incisors) in the older girl. Radiographic examination confirmed the presence of severe enamel hypoplasia and showed thickened, bulbous roots in both erupted and unerupted teeth (Fig. 8-18). Histopathological examination of extracted teeth confirmed the severe enamel hypoplasia, and what remained was also dysplastic. Dentin below the pulp chamber had a cascading appearance resembling that seen in DD type I but elsewhere appeared normal (Fig. 8-19). Roots were grossly thickened by the deposition of a cellular type of cementum. Attempts to promote tooth eruption by surgical incision met with little success, but the connective tissue overlying the tooth was described as thick and densely fibrous. Microscopic sections of the gingiva revealed this same abnormal band of connective tissue lying beneath a thin, normal layer of dermis and showed it to contain multiple areas of ectopic calcification (Fig. 8-20).

Since this defect affects all three primary dental tissues, it might legitimately be described as odontogenesis imperfecta. Most importantly, neither parent had the trait, and they were related as first cousins. These findings, coupled with the fact that the affected sibs were both female, strongly suggests autosomal recessive inheritance, which separates it from any of the other previously described entities of dysplasia, which are all dominant traits.

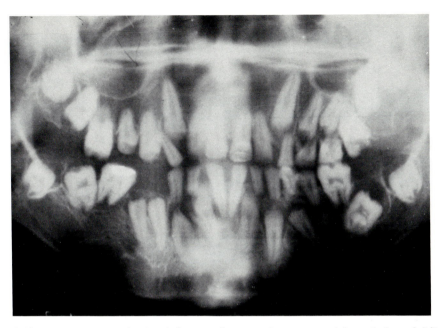

Fig. 8-18. Enamel and dentin dysplasia, recessive type. Severe enamel hypoplasia and failure of eruption. Note bulbous roots. (Courtesy Dr. Minoru Nakata, Tokyo, Japan.)

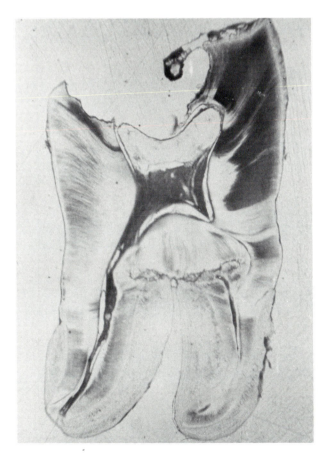

Fig. 8-19. Enamel and dentin dysplasia, recessive type. Abnormal dentin below pulp chamber resembles that of DD type I. (Courtesy Dr. Minoru Nakata, Tokyo, Japan.)

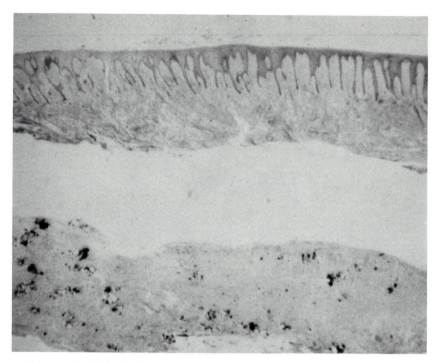

Fig. 8-20. Enamel and dentin dysplasia, recessive type. Note abnormal rete pegs, thin layer of dermis, and, below this, thickened fibrous layer of connective tissue with ectopic calcification. (Courtesy Dr. Minoru Nakata, Tokyo, Japan.)

Hopefully, all cases of hereditary defects of teeth reported in the future will contain adequate clinical, radiographic, histological, and genetic information to permit their complete classification.

Fibrous dysplasia of dentin. Fibrous dysplasia of dentin has been noted in a single family and appears to be limited to the teeth. Other organ systems are not known to be affected. No original publication has appeared as yet, but Witkop[76] has reviewed the disease characteristics obtained by personal contact with the family.

Clinical, radiographic, and histopathological features. No data are available on the primary dentition, since all affecteds examined have been adults. The secondary teeth are clinically normal in color and shape. Radiographs show normal shape to the pulp chambers with occasional small foci of radiolucent areas, some even seen in the root canals. Histopathologically, all of the dentin is abnormal, although its appearance varies from area to area. Large bundles of predentin-like collagen are interspersed with lacunae larger than Tomes' fibers and without the normal tubular form. A dystrophic type of calcification is observed for the remnants of pulp tissue, which are trapped in lacunae of the root dentin. This disorder would seem to represent a dysplasia of collagen in which the matrix is too disorganized for normal mineralization to occur.

Heredity. Witkop comments that fibrous dysplasia of the dentin is inherited as an autosomal dominant trait. Since the single abnormal finding of dysplastic dentin collagen seems to be revealed only by histopathological study of the dentin, it may be that there are many more affected families in the population, but they will be difficult to ascertain and diagnose.

SYNDROMES WITH DISEASE OF DENTIN
Vitamin D–resistant rickets (hereditary hypophosphatemic rickets)

Vitamin D promotes the absorption of calcium and phosphorus from the intestinal tract. Therefore a diet deficient in vitamin D produces a negative calcium balance in the organism, which, in turn, results in an undermineralization of the skeletal system. When such undermineralization is severe enough to produce clinical and radiographic changes, it is called rickets. The organic matrix of bone in a person with rickets is essentially normal and eventually may become normally mineralized if calcium and phosphorus are supplied to this tissue (1) in adequate amounts and (2) in the proper proportion to one another (calcium and phosphorus concentrations are sufficient for mineralization to occur). Thus rickets is the result of a lack of calcification of cartilage and osteoid. Since the organic matrices of bone and dentin are similar, one might expect to see hypomineralization of dentin in children with rickets. Such is actually the case. Experimentally, rats fed diets deficient in vitamin D show an increased width of predentin, irregularities of the mineralization front with odontoblast disorganization, and a marked decrease in alkaline phosphatase activity in the tooth germ.[79, 81]

It was recognized some time ago that certain patients with the classical features of rickets did not respond to vitamin D therapy, which was typically curative for this disorder. Albright, in 1937, first demonstrated that these refractory patients would, however, respond to massive doses of vitamin D, and hence the disease came to be known as vitamin D–resistant rickets (abbreviated as VDRR). The prime features of this disorder are (1) familial occurrences, (2) lowered serum phosphate levels associated with decreased renal resorption of phosphate, and (3) rickets, unresponsive to physiological doses of vitamin D. The widely accepted term in use today, coming from the above description, is familial hypophosphatemic rickets.

Unfortunately, familial does not adequately describe this disorder, since the hereditary basis is well documented as an X-linked dominant trait.

Clinical and radiographic features. Affected children are short of stature and often have significant bowing of the legs, even without other evidence of active bone disease. Bony overgrowth at the site of muscular attachments and around joints may result in limitation of motion. The rachitic rosary of classic vitamin D–dependent rickets may also occur here. Typically, the disease is first recognized in young children about the time they begin to walk. At this time the only abnormalities are a shortened stature, an abnormally low serum phosphate, and an elevated serum alkaline phosphatase. Dental changes may be diagnostic as well, and these are discussed in a separate section. Radiographs of the skeleton show active rickets sometimes with a cystic appearance to the metaphyseal and epiphyseal areas and a coarsened bony trabeculation. The short stature and bowed legs persist into adult life often in spite of treatment, and the radiographic picture in the adult is one of postrachitic deformities and pseudofractures. The serum phosphate levels remain consistently low, and serum alkaline phosphatase activity ranges from normal to high.

Proposed biochemical abnormality. The major blood chemical abnormality is the low phosphate concentration, which may be normal in affected babies during the first few months of life. Harrison[80] has proposed that this is due to the low glomerular filtration characteristic of this age, which allows normophosphatemic levels to be maintained. Nevertheless, hypophosphatemia, at whatever age of onset, is invariably accompanied by increased renal excretion and decreased tubular resorption of phosphate. Renal studies in these patients show that kidney function except for phosphate resorption is completely normal. It appears that a defect in vitamin D metabolism could explain these results, although no specific defect has yet been identified. For example, the conversion of vitamin D, cholecalciferol, to its first product, 25-hydroxycholecalciferol (abbreviated as 25-HCC), takes place in the liver. This conversion is considerably slower in persons with resistant rickets. A lack of 25-HCC could also explain the reduced intestinal calcium absorption in these subjects. However, daily treatment of these subjects with 2500 units of 25-HCC does not correct the serum biochemical abnormalities.[86] Furthermore, 25-HCC can be hydroxylated in the kidney to 1,25-dihydroxycholecalciferol (1,25-DHCC), and since this substance is even more active in mobilizing bone calcium and enhancing the intestinal absorption of calcium, it may be that this next metabolic step is the essential one to consider. Thus the primary defect could still reside in specific kidney cells and be evidenced as a defect in tubular resorption of phosphate. These same kidney cells might also be unable to effect the conversion of 25-HCC to 1,25-DHCC, a deficiency of which produces the secondary effects characteristic of the clinical picture. A review of these biochemical problems relative to vitamin D metabolism has been made by Kolata.[82]

Inheritance. Hypophosphatemic rickets is well established as an X-linked dominant disorder (Fig. 8-21). This means that affected males (assuming they are married to unaffected females) can have *only* normal sons and affected daughters. Furthermore, the low serum phosphate level is the consistent phenotype of this gene defect. Bone disease is more highly variable in severity, and instances of an obligate gene-carrier parent without bone disease who pass on the trait to offspring are known. A probable explanation for the variability in clinical expression of the disease is Lyonization. Thus Stanbury and co-workers[86] comment in a literature review that forty-four out of forty-six hypophosphatemic males have skeletal disease, whereas only fifty-three out of 100 hypophosphatemic females have bone disease. Note that the male:female affected ratio for these same families is 46:100 or close to the 1:2 ratio expected for an X-linked dominant trait.

An autosomal dominant form of this disorder has been suggested by several authors. McKusick,[83] in reviewing these reports, states that "it is certainly possible for more than one genetic variety of vitamin D–resistant rickets to exist."

Further heterogeneity in the diseases classified as rickets is suggested by the report of Dent and associates.[78] In the disease variation described by them, response to vitamin D therapy is considerably better, and the manner of inheritance is probably autosomal recessive.[85] The latter is supported by the observations of five different families showing multiple affected sibs who had normal parents, three instances of which have been consanguineous matings of cousins.

Dental manifestations of familial hypophosphatemic rickets (or VDRR). The clinical,

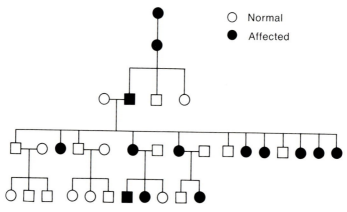

Fig. 8-21. Pedigree of X-linked dominant vitamin D–resistant rickets. Note affected male who has had no affected sons and no completely normal daughters.

radiographic, and histopathological dental features of this disease have been reviewed[77] and are so different as to require a separate discussion. It behooves the dentist to be especially aware of this disorder, since the dental signs and symptoms are largely unknown to the medical profession. Furthermore, these dental changes may produce the first overt symptoms of the disease, which cause the patient to seek dental attention first and subsequently medical evaluation.

Clinical and radiographic features. Both primary and permanent dentitions are involved. The clinical evidence of this involvement may be draining periapical abscesses and fistulae about the primary teeth, but the permanent teeth are less often so affected and often present only a nonvital pulp test on routine examination. Radiographic examination of symptomatic teeth often reveals enlarged pulp chambers and extension of the pulp horns into the cusp tips (Fig. 8-22). Periapical pathological conditions are often seen on these affected teeth. Most important to the dentist is that these clinical and radio-

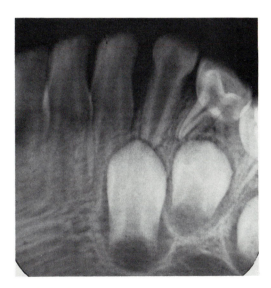

Fig. 8-22. Vitamin D–resistant rickets. Pulp horn of deciduous canine extending to incisal edge. (Courtesy Dr. Carl J. Witkop, Jr.; from Tiecke, R. W., editor: Oral pathology, New York, 1965, McGraw-Hill Book Co. Copyright 1965; used with permission of McGraw-Hill Book Co.)

graphic signs are seen in teeth that do not demonstrate any causative factors such as dental caries, periodontal disease, or fracture.

One of the routine clinical findings with vitamin D–*dependent* rickets is a severe hypoplasia of the incisal and occlusal enamel with radiographs showing dentin changes exemplified by large pulp chambers and delayed closure of root apices. By contrast, enamel changes are usually absent in the vitamin D–*resistant* form of rickets, and the dental changes are confined principally to the dentin.[76, 78]

Histopathology. Both decalcified and ground sections of affected teeth in hypophosphatemic rickets demonstrate the reason for the clinical dental problems. The enamel and dentinoenamel junction (DEJ) are normal. A thin layer of mantle dentin is normal. However, beneath the mantle layer the dentin becomes grossly globular in appearance with the largest globules being nearest to the DEJ and gradually becoming smaller and coalesced as they approach the pulp. In the region of pulp horns, tubular defects of the dentin are noted that extend to the DEJ out in the cusp tips and under the incisal edges (Fig. 8-23). Thus open cracks in the surface enamel may literally extend down into the pulp, offering an avenue for pulpal infection by oral bacteria.

Tracy and associates[87] reported that affected dentin shows a considerable range in severity. However, interglobular dentin was present in all affected teeth examined. These authors were able to show that dentin laid down prenatally was also defective; they described it as prenatal interglobular dentin. This turns out to be a second discriminating feature between the vitamin D–*dependent* and vitamin D–*resistant* disorders, since in the former disease the mother's normal vitamin D metabolism appears to protect the fetus from dental insults. By contrast, a mother affected with hypophosphatemic rickets (VDRR) would not be expected to exert a protective metabolic effect over the fetal dentition. Lyonization is a complication to this conclusion. Since VDRR is an X-linked trait, on the average one would expect to find

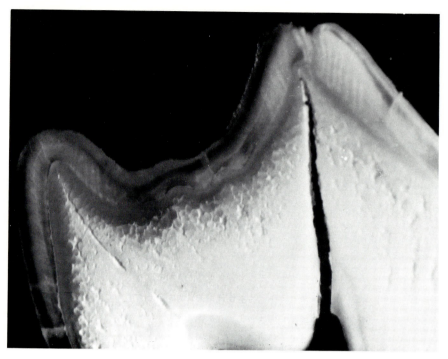

Fig. 8-23. Vitamin D–resistant rickets. Ground section of tooth shows pulpal extension through enamel. (Courtesy Dr. Carl J. Witkop, Jr.; from Tiecke, R. W., editor: Oral pathology, New York, 1965, McGraw-Hill Book Co. Copyright 1965; used with permission of McGraw-Hill Book Co.)

twice as many affected mothers as fathers, and therefore the incidence of prenatal dentin insults in those affected families may be more common than previously suspected.

The proportion of new cases due to a fresh mutation is not known, but sporadic occurrences have been reported. Possibly the presence of prenatal interglobular dentin in the child may be of use in deciding whether an affected child of apparently normal parents represents a new mutation.

Sauk and Witkop[84] have made scanning electron-microscopic studies on teeth from a VDRR-affected male. These studies confirm that the basic dentin defect, which was characterized above by light microscopy study, consists of elongated pulp horns extending into the incisal edge just below the enamel. Sauk and Witkop noted large calcospherites of globular dentin that formed definite anatomical boundaries picturesquely described by them as a "complex of caves and caverns." They suggested that the dentin defect is somehow intimately related to vascularization of the dental pulp.

For all practical purposes one may presume that systemic conditions that interfere with normal mineralization will produce defects in teeth. Thus hyperparathyroidism, vitamin D deficiency, or even diets severely deficient in calcium and/or phosphorus are known to produce dental defects. At a more subtle level are those heritable disorders which interfere with normal mineralization. These include both the vitamin D–dependent and vitamin D–resistant forms of rickets, the Fanconi syndrome (renal rickets), and other renal tubular resorption defects in which elements essential for normal mineralization are lost in the urine. All of these defects should be conceptually separated from those in which there is a primary defect in the mineralization matrix. The various types of dentinogenesis imperfecta and dentin dysplasia, along with osteogenesis imperfecta, fall into this latter category. Interestingly, none of these latter disorders appear to have a recessive mode of inheritance, implying that the genetic defect may reside in a structural protein rather than an enzyme.

Albright's hereditary osteodystrophy

Clinical features. Albright's hereditary osteodystrophy is a symptom complex whose primary problem is a failure of end organ responsiveness to parathyroid hormone (PTH). Chemically, the disease is characterized by hypocalcemia and hyperphosphatemia, which are the same laboratory findings seen in hypoparathyroidism. A group of such hypoparathyroid patients has been described who have an unresponsiveness to PTH and a unique collection of physical stigmata. These persons were unfortunately given the disease designation of pseudohypoparathyroidism (PHP). Patients with PHP actually have increased levels of circulating PTH. They have no identifiable circulating antibodies to the hormone, and the hormone is biologically active. Thus the term PHP is inaccurate. The full syndrome includes the biochemical problems just named plus shortness of stature, brachydactyly, mental retardation, and ectopic soft tissue calcification. To make matters even more confusing, a third group of patients with these same biochemical abnormalities and physical findings was identified who *did* respond appropriately to exogenous PTH. This new disease variation was designated as pseudopseudohypoparathyroidism (PPHP)! We now know that PHP and PPHP are only different severities of the same genetic disorder, which biochemically represents an end-organ unresponsiveness to normal or increased levels of circulating PTH. A review of the pertinent clinical and radiographic findings has been made by Steinbach and Young.[89]

Inheritance. Albright's osteodystrophy is apparently inherited as an X-linked dominant trait. This is evident from the fact that no male-to-male transmission is observed and females are affected twice as often as males. However, hemizygous males are not more severely affected than heterozygous females, as would be expected with Lyonization of an X-linked trait.[83] Perhaps this trait may ultimately prove to be a sex-influenced but autosomal dominant one. As indicated above, both PHP and PPHP occur in the same family, often in a parent-offspring relationship, and therefore must be considered clinical variants of the same basic disorder.

Dental features. This disorder is presented here because there are defects of all the primary dental structures, as follows: (1) a dull, white clinical appearance to enamel with pitting of its surface as evidence of hypoplasia, (2) small crowns and short roots with blunted apices, (3) large pulp chambers, and (4) unusual histopathological changes in the dentin.

These light microscopic changes in the dentin include irregular dentinal tubules that have sharp bends at both the pulpal and dentinoenamel junctions. Ground sections show accentuated incremental lines in the dentin, and the tubular nature of this dentin disappears apically, being replaced by a bone-like tissue.[90] The matrix is irregularly calcified and shows interglobular dentin with unusual vascular channels extending from the peripheral dentin into the cementum. The cementum itself is thick and of the cellular type with a cartilage-like appearance. Pulp chambers are mostly filled with calcified material that shows a whorllike pattern. In reviewing the above findings, Ritchie[88] noted that there is evident similarity with those dental changes observed in idiopathic hypoparathyroidism. Thus the dental alterations of PHP are representative of the overall metabolic picture, which favors ectopic calcification and other mineralization defects and is, therefore, not a primary dental disease in itself. It might be noted that the intrapulpal calcification described in radiographs of affected patients has been noted both in this clinic and in others.[91]

It is possible that the mineralizing defects in this disease are not entirely due to end-organ unresponsiveness to PTH. As noted in the discussion of hypophosphatemic rickets, the vitamin D metabolite, 25-HCC, is converted to the more active vitamin form 1,25-DHCC in the kidney. This step is regulated (at least in part) by parathyroid hormone. Hence, if kidney cells are also unresponsive to PTH action, as bone appears to be, persons with Albright's osteodystrophy would also be vitamin D deficient!

Branchio-skeletal-genital (BSG) syndrome

Abnormalities of dentin appear as part of many syndromes, some as a secondary phenomenon related to prevailing systemic conditions that favor incomplete mineralization, as in vitamin D–resistant rickets, and in other instances for unknown reasons. For example, persons with the BSG syndrome show a completely typical form of dentin dysplasia (type I) along with a clinical constellation of disorders involving various other organ systems. The significant findings as originally reported by Elsahy and Waters[92] are described in the following section.

Clinical and radiographic features. Affected individuals show a severe maxillary hypoplasia, giving them a prognathic or bulldog appearance. Cephalometric measurements confirm that the basic problem is maxillary hypoplasia. The maxillary teeth are grossly misaligned, and radiographs reveal the presence of multiple cystic areas, presumed by the authors to be dentigerous cysts on the basis of both histopathological and radiographic appearance. Dentin histopathology was reported to be typical of that described for dentin dysplasia type I. The authors have erroneously presented a photomicrograph of fibrous dysplasia of dentin, although the patients actually had the DD type I appearing teeth (see Witkop[57] for the correct photomicrograph).

Affected individuals are severely mentally retarded and show primary telecanthus with strabismus, bifid uvula, nasal speech with articulation defects, and penoscrotal hypospadias. Minor skeletal anomalies, including fusion of the second and third cervical vertebrae and Schmorl's nodes in the lumbar vertebrae, were also noted.

This constellation of clinical findings is unique and constitutes a new syndrome. The developmental relationship of the dental findings to those of other tissues is unknown. I have examined what is probably another case of the BSG syndrome in which multiple cystic areas of the jaws were absent.

Heredity. Three males in a single sibship are affected with this syndrome. Another male sib is retarded but without anomalies, and there is a normal male sib. The single female in this sibship is retarded without anomalies. Since a careful examination showed the mother and father to be unaffected, and since they were second cousins, the authors propose autosomal recessive inheritance, although an X-linked recessive trait is also possible with this family pattern. Other heritable dentin defects occur both in isolated and syndromic form (for example, DI types I and II) but it is difficult to see any causal relation between the various clinical anomalies and production of dentin dysplasia, type I in the BSG syndrome. It is possible that isolated DD type I and syndromic dentin dysplasia are structurally the same entity but perhaps produced by different metabolic errors that are not yet distinguishable. More examples of both types of dentin dysplasia are necessary to clarify this point.

DENTAL DISEASES INVOLVING DENTIN AS A POSSIBLE PRIMARY DEFECT

Dens invaginatus (dens in dente)

This developmental anomaly is most often called *dens in dente,* which is descriptive of the radiographic appearance of the condition itself—"a tooth within a tooth." The cause is unknown, but dens invaginatus is presumed to result from an invagination of the enamel organ at an early stage of development,[96] somewhat analogous to the amphibian process of creating a gastrula from a blastula. Several hypotheses have been proposed to explain this invagination, including fusion of two tooth germs, pressure from surrounding tissues, dislocation of enamel organ from the dental papilla, enamel organ defect, and retention of aberrant cells from the inner enamel epithelium. With the exception of the last idea, none of these seems to encompass the current concepts relating to causation of developmental anomalies, for example, cell movement, cell contact, and cell adhesion through specific protein chains in the cell membrane (see discussion of odontodysmorphogenesis on p. 244). Therefore it seems likely that an answer to the cause of dens invaginatus may be slow in coming.

Clinical and radiographic features. Any tooth in the mouth may have an invagination, but the great majority occur in maxillary lateral incisors, about half of the time symmetrically.[95] The presence of a dens invaginatus in these teeth may be suspected by the external appearance of the lingual surface and cingulum. Often the marginal ridges are prominent with a heavy cingulum and a centrally located pit. This pit may be superficial or deep, even extending to the apical foramen. Teeth with a marked invagination usually have a wide-open apical foramen. Thus the final diagnosis is best made radiographically.

Radiographs reveal the presence of a double layer of enamel, one on the outside of the tooth and one on the inside of the invagination (Fig. 8-24). This illustrates that the term *dens in dente* is not strictly accurate, since the defect actually represents an everted tooth within a normally oriented tooth. A double invagination in a single tooth has been reported several times.[94, 95, 100, 101] Hallett[97] has made a descriptive classification based on the depth of the invagination and degree of occlusion of the pulp chamber by the abnormal tooth.

Histological examination shows that the enamel and dentin comprising the outer (or normal) tooth is unaffected, whereas the enamel covering the invaginated tooth is often severely defective.[99] In some areas enamel and dentin both may be defective or even missing.

Epidemiology and genetics. Dens invaginatus of the maxillary lateral incisor varies somewhat in prevalence according to racial background. In Caucasians, the prevalence is variable ranging from about 1%[93] to a re-

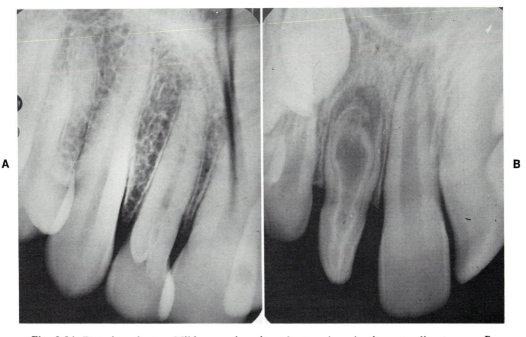

Fig. 8-24. Dens invaginatus. Mild expression, **A,** and severe invagination extending to apex, **B.** (From Shafer, W. G., Hine, M. K., and Levy, B. M.: Textbook of oral pathology, ed. 3. Philadelphia, 1974, W. B. Saunders Co.)

markable high of 49.6%.[97] Undoubtedly, this range reflects different criteria, variable radiograph quality, and population sampling bias more than a true population prevalence range. Grahnen and associates[95] found the incidence in 3000 Swedish children to be 3%. Kong[98] found the incidence in persons of Mongoloid extraction to be 2.5%. Interestingly, within his mixed racial group of 2338 children examined, Kong found the prevalence in Chinese children to be 3.6%, whereas Malays and Indians had a prevalence of about 1.4%. It has been suggested that Negroes are free of this anomaly.[93] From these results it appears that there are differences in racial group prevalence, but more studies, especially on those of Negroid ancestry, are indicated.

There are no pedigrees in the literature showing inheritance of dens invaginatus. However, Grahnen and co-workers,[95] in their study of Swedish schoolchildren, carefully examined the parents and sibs of fifty of the fifty-eight propositi with dens invaginatus for evidence of hereditary transmission of this trait. Of forty-two parents examined, eighteen were affected (Hallett's types II to IV, inclusive), for an incidence of 43%. Of forty-one sibs examined, thirteen were affected for an incidence of 32%. No sex differences were noted for either affected parents or sibs. The authors emphasize that this first-degree relative incidence is significantly higher than the general population incidence for the trait in that area. No differences in heritability were seen if the oral trait was either unilateral or bilateral. Thus dens invaginatus, regardless of severity as judged both by morphology and symmetry, has a high degree of heritability. No pedigrees were shown, but it would appear from the sibship data presented that, where one parent is affected, twelve out of seventeen offspring were affected, a ratio compatible with dominance. No statement can be made regarding autosomal versus sex linkage, but there is at least one family presented with an affected offspring in which both parents are normal, suggesting nonpenetrance. Presumably the basic defect resides in the dental papilla itself, whose cells are pro-

viding incorrect positional information for the odontomorphogenic process.

Dens evaginatus

This developmental anomaly is a rare and unusual trait that has appeared in the dental literature during the past 40 years. A wide variety of names have been used to describe this anomaly,[106] but this section will employ the more popular and descriptive term, *dens evaginatus.*

Evaginated teeth usually occur bilaterally and are most often premolars, although the condition has also been described in molars, canines, and incisors.[102, 103] Mandibular premolars are affected five times more frequently than maxillary premolars.[106]

Clinical and radiographic features. Dens evaginatus involves an outfolding of the enamel organ in such a way that the occlusal surface of the affected posterior tooth has a tuberculated appearance. Radiographs show no abnormality except an occlusal extension of the tubercle with pulp material inside it. Since these evaginations may be fractured off, pulpal exposure often follows, and pulpal necrosis may occur with resultant periapical infection. The degree of pulpal extension into these tubercles is variable.

Epidemiology. This anomaly has been reported among all persons of Mongoloid racial stock, including Chinese, Japanese, Eskimos, Malays, Aleuts, Filipinos, and even American Indians.[106] The paucity of literature on its occurrence in non-Mongoloid races suggests that it is either rare in these groups or almost exclusive to the Mongoloid race.[104] A case of dens evaginatus in a female of Greek ancestry has recently been reported.[105]

The estimated prevalence varies from about 1% to 4% in the various groups of Mongoloids. It also appears to be equally distributed between the sexes,[106] although Merrill[104] has reported a female predilection among Eskimos.

Genetics. No familial cases of dens evaginatus have appeared in the literature. One exception is a family of a father and two daughters mentioned in a discussion of this trait in Chapter 6. Because of the apparent select racial occurrence, it is reasonable to consider that this is a heritable trait and that families showing transmission of the phenotype have simply not been reported as yet. Support for this idea resides in the following facts:

1. With a single exception, all reported cases have occurred in persons of Mongoloid ancestry.

2. These occurrences have been noted in a wide geographic distribution of these Mongoloid groups, literally ranging around the world.

3. Prevalence in so-called mixed-ancestry groups (Malays) is lower than in other so-called pure groups (Chinese, Japanese) and is absent in geographically adjacent and culturally similar groups that have Caucasian background (Malay Indians of European ancestry).

Collectively, these observations suggest a heritable trait, possibly polygenic or autosomal dominant in nature, at least for the most common situation, dens evaginatus in premolars. As noted in a previous section, a somatic mutation affecting positional information of cells in the dental papilla could also account for this trait, in which case one would not expect to see any familial cases. It is difficult to imagine a mutation that occurs only in a select racial group. The lack of any reported difference in sex prevalence is not helpful in formulating a genetic hypothesis. Family studies of relatives of affected probands are clearly indicated. (See Chapter 6 for additional discussion.)

DENTIN DEFECTS IN OTHER SYNDROMES

Dental changes nearly identical to those observed in dentin dysplasia type I have been observed in patients with generalized calcinosis and in the Ehlers-Danlos syndrome. The significance of these observations is presently unknown, but they are included here because of the possible relationship to a heritable, primary disease of dentin.

Ehlers-Danlos syndrome (EDS) is a disease complex presently consisting of at least seven different heritable entities.[110] In each case a specific defect of collagen is probable, although such specificity has been identified only for a few of the different types. Nevertheless, reports are available indicating that dentin and cementum abnormalities exist in the teeth of persons affected with the Ehlers-Danlos syndrome. Barabas[107] has shown abnormal scalloping at the DEJ, irregular dentin, and consistently the formation of intrapulpal calcification. Since there was no classification of the various Ehlers-Danlos subtypes existing at the time of Barabas' report, the teeth he reported on could have come from persons with different types of EDS.

Calcinosis refers to abnormal deposition of calcium within tissues, and two broad categories encompassing the majority of cases are recognized, calcinosis universalis and calcinosis circumscripta. A third rare form, tumoral calcinosis, has been described. In this latter form, calcific deposits are typically periarticular, dense, and irregular and occur in subcutaneous tissue. Hunter and associates[109] reported on a young female with subcutaneous calcific deposits who also demonstrated a significantly elevated serum phosphate with normal calcium and alkaline phosphatase values. Tooth roots showed gross pulp stones in the coronal third of the root, which produced pulpal obliteration and even root expansion in this area. This is a developmental abnormality believed to be due to calcification of the dental papilla. Interestingly, other reports of the same or similar anomaly have occurred in the absence of tumoral calcinosis,[111] in Ehlers-Danlos syndrome,[107] and with calcinosis universalis.[108] The metabolic conditions vary in these disorders, but remarkable similarity of dental pulp response suggests that they have a common basis, probably related to an abnormal calcifying matrix rather than to the calcification process itself.

REFERENCES
Embryology and biochemistry

1. Bachra, B. M.: Calcification of connective tissue, Int. Rev. Connect. Tissue Res. 5:165-208, 1970.
2. Carmichael, D. J., Veis, A., and Wang, E. T.:

Dentin matrix collagen: Evidence for a covalently linked phosphoprotein attachment, Calcif. Tissue Res. **7**:331-344, 1971.

3. Croissant, R., Guenther, H., and Slavkin, H. C.: How are embryonic preameloblasts instructed by odontoblasts to synthesize enamel? In Slavkin, H. C., and Greulich, R. C., editors: Extracellular matrix influences on gene expression, New York, 1975, Academic Press, Inc., pp. 515-521.

4. Eastoe, J. E., Martens, P., and Thomas, N. R.: The amino-acid composition of human hard tissue collagens in osteogenesis imperfecta and dentinogenesis imperfecta, Calcif. Tissue Res. **12**:91-100, 1973.

5. Johnston, M. C., and Pratt, R. M.: The neural crest in normal and abnormal craniofacial development. In Slavkin, H. C., and Greulich, R. C., editors: Extracellular matrix influences on gene expression, New York, 1975, Academic Press, Inc., pp. 773-777.

6. Kollar, E. J., and Baird, G. R.: Tissue interactions in embryonic mouse tooth germs. I. Reorganization of the dental epithelium during tooth germ reconstruction, J. Embryol. Exp. Morphol. **24**:159-171, 1970.

7. Kollar, E. J., and Baird, G. R.: Tissue interactions in embryonic mouse tooth germs. II. The inductive role of the dental papilla, J. Embryol. Exp. Morphol. **24**:173-186, 1970.

8. Ruch, J. V., and Karcher-Djuricic, V.: On odontogenic tissue interactions. In Slavkin, H. C., and Greulich, R. C., editors: Extracellular matrix influences on gene expression, New York, 1975, Academic Press, Inc., pp. 549-551.

Dentinogenesis imperfecta and dentin dysplasia

9. Becks, H.: Histologic study of tooth structure in osteogenesis imperfecta, Dent. Cosmos **73**: 437-454, 1931.

10. Bergman, G., Engfeldt, B., and Sundvall-Hagland, I.: Studies on mineralized dental tissues. VIII. Histologic and microradiographic investigation of hereditary opalescent dentine, Acta Odontol. Scand. **14**:103-117, 1956.

11. Bernard, W. V.: Roentgenographic and histologic differentiation of dentinogenesis imperfecta and dentinal dysplasia, J. Dent. Res. **39**:674-675, 1960.

12. Bixler, D., Conneally, P. M., and Christen, A. G.: Dentinogenesis imperfecta: genetic variations in a six-generation family, J. Dent. Res. **48**:1196-1199, 1969.

13. Blumenkrantz, N., Rosenbloom, J., and Prockop, D. J.: Sequential steps in the synthesis of hydroxylysine and the glycosylation of hydroxylysine during biosynthesis of collagen, Biochim. Biophys. Acta **192**:81-89, 1969.

14. Brookerson, K. R., and Miller, A. S.: Dentinal dysplasia: report of a case, J. Am. Dent. Assoc. **77**:608-611, 1968.

15. Bruszt, P.: Sur deux cas de dysplasia dentinare, Bull. Group. Int. Rech. Sci. Stomatol. **12**:107-119, 1969.

16. Burstone, M. S.: The ground substance of abnormal dentin, secondary dentin and pulp calcifications, J. Dent. Res. **32**:269-279, 1953.

17. Elzay, R. P., and Robinson, C. T.: Dentinal dysplasia: report of a case, Oral Surg. **23**: 338-342, 1967.

18. Glimcher, M. J., and Krane, S. M.: The organization and structure of bone and the mechanism of calcification. In Gould, B. S., editor: Treatise on collagen, vol. 2B, London, 1968, Academic Press Inc. (London), Ltd., pp. 67-251.

19. Grimer, P. T.: An atypical form of hereditary opalescent dentine, Br. Dent. J. **100**:275-278, 1956.

20. Herold, R. C.: Fine structure of tooth dentine in human dentinogenesis imperfecta, Arch. Oral Biol. **17**:1009-1013, 1972.

21. Heys, F. M., Blattner, R. J., and Robinson, H. B. G.: Osteogenesis imperfecta and odontogenesis imperfecta: clinical and genetic aspects in eighteen families, J. Pediatr. **56**:234-245, 1960.

22. Hodge, H. C., and Finn, S. B.: Hereditary opalescent dentin: a dominant hereditary tooth anomaly in man, J. Hered. **29**:359-364, 1938.

23. Hodge, H. C., Lose, G. B., Finn, B., Gachet, F. S., Bassett, S. H., Robb, R. C., van Huysen, G., Robinson, H. B. G., leFevre, M. L., Bale, W. F., and McCoord, A. B.: Correlated clinical and structural study of hereditary opalescent dentin, J. Dent. Res. **15**:316-317, 1936.

24. Hursey, R. J., Witkop, C. J., Miklashek, D., and Sackett, L. M.: Dentinogenesis imperfecta in a racial isolate with multiple hereditary defects, Oral Surg. **9**:641-658, 1956.

25. Ivancie, G. P.: Dentinogenesis imperfecta, Oral Surg. **7**:984-992, 1954.

26. Johnson, D. N., Chaudhry, A. P., Gorlin, R. J., Mitchell, D. F., and Bartholdi, W. L.: Hereditary dentinogenesis imperfecta, J. Pediatr. **54**:786-792, 1959.

27. Lapiere, C. M., and Nusgens, B. V.: Maturation related changes of the protein matrix of bone. In Balazs, E. A., editor: Chemistry and molecular biology of the intercellular matrix, New York, 1970, Academic Press, Inc., pp. 55-80.

28. Listgarden, M. A.: Osteogenesis imperfecta

and dentinogenesis imperfecta, J. Can. Dent. Assoc. **26**:412-416, 1960.

29. Logan, J., Becks, H., Silverman, S., and Pindborg, J.: Dentinal dysplasia, Oral Surg. **15**:317-333, 1962.

30. Lyons, D. C.: Evidence of the hereditary factor in opalescent dentin, J. Am. Dent. Assoc. **27**:1281-1284, 1940.

31. Miller, W. A., Winkler, S., Rosenberg, M. A., Mastracola, R., Fischman, S. L., and Wolfe, R. J.: Dentinogenesis imperfecta traceable through five generations of a part American Indian family, Oral Surg. **35**:180-186, 1973.

32. Morgan, P. H., Jacobs, H. G., Segrest, J. P., and Cunningham, L. W.: A comparative study of glycopeptides derived from selected vertebrate collagens, J. Biol. Chem. **245**:5042-5048, 1970.

33. Munch, J.: Erbliche Schmelzhypoplasie, Zahnaerztl. Prax. **7**:1-4, 1956.

34. Noyes, F. B.: Hereditary anomaly in structure of dentin, J. Dent. Res. **15**:154-155, 1935.

35. Petersson, A.: A case of dentinal dysplasia and/or calcification of the dentinal papilla, Oral Surg. **33**:1014-1017, 1972.

36. Pfluger, H.: Hochgradige mangelhafte schmelzbildung in vier generationen, Dtsch. Zahnaerztl. Wochenschr. **32**:337-349, 1929.

37. Pindborg, J. J.: Dental aspects of osteogenesis imperfecta, Acta pathol. Microbiol. Scand. **24**:47-58, 1947.

38. Pindborg, J. J.: Dentinogenesis imperfecta, Tandlaegebladet **52**:279-296, 1948.

39. Rao, S. R., Witkop, C. J., and Yamane, G. M.: Pulpal dysplasia, Oral Surg. **30**:682-689, 1970.

40. Richardson, A. S., and Fantin, T. D.: Anomalous dysplasia of dentine: report of a case, J. Can. Dent. Assoc. **36**:189-191, 1970.

41. Rushton, M. A.: A case of dentinal dysplasia, Guy's Hosp. Rep. **89**:369-373, 1939.

42. Rushton, M. A.: A new form of dentinal dysplasia: shell teeth, Oral Surg. **7**:543-549, 1954.

43. Rushton, M. A.: Anomalies of human dentine, Br. Dent. J. **98**:431-444, 1955.

44. Rushton, M. A.: The structure of the teeth in a late case of osteogenesis imperfecta, J. Pathol. Bacteriol. **48**:591-603, 1939.

45. Sauk, J. J., Lyon, H. W., Trowbridge, H. O., and Witkop, C. J.: An electron optic analysis and explanation for the etiology of dentinal dysplasia, Oral Surg. **33**:763-771, 1972.

46. Schimmelpfennig, C. B., and McDonald, R. E.: Enamel and dentin aplasia, Oral Surg. **6**:1444-1449, 1953.

47. Sclare, R.: Hereditary opalescent dentine, Br. Dent. J. **84**:164-166, 1948.

48. Shields, E. D., Bixler, D., and El-Kafrawy, A. M.: Heritable dentine defects: dentine dysplasia type II, Arch. Oral Biol. **18**:543-553, 1973.

49. Shokeir, M.: Dentinogenesis imperfecta: severe expression in a probable homozygote, Clin. Genet. **3**:442-447, 1972.

50. Shuttleworth, A., and Veis, A.: The isolation of anionic phosphoproteins from bovine cortical bone via the periodate solubilization of bone collagens, Biochim. Biophys. Acta **257**:414-420, 1972.

51. Spiro, G. R.: The carbohydrate of collagens. In Balazs, E. A., editor: Chemistry and molecular biology of the intercellular matrix, New York, 1970, Academic Press, Inc., pp. 195-215.

52. Toole, B. P., Kang, A. H., Trelstad, R. L., and Gross, J.: Collagen heterogeneity within different growth regions on long bones of rachitic and nonrachitic chicks, Biochem. J. **127**:715-720, 1972.

53. Toto, P. D.: Osteogenesis imperfecta tarda and dentinogenesis imperfecta, Oral Surg. **6**:772-774, 1953.

54. Veis, A., Spector, A. R., and Zarnoscianyk, H.: The isolation of an EDTA-soluble phosphoprotein from mineralizing dentin, Biochim. Biophys. Acta **257**:403-413, 1972.

55. Wilson, G. W., and Steinbrecker, M.: Hereditary hypoplasia of the dentin, J. Am. Dent. Assoc. **16**:866-879, 1929.

56. Winter, G. R., and Maiocco, P. O.: Osteogenesis imperfecta and detinogenesis imperfecta, Oral Surg. **2**:782-798, 1949.

57. Witkop, C. J., Jr.: Hereditary defects of dentin, Dent. Clin. North Am. **19**:25-45, 1975.

58. Witkop, C. J., Jr., MacLean, C. J., Schmidt, P. J., and Henry, J. L.: Medical and dental findings in the Brandywine isolate, Ala. J. Med. Sci. **3**:382-403, 1966.

59. Witkop, C. J., Jr.: Studies of intrinsic disease in isolates with observations on penetrance and expressivity of certain anatomical traits. In Pruzansky, S., editor: Congenital anomalies of the face and associated structures, Springfield, Ill., 1961, Charles C Thomas, Publisher.

60. Witkop, C. J., Jr., and Rao, S.: Inherited defects in tooth structures. In Bergsma, D., editor: Birth defects original articles series. XI. Orofacial structures, vol. 7, no. 7, Baltimore, 1971, The Williams & Wilkins Co. for The National Foundation—March of Dimes.

61. Zellner, R.: Mitteilung uber drei falle von familiaerer genuiner wurzelmissbildung des gesamten gebisses, Dtsch. Zahn. Mund. Kieferheilkd. **26**:277-291, 1957.

Odontodysplasia

62. Abrams, A. M., and Groper, J.: Odontodysplasia: report of three cases, J. Dent. Child. **33**:353-362, 1966.
63. Alexander, W. N., Lilly, G. E., and Irby, W. B.: Odontodysplasia: report of case and review of literature, Oral Surg. **22**:814-820, 1966.
64. Bergman, G., Lysell, L., and Pindborg, J.: Unilateral dental malformation: report of 2 cases, Oral Surg. **16**:48-60, 1963.
65. Chaudhry, A. P., Wittich, H. D., Stickel, F. R., and Holland, M. R.: Odontogenesis imperfecta: report of a case, Oral Surg. **14**: 1099-1103, 1961.
66. Melnick, M., and Shields, E.: Odontodysmorphogenesis and gene mutation. (In press.)
67. Rushton, M. A.: Odontodysplasia: "ghost teeth," Br. Dent. J. **119**:109-113, 1965.
68. Zegarelli, E. T., Kutscher, A. H., Applebaum, E., and Archard, H. O.: Odontodysplasia, Oral Surg. **16**:187-193, 1963.

Hereditary dysplasias of enamel and dentin

69. Helfer, A. R., and Cuttita, J. A.: A case of odontogenesis and/or amelogenesis, J. Clin. Stomat. Conf. **5**:55-56, 1964.
70. Holder, B. C.: Non-development of the enamel: report of a case, J. Am. Dent. Assoc. **15**:761, 1928.
71. Hopewell-Smith, A.: A case of partial dental aplasia, Dent. Cosmos **63**:465-470, 1921.
72. Kimura, O., and Nakata, M.: Personal communication, Tokyo Dental College, 1975.
73. Olson, J. J.: Hereditary aplasia of enamel: report of a case, J. Am. Dent. Assoc. **25**: 830-831, 1938.
74. Schimmelpfennig, C. B., and McDonald, R. E.: Enamel and dentin aplasia, Oral Surg. **6**:1444-1449, 1953.
75. Siirila, H. A., and Heikinheimo, O.: Odontogenesis imperfecta, Suom. Hammaslaak. Toim. **58**:35-47, 1962.

Fibrous dysplasia of dentin

76. Witkop, C. J.: Hereditary defects of dentin, Dent. Clin. North Am. **19**:25-45, 1975.

Vitamin D–resistant rickets

77. Archard, H. O., and Witkop, C. J., Jr.: Hereditary hypophosphatemia (vitamin D resistant rickets) presenting primary dental manifestations, Oral Surg. **22**:184-193, 1966.
78. Dent, C. E., Friedman, M., and Watson, L.: Hereditary pseudo-vitamin D deficiency rickets (pseudo-mangelrachitis), J. Bone Joint Surg. **50B**:708-719, 1968.
79. Ferguson, H., and Hartles, R. L.: The effects of vitamin D on the dentine of the incisor teeth and on the alveolar bone of young rats maintained on diets deficient in calcium or phosphorus, Arch. Oral Biol. **9**:447-460, 1964.
80. Harrison, H. E., Harrison, H. C., Lifscjitz, F., and Johnson, A. D.: Growth disturbance in hereditary hypophosphatemia, Am. J. Dis. Child. **112**:290, 1966.
81. Kiguel, E.: Alkaline-phosphatase activity in developing molars of vitamin D–deficient rats. I. High calcium-phosphorus ratio diet, J. Dent. Res. **43**:71-77, 1964.
82. Kolata, G. B.: Vitamin D: investigations of a new steroid hormone, Science **187**:635-636, 1975.
83. McKusick, V. M.: Mendelian inheritance in man, ed. 4, Baltimore, 1975, The Johns Hopkins University Press.
84. Sauk, J. J., and Witkop, C. J., Jr.: Electron optic analyses of human dentin on hypophosphatemic vitamin D–resistant rickets, Oral Surg. **32**:38-44, 1971.
85. Scriver, C. R.: Vitamin D dependency, Pediatrics **45**:361-363, 1970.
86. Stanbury, J. B., Wyngaarden, J. B., and Fredrickson, D. S.: The metabolic basis of inherited disease, ed. 3, New York, 1972, McGraw-Hill Book Co., pp. 1465-1487.
87. Tracy, W. E., Steen, J. C., Steiner, J. E., and Buist, N. R.: Analysis of dentine pathogenesis in vitamin D–resistant rickets, Oral Surg. **32**:38-44, 1971.

Albright's hereditary osteodystrophy

88. Ritchie, G. MacC.: Dental manifestations of pseudohypoparathyroidism, Arch. Dis. Child. **40**:565-572, 1965.
89. Steinbach, H. L., and Young, D. A.: The roentgen appearance of pseudohypoparathyroidism (PH) and pseudo-pseudohypoparathyroidism (PPH), Am. J. Roentgenol. **97**: 49-66, 1966.
90. Sunde, O. E., and Hals, E.: Dental changes in a patient with hypoparathyroidism, Br. Dent. J. **111**:112-117, 1961.
91. Witkop, C. J., Jr.: Personal communication, 1972.

Branchio-skeletal-genital syndrome

92. Elsahy, N. I., and Waters, W. R.: The branchio-skeletal-genital syndrome, Plast. Reconstr. Surg. **48**:542-550, 1971.

Dens invaginatus

93. Amos, E. R.: Incidence of the small dens in dente, J. Am. Dent. Assoc. **51**:31-33, 1955.
94. Conklin, W. H.: Double bilateral dens invaginatus in the maxillary incisor region, Oral Surg. **39**:949-952, 1975.

95. Grahnen, H., Lindahl, B., and Omnell, K. A.: Dens invaginatus. I. A clinical, roentgenological and genetic study of permanent upper lateral incisors, Odontol. Revy. **10:**115-137, 1959.

96. Gustafson, G., and Sundberg, S.: Dens in dente, Br. Dent. J. **80:**83-88, 111-122, and 144-146, 1950.

97. Hallett, G. E. M.: The incidence, nature and clinical significance of palatal invaginations in the maxillary incisor teeth, Proc. R. Soc. Med. **46:**491-499, 1953.

98. Kong, Y. W.: The prevalence of dens invaginatus in maxillary incisors. Dent. J. Malaysia Singapore **12:**9-14, 1972.

99. Omnell, K. A., Swanbeck, G., and Lindahl, B.: Dens invaginatus. II. A microradiographical, histological, micro x-ray diffraction study, Acta Odontol. Scand. **18:**303-330, 1960.

100. Payton, G., and Morgan, G. A.: Dens in dente, Dent. Radiogr. Photogr. **39:**27-33, 1966.

101. Ulmansky, M., and Hermel, J.: Double dens in dente in a single tooth, Oral Surg. **17:** 92-97, 1964.

Dens evaginatus

102. Allwright, W. C.: Odontomes of the axial core type as a cause of osteomyelitis of the mandible, Br. Dent. J. **129:**324, 1970.

103. Lau, T. C.: Odontome of the axial core type, Br. Dent. J. **99:**219, 1955.

104. Merrill, R. G.: Occlusal anomalous tubercles on premolars of Alaskan Eskimos and Indians, Oral Surg. **17:**484-496, 1964.

105. Sykaras, S. N.: Occlusal anomalous tubercle on premolars of a Greek girl, Oral Surg. **38:** 88-91, 1974.

106. Yip, W. W.: The prevalence of dens evaginatus, Oral Surg. **38:**80-87, 1974.

Ehlers-Danlos syndrome and calcinosis

107. Barabas, G. M.: The Ehlers-Danlos syndrome: abnormalities of the enamel, dentine and cementum and the dental pulp, Br. Dent. J. **126:**509-515, 1969.

108. Hoggins, G. S., and Marsland, E. A.: Developmental abnormalities of the dentine and pulp associated with calcinosis, Br. Dent. J. **92:**305-311, 1952.

109. Hunter, I. P., MacDonald, D. G., and Ferguson, M. M.: Developmental abnormalities of the dentine and pulp associated with tumoral calcinosis, Br. Dent. J. **135:**446-448, 1973.

110. McKusick, V. M.: Heritable disorders of connective tissue, ed. 4, St. Louis, 1974, The C. V. Mosby Co.

111. Petersson, A.: A case of dentinal dysplasia and/or calcification of the dentinal papilla, Oral Surg. **33:**1014-1017, 1972.

9

Heritable disorders affecting cementum and the periodontal structure

DAVID BIXLER

Few diseases primarily involving cementum have been identified. This is somewhat remarkable, since one would expect such a tissue disorder to manifest itself clinically as a tooth that fails to erupt or one that is not stabilized in the alveolar bony socket and is exfoliated prematurely. These conditions are both obvious clinically and do not need a radiographic examination to raise a suspicion of abnormality, as many of the dentin disorders require. Perhaps the current periodontal interest in cementum chemistry in relation to bone formation will uncover new phenotypes involving cementogenesis.

In this chapter the same general approach will be followed as presented in the chapter on heritable diseases of dentin. A review of cementum embryology and biochemistry is presented to stimulate the reader to think of these disorders from an etiological standpoint. Next, the primary disorders of cementum are presented, and finally, those syndromes or disease complexes in which a cementum defect is an accompanying feature are discussed. Some heritable diseases involving the periodontium in which a cementum defect is possible but not established have also been included in this chapter.

CEMENTUM
Embryology

As each enamel organ passes through the bud, cap, and bell developmental stages, this double-layered epithelial lamina progressively encases the mesenchymal condensation of the dental papilla. At this growing rim of the enamel organ, the external dental epithelium becomes continuous with the internal dental epithelium. Once the final crown form has been laid down (note that the inner enamel epithelium gives rise to the enamel) both the inner and outer layers fuse below the level of enamel formation and form a double-layered structure. This is the epithelial root sheath of Hertwig, which initiates root formation and molds its shape.

Before beginning root formation, the root sheath forms the epithelial diaphragm, which is responsible for demarcating each root (Fig. 9-1). In single-rooted teeth, the fused inner and outer epithelia bend at the future cementoenamel junction (CEJ) into a horizontally placed diaphragm that narrows the cervical opening of the crown. Ultimately, elongations of the root sheath occur between the CEJ and the epithelial diaphragm, but most of these intermediately placed cells degenerate, leaving behind the epithelial rests of Malassez. The function of this diaphragm in multirooted teeth is more complex and is best illustrated by a surface view of the diaphragm (Fig. 9-2). Here, it can be seen that in a two-rooted tooth *(top)*, the diaphragm expands so that horizontal flaps are formed that come together in the approximate middle. Thus the dental papilla is apically separated into two parts. A three-rooted tooth *(bottom)* has three diaphragm flaps that meet centrally, thereby dividing the apex of the dental papilla into three segments, each one corresponding to a future root.

Root formation, then, consists of the following sequence of events: (1) elongation of the root sheath by mitosis, (2) formation of the epithelial diaphragm, (3) ingrowth and fusion of the epithelial flaps (Fig. 9-2), and (4) dentin proliferation along the pulpal side of the root sheath (Fig. 9-3).

Histogenesis

The portion of the epithelial root sheath of Hertwig remaining below the CEJ forms a mold against which root dentin is deposited. On the outside, the root sheath lies against connective tissue, some of whose cells will differentiate into the cementoblasts that produce cementum. Breakdown of the root sheath is promoted by connective tissue pro-

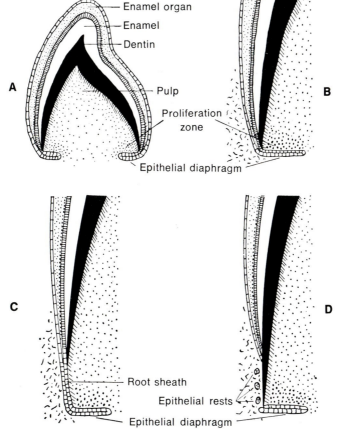

Fig. 9-1. Three stages in root development. **A** and **B,** Early stages in formation of the epithelial diaphragm. **C,** Projected elongation of Hertwig's root sheath. **D,** Epithelial rests remaining after mesenchymal penetration of root sheath. (From Bhaskar, S. N., editor: Orban's oral histology and embryology, ed. 8, St. Louis, 1976, The C. V. Mosby Co.)

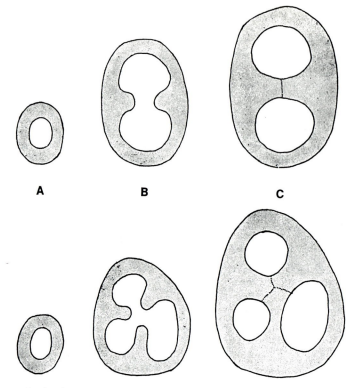

Fig. 9-2. Stages in development of roots on multirooted teeth. Surface views showing **A,** formation of horizontal flaps, **B,** flap proliferation, and **C,** union of flaps that divides cervical opening into two (upper) and three (lower) openings. (From Bhaskar, S. N., editor: Orban's oral histology and embryology, ed. 8, St. Louis, 1976, The C. V. Mosby Co.)

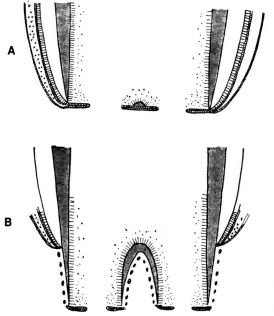

liferation and penetration* such that a physical contact is established between the undifferentiated connective tissue and dentin. Although data are not available, it seems logical to assume that this dentin functions in an inductive fashion to stimulate the differentiation of cementoblasts from these mesenchymal cells, which in turn lay down

*Recall that epithelial remnants of this mesenchymal penetration process are the rests of Malassez.

Fig. 9-3. Two stages in development of two-rooted teeth. **A,** Beginning dentin proliferation at bifurcation. **B,** Root formation in progress. (From Bhaskar, S. N., editor: Orban's oral histology and embryology, ed. 8, St. Louis, 1976, The C. V. Mosby Co.)

the collagenous cementum matrix. This matrix eventually undergoes mineralization characteristic of that seen in other collagenous matrices such as bone and dentin. Two morphological types of cementum are observed, (1) acellular cementum, typically extending from the CEJ toward the apex and (2) cellular cementum, often covering the apical third of the root. These two layers represent different functional states in cementogenesis and may even alternate in deposition as the process of cementum matrix formation by apposition continues. Thus, acellular cementum is the initial product of the cementoblasts and is laid down so slowly that no cells are trapped in its matrix (hence the name, acellular cementum). Cellular cementum, on the other hand, is formed rapidly, mostly on top of the acellular cementum, and does show cementoblasts trapped in its matrix. Many authors associate cellular cementum with the eruptive process. Those cells embedded in the cementum are designated

cementocytes and are analogous to osteocytes.

An interesting developmental anomaly, the so-called Turner tooth, provides some insight into the ability of dental epithelium to form cementum. The Turner tooth is a well-recognized developmental anomaly of the permanent dentition associated with periapical infection of the preceding primary tooth. Clinically, affected teeth have smaller crowns and exhibit developmental defects, in part comprising both loss of enamel and deposition of cementum in these enamel defective areas.[1] This anomaly is evidence that the outer enamel epithelium acts as a physical barrier to prevent the transformation of undifferentiated mesenchymal cells into cementoblasts even in those areas where enamel is normally lacking as in the areas where root cementum is formed. Further support for this idea has been given by Listgarten,[6] who observed that coronal cementogenesis in erupting bovine teeth is dependent on a prior degeneration of the reduced enamel

Table 9-1. Amino acid composition of various dental matrices (residues per 1000 total residues)*

Amino acid	Cementum		Dentin	Bone
	Acellular	Cellular		
Hydroxyproline	90	59	100	90
Aspartic acid	50	38	45	51
Threonine	20	17	17	23
Serine	38	24	33	37
Glutamic acid	81	58	74	75
Proline	106	81	116	127
Glycine	113	329	328	326
Alanine	108	110	112	95
Cystine	1.8	2	0	0
Valine	24	24	25	28
Methionine	16	8	6	8
Isoleucine	15	22	10	12
Leucine	33	40	25	30
Tyrosine	5.2	6.7	6	4.2
Phenylalanine	18	20	16	17
Hydroxylysine	10	11.3	10	5.8
Lysine	21	25	22	19
Histidine	6	8	6	8
Arginine	54	60	50	48

*From Rodriguez, M. S., and Wilderman, M. N.: Amino acid composition of the cementum matrix from human molar teeth, J. Periodontol. **43:**438-440, 1972.

epithelium. This latter process underscores the essentiality of breakdown of the epithelial root sheath for normal cementum apposition to begin against the "exposed" dentin.

Biochemistry

To date, all published studies support the basic concept of cementum as a collagenous matrix which eventually mineralizes. Electron microscopy confirms the collagenous nature of this organic matrix. Furthermore, amino acid analyses of root cementum have also been performed and been found to be similar to other known collagen matrices.[5, 7] Table 9-1 indicates the amino acid composition of cementum (both cellular and acellular) compared to dentin and bone. These results suggest that acellular cementum has only about a third as much glycine as cellular cementum, although the value for cellular cementum is well in accord with that reported for the collagen matrices of dentin and bone. Furthermore, acellular cementum has proportionately more hydroxyproline and proline. From this it appears that these two types of cementum not only represent different functional states but also may consist of more than one type of collagen,* since their apparent amino acid composition is so different. Most importantly, there is a marked resemblance in amino acid content between dentin and cellular cementum, although the latter tissue shows a lower amino acid content (hydroxyproline, proline).

In summary, the evidence supports the idea that cementum consists of a collagenous matrix resembling that of bone and dentin. However, cementum may consist of more than one type of collagen present in different amounts at different times (perhaps both type I and type III are present); the functional significance of this possible difference remains speculative. That the two matrices of bone and cementum are not identical is also apparent from the report of Giansanti,[3] who noted that cementum has an intrinsic collagen bundle width and pattern that is unique and unlike that observed in bone.

---

*See discussion of collagen types in Chapter 8 on dentin; see Table 8-2.

PERIODONTAL LIGAMENT (PDL)

Some of the disorders presented in this chapter are actually diseases of the periodontium in which there may or may not be a primary defect of cementum. Thus a few comments about development of the periodontal ligament are pertinent.

Embryology and histogenesis

The periodontal ligament is derived from the dental follicle or sac, which is enveloping the developing tooth germ. Three zones are recognizable around this tooth germ, the center zone with its collagenous fibers relating to bone, an inner zone in which the fibers are intimately related to cementum, and an intermediate zone with unoriented fibers.

The main elements of the PDL are the principal fibers, all of which are attached to cementum. These are collagenous in nature—no elastic elements are seen in the PDL—and are subdivided into three groups depending on their anatomical origin: gingival, transseptal (between adjacent teeth), and alveolar. The collagenous fibers in the latter two groups run in different directions thereby ensuring that no matter from which direction a force is applied to the tooth, some fiber groups are available to counteract it. Bony attachment is secured by the formation of new bone around the ends of these fibers. In contrast to the bone attachment, the cementum attachment is accomplished by connection of the collagen fibers to the cementoblasts themselves, which show irregular cell surface projections that fit around these fibers. As described in the previous paragraphs on cementum, mesenchymal cells are induced to differentiate into cementoblasts, and these cells manufacture collagen fibrils, which make up the cementum matrix. By comparison, the collagenous fibers of the periodontal ligament are produced from mesenchymal cells of the dental sac, which penetrate the precementum and become attached to the cementoblasts. These are called Sharpey's fibers. When calcification of precementum finally occurs, Sharpey's fibers are firmly anchored in the cementum.

Biochemistry

Little is known about the biochemistry of the PDL, although it has been reported to contain about equal amounts of collagen and other noncollagenous proteins.[4] Furthermore, it appears that soluble collagen is present in greater amounts in the PDL that is associated with erupting teeth, which is probably a reflection of greater metabolic activity in collagen synthesis. As noted in the chapter on dentin, different types of collagen are now recognized to be associated with different functional needs (for example, type I collagen in bone versus type II in cartilage). Several diseases of the periodontium are reviewed in this chapter, and it seems a reasonable explanation for some of them that a predominant replacement of one type of collagen by another could alter primary function of the PDL, which, in turn, could produce a so-called periodontal disease. These thoughts seem especially appropriate in considering the cause of diseases such as periodontosis or Papillon-Lefèvre syndrome.

Collagen in the PDL has been shown to be predominantly type I $(a_1I)_2a_2$, although approximately 16% is type III $(a_1III)_3$.[2] This can be compared to only about 5% type II collagen found in cementum.[2]

PRIMARY DISEASES OF CEMENTUM
Taurodontism

Clinical and radiographic features. The term *taurodontism* (bull-like teeth) has been applied to the dental condition in which the body of the tooth is enlarged and the roots are reduced in size. Most teeth in modern man are classified as cynodont (doglike teeth), in which the pulp chambers are relatively small, there is a definite constriction at the cementoenamel junction, and the distance from the root furcation to the CEJ in multirooted teeth is *less* than the occlusocervical distance. Obviously, then, taurodont teeth would show a greater distance from the furcation to the CEJ, and the pulp chamber then is located in a more apical direction than in cynodont teeth (Fig. 9-4).

The anatomical definition of a taurodont tooth has received considerable attention, as noted by Mena[16] in his review of this problem. Most authors have had difficulty defining the end of the crown and the beginning of the root because of a lack of cervical constriction in those teeth and because enamel may extend well down on what would normally be called the root surface. Radiographs have reduced this problem considerably, and today's definition relates primarily to radiographic differences in the pulp chambers of taurodont and cynodont teeth. Typically, the cynodont tooth has a crown pulp of smaller dimension in the coronal-apical direction. However, exceptions appear to exist in which the cynodont pulp chamber is larger and the divided root is insignificant, more like that seen in the taurodont tooth.[12]

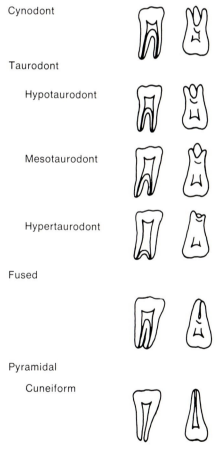

Cynodont

Taurodont

    Hypotaurodont

    Mesotaurodont

    Hypertaurodont

Fused

Pyramidal

    Cuneiform

Fig. 9-4. Types of molar teeth illustrating the six basic root configurations. (From Ackerman, J. L., et al.: Am. J. Phys. Anthropol. **38:**681-694, 1973.)

Thus there appears to be a more or less continuous variation in the two phenotypes with some overlap in their distributions.[8]

In classifying taurodont teeth it is important to consider three elements: (1) size of pulp chamber, (2) size of roots, and (3) position of body (that portion between occlusal enamel and root furcation) relative to the alveolar margin. Concerning the latter, the body of all taurodont teeth is located *below* the alveolar margin. Using the above criteria, the classification of Shaw[17] is useful (Fig. 9-4). Also, since the degree of taurodontism, when present in all three permanent molars, typically increases from the first to the third molar, Shaw suggested using the second molar as an average by which to classify all three. However, taurodontism may also occur in premolars.

Epidemiology. The racial distribution of taurodont teeth is unique with a high frequency recorded in Caucasoid hominoids but a low frequency in modern Caucasians.[12, 15, 18] It is frequently found today in the modern representatives of the Mongoloid and Capoid races, such as Eskimos, Aleuts, and American and Guatemalan Indians.[19] It has been proposed that all peoples who show this trait today trace ancestry to Neanderthal man (taurodontism was a common occurrence in Neanderthal man), who purportedly gave rise to a proto-Mongoloid race. Regardless of the anthropological significance of taurodontism, the racial distribution of this trait today suggests a genetic control; however, as will be explored subsequently, a definitive mode of inheritance may not be recognizable.

Embryology. In the introductory section of this chapter, development of the root sheath of Hertwig and the epithelial diaphragm was described. It has been proposed that the defect in taurodont teeth results from a failure of the epithelial diaphragm to invaginate at the proper horizontal level.[12] The net result would be a persistence of the primitive state of flattened diaphragms and thereby an elongated pulp chamber. This could also account for the failure to form definitive root canals in taurodont teeth except possibly in the apical third. The

dentin in taurodont teeth is routinely reported as normal, and its formation takes place as usual in that region where odontoblasts are in contact with Hertwig's root sheath. An alternative explanation for taurodontism has been offered.[13] That is, a failure of the epithelial root sheath to elongate could also leave the diaphragm at the wrong horizontal level, as originally proposed by Hamner and associates.[12] This suggests a mitotic failure. Unfortunately, application of either of these theories should produce teeth with shortened coronal-apical dimensions, a finding not always observed in taurodontia. Thus the etiologic process remains undefined.

There is no clear-cut differentiation of taurodont and cynodont teeth except at the extremes of their individual morphology. Most authors recognize subtypes such as hypertaurodont, mesotaurodont, and hypotaurodont (Fig. 9-4). The latter category becomes difficult to distinguish from normal variation in cynodont teeth, and the trait is not so much a discrete as a continuous one. The variable phenotype might be explained in part as delayed timing for diaphragm invagination; the longer the delay with ongoing crown formation, the greater the severity of the taurodont phenotype.

Inheritance

Isolated and familial cases. Taurodontism has appeared in multiple family members both as an isolated trait and as part of a heritable syndrome. As an isolated trait, Goldstein and Gottlieb[11] have reported two families who showed a dominant mode of transmission, a mother and five of her children in one instance and a father-daughter occurrence in the other. Fischer[9] reported twelve affected members in a single family (five males and seven females) covering three generations. In this family dominant inheritance also was apparent. Gamer and Zusman[10] described a dominant mode of transmission in their family in which a mother passed the trait to her son. Mena[16] described a Negro family in which five out of seven sibs were affected, the mother was normal, and the father was edentulous. Dominant inheritance was indicated here too but not confirmable. Lehtinen[14] noted taurodont teeth in three of five sibs. One parent had normal teeth, but the other was edentulous and could not be classified.

In all of the foregoing familial cases, varying degrees of severity (hypotaurodont to hypertaurodont) have been noted, even in the same mouth. Furthermore, which teeth are affected appears to be somewhat variable with first permanent molars typically affected but often with affected second deciduous molars and occasionally the second permanent molars showing the trait. Variable expression seems to be the common situation. It might be noted that only nine sporadic cases were reviewed by Goldstein and Gottlieb[11] (at least two of those appeared as part of a syndrome complex), and the total number of sporadic cases reported is then only a few more than the familial ones (twelve to five). Too few data are available to specify a mode of inheritance, but both dominant and multifactorial inheritance are possible, the latter suggested as a likely explanation for what appears to be a continuously variable trait.[8, 20]

Syndromic cases. In addition to the above cases, several reports have appeared in the literature with the authors describing patients with multiple developmental anomalies, among which taurodontism was also present.

Goldstein and Gottlieb[11] showed taurodontism present in sibs affected with orofaciodigital syndrome type II (Mohr syndrome), a recessively inherited trait. Stenvik and co-workers[31] described the trait in three of four sibs who had facies resembling that seen in anhidrotic ectodermal dysplasia. Hypodontia was also present, but the authors did not comment specifically on the presence of other findings usually seen in anhidrotic ectodermal dysplasia. Other cases with this same association of oligodontia, sparse hair, and taurodont teeth have been reported by Stoy[18] and Moller and associates.[27] The findings in these latter reports are compatible with autosomal recessive inheritance.

X-chromosome aneuploidy with taurodontism has been noted by Stewart[32] in two different males and by Keeler[24] in six patients

also with Klinefelter's syndrome. Stewart also refers to other cases of this syndrome with taurodontism personally known to him, which suggests this chromosomal syndrome complex is not a chance occurrence and may have an unknown developmental significance. Taurodontism in other aneuploid chromosome states has not been reported.

Two authors have noted the simultaneous occurrence of amelogenesis imperfecta with taurodent teeth. Crawford[21] described a hypoplastic form of amelogenesis imperfecta (reduced amount of enamel but of normal radiodensity) in a large family of fifteen affecteds in four generations. Taurodontism was documented in only two of the fourth-generation children, so it is impossible to say with certainty that these two conditions were consistently linked in this family. It should be recalled that some of the hypoplastic forms of amelogenesis imperfecta are autosomal dominant traits themselves. Winter and co-workers[33] reported a four-generation family of multiple affecteds who had an amelogenesis imperfecta characterized by hypomaturation (normal enamel thickness but reduced radiodensity) and hypoplasia appearing as random pitting on the surface. Interglobular dentin was also described. These observations were made in two sibs and a male cousin who also showed taurodontism. In this report the evidence linking taurodontism and amelogenesis is more substantial. Some of the enamel defects described in these teeth are unique, and one might conjecture that a basic developmental defect of the inner enamel epithelium could account for both the amelogenesis and root sheath defects seen in this family as a monogenic trait.

Ackerman and associates[20] described taurodontism in some molar teeth, although other molars had fused or pyramidal-shaped single roots (Fig. 9-4). This heritable trait occurred in twenty members of a large English-German family. The authors note that fused roots are relatively uncommon in first permanent molars (0.2% to 0.3%) but common in second molars (15% to 22%) and third molars (19% to 38%). Also, they accept the premise of others that pyramidal-shaped roots represent the most severe expression of the trait, fusion of roots. Robbins and Keene[28] have suggested autosomal dominant inheritance for pyramidal-shaped roots alone. In the family of Ackerman and co-workers,[20] nine of twenty persons examined had taurodont teeth while fused or pyramidal roots coexisted in seven of these nine persons. The proband's sibship consisted of six children, all affected, and the two parents were also both affected! Assuming a dominant mode of inheritance, the unusual finding of an affected by affected mating raises the possibility of a homozygous affected occurring in this sibship. In fact, three of the six affected children have *all* of their molar teeth with the pyramidal root structure—"a most unusual phenomenon," to quote the authors. These affecteds might represent the homozygous phenotype.

The presence of all three root phenotypes (taurodont, pyramidal, and fused) in the same family and even in the same person is a strong argument for common genetic causation. Such was suggested earlier by Kallay[23] in his description of pyramidal root structure in the teeth of Neanderthal man, an early man already known to have a high frequency of taurodont teeth. These subsequent reports make the genetic conclusion inevitable. The one possible qualification to this conclusion lies in the fact that affecteds in the family of Ackerman and associates[20] had a syndrome consisting of dental anomalies (as described) and other defects of skin, bone, and eye. It is conceivable, then, although still unlikely, that the observed root variations were only secondary manifestations of a primary gene defect involving multiple tissues and therefore were related to each other only secondarily. The conclusion that taurodont, pyramidal, and fused-root teeth are variations of a single heritable trait seems valid.

In 1972, Lichtenstein and co-workers[25] reported a large kindred of 102 affected persons in six generations with a syndrome of kinky or curly hair, enamel hypoplasia, taurodontism, and sclerotic bones. They called this the trichodentoosseous syndrome (TDO). Of the ten affecteds carefully studied by the authors, each one had the curly hair and dental and bone changes. The dental findings are unique and are presented here because of the regular finding of taurodont teeth in the affecteds. The following summarizes these dental manifestations:

1. Enamel hypoplasia and hypocalcification. The combined enamel problems could descriptively fall into the enamel hypomaturation category. Affected persons have shown both hypoplasia and hypocalcification on different areas of the same tooth and on different teeth in the same person.

2. Multiple periapical abscesses apparently related to carious exposure of the dental pulp.

3. Taurodontism and enlargement of pulp chambers (Fig. 9-5). Crawford[21] has reviewed the general classification of the root form of human teeth and described a family with taurodontism and amelogenesis, probably representing the TDO syndrome. The remarkable feature in the TDO syndrome is the occurrence of taurodontism in several of the deciduous teeth.[22]

4. Other radiographic abnormalities. These consisted of radiolucent zones around the crowns of impacted teeth, delayed closure of root apices, and the appearance of a condensing osteitis type of lesion around the root apices of the taurodont teeth (Fig. 9-5). Also noted is a severe enamel hypoplasia (Fig. 9-6). Jorgenson and Warson[22] propose that these dental defects can be explained by a basic defect in the enamel epithelium. An epithelial defect could explain the curly hair, possibly as an increase in sulfhydryl bonds in the keratin polypeptide chain, but this does not appear to account for the skeletal problems of delayed maturation and increased bone density. Here, a mesenchymal defect is suggested. Melnick and Shields[26] have reported a kindred with TDO syndrome in which both light microscopic and scanning electron microscopic (SEM) studies were made on teeth from the affecteds. They reported that the enamel present is uniformly reduced in thickness. SEM study showed two randomly dis-

tributed enamel defects: pits and deep depressions (Fig. 9-7). No dentin abnormalities were observed. Remarkably, a band of dense, fibrous connective tissue was noted to bridge the apical foramen and constrict the apical vessels and nerves in each tooth studied (Fig. 9-8). This bilaminar membrane covered the root almost up to the CEJ and bore a striking physical resemblance to von Korff's fibers, which are produced by the dental papilla at the time of dentin matrix formation. The authors propose that this membrane represents the cushioned hammock ligament seen in early root development adjacent to epi-

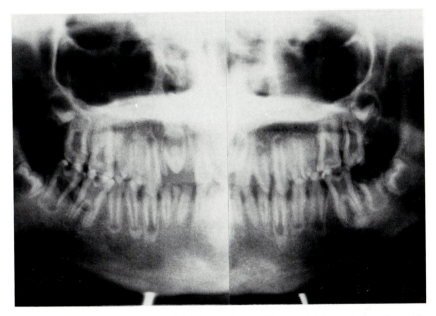

Fig. 9-5. Radiographic appearance of TDO syndrome. Note multiple apical radiopacities and taurodontism. (Courtesy Dr. Michael Melnick, Indianapolis, Ind.)

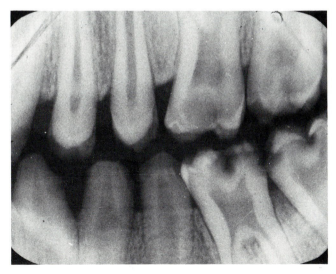

Fig. 9-6. Permanent teeth in TDO syndrome showing marked hypoplasia of enamel. (Courtesy Dr. Michael Melnick, Indianapolis, Ind.)

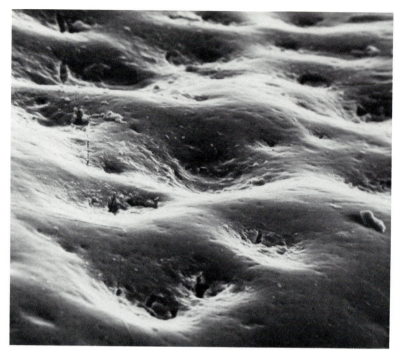

Fig. 9-7. Scanning electron microscope picture of surface enamel in TDO syndrome showing pits and deeper depressions. (Courtesy Dr. Michael Melnick, Indianapolis, Ind.)

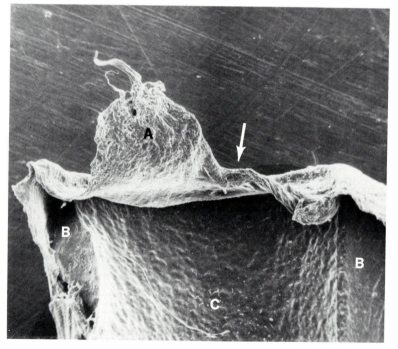

Fig. 9-8. A, SEM picture of fibrous membrane covering root of hemisected tooth in TDO syndrome. **B** and **C,** Lateral and posterior walls of split root canal. *Arrow* points to apical foramen covered by membrane. (Courtesy Dr. Michael Melnick, Indianapolis, Ind.)

thelial diaphragm. They also conclude that the primary defect in the TDO syndrome, which can account for the enamel, pulp chamber and root findings, is a failure in the inductive capability of the odontoblasts.

Other families with the TDO syndrome have been reported by Robinson and associates[29] and by Winter and co-workers.[33] In the latter paper, the authors noted the presence of a laminated, hyaline membrane–like structure on the surface of unerupted teeth, which Rushton[30] has described as the result of an apposition of a noncollagenous, cuticle-like material by the reduced enamel epithelium. Its relationship to the membrane described by Melnick and Shields is unknown.

Familial juvenile periodontosis (Gottlieb syndrome)

Periodontosis is defined by Baer[34] as a disease of the periodontium occurring in an otherwise healthy adolescent characterized by rapid loss of alveolar bone about several teeth of the permanent dentition (Fig. 9-9). Two major forms of periodontosis have been proposed, although only clinical evidence is available to support this dichotomy at present. In one form, molars and incisors are the only teeth affected, whereas the other form shows a more generalized involvement of most of the permanent and even the primary dentition (Fig. 9-10). A third form involving only the deciduous teeth has been proposed but has

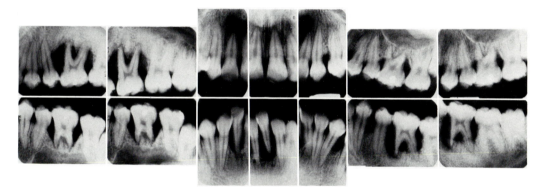

Fig. 9-9. Radiographs of juvenile periodontosis showing severe molar-incisor type bone loss. (Courtesy Dr. Michael Melnick, Indianapolis, Ind.)

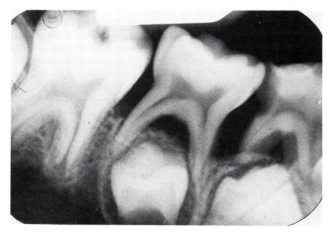

Fig. 9-10. Bone loss around deciduous molars of youngest sib of individual in Fig. 9-9. (Courtesy Dr. Michael Melnick, Indianapolis, Ind.)

little evidence to support its existence. Most authors believe the age of onset lies in the circumpubertal period,[34] but cases of earlier onset involving the deciduous teeth have been reported.[38-41]

The cause of juvenile periodontosis is obscure. Histopathological studies of affected teeth in the early stages of disease show degeneration of the periodontal fibers without presence of an obvious inflammatory process. In the next stage is seen a proliferation of the epithelial attachment with eventual separation of this attachment from the root. This leads to formation of deep periodontal pockets, and a secondary inflammatory process typically ensues. Since alveolar bone appears to form normally before the onset of the disease, and since all teeth erupt in their normal time and sequence, it has been presumed that these normal events preclude the possibility of a primary and/or congenital defect of the bone.[34] Measurements of the periodontal membrane in affected teeth have indicated a normal width with adequate attachment of the periodontal membrane fibers to the cementum.[35] Also, the cementum has been described as thin but not abnormal and showing areas of resorption. However, the loss of alveolar trabeculae in the absence of inflammation is often striking[35, 43] with vertical placement of collagen fibers observed in many of the affected areas. Collectively, these findings suggest that the collagenous fibers that comprise the periodontal apparatus somehow fail either to establish or to maintain their alveolar connection, and the net result is a resorption of alveolar bone such as is often noted in recent surgical extraction sites.

A large number of metabolic parameters have been evaluated in affected persons in a search for a more generalized systemic disease component. Elevated serum alkaline phosphatase levels have been noted by some authors,[41] but this has not been a confirmed finding. A disturbance in citric acid metabolism, which is intimately associated with bone formation and resorption, has been reported by Tsunemitsu and associates.[44] The significance of these observations is unknown.

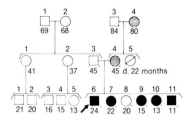

● Examined, affected, age 20   ⊖ Probably affected
○ Reported unaffected   ◒ Examined, unaffected

Fig. 9-11. Pedigree of family with juvenile periodontosis compatible with X-linked dominant inheritance. (Courtesy Dr. Michael Melnick, Indianapolis, Ind.)

Reisel[42] believes this disorder to be an early manifestation of a more generalized disorder, juvenile skeletal osteoporosis. The one thing that seems clear is that more detailed metabolic studies of affected families will be necessary before an etiological definition can be attempted. A primary defect of collagen seems likely.

Inheritance. There is a clear familial pattern to this trait. It has been reported in twins, parents and offspring, siblings, first cousins, uncles, and nephews.[36, 37, 40, 41] Melnick and co-workers[41] performed a segregation analysis of the families reported in the literature in which a total of nineteen sibships were available. A dominant trait with 78% penetrance is the model that best fits the data (Fig. 9-11). However, since a preponderance of female affecteds was noted (thirty-one females to thirteen males), this led the authors to conclude that it is an X-linked trait, a conclusion also supported by a failure to find a single example of male-to-male transmission of the trait in any of the pedigrees. Interestingly enough, in the report by Melnick and associates,[41] all the major types of periodontosis that have been suggested, that is, molar-incisor type, generalized type, and deciduous dentition–only type, have appeared in a *single* family, which strongly suggests these are not separate entities but are variations in the expression of a single gene (Figs. 9-9 and 9-10).

Hereditary multiple cementoses
(gigantiform cementoma)

This is a rare condition that is diagnosed by radiographic appearance of the jaws. Lesions appear as diffuse, radiopaque masses occurring in a periapical position. The same picture has been seen rather commonly in adult Negro females and has been suggested to be a chronic, diffuse sclerosing osteomyelitis.[48] Histological sections of such lesions show them to consist of dense, highly calcified, acellular cementum that is poorly vascularized. Whether this represents a response to chronic inflammation or is a distinct heritable entity is open to question. Agazzi and Belloni[45] observed lesions resembling those just described occurring in all four jaw quadrants of multiple persons in a single family. These lesions had an early age of onset but developed slowly. The hereditary pattern suggested to the authors was autosomal dominant. Possibly the report of Lyons[46] has described the same entity.

Schmidseder and co-workers[47] reported the occurrence of multiple odontogenic tumors in a father, his two sons, and a daughter. Histopathological study resulted in them being classified as ameloblastic fibromas with both ectodermal and mesodermal components to the tumors. This autosomal dominant trait seems to represent a different entity and is only mentioned in passing here.

Additional well-documented family studies will be necessary before it can be said that multiple cementoses is a primary hereditary trait of cementum.

SYNDROMES INVOLVING CEMENTUM
Diseases of hypophosphatasia

Hypophosphatasia is a disease complex involving the skeletal system in which bone fails to mineralize properly. The precise cause is unknown, but it appears to be intimately associated with the enzyme alkaline phosphatase and the ability of bone matrix to calcify. It is included in this chapter not only because of the accompanying cementum defect but also because premature loss of deciduous incisors appears to be an invariant clinical feature of this disorder. The following list is a classification of conditions that lead to premature loss of the primary teeth for the purposes of differential diagnosis:

Toxicities
  Mercury poisoning
  Radiation
Metabolic errors
  Scurvy
  Acatalasia
  Hypophosphatasia
  Juvenile diabetes
  Gaucher's disease
Malignancies
  Leukemia
  Neutropenia
  Histiocytoses X
  Wiskott-Aldrich syndrome
Dentally related
  Dentin dysplasia type I
  Juvenile periodontosis (Gottlieb syndrome)
  Papillon-Lefèvre syndrome

Clinical and biochemical features. There are several well-documented summaries of this disease in the literature[53, 54, 67] that demonstrate that the diagnosis may be made from combinations of the following findings: (1) low serum alkaline phosphatase levels, (2) characteristic histological and radiographic bone lesions, which closely resemble those seen in rickets, (3) increased amounts of phosphorylethanolamine (PEA) in both urine and plasma, and (4) premature loss of deciduous incisors.

Rathbun[68] is credited with naming this disorder and giving it a clinical description, although there are earlier literature reports probably of the same entity. Sobel and associates[71] noted that premature loss of deciduous incisors is an integral part of the syndrome and made the significant observation that serum from their affected patient did not inhibit the normal activity of the alkaline phosphatase bone enzyme. Rasmussen[67] and, later, Fraser and co-workers[56] established that PEA was excreted in increased amounts and probably represented an integral feature of the disease. The relationship of increased urinary PEA excretion to the biochemical pathogenesis of hypophosphatasia is still under debate today.

Fraser and Yendt[55] reported that the cartilage of rachitic rats would calcify in the serum from hypophosphatasia patients but that cartilage from the same persons would not calcify in sera taken from normal persons. Thus the basic defect is in the matrix itself and not in the circulating or interstitial fluids that bathe bone. The currently popular biochemical explanations of the disorder resolve into three modalities: (1) alkaline phosphatase acts as a liberator of inorganic phosphate in support of the de novo nucleation theory,[57] (2) alkaline phosphatase acts as an essential phosphate ion transferase, a modification of the Gutman theory,[58] and (3) alkaline phosphatase acts as a pyrophosphatase to remove bone crystal poisons.[63]

At least three clinical forms of the disease are recognizable, first delineated by Fraser[54]: (1) infantile type, characterized by severe skeletal disease at birth (neonatal?) and higher than 50% mortality, (2) childhood type, a self-limiting disease of moderate severity appearing after 6 months of age, and (3) adult type, characterized by an early adult–onset osteoporosis and bone fragility. In each case premature loss of deciduous incisors and decreased serum alkaline phosphatase activity are noted. The earlier the onset, the more severe will be the rachiticlike bone changes observed radiographically.

A fourth clinical type has been recognized that has a different genetic mode of inheritance from the above three types and thereby is clearly a different disorder.[51, 70] It is characterized by (1) low serum alkaline phosphatase activity, (2) premature loss of deciduous incisors, and (3) absence of bone lesions. This disorder is much milder than any of the foregoing types, and the serum enzyme levels, although definitely reduced, are not nearly so low. Note the absence of skeletal disease in this type.

Genetics. A simple autosomal recessive mode of inheritance has been repeatedly demonstrated for the various types of hypophosphatasia that show (1) markedly decreased serum alkaline phosphatase activity,

(2) increased urinary excretion of PEA, (3) rachitic-like bone diseases, and (4) premature loss of deciduous incisors. Thus the genetic data do not distinguish between the types classified by Fraser as infantile, childhood, and adult. This does not mean, however, that there is not heterogeneity within this grouping, and most workers believe there is more than a single type of hypophosphatasia. Indirect support for this comes from the observation that in some families, the heterozygous gene carriers (normal parents who have had at least two affected children) can be shown to have a serum alkaline phosphatase activity lower than normal but intermediate between that of the affected and the normal.[57] However, numerous other families have not shown this result. In addition, a similar problem has been observed when testing heterozygotes for PEA excretion.[59] A tentative interpretation of these results has been nonpenetrance, but it seems more likely that there is more than one disease entity in the entire group, all with a recessive mode of inheritance.[66]

Only one early report has suggested that there may be a dominantly inherited form of hypophosphatasia.[70] However, we have recently seen four families at Indiana University with this problem and are aware of one other.[64] Each of these latter families is unusual in that they have no bone disease, have a definite lowering of serum alkaline phosphatase (but not so severe as in the recessive form), and show premature incisor loss. In our families there has been no example of nonpenetrance, and the clinical picture is remarkably consistent (Fig. 9-12). The patient's initial disease complaint is typically made to a dentist who is asked to explain the child's early loss of deciduous incisors, usually before 3 years of age. The presence of two genetic forms of hypophosphatasia, one recessive and the other dominant, make it clear that at least two genes are involved in this disease complex, and the variability in clinical phenotype of the recessive form suggests additional genes, allelic or otherwise.

The problem of heterogeneity will not be resolved until a clear biochemical definition of the problem has been made. Along this line, it has been suggested that because serum alkaline phosphatase activity represents a mixture of isozymes from bone, liver, and intestine,[49] variation in the isozymes themselves may help to explain the spectrum of clinical disease.[69] We have noted and reported electrophoretic variation in one of our dominant families as a first approach to this idea.[51] A recent report by Hosenfeld and Hosenfeld[60] has also described isozyme electrophoretic variation in this disease complex.

Dental features. As noted above, skeletal disease is a cardinal feature of the autosomal recessive disorder, and in light of the ob-

servations of Fraser and Yendt,[55] who demonstrated that the calcification defect is inherent in the bone matrix, one might consider all type I collagenous matrices at potential risk. Such is probably true. Dentin appears grossly defective by histopathological studies with wide zones of predentin and large pulp chambers, reduced numbers of odontoblasts but with enlarged dentinal tubules, and abundant interglobular dentin.[50, 61]

Many authors have commented that premature exfoliation (Figs. 9-13 and 9-14) is due to a failure to form cementum on the shed teeth.[50, 52, 61, 65] Histopathological studies confirm that the degree of cementum aplasia is related to the severity of the overall disease itself.[52] Since the deciduous incisors are by far the most severely affected, it appears that whatever the biochemical defect is, it exerts its greatest influence prenatally and during the first year of life.[65] However, even the teeth of affected persons that are *not* exfoliated do not have normal amounts of cementum, thereby illustrating both the qualitative and quantitative disease aspects.[50] Furthermore, it has been shown that the collagen fibrils in the cementum may show no particular attachment to the periodontal ligament and may even be seen running parallel to the root surface.[62] Where cementum is absent, the periodontal ligament fibers approach but do not attach to the dentin. Histopathological studies of exfoliated teeth

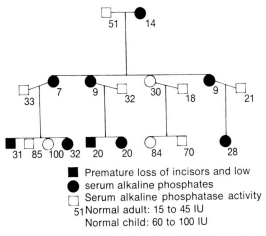

Fig. 9-12. Pedigree of family with autosomal dominant inheritance of mild form of hypophosphatasia.

- ■ Premature loss of incisors and low
- ● serum alkaline phosphates
- □ Serum alkaline phosphatase activity
- 51 Normal adult: 15 to 45 IU
-    Normal child: 60 to 100 IU

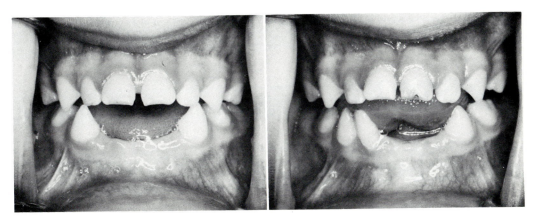

Fig. 9-13. Hypophosphatasia, childhood type with recessive inheritance. Twin sisters, age 3, showing premature incisor loss.

show accentuated incremental lines in post-natal dentin, indicating a severe metabolic disturbance in the first 6 months.[61]

In a general way, one may summarize this disorder by saying that the bone, dentin, and cementum defects are histologically similar and reflect a severe calcification dis-turbance. Thus the cementum (and dentin) defects are part of the overall metabolic disturbance in mineralized tissue and do not comprise a primary cementum defect. Nevertheless, the diagnostic importance of early deciduous incisor loss is great enough to justify separate consideration in this chapter.

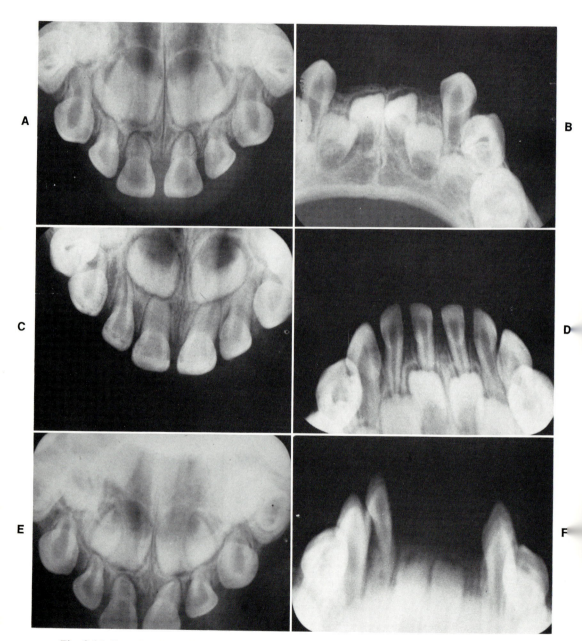

Fig. 9-14. Dental radiographs of twin sisters in Fig. 9-13. **A** and **B,** First twin; **E** and **F,** second twin; **C** and **D,** radiographs of normal child of same age for comparison.

Papillon-Lefèvre syndrome (palmar-plantar hyperkeratosis with premature periodontoclasia)

This syndrome has the principal clinical signs of (1) hyperkeratosis of the palms and soles (Fig. 9-15) and (2) premature destruction of the periodontal ligament of both deciduous and permanent teeth. The hyperkeratotic skin changes appear early in life, usually between the first and fourth years, and are closely associated in time with the appearance of obvious periodontal involvement of the deciduous teeth. In fact, several authors have positively correlated the severity of these two clinical signs.[73, 74] This is a generalized systemic disease as indicated by the fact that hyperkeratotic plaques also appear on eyelids, cheeks, labial commissures, and the extremities. Gorlin and associates[74] suggest that a third clinical sign, calcification of the dura, should be added to the two

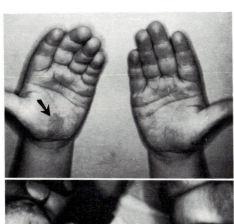
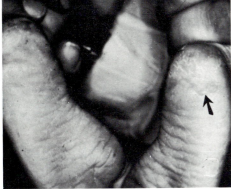

Fig. 9-15. Papillon-Lefèvre syndrome: hyperkeratosis of palms and soles. (From McDonald, R. E.: *Dentistry for the child and adolescent,* ed. 2, St. Louis, 1974, The C. V. Mosby Co.)

signs above, making this disease complex a triad.

Oral and clinical features. Development and eruption of the deciduous teeth occur in normal sequence and timing. Concurrent with the palmar-plantar signs of hyperkeratosis, the gingiva become red, boggy, and swollen and bleed easily. A severe, fetid oral odor develops, and at about the time that the last deciduous molar erupts, destruction of the periodontal ligament can be demonstrated. This is evidenced clinically by the formation of deep pockets and radiographically by the loss of alveolar bone (Fig. 9-16). The teeth become mobile and by 4 or 5 years of age are shed. Remarkably, once the teeth are lost, the intraoral inflammatory processes subside, and the gingiva return to normal. Once the permanent teeth erupt, the inflammatory process is repeated with the usual accompaniment of more severe gingival and alveolar bone changes. Again, with the ultimate loss of these teeth (usually by the sixteenth year) the oral conditions return to normal.

Although not falling into this timing sequence, third molars suffer the same fate on their eruption.[72] A detailed, long-range follow-up covering a 50-year span has been made by Carvel[72] on two affected sisters. This report also provides interesting comments on the dermatological manifestations and their medical management.

Histopathological examination of the gingiva shows the picture of periodontitis—chronic inflammation with destruction of the epithelial attachment and degeneration of the periodontal fibers.[73, 74] This appearance should be contrasted to that observed in the periodontium of patients with juvenile periodontosis (Gottlieb's syndrome), in which there is actually a connective tissue proliferation in the affected areas and the periodontal membrane is relatively normal in width and appearance.

Decalcified sections of teeth from persons affected with Papillon-Lefèvre syndrome have failed to reveal any obvious abnormalities of either the dentin or cementum.

Hereditary features. Detailed studies by

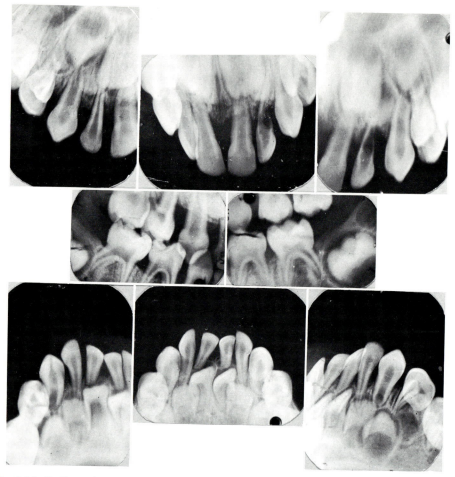

Fig. 9-16. Radiographs of child affected with Papillon-Lefèvre syndrome showing severe bone loss. (From McDonald, R. E.: Dentistry for the child and adolescent, ed. 2, St. Louis, 1974, The C. V. Mosby Co.)

numerous authors have documented the following features:

1. Both parents of affected children are clinically normal themselves.

2. Where there is more than one affected in a single sibship, all affecteds show the same clinical signs and symptoms and disease pathogenesis.

3. The parental consanguinity rate in this disorder is much higher than that observed in the general population.

Collectively, these features support autosomal recessive inheritance. Gorlin and co-workers[74] have attempted to estimate the gene frequency from the parental consan-guinity rate and calculate it to be somewhere between 0.001 and 0.002. This would make the heterozygous (gene carrier) frequency in the general population about three per 1000 persons. This result indicates that the chance of a homozygous affected person having an affected child himself is unlikely, since only three out of every possible 1000 mates will, by chance, be a heterozygous gene carrier. The increased consanguinity rate observed here also emphasizes the genetic principle of increasing homozygosity at a given genetic locus by inbreeding.

There is little to indicate the nature of the fundamental defect leading to this clinical disease. Since the mode of inheritance is clearly recessive, an enzyme defect is suggested, but at this point it is difficult to reconcile the apparently different tissue effects—hyperkeratosis of the skin and oral periodontal destruction. If calcification of the dura proves to be an important feature of this disorder, a basic defect in collagen is suspect, and the skin defect then may be the result of a faulty dermis-epidermis interaction.

Epidermolysis bullosa dystrophica

Evidence has been slowly accumulating over the past 10 to 12 years that this disease is actually a disorder of mesodermal rather than ectodermal tissue. In fact, Cooke[76] has suggested that the term *dermolysis bullosa dystrophica* is more appropriate.

Clinical features. The primary disease process affects skin and is characterized by the development of vesicles and bullae, occasionally involving mucous membranes as well. These lesions appear both spontaneously and in response to minor trauma. Also noted are defects in the cementum and periodontal ligament. It should be emphasized that there are several different diseases in the category of epidermolysis bullosa and that the dystrophic type is only one of these. To further complicate matters, at least two dystrophic types exist, based on their mode of inheritance. The dominantly inherited type, in which lesions appear at *birth* or soon after, is often relatively mild in expression, showing only thin, atrophic skin scars and sometimes involving the mucous membranes and nails. The recessively inherited form is typically more severe and destructive with mucosal and even corneal and conjunctival involvement.

The molecular defect is unknown, but presumably, a defect in collagen metabolism is involved. Bauer and associates[75] have demonstrated elevated collagenase enzyme activity in both the dystrophic skin lesions and the unaffected skin of persons who have the recessive type.

Dental features. Because of the fact that almost all patients with this disorder receive corticosteroids for treatment of their skin lesions, any description of dental or oral conditions for these patients is subject to qualification considering this treatment. Nevertheless, teeth removed from affected persons has revealed that the acellular cementum shows a fibrous character.[77] Cellular cementum appears to have an increased thickness, a finding most prominent on teeth that normally show little or no cellular cementum, such as incisors. There is also poor calcification of the cementum that is formed. These same findings have been made both in patients who were and who were not receiving corticosteroids, with those in the former category showing the milder defects. Hitchin[77] also noted that there is rapid destruction of the periodontal ligament collagen fibers with a resultant compensating overproduction of the more cellular type of cementum. This cementum does not calcify properly.

HERITABLE DISORDERS INVOLVING TOOTH ERUPTION

Elsewhere in this chapter have been listed those diseases involving premature exfoliation of teeth. Premature tooth loss can be due to defective cementogenesis (hypophosphatasia) or other periodontium defects (juvenile periodontosis, Papillon-Lefèvre syndrome). On the other hand, failure to erupt represents a complex and different kind of developmental anomaly for teeth. Consistent with previously described heritable traits, this problem may occur as an isolated defect (both sporadic and familial), or it may be a part of heritable syndromes. The following section discusses examples in both categories.

Eruption failure as a heritable trait

Markedly delayed eruption or even complete failure of permanent teeth to erupt has been noted by many authors. Discounting an ectopic position of the tooth germ as an explanation for this problem (for example, impaction), eruption failure has been most commonly noted for those succedaneous permanent teeth in which the deciduous tooth has not been shed. The clinical description often given for this clinical situation is a *submerged tooth.* Thus this problem could better be considered a primary failure of exfoliation of the deciduous tooth.

Of all deciduous molars, the submerged condition affects the mandibular second molar most often and the maxillary first molar least often. The prevalence has been estimated at 2.5% of children.[79] Darling and Levers[78] have reviewed the subject thoroughly and suggest that the apparent submersion is due to ankylosis between the deciduous molar root and surrounding alveolar bone, a demonstrable condition in 18% of such affected teeth. Some authors have suggested congenital absence of the permanent successor as an explanation for failure to shed the deciduous molar. However, only 20% of submerged teeth examined by Darling and Levers fitted that category. Most importantly, Via[82] has studied families with submerged teeth. Since this is a temporally related phenomenon, identification of the phenotype in different generations is almost impossible. However, Via reported that the incidence of submerged deciduous teeth in sibs of propositi with this phenotype was about 44%, or more than twenty times higher than he observed in sibs in the general population. Thus the submerged tooth appears to have a strong heritable component, although at this stage a mode of inheritance cannot be specified. The reason for failure to erupt, as suggested by Darling and Levers, is ankylosis of the deciduous tooth created by bone deposition in the dentin defects created during the normal process of root resorption. The genetic control for this aberrant process remains obscure.

Since these submerged teeth actually have already erupted, it is inaccurate to describe this condition as a failure of eruption, although this description of submerged teeth is in wide usage.

Bony ankylosis may also be a cause for failure of the permanent teeth to erupt. Shokeir[81] has described a heritable phenotype characterized by a failure of all of the permanent teeth to erupt, apparently due to bony ankylosis. No other systemic defect in affecteds has been noted. The condition was observed in a father and two of his five off-

spring, one of whom was an affected male, making autosomal dominant inheritance likely. In each person, the deciduous teeth were delayed in being shed, and the permanent teeth, with or without predecessors, remained unerupted. Interestingly, multiple dentigerous cysts were noted in one of these affected children. No histopathological examination of the unerupted teeth was reported, so ankylosis remains a speculative explanation for their failure to erupt. This family should probably not be considered as having the same disorder as that reported by Via on heritability of the submerged tooth.

Eruption failure in syndromes

Cleidocranial dysplasia. Failure of tooth eruption has also been reported as part of heritable syndromes, most notably in cleidocranial dysplasia and cryptodontic brachymetacarpalia, and to a lesser degree in the diseases incontinentia pigmenti and focal dermal hypoplasia. Only the first two examples will be discussed here.

As a result of the Paris Conference held in 1969 on nomenclature of bone disorders,[80] this disorder was reclassified from a dysostosis to a dysplasia, hence the name usage employed here. A thorough discussion of cleidocranial dysplasia is found elsewhere in this volume. The following paragraphs are limited to one aspect of this autosomal dominant trait, the failure in eruption of the permanent succedaneous teeth and delayed eruption of the remaining permanent ones (first to third molars).

One of the cardinal clinical signs of cleidocranial dysplasia is the eruption failure of succedaneous permanent teeth (Fig. 9-17). Many reports allude to the presence of multiple supernumerary teeth in the jaws of affected persons, but it now seems clear that at least some of these observations were related to the presence of normal but unerupted teeth. However, it has been confirmed that supernumerary teeth as well as odontomas occur with increased frequency in affecteds. The reason for the eruptive failure remains unclear. Smith and Sydney[88] have made detailed histological observations on the teeth

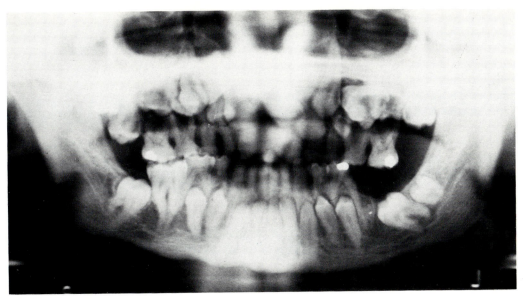

Fig. 9-17. Cleidocranial dysplasia in 25-year-old man. Note marked failure of eruption of permanent teeth.

of a patient with cleidocranial dysplasia and have observed an almost complete lack of cellular cementum on both the erupted deciduous and unerupted permanent teeth. They concluded from this that cellular cementum formation must not be the only essential factor involved in normal tooth eruption and that the dental space acquired by the eruption process must then be maintained by apposition of alveolar bone.

Formicola and co-workers[85] have shown with the rat molar that acellular cementum covers the coronal two thirds of the root and is formed before eruption. This cementum they designated *preeruptive*. On the other hand, cellular cementum covers the apical third of the root and has cementoblasts trapped in it. The authors designate this latter type as *posteruptive* cementum, since it is only seen in teeth that are completing or have completed the eruptive process. The essential difference between these two types appears to be their rate of formation, since in preeruptive cementum the formation rate is slow. By contrast, posteruptive cementum forms rapidly, traps cementoblasts, and thereby produces a tissue more closely resembling the Haversian system seen in bone. From this

one would conclude that preeruptive cementum formation in patients with cleidocranial dysplasia is satisfactory but that posteruptive or cellular cementum formation is defective, which accounts for the poor eruptive performance of these teeth.

It has been suggested by several authors[83, 87] that surgical exposure of these permanent teeth provides little or no encouragement to eruption. This has not been our experience at Indiana University. Incisors and premolars have been surgically uncovered in a series of children with cleidocranial dysplasia whose root formation was less than half completed. A slow but steady eruption was observed provided that the surgical area was kept open and not allowed to scarify.[86] This would suggest that the eruptive force is present in these teeth but greatly diminished and that even a slight obstacle to eruption may completely prevent eruption. Support for this idea comes from the studies of di Biase,[84] who has described the effects of surgical exposure on teeth that are failing to erupt. The patients with these teeth were orthodontic cases and did not have any known syndromes. He noted that in teeth that are not erupting there is a superficial outer layer of epithelium and connective tissue that is readily incised. Below this is a fleshy, fibrous layer of dense connective tissue that is tough and resistant to surgery, which appears to be unique to the tooth that fails to erupt. On the basis of histochemical and histopathological findings, di Biase concluded that eruption failure is attributable to a lack of union between the dental follicle and the oral mucosa with subsequent fibrous tissue formation in this hiatus acting as a barrier to eruption.

It is most interesting to note that the failure of eruption noted by Kimura and Nakata (p. 246) on two patients with a heritable enamel and dentin dysplasia was also characterized by the presence of a thick fibrous band between the dental follicle and the oral epithelium (Fig. 8-20).

Cryptodontic brachymetacarpalia. In 1971, Gorlin and associates[90] reported a family of seven affecteds in four generations who had shortened metacarpals and metatarsals, impacted teeth, and short terminal thumbs and clavicles. Affected individuals have a marked similarity to patients with Albright's hereditary osteodystrophy or pseudohypoparathyroidism, which is an X-linked trait. The authors believed that the latter diagnosis was ruled out by male-to-male transmission of the trait in their family. In addition, their patients had normal somatic and mental growth and did not have either ectopic calcification or biochemical abnormalities in serum calcium, phosphorus, and responsiveness to parathyroid hormone. They also point to other reported instances of PHP in which male-to-male transmission occurred and suggest that these cases may represent the cryptodontic brachymetacarpalia syndrome instead.[89, 91, 92] However, radiographic documentation of the unerupted teeth for these other cases is not available. Furthermore, no histopathology of the unerupted teeth has been studied, so a cause for the eruption failure remains speculative.

These heritable disorders affecting tooth eruption and exfoliation may ultimately be most helpful in providing answers to the question of why and how teeth erupt.

REFERENCES
Cementum and periodontal ligament

1. Bauer, W. H.: Effect of periapical processes of deciduous teeth on the buds of permanent teeth, Am. J. Orthod. Oral Surg. **32**:232-241, 1946.
2. Butler, W. T., Birkedal-Hansen, H., and Taylor, R. E.: Proteins of the periodontium: the chain structure of the collagens of bovine cementum and periodontal ligament. In Slavkin, H. C., and Greulich, R. C., editors: Extracellular matrix influences on gene expression, New York, 1975, Academic Press, Inc., pp. 371-377.
3. Giansanti, J. S.: The pattern and width of the collagen bundles in bone and cementum, Oral Surg. **30**:508-514, 1970.
4. Guis, M. B., and Sloatweg, R. N.: A biochemical study of collagen in the periodontal ligament from erupting and non-erupting bovine incisors, Arch. Oral Biol. **18**:253-263, 1973.
5. Levine, P. T., Glimcher, M. J., and Bonar, L. C.: Collagenous layer covering the crown enamel of unerupted permanent teeth, Science **146**:1676, 1964.
6. Listgarten, M. A.: A light and electron microscopic study of coronal cementogenesis, Arch. Oral Biol. **13**:93-114, 1968.
7. Rodriguez, M. S., and Wilderman, M. N.: Amino acid composition of the cementum matrix from human molar teeth, J. Periodontol. **43**:438-440, 1972.

Taurodontism

8. Blumberg, J. E., Hylander, W. L., and Goepp, R. A.: Taurodontism: a biometric study, Am. J. Phys. Anthropol. **34**:243-256, 1971.
9. Fischer, H.: Die "primatischen" Molaren von Krapina/Kroatien im Lichte rezenter Funde, Dtsch. Zahnaertzl. Z. **16**:8-15, 1961.
10. Gamer, S., and Zusman, S.: Taurodontism in a 15 year old boy and his mother, J. South. Calif. Dent. Assoc. **35**:441-444, 1967.
11. Goldstein, E., and Gottlieb, M. A.: Taurodontism: familial tendencies demonstrated in eleven of fourteen case reports, Oral Surg. **36**:131-144, 1973.
12. Hamner, J. E., Witkop, C. J., and Metro, P. S.: Taurodontism, report of a case, Oral Surg. **18**:409-418, 1964.
13. Kovacs, I.: Contribution to the ontogenetic morphology of roots of human teeth, J. Dent. Res. (Supp.) **46**:865-874, 1967.
14. Lehtinen, R.: Taurodontism: a report of a case with familiar occurrence, Suom. Hammaslaak. Toim. **67**:71-73, 1971.
15. Lysell, L.: Taurodontism: a case report and a summary of the literature, Odontol. Revy **13**:158-174, 1962.

16. Mena, C. A.: Taurodontism, Oral Surg. **32:** 812-823, 1971.

17. Shaw, J. C. M.: Taurodont teeth in South African races, J. Anat. **62:**476-498, 1928.

18. Stoy, P. J.: Taurodontism associated with other dental abnormalities, Dent. Pract. Dent. Rec. **10:**202-205, 1960.

19. Witkop, C. J.: Manifestation of genetic diseases in the human pulp, Oral Surg. **32:**278-316, 1971.

Taurodontism in syndromes

20. Ackerman, J. L., Ackerman, L. L., and Ackerman, A. B.: Taurodont, pyramidal and fused roots associated with other anomalies in a kindred, Am. J. Phys. Anthropol. **38:**681-694, 1973.

21. Crawford, J. L.: Concomitant taurodontism and amelogenesis imperfecta in the American Caucasian, J. Dent. Child. **37:**171-175, 1970.

22. Jorgenson, R. J., and Warson, R. W.: Dental abnormalities in the tricho-dento-osseous syndrome, Oral Surg. **36:**693-700, 1973.

23. Kallay, J.: A radiographic study of the Neanderthal teeth from Krapina, Croatia. In Brothwell, D. R., editor: Dental anthropology, New York, 1963, The Macmillan Co.

24. Keeler, C.: Taurodont molars and shovel incisors in Klinefelter's syndrome, J. Hered. **64:** 234-236, 1973.

25. Lichtenstein, J., Warson, R., Jorgenson, R., Dorst, J. O., and McKusick, V. M.: The tricho-dento-osseous (TDO) syndrome, Am. J. Hum. Genet. **24:**569-582, 1972.

26. Melnick, M., and Shields, E.: Etiopathogenesis of the TDO syndrome based upon scanning electron microscopy studies. (In press.)

27. Moller, K. T., Gorlin, R. J., and Wedge, B.: Oligodontia, taurodontia and sparse hair growth—a syndrome, J. Speech Hear. Res. **38:** 268-271, 1973.

28. Robbins, I. M., and Keene, H. J.: Multiple morphologic dental anomalies, Oral Surg. **17:** 683-690, 1964.

29. Robinson, G. C., Miller, J., and Worth, H. M.: Hereditary enamel hypoplasia: its association with characteristic hair structure, Pediatrics **37:**498-502, 1966.

30. Rushton, M. A.: The surface of the enamel in hereditary enamel hypocalcification, Br. Dent. J. **112:**24-27, 1962.

31. Stenvik, A., Zachrisson, B., and Svatun, B.: Taurodontism and concomitant hypodontia in siblings, Oral Surg. **33:**841-845, 1972.

32. Stewart, R. E.: Taurodontism in X-chromosome aneuploid syndromes, Clin. Genet. **6:**341-344, 1974.

33. Winter, G. B., Lee, K. W., and Johnson, N. W.: Hereditary amelogenesis imperfecta: a rare autosomal dominant trait, Br. Dent. J. **127:**157-164, 1970.

Juvenile periodontosis (Gottlieb syndrome)

34. Baer, P. N.: The case for periodontosis as a clinical entity, J. Periodontol. **42:**516-520, 1971.

35. Baer, P. N., Stanley, H. R., Brown, K., Smith, L., Gamble, J., and Swerdlow, H.: Advanced periodontal disease in an adolescent (periodontosis), J. Periodontol. **34:**533-539, 1963.

36. Benjamin, S. D., and Baer, P. N.: Familial patterns of advanced bone loss in adolescence (periodontosis), Periodontics **5:**82-88, 1967.

37. Butler, J. H.: A familial pattern of juvenile periodontosis (periodontosis). J. Periodontol. **40:**115-118, 1969.

38. Fourel, J.: Periodontosis: a periodontal syndrome, J. Periodontol. **43:**240-255, 1972.

39. Fourel, J.: Periodontosis, juvenile periodontosis or Gottlieb syndrome? Report of 4 cases, J. Periodontol. **45:**234-237, 1974.

40. Jorgenson, R. J., Levin, L. S., Hutcherson, S. T., and Salinas, C. F.: Periodontosis in sibs, Oral Surg. **39:**396-402, 1975.

41. Melnick, M., Shields, E. D., and Bixler, D.: Periodontosis: a phenotypic and genetic analysis, Oral Surg. **41:**32-43, 1976.

42. Reisel, J. H.: Clinical osteoporosis and periodontal disease, Ned. Tijdschr. Tandheelkd. **78:**132-135, 1971.

43. Shafer, W. G., Hine, M. K., and Levy, B.: A textbook of oral pathology, ed. 3, Philadelphia, 1974, W. B. Saunders Co., pp. 747-748.

44. Tsunemitsu, A., Honjo, K., Kani, M., and Matsumura, T.: Citric acid metabolism in periodontosis, Arch. Oral Biol. **9:**83-86, 1964.

Hereditary multiple cementoses

45. Agazzi, C., and Belloni, L.: Gli odontomi duri dei mascellari, Arch. Ital. Otol. (Supp. 16) **64:**3-102, 1953.

46. Lyons, D. C.: Multiple osteomas of the maxilla and mandible, Oral Surg. **8:**738-742, 1955.

47. Schmidseder, R., and Hausamen, J.-E.: Multiple odontogenic tumors and other anomalies, Oral Surg. **39:**249-258, 1975.

48. Shafer, W. G., Hine, M. K., and Levy, B.: Textbook of oral pathology, ed. 3, Philadelphia, 1974, W. B. Saunders Co.

Hypophosphatasia

49. Aminoff, D., Austrins, M., and Zolfaghari, S. P.: Plasma alkaline phosphatase isozymes: isolation and characterization of isozymes, Biochim. Biophys. Acta **242:**108, 1971.

50. Beumer, J., Trowbridge, H. O., Silverman, S., and Eisenberg, E.: Childhood hypophospha-

tasia and the premature loss of teeth, Oral Surg. 35:631-640, 1973.

51. Bixler, D., Poland, C. P., Brandt, I. K., and Nicholas, N. J.: Autosomal dominant hypophosphatasia without skeletal disease, American Society of Human Genetics 26th Annual Meeting, Portland, Ore., 1974.

52. Bruckner, R. J., Rickles, N. H., and Porter, D. R.: Hypophosphatasia with premature shedding of teeth and aplasia of cementum, Oral Surg. 15:1351-1359, 1962.

53. Currarino, G., Neuhauser, E., Reyersback, G., and Sobel, E.: Hypophosphatasia, Am. J. Roentgenol. 78:392, 1957.

54. Fraser, D.: Hypophosphatasia, Am. J. Med. 22:730, 1957.

55. Fraser, D., and Yendt, E. R.: Metabolic abnormalities in hypophosphatasia, Am. J. Dis. Child. 90:552, 1955.

56. Fraser, D., Yendt, E. R., and Christie, F. H.: Metabolic abnormalities in hypophosphatasia, Lancet 1:286, 1955.

57. Glimcher, M. J., and Krane, S. M.: Studies of the interactions of collagen and phosphate. I. The nature of inorganic orghophosphate binding. In Lacroix, P., and Budy, A. M., editors: Radioisotopes and bone, Oxford, England, 1962, Blackwell Scientific Publications, Ltd., pp. 393-418.

58. Gutman, A. B., and Yu, R. F.: Concept of role of enzymes in endochondral calcification, Re. Conf. Metabolic Interrelations, vol. 2, New York, 1950, Josiah Macy Foundation, p. 167.

59. Harris, H., and Robson, E. B.: A genetical study of ethanolamine phosphate excretion in hypophosphatasia, Hum. Genet. 23:421, 1958.

60. Hosenfeld, D., and Hosenfeld, A.: Qualitative and quantitative examinations of the isoenzymes of serum alkaline phosphatase in hypophosphatasia, Klin. Paediatr. 185:437-443, 1973.

61. Kjellman, M., Oldfelt, V., Nordenram, A., and Olow-Nordenram, M.: Five cases of hypophosphatasia with dental findings, Int. J. Oral Surg. 2:152-158, 1973.

62. Listgarten, M. A., and Houpt, M.: Ultrastructural features of the root surface of deciduous teeth in patients with hypophosphatasia, J. Periodont. Res. (Supp.) 4:34-35, 1969.

63. Neuman, W. F., diStefano, V., and Mulryan, B. J.: Surface chemistry of bone. III. Observations on role of phosphatase, J. Biol. Chem. 193:227, 1951.

64. Opitz, J.: Personal communication, 1971.

65. Pimstone, B., Eisenberg, E., and Silverman, S.: Hypophosphatasia: genetic and dental studies, Ann. Intern. Med. 65:722-729, 1966.

66. Poland, C. P., Eversole, L. R., Bixler, D., and

Christian, J. C.: Histochemical observations of hypophosphatasia, J. Dent. Res. 51:333-338, 1972.

67. Rasmussen, K.: Phosphorylethanolamine and hypophosphatasia, Dan. Med. Bull. 15:1, 1968.

68. Rathbun, J. C.: Hypophosphatasia, a new developmental anomaly, Am. J. Dis. Child. 75:822, 1948.

69. Scriver, C. R., and Cameron, D.: Pseudohypophosphatasia, N. Engl. J. Med. 281:604, 1969.

70. Silverman, J. L.: Apparent dominant inheritance of hypophosphatasia, Arch. Intern. Med. 110:191-198, 1962.

71. Sobel, E. H., Clark, L. C., Fox, R. P., and Robinow, M.: Rickets, deficiency of "alkaline" phosphatase activity and premature loss of teeth in childhood, Pediatrics 11:309, 1953.

Papillon-Lefèvre syndrome

72. Carvel, R. I.: Palmar-plantar hyperkeratosis and premature periodontal destruction, J. Oral Med. 24:73-82, 1969.

73. Galanter, D. R., and Bradford, S.: Hyperkeratosis palmoplantaris and periodontosis: the Papillon-Lefèvre syndrome, J. Periodontol. 40:40-47, 1969.

74. Gorlin, R. J., Sedano, H., and Anderson, V. E.: The syndrome of palmar-plantar hyperkeratosis and premature periodontal destruction of the teeth, J. Pediatr. 65:895-908, 1964.

Epidermolysis bullosa dystrophica

75. Bauer, E. A., Gedde-Dahl, T., and Eisen, A. Z.: Rose of human skin collagenase in dystrophic epidermolysis bullosa, Clin. Res. 22:326A, 1974.

76. Cooke, B. E. D.: The oral manifestation of bullous lesions, J. R. Coll. Surg. Edinb. 15:129-136, 1970.

77. Hitchin, A. D.: The defects of cementum in epidermolysis bullosa dystrophica, Br. Dent. J. 135:437-442, 1973.

Heritable disorders involving tooth eruption

78. Darling, A. I., and Levers, B. G. H.: Submerged human deciduous molars and ankylosis, Arch. Oral Biol. 18:1021-1040, 1973.

79. Dixon, D. A.: Observations on submerging deciduous molars, Dent. Pract. Dent. Rec. 13:306-316, 1963.

80. McKusick, V. M., and Scott, C. I.: A nomenclature for constitutional disorders of bone, J. Bone Joint Surg. 53A:978-986, 1971.

81. Shokeir, M. H.: Complete failure of eruption of all permanent teeth: an autosomal dominant disorder, Clin. Genet. 5:322-326, 1974.

82. Via, W. F.: Submerged deciduous molars: familial tendencies, J. Am. Dent. Assoc. 69:127-129, 1964.

Cleidocranial dysplasia

83. Archer, W. H., and Henderson, S. C.: Cleidocranial dysostosis, Oral Surg. **4:**1201-1213, 1951.
84. di Biase, D. D.: Mucous membrane and delayed eruption, Dent. Pract. **21:**241-249, 1971.
85. Formicola, A. G., Krampf, J. I., and Witte, E. T.: Cementogenesis in developing rat molars, J. Periodontol. **42:**766-773, 1971.
86. Hutton, C. E., Garner, L., and Bixler, D.: Surgically promoted eruption of permanent teeth in children with cleidocranial dysplasia (personal communication), 1976.
87. Kalliala, E., and Taskinen, P. J.: Cleidocranial dysostosis, Oral Surg. **15:**808-822, 1962.
88. Smith, N. H., and Sydney, N. S. W.: A histologic study of cementum in a case of cleidocranial dysostosis, Oral Surg. **25:**470-478, 1968.

Cryptodontic brachymetacarpalia

89. Geominne, L.: Albright's hereditary polyosteochondrodystrophy (pseudopseudohypoparathyroidism with diabetes, hypertension, arteritis and polyarthrosis), Acta Genet. Med. (Roma) **14:**226-281, 1965.
90. Gorlin, R. J., Sedano, H. O., and Vickers, R. A.: Cryptodontic brachymetacarpalia. In Bergsma, D., editor: Birth defects original article series. XI. Orofacial structures, vol. 7, no. 7, Baltimore, 1971, The Williams & Wilkins Co. for the National Foundation–March of Dimes.
91. Hermans, P. E., Gorman, C. A., Martin, W. J., and Kelly, P. J.: Pseudopseudohypoparathyroidism (Albright's hereditary osteodystrophy): a family study, Mayo Clin. Proc. **39:**81-91, 1964.
92. Minozzi, M. I., Faggiano, M., Blanco, A., Bizzi, G., and Calizianni, A.: On a case of Albright's hereditary osteodystrophy, of the normocalcemic type, with documented male-to-male transmission, Folia Endocrinol. (Roma) **16:**168-188, 1963.

10

Genetic disorders affecting the dental pulp

DAVID G. GARDNER

The dental pulp, the layman's "nerve of the tooth," develops from a condensation of mesenchymal tissue called the dental papilla. It is, of course, more than a nerve, being composed of loose connective tissue with associated blood vessels and both myelinated and nonmyelinated nerve fibers. The nerve fibers are almost entirely sensory and are part of the peripheral nervous system. There are also present a few autonomic nerve fibers concerned with vasoconstriction and dilatation but no motor fibers. The dental pulp provides sensation to the tooth and the means by which tissue fluid and metabolites reach the odontoblasts and their product, dentin. The success of modern root canal therapy is ample proof that the tooth can function well without its pulp; however, the tooth obviously loses its sensation, the ability to form further dentin, and the dentin itself becomes drier and relatively brittle.

Dentin also develops from the dental papilla, and its cells, the odontoblasts, lie at the periphery of the pulp. They can, in fact, be considered part of it. It follows that dentin and dental pulp are so intimately related that they should be considered one anatomical unit, namely the dentinopulpal complex.

From this discussion one can justifiably conclude that there are probably no disorders that affect the dental pulp exclusively and that all disorders affecting dentin must also indirectly affect the dental pulp. If a disturbance in dentinogenesis results in more dentin than normal being formed, then the pulp is correspondingly decreased in volume. Dentinogenesis imperfecta and dentin dysplasia are examples of such conditions. On the other hand, the dental pulp is correspondingly larger in those conditions in which an abnormally small amount of dentin is formed. This situation is found, for example, in vitamin D–resistant rickets and in taurodontism. Again, some diseases, such as hypophosphatasia and dentin dysplasia, are characterized by defects in the dentin that result in bacteria invading the dental pulp with subsequent pulpitis and pulpal necrosis.

Despite the obvious interrelationship of dental pulp and dentin, there are various genetic systemic disorders that might be expected to affect the dental pulp, rather than dentin. They include those inherited conditions which affect peripheral sensory nerves, connective tissue, or small blood vessels, as well as those genetic disorders characterized by the accumulation of various materials throughout the tissues of the body.

HISTORICAL NOTES AND LITERATURE REVIEW

The little that is known about the effect of inherited systemic disorders on the dental

I am grateful to Drs. M. D. Haust and J. C. E. Kaufmann for their helpful suggestions during the preparation of this chapter. This work was supported in part by grant MA-3613 of the Medical Research Council of Canada.

pulp has been reviewed recently by Witkop.[84] There are a number of reasons for this lack of information.

1. Most of the conditions are rare.

2. The dental pulp is not examined at autopsy by medical pathologists and seldom by oral pathologists.

3. The dental pulp is rarely biopsied, although this procedure has been advocated in two neurological disorders, metachromatic leukodystrophy[24, 26] and Fabry's disease,[19] and might conceivably be useful in other disorders.

4. Even when teeth are extracted from patients with various inherited disorders, the dental pulps are not generally examined pathologically.

5. The removal of dental pulps from pa-

Table 10-1. Primary defects of dentin*

Disorder	Mode of inheritance	Effects on dental pulp
Dentinogenesis imperfecta associated with osteogenesis imperfecta (DI type I)	Autosomal dominant	Expressivity varied; characteristically pulp chambers and canals almost totally obliterated; however, some teeth may exhibit normal pulp chambers and canals; deciduous teeth more severely affected than permanent teeth; permanent incisors and first molars more severely affected than teeth that erupt later
Hereditary opalescent dentin (DI type II) (not associated with osteogenesis imperfecta)	Autosomal dominant	Similar to DI type I; pulp chambers and canals almost totally obliterated; normal-sized pulp chambers sometimes seen, usually in deciduous dentition, but less commonly than in DI type I; occasionally shell teeth are found in deciduous teeth; deciduous teeth more severely affected than permanent teeth; permanent incisors and first molars more severely affected than teeth that erupt later
Dentinogenesis imperfecta type III (brandywine type)	Autosomal dominant	Considerable variation, ranging from normal to severely affected teeth similar to those seen in DI types I and II to shell teeth; multiple pulp exposures observed in deciduous teeth
Dentin dysplasia type I (radicular dentin dysplasia)	Probably autosomal dominant	Pulp chambers are usually obliterated in deciduous dentition and appear as crescent-shaped remnants in permanent teeth; root canals usually absent; pulp chambers obliterated by numerous, often large, denticles that fuse with primary dentin, resulting in "stream flowing around boulders" effect
Dentin dysplasia type II (coronal dentin dysplasia) (pulpal dysplasia)	Autosomal dominant	Pulp chambers of all teeth in both dentitions are large, bulbous, or flame-shaped and contain numerous pulp stones; in older affecteds, chamber becomes reduced and may become obliterated; pulp stones generally do not fuse with primary dentin; pulp horns often extend to dentinoenamel junction
Atypical dentin dysplasia with characteristic facies (fibrous dysplasia of dentin)	Autosomal dominant	Complete obliteration of pulp chambers and canals by atypical fibrotic dentin

*See references by Shields and associates[67] and Witkop.[84, 85]

tients with inherited systemic disorders cannot be justified for purely research reasons. The procedure can be justified if it may contribute to the diagnosis of the patient's condition.

GENETIC DISORDERS AFFECTING THE DENTIN AND THEREFORE THE DENTAL PULP

The primary defects of dentin also affect the dental pulp because of the close relationship between the two tissues. These conditions have been discussed in detail in Chapter 8. Their effect on the dental pulp is summarized in Table 10-1.

Certain types of anomalous teeth with genetic overtones, such as dens invaginatus

(dens in dente), dens evaginatus, and taurodontism have also been described in Chapter 8. In the first of these disorders the morphology of the pulp chamber and canal is markedly altered by the invagination, the enamel of which is often defective. The result is that pulpal infection is common in these teeth. This is also true of dens evaginatus. In this condition a narrow strand of dental pulp extends into the occlusal tubercle, which tends to fracture off during mastication, resulting in exposure of the pulpal extension and subsequent pulpal infection. In the third disorder, taurodontism, the pulp chamber is abnormally large, its floor being positioned considerably further toward the apex than normal. Furthermore, the normal constriction of

Table 10-2. Systemic disorders affecting dentin and therefore the dental pulp

Disorder	Mode of inheritance	Effects on dental pulp
Hypophosphatasia	Autosomal recessive	Delayed closure of apices; large pulp chambers; low alkaline phosphatase activity in pulp tissue
Hypophosphatemic vitamin D–resistant rickets	X-linked recessive	Unusually large pulp chambers; pulp horns extend to dentinoenamel junction; enamel over these pulp horns is often hypoplastic, resulting in pulpitis and abscessed teeth
de Toni-Debré-Fanconi syndrome[84] (osteomalacia, renal glycosuria, aminoaciduria, and hyperphosphaturia)	Sometimes acquired. Other cases are probably autosomal recessive	Similar to those in hypophosphatemic vitamin D–resistant rickets
Vitamin D–dependent rickets[85]	Autosomal recessive	Similar to those in hypophosphatemic vitamin D–resistant rickets
Progeria[3, 25]	Autosomal recessive	Abnormally large amounts of irregular dentin seen for age of child; increased quantities of collagen in pulps of some teeth
Otodental syndrome (globodontia)[28, 86]	Possibly autosomal dominant	Large pulp chambers, which may appear duplicated
Trichodentoosseous syndrome[61, 39]	Autosomal dominant	Multiple taurodont teeth (which see); sometimes high pulp horns present that extend to the dentinoenamel junction; rapid attrition through thin enamel may result in pulpal exposure and necrosis[85]
Ehlers-Danlos syndrome[7]	Autosomal dominant	Similar changes to those seen in dentin dysplasia (type I) present in some patients
Tumoral calcinosis[38]	Familial	Calcifications in pulp chamber and root canal have been reported
Brachio-skeletal-genital syndrome[85] (Unger-Trott syndrome)	Familial	Similar to those in dentin dysplasia (type I)

the pulp at approximately the level of the cementoenamel junction is absent.

There are also several inherited systemic disorders that affect the dentin and consequently the dental pulp. These conditions are summarized in Table 10-2. Hypophosphatemic vitamin D–resistant rickets and the de Toni-Debré-Fanconi syndrome are only two of the metabolic disorders that result in rachitic disease and are refractory to normal doses of vitamin D. Other such disorders include cystine storage disease, the Abderhalden-Kaufmann-Lignac syndrome, and the familial aminoacidurias.[84] The teeth do not appear to have been studied in these latter diseases, but they might be expected to be similarly affected. Again, Cockayne's syndrome[15] and the Neill-Dingwall[52] syndrome also exhibit premature senility. It is possible that the teeth in these conditions exhibit similar changes to those found in progeria, but this has not yet been reported.

GENETIC DISORDERS AFFECTING THE VARIOUS COMPONENTS OF THE DENTAL PULP

In this section the genetic disorders that have been shown to affect the nerves, blood vessels, or connective tissue of the dental pulp will be discussed. However, little work has been done in this area. An additional aim, consequently, will be to point out those disorders or groups of disorders that might logically be expected to affect the dental pulp. It is hoped that this information will serve to encourage further work in this aspect of oral pathology.

Genetic disorders affecting the nerve fibers

Sensory nerve fibers are an important component of the dental pulp and are part of the peripheral nervous system. Therefore any genetic disorder that affects the sensory fibers of the peripheral nervous system might be expected to affect the nerve fibers of the dental pulp. Metachromatic leukodystrophy is an example of such a disease that in fact does so. However, it should be remembered that the peripheral nervous system is extensive and that the nerves of the pulp obviously represent only a small sample of it. As such, they may conceivably not be involved in a particular patient to the same extent as another peripheral nerve from elsewhere in that patient.

Furthermore, some conditions that affect the peripheral nerves are also associated with the accumulation of metabolites in various tissues. The lipidoses are prime examples of this situation. Consequently, such a disease might be expected to exhibit accumulation of the appropriate metabolite in the connective tissue of the pulp, in addition to involving its nerve fibers.

There are four main groups of hereditary neurological disorders that could affect the peripheral nerves of the dental pulp. These are the leukodystrophies, lipidoses, the ceroid-lipofuscinoses, and the genetic or familial polyneuropathies. In addition, there are a number of hereditary systemic conditions that have peripheral neuropathy as one of their manifestations. Diabetes mellitus is an important disease with genetic aspects that does so. Pathology of the peripheral nervous system is one aspect of neuropathology evoking much interest at the present time with the result that studies on the peripheral nerve involvement in a wide variety of conditions have been reported recently. Presumably, the peripheral nerves of the pulp may also be involved in these diseases.

The leukodystrophies. The leukodystrophies are an important group of relatively rare inherited disorders characterized primarily by disturbances in myelin formation, hence the reference to white matter (leuko-) in the name, leukodystrophy. Poser[58] believes that the materials that accumulate in these enzymatic disorders originate from compounds that cannot be used in the anabolism of myelin, as opposed to products that result from disintegration of myelin but which cannot be removed because of defective catabolism.

The leukodystrophies as classified by Norman[53] are as follows:

Metachromatic leukodystrophy
Globoid cell leukodystrophy (Krabbe's disease)
Sudanophilic leukodystrophy
Pelizaeus-Merzbacher disease

Sudanophilic leukodystrophy—cont'd
    Seitelberger type
    Lowenberg-Hill type
Leukodystrophies with mixed prelipoid and
    sudanophil deposits
Leukodystrophy with deposits resembling Rosenthal fibers (Alexander type)
Spongy degeneration of the white matter (Canavan type)

Adrenoleukodystrophy should now be added to this classification as a form of sudanophilic leukodystrophy.[12] In one of these disorders, metachromatic leukodystrophy, biopsy of the dental pulp has been advocated as a diagnostic procedure.[24, 26] Of the others, Krabbe's disease involves peripheral nerves and therefore is the most logical one in which to expect changes in the peripheral nerves of the dental pulp. The remainder are rare, and their pathological changes, with the exception of adrenoleukodystrophy, are apparently confined to the central nervous system.

Metachromatic leukodystrophy. Metachromatic leukodystrophy is a rare autosomal recessive disorder characterized by progressive degeneration of the nervous system. The commonest form is the late infantile type, but there is also a juvenile form, which may really be the same disease with a later age of onset. Metachromatic leukodystrophy has also been described in adults.

The clinical features in the late infantile form commence around 20 months of age and consist of cerebral dysfunction resulting in mental and motor-sensory disturbances. In the early stages of the disease the child is often thought to be mentally retarded or to suffer from cerebral palsy or a cervical cord tumour. However, the progressive nature of the disorder soon becomes apparent. The patient gradually loses his ability to walk, stand, crawl and eventually becomes paralyzed. There is also progressive mental degeneration, and the child becomes blind, deaf, loses contact with the external environment, and finally dies.

Metachromatic leukodystrophy is characterized by the breakdown of myelin and the accumulation of cerebroside-sulfuric acid esters (sulfatides) in the white matter of the central nervous system, in the peripheral nerves, and in various organs. The basic biochemical defect is a specific deficiency of arylsulfatase A, one of the enzymes required in the degradation of sulfatides.

Histologically, the accumulation of sulfatides in various tissues can best be demonstrated by the finding of abnormal amounts of metachromatic lipid in frozen sections. The most reliable method of doing this is that of von Hirsch and Pieffer.[55, 81] I have summarized this procedure previously, as follows:

Free floating sections are immersed for ten minutes in a freshly prepared and filtered solution consisting of 99 parts 0.5 per cent aqueous cresyl violet or cresylecht violet and one part glacial acetic acid. They are then rinsed in distilled water and mounted in glycerine. Because this stain fades within a few days, the findings should be recorded immediately by color photomicrography.

The nature of the brown metachromasia should be confirmed by placing additional sections in a mixture composed of equal parts of methyl alcohol and chloroform for ten minutes and one hour respectively before staining. This procedure removes the sulfatides and therefore unmasks a red metachromasia produced by the retention of lipids of higher polarity.*

The diagnosis of metachromatic leukodystrophy can now be confirmed by a variety of clinical tests. These include the demonstration of arylsulfatase A deficiency in urine, the demonstration of high levels of sulfatides in urine, and the demonstration of abnormal amounts of sulfatides in biopsies of peripheral nerves and other tissues. The sural nerve has been the most frequently biopsied nerve for this purpose.

In 1965, Gardner and Zeman[26] recommended biopsy of the dental pulp as a diagnostic procedure in metachromatic leukodystrophy. They demonstrated increased quantities of sulfatides as brown metachromatic granules within the cytoplasm of the Schwann cells of the peripheral nerves of the dental pulp in patients with this disorder (Fig.

---

*From Gardner, D. G.: Pulpectomy as a diagnostic procedure in metachromatic leukodystrophy, Oral Surg. 23:379-384, 1967.

10-1). The advantages of biopsy of the dental pulp as opposed to biopsies of other peripheral nerves or rectal mucosa include the simplicity of the operation, which can be performed on an outpatient basis, the lack of complications, and the low cost of the procedure. The pulp can be obtained either by pulpectomy, usually of a deciduous tooth, or by extraction. The latter procedure can be justified in the diagnosis of a child with a progressive dengenerating condition.

The extirpated pulp is fixed in 10% formalin and then frozen onto a piece of any readily available tissue to ensure that the microtome knife clears the freezing disk. Sections are cut at 15 μm or less and stained and studied as just described.

Recently, Olsson and Sourander[55] have suggested that the reliable diagnosis of metachromatic leukodystrophy by peripheral nerve biopsy requires the demonstration of sulfatide accumulations in typical phagocytes. This more stringent criterion can, of course, be applied to dental pulp biopsies.

Globoid cell leukodystrophy (Krabbe's disease). Globoid cell leukodystrophy,[77] an autosomal recessive disorder, usually commences in infancy, with the patients dying before they are 2 years old. During their illness they exhibit retarded development, spastic quadriparesis, cortical blindness, and deafness. The histopathological feature pathognomic of the disorder is the presence of groups of histiocytes, called globoid cells, in the demyelinated area of the central nervous system. Some of these cells, which tend to occur around small blood vessels, are large and multinucleated.

The peripheral nervous system is also affected.[11, 21, 77] Degenerative changes are found in both the axons and myelin sheaths, and there is endoneurial fibrosis. Histiocytes occur around endoneurial blood vessels or elsewhere

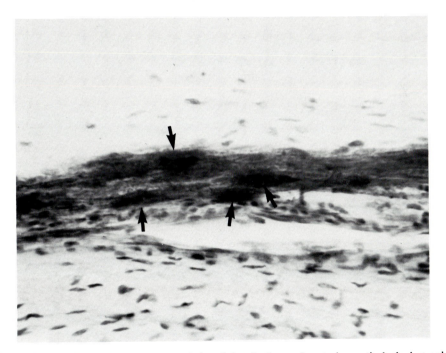

Fig. 10-1. Dental pulp from patient with late infantile form of metachromatic leukodystrophy. There are marked accumulations of brown metachromatic material, *arrows,* within Schwann cells of peripheral nerve. This appearance is diagnostic of metachromatic leukodystrophy. In contrast, only finely distributed brown metachromatic granules are found in normal myelin sheaths. (Frozen section of formalin fixed material; acidified cresyl violet stain.) (From Gardner, D. G., and Zeman, W.: Dev. Med. Child. Neurol. 7:620-621, 1965.)

in the endoneurium. Although globoid cells are not found in the peripheral nerves, ultrastructural inclusions similar to those in the globoid cells of the brain are present in the cytoplasm of the histiocytes, in the proliferating endoneurial connective tissue, and around small blood vessels.

It is highly probable that the peripheral nerves of the dental pulp are affected in Krabbe's disease, but this has not yet been confirmed.

The lipidoses. The one characteristic that identifies this group of disorders is damage to the cell bodies of the neurons of the gray matter with storage of complex lipids in the perikymata of these cells. In contrast, the basic injury in the leukodystrophies is to myelin and white matter. There is, however, some overlap between the pathological lesions of these two groups of disorders.

Table 10-3 lists the lipidoses together with the changes in the peripheral nerves in each disease. Only in Fabry's disease[19] has the dental pulp been studied in any detail. However, the typical foam cell has been found in the dental pulp in one case of Niemann-Pick disease.[75]

Fabry's disease. Fabry's disease[78] is a rare inherited disorder of glycosphingolipid metabolism. The basic defect lies in the lack of an α-galactosyl hydrolase, which is necessary for the breakdown of galactogalactoglucosyl ceramide, a trihexosyl ceramide. The result is accumulation of this birefringent lipid in

Table 10-3. The lipidoses

Disorder	Clinical findings	Mode of inheritance	Peripheral nerve changes	Remarks
Gangliosidoses[54]				
GM$_2$ gangliosidosis I (Tay-Sachs disease)	Seizures, mental retardation, blindness, abnormal muscle tone and postures; relentlessly progressive; cherry red spot in macula	Autosomal recessive	Almost total destruction of myelin sheaths associated with crowding of Schwann cell nuclei; frequent occurrence of irregular, elongated thickenings of axons[42]	Previously considered infantile form of amaurotic familial idiocy (AFI)
GM$_2$ gangliosidosis II (Sandhoff's disease)		Autosomal recessive		
GM$_2$ gangliosidosis III (juvenile GM$_2$ gangliosidosis)	All five gangliosidoses involve progressive mental and motor deterioration; onset is in childhood, and disorders are fatal	Autosomal recessive		
GM$_1$ gangliosidosis I* (generalized gangliosidosis)		Autosomal recessive		

*The GM$_1$ gangliosidoses have been classified as mucolipidoses by Spranger and Wiedemann[80] and are consequently also listed in Table 10-8.

plasma and most tissues, including heart, kidney, and eye.

The clinical features generally appear in childhood or adolescence and are caused by the lipid deposition in the tissues. They are characterized by periodic febrile crises, severe pain in the extremities, corneal opacities, and telangiectatic lesions on the skin, oral mucosa, and conjunctiva. This last manifestation accounts for one synonym for the disorder, *angiokeratoma corporis diffusum.* The patients usually die in adulthood from renal failure or cardiac or cerebrovascular disease.

Fabry's disease is an X-linked disorder. Affected males are hemizygous for the allele and exhibit the complete disease complex. Males obviously cannot be heterozygous for an X-

linked trait. Females may be heterozygous for the gene and exhibit the features of Fabry's disease, generally in an attenuated form; corneal changes are the commonest manifestation in such individuals. The phenotype in the heterozygous female varies considerably because of the Lyon effect. There do not appear to be any reports of homozygous females in this disease.

The diagnosis of Fabry's disease is generally suspected by finding the characteristic cutaneous and corneal lesions in members of families known to harbor the disorder. It can be confirmed by a skin biopsy in which the characteristic birefringent lipid is detected in the blood vessels or by finding doubly refractile lipid bodies in urinary sedi-

Table 10-3. The lipidoses—cont'd

Disorder	Clinical findings	Mode of inheritance	Peripheral nerve changes	Remarks
GM$_1$ gangliosidosis II* (juvenile GM$_1$ gangliosidosis)		Autosomal recessive		
Gaucher's disease (three types)	Hepatosplenomegaly, bone pain, and pathological fractures; neurological signs in some patients	Autosomal recessive		"Gaucher cells" accumulate in spleen, liver, lymph nodes, and bones
Niemann-Pick disease (five types)	Hepatosplenomegaly, severe neurological disturbances in many, but not all, cases	Autosomal recessive	Axon degeneration and inclusions in satellite cells[6]	Typical foam cell has been demonstrated in dental pulp of a patient with this disease[75]
Fabry's disease (angiokeratoma corporis diffusum)	Periodic febrile crises, pain in extremities, corneal opacities, telangiectasia	X-linked recessive	Axon degeneration in large unmyelinated nerve fibers; stored ceramide trihexosides seen under EM as inclusions in capillary endothelia and their pericytes as well as in perineurial sheath cells[6]	Dental pulp in hemizygotes and heterozygotes for Fabry gene has been well studied[19]; see text

ment. Heterozygotes, as well as homozygotes, can be identified by the biochemical detection of increased levels of trihexosyl ceramide in plasma, urinary sediment, or cultured fibroblasts. The level of α-galactosyl hydrolase activity can also be determined in plasma, leukocytes, or cultured fibroblasts.

In a recent interesting paper, Desnick and her colleagues[19] reported on their observations in the dental pulp of one male (hemizygote) with Fabry's disease compared to the dental pulps of two heterozygous females and of normal patients. Their investigation involved histochemical studies on frozen sections of formalin-fixed tissue and biochemical techniques. The dental pulp of the hemizygote exhibited extensive deposition of diastase-resistant PAS-positive material in blood vessel walls or scattered throughout the pulp tissue with some concentration near arterioles (Fig. 10-2). This material stained positively with a PAS method modified specifically to stain neutral glycosphingolipids and gangliosides[1] and was dissolved by lipid solvents. Only small amounts of PAS-positive, lipid-soluble material were found in the dental pulps of the heterozygotes and the normal individuals. Compared to the pulps from the heterozygotes and the controls, the dental pulp of the hemizygote showed only a moderate increase in staining intensity with Sudan Black B, a stain used to demonstrate lipids. Witkop,[84] one of Desnick's co-workers, has stated previously that the PAS-positive material in the dental pulp of the patient with Fabry's disease showed the typical Maltese cross pattern under polarized light.

The biochemical investigations consisted of studying the extracted total lipids from the dental pulp by various forms of chromatography. The pulp tissue from the hemizygote contained significantly more total fractionated lipid and markedly higher concentrations of trihexosyl ceramide, the specific neutral glycosphingolipid that accumulates in the tissues in Fabry's disease, than that of the hemizygotes or controls.

Desnick and associates[19] concluded that examination of the dental pulp by these histochemical and biochemical techniques provides

Table 10-4. The ceroid-lipofuscinoses

Disorder	Clinical findings	Mode of inheritance	Peripheral nerve changes	Remarks
Jansky-Bielschowsky type	Similar to Tay-Sachs disease	Autosomal recessive	Characteristic cytoplasmic inclusions detected in skin biopsies; suggested as means of diagnosis[20]	Previously considered the late infantile form of AFI (Bielschowsky-Jansky)
Spielmeyer-Sjögren type	Onset is about 1 to 8 years of age; more slowly progressive than Tay-Sachs; seizures and dementia develop late	Autosomal recessive	Extensive destruction of myelin sheaths; sometimes segmental demyelination; extensive fragmentation of axons in some cases[42]; characteristic cytoplasmic inclusions detected in skin biopsies; suggested as means of diagnosis[20]	Previously considered the juvenile form of AFI (Batten-Mayou; Spielmeyer-Vogt)
Adult AFI (Kufs')	Onset is after 20 year of age; no blindness; no dementia	Autosomal recessive or dominant		Rare disorder, previously considered the adult form of AFI (Kufs')

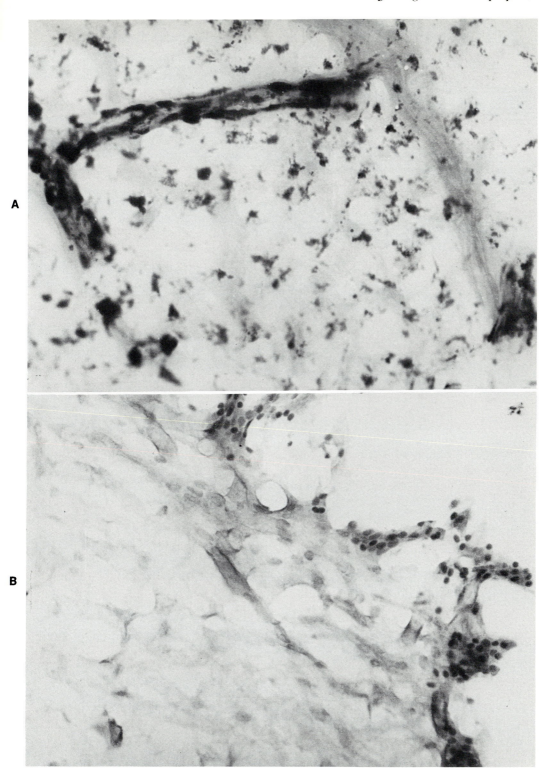

Fig. 10-2. Dental pulp from patient with Fabry's disease, **A**, compared to that from unaffected person, **B**. There is extensive deposition of PAS-positive material within pulp from patient with Fabry's disease. (Modified PAS stain.) (From Witkop, C. J., Jr.: Oral Surg. **32:**278-316, 1971.)

a reliable method for confirming the diagnosis of the hemizygote state in Fabry's disease. They could not, however, distinguish between the two heterozygotes and normal controls by their methods.

The ceroid-lipofuscinoses. The ceroid-lipofuscinoses were previously classified as forms of amaurotic familial idiocy (**AFI**) but have now been shown to be caused by the storage of lipopigments in the nervous system and other tissues. They have been well reviewed by Zeman.[87] Changes in small peripheral nerves have been reported in two members of this group,[20, 30, 47] and it is probable that these structures in the dental pulp are also affected. There have been no studies reported confirming this, however. The ceroid-lipofuscinoses are summarized in Table 10-4.

The genetically determined neuropathies. The genetically determined neuropathies, a group of chronic familial disorders, is characterized by the degeneration of the peripheral nerves alone or of the peripheral nerves together with parts of the central nervous system. These diseases are usually noted first in childhood or adolescence and exhibit a slowly progressive polyneuropathy, first of the lower extremities and later of the hands and arms. A number of trophic changes are generally found, including muscle wasting, anesthesia of distal parts, and ulcers. The peripheral nerve changes have been well documented, but the potential manifestations in the dental pulp have apparently not yet been studied. The genetically determined neuropathies are summarized in Table 10-5.

Table 10-5. The genetically determined neuropathies

Disorder	Clinical findings	Mode of inheritance	Peripheral nerve changes	Remarks
Progressive peroneal atrophy (Charcot-Marie-Tooth disease)[37]	Slowly progressive paresis affecting mainly distal muscles of legs; stork leg appearance; slight sensory changes with absent tendon reflexes	Autosomal dominant	Fibrosis replacing absent nerve fibers; axonal degeneration[6, 36]	
Hypertrophic interstitial neuropathy (Dejerine-Sottas disease)[36]	Lower motor paresis combined with sensory loss causing areflexia and ataxia; usually slowly progressive; there may be alternating relapses and remissions	Autosomal dominant	Peripheral nerves are considerably thickened because of concentric proliferation of connective tissue and Schwann cell processes resulting in typical onion bulb appearance; endoneurial space distended by PAS-positive metachromatic with toluidine blue material; depletion of myelin and probably of axons[22, 43, 79, 82]	

Table 10-5. The genetically determined neuropathies—cont'd

Disorder	Clinical findings	Mode of inheritance	Peripheral nerve changes	Remarks
Phytanic acid storage disease (Refsum's syndrome)[74]	Ataxia, retinitis pigmentosa, changes in skin and bones	Autosomal recessive		Accumulation in tissues, especially in liver and kidney, of lipid, phytanic acid
Hereditary sensory neuropathy (Denny-Brown)[18, 32, 36]	Severe peripheral sensory loss, loss of deep reflexes, severe trophic disorders of all four extremities	Autosomal dominant	Reduction in number of nerve fibers[18]; marked demyelination[32]	
Portuguese polyneuritis familial type of amyloidosis (Andrade's disease)[4, 16, 34]	Generalized amyloidosis with major involvement of nervous system	Autosomal dominant	Classic amyloid in peripheral nerves	Hereditary amyloid neuropathies are a group of disorders, of which Portuguese type is prototype[16]
Tangier disease (hereditary high-density lipoprotein deficiency)[23]	Grossly enlarged yellow tonsils; splenomegaly; neurological abnormalities	Autosomal recessive	Gross loss of unmyelinated and myelinated axons, extensive accumulation of lipid within Schwann cells, excessive endoneurial collagenization[40]	
Abetalipoproteinemia (acanthocytosis) (Bassen-Kornzweig syndrome)[23]	Steatorrhea, abdominal distension, poor growth pattern, retinitis pigmentosa, and ataxia	Probably autosomal recessive	Small increase in quantity of endoneural connective tissue and of Schwann cell nuclei, extensive demyelination[41, 65, 68]	
Ataxia telangiectasia[76]	Progressive cerebellar ataxia, cutaneous telangiectases, involuntary movements, mental retardation, small stature	Autosomal recessive	Schwann cell nuclei enlarged; denervation atrophy of skeletal muscles[76]	
Congenital sensory neuropathy (Winklemann)[29, 44, 83]	Incomplete distribution of sensory loss involving pain, temperature, and touch; nonprogressive disorder	Mostly sporadic, occasionally dominant or autosomal recessive	No myelinated fibers or sensory end organs	

Continued.

Table 10-5. The genetically determined neuropathies—cont'd

Disorder	Clinical findings	Mode of inheritance	Peripheral nerve changes	Remarks
Acute intermittent porphyria (Swedish genetic porphyria)[17]	Acute illness often follows use of barbiturates or sulphonamides; during attack, patient exhibits severe pain, great increase in urinary porphyrin, and is highly emotional; peripheral neuritis and death may occur	Autosomal dominant	Neuropathy is chiefly motor; sensory disturbances occur in half the cases, however; extensive peripheral nerve degeneration affecting axons and myelin[37]; peripheral nerve changes appear to be variable[60]	
Riley-Day syndrome (familial dysautonomia)[2]	Emotional lability, insensitivity to pain, absence of tears, postural hypotension, hypoactive corneal and tendon reflexes, absence of fungiform papillae on tongue	Autosomal recessive	One case, sural nerve only; marked reduction in number of unmyelinated fibers; no myelinated fibers greater than 12 μm in diameter; nerve fibers 6 μm to 12 μm in diameter show abnormally short internodal length[2]	
Diabetes mellitus[59]	Metabolic disorder characterized by hyperglycemia, glycosuria, polyuria, weight loss; numerous clinical manifestations in cases of long duration, many on vascular basis	Predisposition to develop diabetes is inherited—probably multifactorial pattern[59]	Marked reduction in number of myelinated fibers[5]; segmental demyelination; hyperplasia of basement membrane and changes in Schwann cell cytoplasm[6]	Changes in peripheral nerves of dental pulp have not yet been reported; however, vascular changes have been found in pulp[63]
Friedreich's ataxia (hereditary spinal ataxia)	Onset usually between 7 and 15 years; patients develop ataxia, dysarthria, loss of deep tendon reflexes, pes cavus	Autosomal recessive	Depletion of myelinated nerve fibers with presence of fine unmyelinated axons[37]	

Other disorders. In addition to the leukodystrophies, the lipidoses, the ceroid-lipofuscinoses, and the genetically determined neuropathies, there are a number of inherited disorders that exhibit peripheral nerve changes as a relatively minor feature. These disorders may also affect the peripheral nerves of the dental pulp, although this has not yet been confirmed. They are summarized in Table 10-6.

Congenital insensitivity to pain. A number of interesting conditions exhibiting congenital insensitivity to pain have recently been reviewed by MacEwen and Floyd.[45] Some of the inherited ones, such as congenital sensory neuropathy,[29, 44, 83] familial dysautonomia,[2]

Table 10-6. Other genetic disorders exhibiting changes in peripheral nerves

Disorder	Clinical findings	Mode of inheritance	Peripheral nerve changes
Lafora's disease[64, 66] (myoclonus body disease)	Myoclonic epilepsy, progressive motor and mental deterioration, amaurosis	Autosomal recessive	Round, diastase resistant, PAS-positive "Lafora bodies" within axis cylinders of spinal nerves[64]
Cockayne's syndrome[48]	Cachectic dwarfism, characteristic facies, photosensitivity, mental retardation, contractures of joints	Autosomal recessive	Overall loss of myelinated fibers (segmental demyelination)[57]; electron-dense bodies in Schwann cells[62]
Wilson's disease (hepatolenticular degeneration)[9]	Degenerative changes in brain, cirrhosis of liver, Kayser-Fleisher rings	Autosomal recessive	Primary demyelination and secondary changes in axons[50]

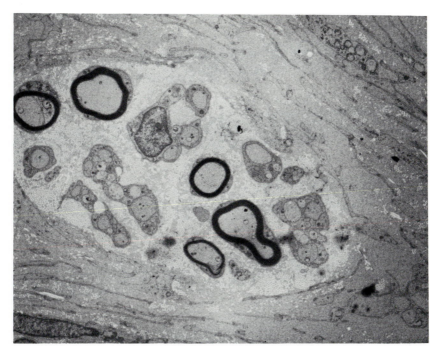

Fig. 10-3. Electron micrograph of cross section of peripheral nerve within dental pulp of patient with congenital indifference to pain. Nerve is normal in this condition but would be expected to be abnormal in certain other disorders characterized by congenital analgesia. Examination of dental pulp in such patients should therefore be of diagnostic importance. (×4300.) (Courtesy J. P. Sapp, London, Ontario, Canada.)

and hereditary sensory neuropathy[18, 32, 36] have been mentioned previously in this chapter. Another condition, familial sensory neuropathy with anhidrosis,[57, 80] apparently does not exhibit peripheral nerve changes, although there is loss of the dorsolateral tract and dorsal root fibers. Of this group of diseases, perhaps the most familiar is that known as congenital indifference to pain.[8, 46] This condition is not inherited, although D trisomy mosaicism has been described in two cases.[10]

Congenital sensory neuropathy, familial

dysautonomia, and hereditary sensory neuropathy exhibit morphological changes in peripheral nerve; others, like congenital indifference to pain, do not. Patients with these conditions bite their tongues and lips with resultant marked mutilation, and consequently, it is often necessary to extract the teeth. In such cases the peripheral nerves of the dental pulps of the extracted teeth should be examined under the electron microscope, a procedure that can be of diagnostic importance. Fig. 10-3 illustrates nerve fibers from the dental pulp in a case of congenital indifference to pain. They are normal, as would be expected in this disorder. However, this electron micrograph does illustrate the potential value of the ultrastructural examination of the dental pulp in children exhibiting congenital analgesia.

Genetic disorders affecting the connective tissue

Connective tissue represents the second major component of the dental pulp. Like connective tissues elsewhere in the body, it consists of cells and intercellular material. In turn, the latter is composed of fibers and ground substance, both of which are products of the cells.

The genetic disorders of connective tissue are reviewed in this section with regard to their effect or potential effect on the connective tissue of the dental pulp. The so-called storage diseases are also discussed here because any stored metabolites in the dental pulp would be expected to be found mainly in the connective tissue.

The fibrous component. The dental pulp consists of loose connective tissue with relatively few collagen fibers. Reticulin fibers, generally considered to be precollagenous, are also present.

An obvious approach to the study of the effect of genetic disease on the collagen of the dental pulp would be to explore whether the quantity or quality of collagen has been altered. There appears to have been no work reported in this area.

There are a number of heritable connective tissue disorders that may affect collagen itself.

These are discussed in detail in McKusick's monograph.[49] However, little is known about whether the collagen is in fact altered. Consequently, at our present stage of knowledge there appears to be little reason to investigate qualitatively the collagen of the dental pulp in these conditions.

At first glance, studying the relative amount of collagen in the dental pulp in these conditions appears to be a simple task. However, there are a number of complicating factors. First, it is necessary to know what constitutes the normal quantity of collagen in dental pulps at different ages, since this varies considerably. Stanley and Ranney[73] have shown that the amount of collagen in the dental pulp is related not so much to age as to the amount of irregular dentin that has formed in the particular tooth. A tooth that exhibits irregular dentin should also exhibit increased quantities of collagen. The quantity of irregular dentin in a particular tooth depends on such irritations as caries and restorative treatment and attrition as well as age. Stanley and Ranney[73] have also shown that the anterior teeth exhibit more collagen in their dental pulps than do posterior teeth and that radicular pulp tissue has more collagen than coronal pulp tissue. Moreover, the size of the pulp cavity decreases with age. It follows that the same amount of collagen confined to a smaller volume would give an apparent increase in the amount of collagen present. Finally, artifactual changes caused by suboptimal fixation of the dental pulp tend to result in the aggregation of the normally dispersed collagen fibers, producing an apparent focal increase in the quantity of collagen.

The ground substance. The main organic components of the histologist's ground substance are the high-molecular-weight mucopolysaccharides (glycosaminoglycans). There are two groups of inherited disorders involving these substances, the mucopolysaccharidoses and the mucolipidoses. Glycosaminoglycans are stored in increased amounts in the tissues in these disorders. Furthermore, the relative proportions of the specific glycosaminoglycans found in the various tissues often differ from normal; the actual composition of the glycosaminoglycans is not altered.

The mucopolysaccharidoses. The muco-polysaccharidoses are a group of inherited disorders of glycosaminoglycan metabolism, the prototype of which is the Hurler syndrome (MPS I). These disorders have recently been reviewed by Haust[30] and by McKusick[49] and are summarized in Table 10-7. They are characterized by the accumulation of glycosaminoglycans in tissues and organs other than brain and by mucopolysacchariduria. In many, gangliosides are present in the neurons. The mucopolysacchari-doses are all autosomal recessive conditions except MPS II, which is X-linked recessive.

In all of these disorders the accumulated glycosaminoglycans can be demonstrated histochemically within various tissues. These substances are stored both intracellularly and extracellularly. In MPS IV, the Morquio syndrome, the stored glycosaminoglycans are confined largely to liver and cartilage. However, in the other mucopolysaccharidoses they are found in fibrous connective tissue, among other sites. Therefore, accumulating glycosaminoglycans could be expected to be stored also within the dental pulp in all of the muco-polysaccharidoses except MPS IV.

The histochemical techniques used are not completely specific, and it is therefore prudent to identify the substances stained only collectively as acid mucopolysaccharides. Moreover, quantitative studies are not possible. Vacuolated cells, considered to be of fibroblastic origin, are found within various tissues, including fibrous connective tissue, in all the disorders except MPS IV. These cells have been called *gargoyle cells.* If special precautions are employed to avoid aqueous solutions, it is possible to demonstrate granules of metachromatic material within the cytoplasm of many of these cells.

There are no reports concerning the morphology of the dental pulp in any of the mucopolysaccharidoses. However, Gardner and Haust have recently completed preliminary studies on the dental pulp in the Hurler syndrome (MPS I). Similar investigations in other mucopolysaccharidoses except MPS IV should prove rewarding.

MUCOPOLYSACCHARIDOSIS I. THE HURLER SYNDROME. The Hurler syndrome, an autosomal recessive disorder, manifests itself in infancy or early childhood and is characterized by mental retardation, dwarfism, a large, deformed head, a typical facial appearance, progressive corneal clouding, hernias, skeletal abnormalities, flexion contractures, and hepatosplenomegaly. The diagnosis is confirmed by the identification of increased quantities

Table 10-7. The mucopolysaccharidoses*

Disorder	Clinical findings	Mucopolysacchariduria
MPS I (Hurler)	Typical facies, mental retardation, clouding of cornea, death by 10 years of age	Dermatan sulfate Heparan sulfate
MPS II (Hunter)	Facies are not as coarse as in MPS I; no clouding of cornea; most die before 20 years of age	Dermatan sulfate Heparan sulfate
MPS III (Sanfilippo)	Somatic changes are milder; profound mental retardation	Heparan sulfate
MPS IV (Morquio)	Dwarfed, normal intelligence, characteristic bone and dental changes	Keratan sulfate (chondroitin 4/6 sulfate may also be excreted)
MPS V (Scheie)	No mental retardation; corneal clouding, characteristic facies	Dermatan sulfate Heparan sulfate
MPS VI (Maroteaux-Lamy)	Retarded growth; facies resemble other mucopolysaccharidoses; normal intellect; severe osseous abnormalities	Dermatan sulfate

*Modified from McKusick, V. A.: Heritable disorders of connective tissue, ed. 4, St. Louis, 1972, The C. V. Mosby Co.

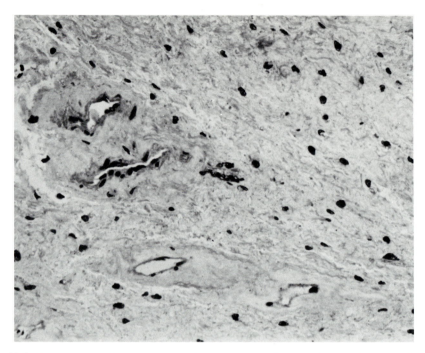

Fig. 10-4. Dental pulp taken at autopsy from case of Hurler's syndrome (MPS I). There is marked hyalinization around blood vessels. (1 μm section. Toluidine blue stain. ×280.) (Courtesy M. D. Haust, London, Ontario, Canada.)

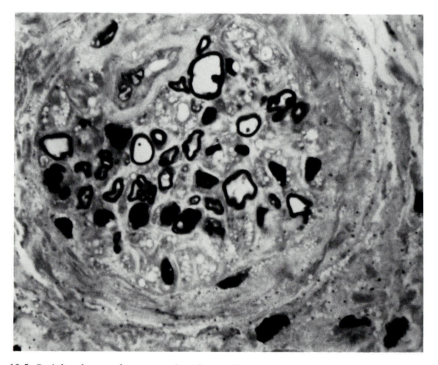

Fig. 10-5. Peripheral nerve from same dental pulp illustrated in Fig. 10-4. Numerous vacuolated cells are present within nerve bundle. (1 μm section; toluidine blue stain; ×1125.) (Courtesy M. D. Haust, London, Ontario, Canada.)

of dermatan sulfate and heparan sulfate in the urine.

Gardner and Haust observed several interesting features in 1 μm thick plastic embedded sections of dental pulp, stained with toluidine blue. The two most prominent findings were a hyaline thickening around the blood vessels (Fig. 10-4) and the presence of vacuolated cells in the peripheral nerves (Fig. 10-5). These vacuolated cells were also present in the connective tissue of the pulp and in the hyalinized material surrounding the blood vessels. The glycosaminoglycans of the tissues in the Hurler syndrome are markedly soluble in water; they were consequently almost entirely lost in the preparation of the aqueous toluidine blue–stained sections. This accounted for the vacuoles observed in this study. A small amount of granular material, apparently representing retained acid mucopolysaccharide, was present in the connective tissue.

Frozen sections of the second dental pulp were stained by the method of Haust and Landing.[31] This procedure involves fixation of the frozen sections in a mixture of equal parts of tetrahydrafuran and acetone for at least 20 to 30 minutes. The fixed sections

Table 10-8. The mucolipidoses

Disorder	Clinical findings	Pathological findings	Potential changes in dental pulp
Mucolipidosis I (lipomucopolysaccharidosis)	Mild Hurler-like symptoms with moderate mental retardation	Coarse refractile inclusions in cultured fibroblasts; increased quantities of metachromatic lipids in peripheral nerves	Should be reflected in fibroblasts and nerves of dental pulp
Mucolipidosis II (I cell disease)	Severe clinical and radiological signs resembling Hurler's syndrome; hyperplastic gingiva	Coarse refractile inclusions in cultured fibroblasts	Should be reflected in fibroblasts from dental pulp
Mucolipidosis III (pseudo-Hurler polydystrophy)	Mild mental retardation; mild Hurler-like facies in some patients	Little pathological information available	
Fucosidosis	Progressive neurological deterioration; mild Hurler-like facies	Accumulation of fucose-containing lipids	Dental pulp may be affected
Mannosidosis	Hurler-like facies; psychomotor development is slow	Accumulation of mannose-containing glycoproteins	Dental pulp may be affected
Juvenile sulfatidosis, Austin type	Combination of metachromatic leukodystrophy and Hurler-like symptoms	Increased quantities of metachromatic lipids in peripheral nerves	Should be reflected in nerves of dental pulp
GM_1 gangliosidosis I*	Resembles MPS I; hyperplastic gingiva	Generalized accumulation of GM_1 ganglioside; visceral and mesenchymal storage of mucopolysaccharide	Dental pulp may be affected
GM_1 gangliosidosis II*	Progressive mental deterioration; does not resemble MPS I clinically	Accumulation of GM_1 ganglioside in brain; visceral storage of mucopolysaccharide	Dental pulp may be affected

*The GM_1 gangliosidoses are perhaps more properly included in the lipidoses and consequently have also been listed in Table 10-3.

are then stained in 0.5% toluidine blue in 25% acetone at pH 2. The acid mucopolysaccharides stored in the mucopolysaccharidoses are consistently demonstrated by this method because no aqueous medium is involved. The dental pulp fixed and stained in this manner exhibited abundant extracellular metachromatic material. In addition, many of the cells contained granules of a similar nature. This metachromatic material represents the acid mucopolysaccharides stored in this disorder.

The mucolipidoses. The mucolipidoses are a group of rare inherited disorders, listed in Table 10-8, that share some of the features of both the mucopolysaccharidoses and the sphingolipidoses. In the past they have often been described as variants of the Hurler syndrome. The mucolopidoses are characterized by the accumulation of excessive amounts of acid mucopolysaccharides, sphingolipids, and/or glycolipids in various tissues. An excellent review of this group of storage diseases is that of Spranger and Wiedemann.[70] The mode of inheritance of these conditions has not yet been completely worked out, but the available evidence supports their being autosomal recessive. There have been no reports concerning changes in the dental pulp in these disorders. However, it probably is affected.

The cellular component. The work of Gardner and Haust on the Hurler syndrome shows that the cells of the dental pulp may be affected by genetic disease. No further information is available on this matter.

The storage diseases. The term *storage diseases* is applied to a wide variety of inherited disorders in which specific metabolites accumulate in the tissues. These diseases are discussed in detail in such reference works as Stanbury and associates[71] and Hers and van Hoof.[33] It is probable that in most, if not all, of the storage disorders, chemical analysis of the dental pulp would reveal elevated quantities of the appropriate metabolite. In fact, chemical analysis of the dental pulp has been reported in only one such condition, Fabry's disease.[19] The amount of the metabolite concerned, a trihexosyl ceramide, was increased in the dental pulp of a patient with this condition.

Again, many of the storage diseases exhibit typical histological, ultrastructural, and histochemical features that might be expected to be found in the dental pulps of affected persons. As noted previously, the characteristic histochemical features of metachromatic leukodystrophy, the Hurler syndrome and Krabbe's disease, and the typical cells of the Niemann-Pick disease have been found in the dental pulp of patients with these disorders. There are many other storage diseases that could be similarly studied.

In addition to the above disorders a number of other storage diseases have been discussed briefly in this chapter, including the lipidoses, ceroid-lipofuscinoses, mucopolysaccharidoses, and mucolipidoses. Study of dental pulp tissue in these conditions and in hemachromatosis, the glycogen storage diseases, Wilson's disease, Lesch-Nyham syndrome, and alcaptonuria should prove interesting.

Genetic disorders affecting the blood vessels

The blood vessels are the third component of the dental pulp that could be affected by genetic diseases. However, there are no inherited disorders that affect the peripheral blood vessels primarily, and the only disease with genetic implications that affects peripheral blood vessels is diabetes mellitus. There are a few conditions, for example, von Hippel–Lindau and Riley's syndromes, that have hemangiomas as one of their components. Conceivably, if a hemangioma occurred on the alveolar ridge and gingiva, it might affect the pulps of adjacent teeth. In fact, extensive angiomatous tissue has been reported in the dental pulp in one case of Sturge-Weber syndrome,[72] a disorder that is sometimes familial but more often sporadic. Nevertheless, the study of the small vessels of the dental pulp in genetic disorders does not appear to be a potentially rewarding area for research.

Diabetes mellitus. Diabetes mellitus is a disorder of carbohydrate metabolism. Predisposition to diabetes, rather than the disease itself, is inherited, probably in a multifactorial pattern.[59]

Generalized microangiopathy, consisting of marked thickening of the basement membranes of capillaries and small blood vessels, is common in diabetics. Russell[63] has demonstrated similar alterations in the dental pulp in patients with this disorder. He described the changes that he found as PAS-positive mural thickening of the vessels of the pulp. He also concluded that calcifications were more common in the dental pulp of diabetics than in nondiabetics and stated that these calcifications were often sickle-shaped and embraced the vessels.

CHROMOSOMAL ANALYSIS OF DENTAL PULP CELLS IN TISSUE CULTURE

Aneuploidy is a term used to designate deviations from the normal diploid number of chromosomes that are not multiples of this number, which in humans is forty-six. Proportionately more bone marrow cells lacking the Y chromosome are found in males as they become older.[56] Aneuploidy in the human has also been found in the cells of the endometrium,[35] in amniotic fluid, and in fibroblasts and peripheral lymphocytes.[14]

Armed with this information, Cervenka and Ballin[14] attempted to grow the cells of the dental pulp in tissue culture. They were interested in establishing the growth potential of dental pulp cells in vitro, in determining whether aneuploidy occurs in these cells and, if so, whether this feature occurs proportionately more often with increasing age of the patient. These investigators were able to grow two types of cells from the dental pulp, fibroblasts and epithelial-like cells that they believed to have originated from odontoblasts. They concluded that the cells of the dental pulp generally grow poorly in tissue culture and that their mitotic index is lower than that of cutaneous fibroblasts or peripheral lymphocytes. Moreover, there were proportionately more aneuploid cells in pulps from males 48 years old and older than in those from males 24 years old and younger. Cervenka and Ballin did not study sufficient dental pulp from females to make a similar comparison for that sex. The missing chromosomes were from groups B, C, D, and G.

METHODS OF STUDYING THE DENTAL PULP

The manner in which the dental pulp is obtained and subsequently handled is important if maximum information is to be obtained from the tissue. The particular methods to be used in processing the tissue depend on the nature of the disease being studied; consequently some knowledge of the disease in question is required so that the appropriate choice may be made. In this section some suggestions will be made concerning the obtaining of pulp tissue for investigation and its subsequent processing.

Obtaining the tissue

Dental pulp tissue may be obtained at autopsy or from a living patient.

Tissue taken at autopsy is not ideal because there is usually some delay between the death of the patient and commencement of the postmortem examination. This delay may result in autolysis and is particularly detrimental in electron microscopy. Nevertheless, autopsy material is a valuable source for research into human disease. The point is simply that the less time allowed to elapse between the death of the patient and the obtaining of tissue the better. No tissue should be removed from a body without the authorization of the pathologist in charge of the case.

The removal of dental pulp tissue from the living patient solely for scientific research cannot be justified. However, it is acceptable if it may aid in the diagnosis of the patient's condition or identify him as a heterozygote for a pathological gene. Research involving removal of tissue from living patients should be cleared through appropriate hospital or university committees on research involving human subjects. Because of the justifiable restrictions concerning research on human subjects, the main source of dental pulp from patients with interesting disorders is from teeth that have to be extracted in connection with dental treatment, for example, for periodontic or orthodontic reasons. The removal of impacted teeth is another possible source.

A pulpectomy may be performed for diagnostic purposes in a living patient. Ideally a single-rooted tooth with a large pulp canal should be chosen to obtain as much pulp tissue as possible. Care must be taken not to damage the pulp unduly. A barbed broach should be introduced carefully to the apex of the tooth and the pulp removed in one piece. The pulp should then be removed immediately from the instrument and placed in the fixative or frozen in dry ice, depending on investigations to be performed. Barbed broaches rust, thereby damaging the tissue, and consequently the temptation to place the barbed broach with the pulp still attached into the fixative should be avoided.

In some cases the investigator may wish to study the dental pulp in situ using the light microscope. No special precautions in respect of fixation are necessary with incompletely developed teeth having open apices. However, in other teeth special techniques are required to ensure that the pulp is fixed adequately. Poorly fixed dental pulp exhibits various artifacts that make any changes found difficult to interpret. Stanley[72] has discussed this problem in some detail. Adequate fixation of the dental pulp can be obtained by snipping off part of the root with rongeurs. This procedure must be done as soon as the extraction is performed and may have to be midway up the root in teeth with narrow canals if the resulting opening is to be sufficiently large to allow adequate access of the fixative. An alternative method of ensuring that the fixative reaches the pulp tissue is to remove an area of dentin from the cervical third of the root using a high-speed handpiece. This procedure should be carried out until pulp tissue can be seen through a thin layer of remaining dentin. This method has the advantage of allowing the fixative to permeate both coronally and apically.

In those cases in which only the dental pulp is to be studied, it can be readily obtained by fracturing the extracted tooth mechanically and dissecting out the pulpal tissue in one piece. In deciduous molars the floor of the pulp chamber can be easily removed, allowing ready access to the dental pulp, which can then be removed intact.

Control tissue should be obtained from teeth that have been extracted during dental treatment from apparently healthy people, preferably of ages similar to those having the disease being studied.

Fixation of the tissue

The choice of whether to fix the tissue or to freeze it immediately in dry ice depends on the nature of the investigation planned, as does the selection of the actual fixative.

Light microscopy. Ten percent phosphate-buffered formalin is a good standard fixative for light microscopy but is not suitable for any study involving water-soluble material. This problem occurs, for example, with the glycosaminoglycans, which are normally somewhat soluble in water, and markedly so in the mucopolysaccharidoses. In these disorders, for example, the Hurler and Hunter syndromes, the tissue should be frozen. This is also true when histochemical studies of enzymes are planned. The dental pulp tends to curl up if it is simply placed in a bottle of fixative. This complicates the further processing and examination of the tissue and can be avoided by placing the pulp on a piece of card and floating the card into the fixative.

Electron microscopy. A standard procedure in electron microscopy is to cut the tissue into 1 or 2 mm cubes and then fix it for at least 2 hours in 4% glutaraldehyde that has been chilled to 4° C. In our laboratories we buffer the glutaraldehyde with 0.1M sodium cacodylate.

Orienting the tissue for electron microscopy

Orientation of the tissue is not important if the planned investigation is concerned only with the connective tissue of the pulp. The pulp tissue should simply be diced into 1 or 2 mm cubes as just described. However, orientation is more critical if the study involves the blood vessels or nerves of the pulp. In this case the coronal part of the pulp should be divided from the radicular pulp tissue. The radicular pulp can then be cut into approximately 5 mm lengths and fixed. The diameter of the radicular pulp is around 1 or 2 mm, so fixation of these strips will be adequate. Later, sections can be obtained by cutting across these strips of pulp tissue. This technique ensures good cross sections of nerve fibers and blood vessels. Axons, myelin sheaths, and Schwann cells can be readily studied (Fig. 10-3). Longitudinal sections of nerves and blood vessels can be obtained but with more difficulty. This method also leaves the coronal pulp available for histochemical or biochemical studies, an important consideration if only one dental pulp is available.

Special procedures for myelin and the sphingolipids

Myelin and its sphingolipid constituents are not soluble in aqueous fixatives, but they are lost in the subsequent histological techniques by which paraffin sections are produced. This property is obviously important whenever one wishes to study the leukodystrophies and lipidoses or the state of myelination of the nerve fibers. In these cases frozen sections of tissue that has been previously fixed in formalin, or frozen sections of fresh tissue, should be used.

Freezing the tissue

As mentioned previously, in some studies the tissue should be frozen rather than placed in an aqueous fixative. This is particularly true in histochemical studies of enzymes and of the mucopolysaccharidoses. Freezing the tissue is also a satisfactory method of preserving tissue for chemical analysis.

A convenient portable method of freezing tissue in a dental operatory or at autopsy is the use of dry ice in an insulated container. The tissue is placed in the bottom of a specimen jar that has been chilled on the dry ice for 10 minutes. The inferior surface of the specimen freezes as soon as it contacts the bottom of the jar, so it is important that the specimen is oriented carefully during this procedure. It is also essential that the specimen not be allowed to thaw during storage and thereby deteriorate. The jar containing the specimen can be placed in the cryostat when sections are to be prepared, at which time the specimen can be readily dislodged from the bottom of the jar with a wooden applicator stick.

Tissue culture

Dental pulp tissue can be cultured in a suitable medium, although Cervenka and Ballin[14] have shown that the cells of this tissue grow slowly. The pulp should be removed from the tooth, diced under sterile conditions, and then placed in tubes or flasks, which are incubated at 38° C. Cervenka and Ballin[14] used TC 199 medium* and 20% fetal calf serum. Gerstner[27] has written an interesting article on the growth of rodent dental pulp in tissue culture.

SUMMARY

The dental pulp is necessarily affected in the primary inherited disorders of dentin and in those systemic genetic conditions which affect that tissue. Moreover, there is a wide variety of inherited systemic conditions that probably affect the various components of the dental pulp. However, little work has been done in this field. An attempt has therefore been made in this chapter to suggest which inherited systemic conditions might be expected to affect the dental pulp in the hope that further research will be stimulated in this area of oral disease.

---

*Difco Laboratories, Inc., Detroit, Mich.

REFERENCES

1. Adams, R. D., and Sidman, R. L.: Introduction to neuropathology, New York, 1968, McGraw-Hill Book Co.
2. Aguayo, A. J., Nair, C. P. V., and Bray, G. M.: Peripheral nerve abnormalities in the Riley-Day syndrome, Arch. Neurol. 24:106-116, 1971.
3. Album, M. M., and Hope, J. W.: Progeria, report of a case, Oral Surg. 11:985-998, 1958.
4. Andrade, C.: A peculiar form of peripheral neuropathy, Brain 75:408-427, 1952.
5. Appenzeller, O., and Lewis, J. A.: Peripheral neuropathies, Med. Times 97:160-175, 1969.
6. Babel, J., Bischoff, A., and Spoendlin, H.: Ultrastructure of the peripheral nervous system and sense organs, St. Louis, 1970, The C. V. Mosby Co., pp. 99-159.
7. Barabas, G. M.: The Ehlers-Danlos syndrome: abnormalities of enamel, dentine, cementum and the dental pulp: a histologic examination of 15 teeth from 6 patients, Br. Dent. J. 126: 509-515, 1969.

8. Baxter, D. W., and Olszewski, J.: Congenital universal insensitivity to pain, Brain 83:381-393, 1960.

9. Bearn, A. G.: Wilson's disease. In Stanbury, J. B., Wyngaarden, J. B., and Fredrickson, D. S., editors: The metabolic basis of inherited disease, ed. 3, New York, 1972, McGraw-Hill Book Co., pp. 1033-1050.

10. Becak, W., Becak, M. L., and Schmidt, B. J.: Chromosomal trisomy of group 13-15 in two cases of generalized congenital analgesia, Lancet 1:644-645, 1963.

11. Bischoff, A., and Ulrich, J.: Peripheral neuropathy in globoid cell leucodystrophy (Krabbe's disease), Brain 92:861-870, 1969.

12. Blaw, M. E.: Melanodermic type leukodystrophy (adreno-leukodystrophy). In Vinken, P. J., and Bruyn, G. W., editors: Handbook of clinical neurology, vol. 10, Amsterdam, 1970, North-Holland Publishing Co., pp. 128-133.

13. Carpenter, S., Karpati, G., and Andermann, F.: Specific involvement of muscle, nerve and skin in late infantile and juvenile amaurotic idiocy, Neurology (Minneap.) 22:170-186, 1972.

14. Cervenka, J., and Ballin, R.: Tissue culture and chromosomal analysis of dental pulp cells, J. Dent. Res. 53:768, 1974.

15. Cockayne, E. A.: Dwarfism with retinal atrophy and deafness, Arch. Dis. Child. 11:1-8, 1936.

16. Cohen, A. S.: Inherited systemic amyloidosis. In Stanbury, J. B., Wyngaarden, J. B., and Fredrickson, D. S., editors: The metabolic basis of inherited disease, ed. 3, New York, 1972, McGraw-Hill Book Co., pp. 1273-1294.

17. Dean, G.: The porphyrias. In Minckler, J., editor: Pathology of the nervous system, vol. 1, New York, 1968, McGraw-Hill Book Co., pp. 1134-1139.

18. Denny-Brown, D.: Hereditary sensory radicular neuropathy, J. Neurol. Neurosurg. Psychiatry 14:237-252, 1951.

19. Desnick, S. J., et al.: Fabry's disease (ceramide trihexosidase deficiency): diagnostic confirmation by analysis of dental pulp, Arch. Oral Biol. 17:1473-1479, 1972.

20. Dolman, C. L., MacLeod, P. M., and Chang, E.: Skin punch biopsies and lymphocytes in the diagnosis of lipidoses, Can. J. Neurol. Sci. 2:67-73, 1975.

21. Dunn, H. G., Lake, B. D., Dolman, C. L., and Wilson, J.: The neuropathy of Krabbe's infantile cerebral sclerosis (globoid cell leucodystrophy), Brain 92:329, 1969.

22. Dyck, P. J., Ellefson, R. D., Lais, A. C., et al.: Histologic and lipid studies of sural nerves in inherited hypertrophic neuropathy: preliminary report of a lipid abnormality in nerve

and liver in Déjérine-Sottas disease, Mayo Clin. Proc. 45:286-327, 1970.

23. Fredrickson, D. S., Gotto, A. M., Jr., and Levy, R. I.: Familial lipoprotein deficiency (abetalipoproteinemia, hypobetalipoproteinemia, and Tangier disease). In Stanbury, J. B., Wyngaarden, J. B., and Fredrickson, D. S., editors: The metabolic basis of inherited disease, ed. 3, New York, 1972, McGraw-Hill Book Co., pp. 493-530.

24. Gardner, D. G.: Pulpectomy as a diagnostic procedure in metachromatic leukodystrophy, Oral Surg. 23:378-384, 1967.

25. Gardner, D. G., and Majka, M.: The early formation of irregular secondary dentine in progeria, Oral Surg. 28:877-884, 1969.

26. Gardner, D. G., and Zeman, W.: Biopsy of the dental pulp in the diagnosis of metachromatic leukodystrophy, Dev. Med. Child. Neurol. 7:620-621, 1965.

27. Gerstner, R.: Tissue cultures of pulpal elements, Oral Surg. 32:473-486, 1971.

28. Gundlach, K. K. H., Witkop, C. J., Jr., Streed, W. J., and Sauk, J. J., Jr.: Globodontia: a new inherited anomaly of tooth form (abstract), 28th Annual Meeting of the American Academy of Oral Pathology, 1974, New Orleans.

29. Haddow, J. E., Shapiro, S. R., and Gall, D. G.: Congenital sensory neuropathy in siblings, Pediatrics 45:651-655, 1970.

30. Haust, M. D.: The genetic mucopolysaccharidoses (GMS). In Richter, G. W., and Epstein, M. A., editors: Int. Rev. Exp. Pathol. 12:251-314, 1973.

31. Haust, M. D., and Landing, B. H.: Histochemical studies in Hurler's disease: a new method for localization of acid mucopolysaccharide, and an analysis of lead acetate "fixation," J. Histochem. Cytochem. 9:79-86, 1961.

32. Heller, I. H., and Robb, P.: Hereditary sensory neuropathy, Neurology (Minneap.) 5:15-29, 1955.

33. Hers, H. G., and van Hoof, F., editors: Lysosomes and storage diseases, New York, 1973, Academic Press, Inc.

34. Horta, J. S., Filipe, I., and Duarte, S.: Portuguese polyneuritic familial type of amyloidosis, Pathol. Microbiol. (Basel) 27:809-825, 1964.

35. Hughes, E. C., and Csermely, T. V.: Chromosomal constitution of human endometrium, Nature 209:326, 1966.

36. Hughes, J. T.: Neuritis, neuropathy and neuralgia. In Minckler, J., editor: Pathology of the nervous system, vol. 3, New York, 1972, McGraw-Hill Book Co., pp. 2700-2714.

37. Hughes, J. T., Brownell, B., and Hewer, R. L.: The peripheral sensory pathway in Friedreich's ataxia: an examination by light and

electron microscopy of the posterior nerve roots, posterior root ganglia, and peripheral sensory nerves in cases of Friedreich's ataxia, Brain **91**:803-818, 1968.

38. Hunter, I. P., Macdonald, D. G., and Ferguson, M. M.: Developmental abnormalities of the dentine and pulp associated with tumoral calcinosis, Br. Dent. J. **135**:446-448, 1973.

39. Jorgenson, R. J., and Warson, R. W.: Dental abnormalities in trichodento-osseous syndrome, Oral Surg. **36**:643-700, 1973.

40. Kocen, R. S., King, R. H. M., Thomas, P. K., and Haas, L. F.: Nerve biopsy findings in two cases of Tangier disease, Acta Neuropathol. (Berl.) **26**:317-327, 1973.

41. Kornzweig, A. L., and Bassen, F. A.: Retinitis pigmentosa, acanthocytosis and heredodegenerative neuromuscular disease, Arch. Ophthalmol. **58**:183-187, 1957.

42. Kristensson, K., and Olsson, Y.: Peripheral nerve changes in Tay-Sachs and Batten-Spielmeyer-Vogt disease, Acta Pathol. Microbiol. Scand. **70**:630-632, 1967.

43. Krücke, W.: Die mucoide Degeneration der peripheren Nerven, Virchows Arch. (Pathol. Anat.) **304**:442-463, 1939.

44. Linarelli, L. G., and Prichard, J. W.: Congenital sensory neuropathy. Complete absence of superficial sensation, Am. J. Dis. Child. **119**:513-520, 1970.

45. MacEwen, G. D., and Floyd, G. C.: Congenital insensitivity to pain and its orthopedic implications, Clin. Orthop. **68**:100-107, 1970.

46. Magee, K. R.: Congenital indifference to pain, Arch. Neurol. **9**:635-640, 1963.

47. Martin, J. J., and Jacobs, J. J.: Skin biopsy as a contribution to diagnosis in late infantile amaurotic idiocy with curvilinear bodies, Eur. Neurol. **10**:281-291, 1973.

48. McDonald, W. B., Fitch, K. D., and Lewis, I. C.: Cockayne's syndrome: a heredofamilial disorder of growth and development, Pediatrics **25**:997-1007, 1960.

49. McKusick, V. A.: Heritable disorders of connective tissue, ed. 4, St. Louis, 1972, The C. V. Mosby Co.

50. Miyakawa, T., et al.: A biopsy case of Wilson's disease: pathological changes in peripheral nerves, Acta Neuropathol. (Berl.) **24**:174-177, 1973.

51. Moosa, A., and Dubowitz, V.: Peripheral neuropathy in Cockayne's syndrome, Arch. Dis. Child. **45**:674-677, 1970.

52. Neill, C. A., and Dingwall, M. M.: A syndrome resembling progeria; a review of two cases, Arch. Dis. Child. **25**:213-221, 1950.

53. Norman, R. M.: Lipid diseases of the brain. In Williams, D., editor: Modern trends in neurology, London, 1962, Butterworth & Co. (Publishers), Ltd., pp. 173-199.

54. O'Brien, J. S., et al.: Ganglioside storage diseases, Fed. Proc. **30**:956-969, 1971.

55. Olsson, Y., and Sourander, P.: The reliability of the diagnosis of metachromatic leucodystrophy by peripheral nerve biopsy, Acta Paediatr. Scand. **58**:15-24, 1969.

56. Pierre, R. V., and Hoagland, H. C.: 45, X cell lines in adult men: loss of Y chromosome, a normal aging phenomenon? Mayo Clin. Proc. **46**:52-55, 1971.

57. Pinsky, L., and di George, A. M.: Congenital familial sensory neuropathy with anhidrosis, J. Pediatr. **68**:1-13, 1966.

58. Poser, C. M.: Diseases of the myelin sheath. In Minckler, J., editor: Pathology of the nervous system, vol. 1, New York, 1968, McGraw-Hill Book Co., pp. 767-821.

59. Renold, A. E., Stauffacher, W., and Cahill, G. F., Jr.: Diabetes mellitus. In Stanbury, J. B., Wyngaarden, J. B., and Fredrickson, D. S., editors: The metabolic basis of inherited disease, ed. 3, New York, 1972, McGraw-Hill Book Co., pp. 83-118.

60. Ridley, A.: The neuropathy of acute intermittent porphyria, Q. J. Med. **38**:307-333, 1969.

61. Robinson, G. C., Miller, J. R., and Worth, H. M.: Hereditary enamel hypoplasia: its association with characteristic hair structure, Pediatrics **37**:498-502, 1966.

62. Roy, S., Srivastava, R. N., Gupta, P. C., and Mayekar, G.: Ultrastructure of peripheral nerve in Cockayne's syndrome, Acta Neuropathol. (Berl.) **24**:345-349, 1973.

63. Russell, B. G.: The dental pulp in diabetes mellitus, Acta Pathol. Microbiol. Scand. **70**:319-320, 1967.

64. Schwarz, G. A., and Yanoff, M.: Lafora's disease, Arch. Neurol. **12**:172-188, 1965.

65. Schwartz, J. F., Rowland, L. P., Eder, H., Marks, P. A., Osserman, E. F., Hirschberg, E., and Anderson, H.: Bassen-Kornzweig syndrome: deficiency of serum β-lipoprotein: a neuromuscular disorder resembling Friedreich's ataxia, associated with steatorrhea, acanthocytosis, retinitis pigmentosa, and a disorder of lipid metabolism, Arch. Neurol. (Chicago) **8**:438-454, 1963.

66. Seitelberger, F.: Myoclonus body disease. In Minckler, J., editor: Pathology of the nervous system, vol. 1, New York, 1968, McGraw-Hill Book Co., pp. 1121-1134.

67. Shields, E. D., Bixler, D., and El-Kafrawy, A. M.: A proposed classification for heritable human dentine defects with a description of a new entity, Arch. Oral Biol. **18**:543-553, 1973.

68. Sobrevilla, L. A., Goodman, M. L., and Kane, C. A.: Demyelinating central nervous system disease, muscular atrophy and acanthocytosis (Bassen-Kornzweig syndrome), Am. J. Med. **37**:821-828, 1964.

69. Sourander, P., and Olsson, Y.: Peripheral neuropathy in globoid cell leucodystrophy (Morbus Krabbe), Acta Neuropathol. (Berl.) **11**:69-81, 1968.

70. Spranger, J. W., and Wiedemann, H. R.: The genetic mucolipidoses, Humangenetik **9**:113-139, 1970.

71. Stanbury, J. B., Wyngaarden, J. B., and Fredrickson, D. S., editors: The metabolic basis of inherited disease, ed. 3, New York, 1972, McGraw-Hill Book Co.

72. Stanley, H. R.: The effect of systemic diseases on the human pulp, Oral Surg. **33**:606-648, 1972.

73. Stanley, H. R., and Ranney, R. R.: Age changes in the human dental pulp. I. The quantity of collagen, Oral Surg. **15**:1396-1404, 1962.

74. Steinberg, D.: Phytanic acid storage disease (Refsum's syndrome). In Stanbury, J. B., Wyngaarden, J. B., and Fredrickson, D. S., editors: The metabolic basis of inherited disease, ed. 3, New York, 1972, McGraw-Hill Book Co., pp. 833-853.

75. Stewart, R. E.: Dental pulp biopsy in the diagnosis of neurological disorders in childhood, J. Hosp. Dent. Pract. **4**:13-17, 1970.

76. Strich, S. J.: Pathological findings in three cases of ataxia-telangiectasia, J. Neurol. Neurosurg. Psychiatry **29**:489-499, 1966.

77. Suzuki, K., and Suzuki, Y.: Galactosyl ceramide lipidosis: globoid cell leucodystrophy (Krabbe's disease). In Stanbury, J. B., Wyngaarden, J. B., and Fredrickson, D. S., editors: The metabolic basis of inherited disease, ed. 3, New York, 1972, McGraw-Hill Book Co., pp. 760-782.

78. Sweeley, C. C., Klionsky, B., Krivit, W., and Desnick, R. J.: Fabry's disease: glycosphingolipid lipidosis. In Stanbury, J. B., Wyngaarden, J. B., and Fredrickson, D. S., editors: The metabolic basis of inherited disease, ed. 3, New York, 1972, McGraw-Hill Book Co., pp. 663-687.

79. Thomas, P. K., and Lascelles, R. G.: Hypertrophic neuropathy, Q. J. Med. **36**:223-238, 1967.

80. Vasella, F., et al.: Congenital sensory neuropathy with anhidrosis, Arch. Dis. Child. **43**:124-130, 1968.

81. von Hirsch, T., and Peiffer, J.: A histochemical study of the pre-lipid and metachromatic degenerative products in leucodystrophy. In van Bogaert, L., Cummings, J. N., and Lowenthal, A., editors: Brain lipids and lipoproteins, and the leucodystrophies: Proceedings of the Neurochemistry Symposium, Seventh International Congress of Neurology, Rome, 1961, Amsterdam, 1963, Elsevier Publishing Co., p. 134.

82. Webster, H. D., et al.: The role of Schwann cells in the formation of "onion bulbs" found in chronic neuropathies, J. Neuropath. Exp. Neurol. **26**:276-299, 1967.

83. Winklemann, R. K., Lambert, E. H., and Hayles, A. B.: Congenital absence of pain, Arch. Dermatol. **85**:325-339, 1962.

84. Witkop, C. J., Jr.: Manifestations of genetic diseases in the human pulp, Oral Surg. **32**:278-316, 1971.

85. Witkop, C. J., Jr.: Hereditary defects of dentin, Dent. Clin. North Am. **19**:25-45, 1975.

86. Witkop, C. J., Jr., Gundlach, K. K. H., Streed, W. J., and Sauk, J. J., Jr.: Globodontia in the otodental syndrome, Oral Surg. **41**:472-483, 1976.

87. Zeman, W.: Studies in the neuronal ceroid-lipofuscinoses, J. Neuropathol. Exp. Neurol. **33**:1-12, 1974.

11

Oral manifestations of immunological disorders and transplantation genetics

G. R. RIVIERE

The immune system is of immense biological importance. It is the body's strongest defense against bacteria, viruses, and fungi that gain access to the internal milieu and is probably the most important means of protection against the constant threat of spontaneous and environmentally induced neoplasms. Without such discriminating immune functions man could not survive. The need to preserve the intergrity of self is of fundamental importance to all living creatures and was probably the drive for the evolution of the immune system. Thus the most primitive immunological characteristic, the ability to recognize and react against nonself, can be found as far back as the phylogenetically remote sea coral.[108] The higher up the evolutionary tree an animal is found (Fig. 11-1), the more complex and diversified is its immunological capacity.[70, 107]

The immune system has evolved through and is preserved in the genome. Included are genes that define individuality, determine responsiveness, and code for immunologic medi-

I am indebted to Professors W. H. Hildemann, Carl Cohen, and John Cantrell for their valuable discussions. Recognition is due Mr. John McCormick, who made the excellent drawings, and Ms. Myra Rouse and Mrs. Dorothy Pinneo, who typed the manuscript. Mr. James Derkowski is heartily thanked for his continued support throughout the preparation of this chapter.

ators. Although the number of genes comprising the immune system is unknown, it is probably large. Eventually they may be found throughout the genome, but to date only a few have been identified with specific chromosomes,[124] including the X-chromosome.[82, 161] Aberrations in the inheritance of these genes or alterations in the function of the gene products put the host at a great disadvantage. Recent advances in immunotherapy have extended the life span of many who suffer immunological diseases, but most retain a lifelong susceptibility to the environment.

Although the reader is assumed to have some knowledge of immunology, the first part of this chapter will review in a concise manner those concepts which are of fundamental importance to the understanding of immunobiology. The second and third parts relate immunological disorders and transplantation genetics, respectively, to dentistry. No attempt has been made to cite every source of information, but rather reference is made to current works and review articles relevant to the topic at hand. It is hoped that they will be useful to the reader to pursue areas of interest.

REVIEW OF IMMUNE SYSTEMS
Foreignness

Immune responsiveness connotes one essential fact: the host can differentiate between

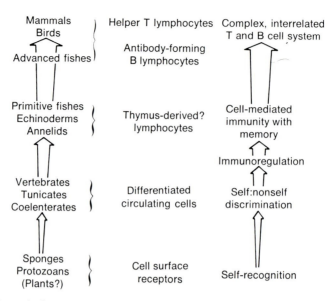

Fig. 11-1. Immunological competence is not limited to mice and men. Indeed, many evolutionarily simple life forms utilize immunological systems to cope with their particular environmental niches. In general, organisms first acquire self-recognition and later, phylogenetically, learn to discriminate between self and nonself. Thymic lymphocytes and cell-mediated immunity are thought to arise before B lymphocytes and humoral immunity. Man's complex system has evolved through summation of these rudimentary forms. (Modified from Hildemann, W. H.: Nature **250:**119, 1974.)

self and the rest of the universe. Recognition of foreignness is the essence of immunological competence and occurs at the molecular level. Since all biological substances are composed of the same chemical building blocks, it is the composition and molecular arrangement of the chemicals that makes nonself foreign. Any biological or synthetic nonself substance that has the potential to stimulate the immune system is called an antigen. There is a lower limit to the size of antigens required to initiate an immune response. This can be demonstrated using small simple chemicals called haptens, such as dinitrophenol (DNP), that will not elicit the formation of antibodies alone but will do so if complexed to a larger carrier molecule such as albumin.

Naturally occurring antigens such as bacteria, viruses, and fungi are composed of a myriad of antigenic units, each of which can stimulate a distinct population of specific antibodies. However, foreign does not necessarily mean exogenous. Self-derived neoplastic cells are antigenic even though they may be mistaken for normal by a susceptible host. Some normal body constituents will also elicit an immune response under unusual conditions, such as when lens protein, spermatozoa, or brain tissue are displaced from their anatomically sequestered body compartments and contact the immune system. Normal tissues can become antigenic as the result of traumatic alteration of their chemical structure. Tissue can also be damaged immunologically as a consequence of its close physical association with, or molecular resemblance to, inciting antigens.

Self-distinction

The individual presumably does not inherit immunological self-awareness, it must be acquired during ontogeny. As far as is known, recognition of foreignness and tolerance of self is strictly a function of lymphocytes, but how they make the critical decision is unknown. The classic concept of clonal selection[37] proposed that self-reactive cell clones were eliminated during fetal development,

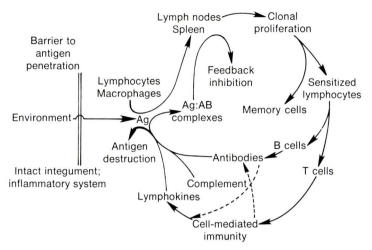

Fig. 11-2. Antigen, having gained access to the internal milieu, is recognized as foreign by the immune system. Antigen-reactive clones of B and T lymphocytes are stimulated to reproduce their own kind, resulting in sensitized lymphocytes, whose mediator systems react specifically with inciting antigen. In some cases, T and B cell systems interact to effect antigen removal. After antigen degradation, soluble antigen-antibody complexes (Ag:Ab) are formed that may act to turn off response cycle. Memory lymphocytes are generated to assure prompt responsiveness should the antigen be encountered again.

producing a permanent state of self-tolerance. It is thought that tissues anatomically sequestered from the immune system during that critical but transient period do not cause the elimination of clones that would react against them. Hence, autoimmunity is possible in later life if the occult tissues are exposed. With this exception, the theory postulates that an adult should have no self-reactive lymphocytes.

Recent experiments have demonstrated, however, that some mature lymphocytes do indeed recognize even accessible self-antigens under in vitro laboratory conditions.[146] Thus self-identification may well involve additional processes that operate throughout the life of the individual. Potential self-reactive lymphocytes may be continually inactivated by soluble self-marker antigens[34] acting on cell membranes. Histocompatibility antigens, commonly associated with cell membranes, have also been found in a soluble form in plasma[9, 18] and may be important in this regard as self-markers. Recent evidence suggests that specific antibody may also play a role in clonal depletion of self-reactive lymphocytes.[132, 211] Whatever the mechanism, the body does not usually react against itself in a detrimental way but can recognize and respond to a seemingly limitless variety of foreign substances.

Responsiveness

Immunological responsiveness means the formation of mediators after antigenic challenge (Fig. 11-2). Only a small part of the total lymphocyte population is stimulated initially, but by rapid cell proliferation these specifically sensitized cells increase their absolute numbers. The type of antigen and the manner in which it is presented to the immune system dictate the nature of the response. B lymphocytes, which are derived from bone marrow precursor cells and which may complete their differentiation in the mammalian liver,[20, 175] are found in the circulation and throughout the peripheral lymphoid system. Once stimulated, they effect a response indirectly through their soluble protein products, the antibodies. Other lymphocytes, called T cells, have completed their differentiation by passage through the thymus. They respond in a more direct manner and effect their role through the release of chemical mediators. Once the offending antigen(s) have been eliminated or neutralized, the immune response is terminated by what may be feedback inhibition by antibodies. However, some long-lived cells of both types persist, carrying information probably within their genomes, which enables them to respond even more rapidly and effectively to a subsequent challenge by the same antigen(s). These cells are called *memory lymphocytes,* and the subsequent challenge is called the *anamnestic* or *secondary* response.

Antibody formation

Essentially all naturally occurring antigens elicit the formation of antibodies. Antibodies are the predominant mediator system involved with antigens that persist within the circulatory system such as bacteria and their soluble products. Approximately 35% of lymphocytes in peripheral blood are antibody-producing B lymphocytes. Antigens composed of homologous repeating units probably stimulate B lymphocytes in spleen and germinal centers of lymph nodes directly, whereas more complex antigens seem to first require processing by macrophages and the help of T lymphocytes before presentation to the B cells. The stimulation occurs first at the cell membrane through antigen receptors, which are probably antibodies themselves. The intracellular processes involved in the induction of antibodies are unknown but probably include RNA-antigen unit complexes and de-repression of antibody structural genes.[207]

The basic antibody unit consists of four polypeptide chains, two heavy (about 430 amino acids each) and two light (about 220 amino acids each), bound together primarily by disulfide linkages.[166, 177] Carbohydrate is found on the heavy chains distal to the antigen combining site. An additional protein, J chain, is associated with the polymeric serum antibodies, IgM and IgA. In addition to J chain, secretory IgA carries another protein component, called *secretory piece.* Early estimates of one gene for each polypeptide chain and associative proteins (J chain and secretory piece) as well as carbohydrate moiety enzymes have been amended on the

basis of more recent data.[60, 132] Thus several genes coding for different polypeptide chains may be required to form a single antibody molecule.

Roughly the first 110 residues from the N-terminal end of both pairs of polypeptide chains, heavy and light, are extremely variable, whereas the remaining units show a great deal of constancy within each group. It is thought that for each heavy class and light chain type there may be a set of related genes that code for the constant region.[130] Differences among the gene products of these sets account for subgroups within the major heavy chain classes and light chain types. On the other hand, a controversy of long standing exists regarding the variable V region genes.[46] It is generally agreed that the variability is related to antigen specificity. That is, basic V region genes code for antibody combining site regions that bind a defined group or type of antigen. Somatic mutation of these V region genes subsequent to antigen stimulation produces combining sites of increasing avidity and specificity. This implies a genetic mechanism that permits unusually high inducible mutation frequencies within the variable region(s), but conserves the genetic structure of the constant region genes. There is also disagreement on the number of germ-line genes inherited. Whatever the mechanisms, the individual does inherit the ability to synthesize proteins that specifically and effectively bind to foreign substances.

The antibody population formed in response to a particular antigen is heterogenous. More than one of the five groups of serum antibodies (IgA, IgD, IgE, IgG, and IgM) are usually represented and furthermore, there are differences among classes of antibodies made in response to a given antigen. Not only are there heavy and light chain differences but also differences in the combination of light chains (κ or λ) with heavy chains ($\propto$, δ, ε, γ, μ), that is, either light chain type can combine with any heavy chain type.

Generally during the primary response, IgM precedes IgG formation, but IgG predominates in late primary and in the secondary response. Just how an individual antibody-forming B lymphocyte knows which structural gene to turn on and for how long and which sets of gene products will combine to make the molecule is unknown. A given cell is thought to express the allele for only one type of heavy and light chain at a time, although it probably has the genetic capacity to make them all.[223] Regulatory mechanisms controlling sequential action of immune response genes may well function in a manner akin to the operon concept described for bacteria. These immune response genes, discussed further in the transplantation genetics section, may be decisive in both structural and regulatory roles.

Most students and practitioners of the dental sciences are aware of the secretory IgA (sIgA) system. It is the major antibody component of the nonvascular secretions and is formed locally in response to local antigenic challenge.[221] The molecules are dimers of the basic unit, two identical pairs of alpha heavy chains and either kappa or lambda light chains, as well as two associated peptides. The first peptide, J chain, is a relatively small protein, which is synthesized by the B lymphocytes and appears to function in formation and stabilization of the dimers.[226] The second peptide, secretory piece, is formed by epithelial cells and is thought necessary for the secretion of the antibody molecule from the tissue to the external fluids. Either or both of these associative peptides may be responsible for sIgA's resistance to in vivo degradation. Secretory IgA does not react with the complement system in a conventional manner, but it probably functions to prevent the ingress of antigens into the body by mechanisms other than cytolysis. IgA has also been implicated in the pathogenesis of some forms of cancer.[171]

Specificity

Specificity is the hallmark of the immune system. Specificity means that once an antigen is identified, the ensuing immune response is made essentially only against that chemical configuration. The progeny of the stimulated clone of lymphocytes produce antibodies of progressively greater capacity to bind to antigen. Some other antigens similar to the inciting antigens will also react with the resultant antibodies, but as the immune response proceeds, the antibodies react with fewer cross-reacting antigens because the avidity and specificity of the antibodies also increases. It should be noted that the relative strength of the cross reaction depends on the resemblance of the cross-reacting antigen to the original. In the main, the immune response can differentiate with amazing clarity between antigenic units. For example, individuals of blood type A form antibodies to erythrocytes of blood group B even though the respective antigens differ by only one hydroxyl group.[106] This acquired information is retained by the long-lived memory cells so that subsequent challenges by the same antigen(s) are met with a rapid and efficient immune response.

Amplification

The interaction of antibody with antigen produces a complex that is more easily phagocytized by the reticuloendothelial system. Moreover, bound antibody can inactivate viruses and neutralize bacterial enzymes and toxins. However, in most cases the antibodies need help in destroying and removing antigen. The effect of antibody on antigen is amplified primarily by a group of eleven serum proteins called the complement (C) system.[152] They are activated by antigen-antibody complexes and interact with one another and the antigen-antibody complex in a sequential manner.[191] At various points nonspecific chemical mediators and events are produced that heighten the immune reaction. Included are increased phagocytosis, immune adherence, anaphylatoxin, neutrophil chemotaxis, histamine release, and cytolysis. IgM and most subgroups of IgG fix complement to their carbohydrate-containing COOH-end constant region. IgA and IgE do not fix complement by this classical pathway but may fix complement by alternate means.[25, 95, 114] The site of synthesis of the complement components is not yet known, although many organ systems have been implicated.[56]

Delayed hypersensitivity

Delayed hypersensitivity, in contrast to humoral immunity (B cells), is mediated by a second type of lymphocyte, the T cell or thymus-derived lymphocyte. T cells also arise in the bone marrow but mature in the thymus, where they acquire innate surface proteins and immunological characteristics that serve to differentiate them from the B lymphocytes. T cells constitute about 65% of the peripheral blood lymphocytes and occupy the medullary area of lymph nodes. The T cells appear to be the primary mediators of defense against pathogens such as fungi and viruses, which become intimately associated with cellular components of tissue. They are also the cells responsible for immunological surveillance against cancer and are the prime cause of foreign tissue graft rejection. T cells probably do not form antibody, although many believe their cell surface antigen receptors are antibody-like.[157, 190] Furthermore, β_2-microglobulin, a small protein found on the surface of lymphocytes, is similar in amino acid sequence to certain portions of antibody molecules. When these peptides are blocked, T-cell function is inhibited.[12] β_2-Microglobulin is also thought to be intimately associated with histocompatibility antigens.[178] Whatever the mechanism, T cells also recognize foreignness and respond to it in much the same way as B cells, that is, by proliferation and differentiation resulting in specificity for antigen. These lymphocytes act directly on the immunological targets by the local release of nonspecific chemical substances that have varied effects. Some chemicals recruit more defense cells to the site (chemotactic factors), others prevent cells from leaving (macrophage migration inhibition factor, MIF), others impart specificity on nonsensitized cells by the transfer of informational subunits (transfer factor), and some damage the target directly (lymphotoxin).

T lymphocytes, perhaps in conjunction with macrophages, also interact with B lymphocytes by breaking down complex antigens into homologous repeating units, which can then stimulate an antibody response. Further interactions between the two systems are evident by the phenomenon called antibody-dependent cell-mediated lympholysis.[42, 160, 230] In this case, specific antibody makes nonsensitized B cells cytotoxic, which helps the T lymphocytes effect their mission. Further examples of the interaction of the major components of the immune system will no doubt appear. Perhaps the most meaningful yet least understood example is the role of antibody in the regulation of immunological responses.

Biological control

Some means of controlling the immune response must exist, lest the proliferation of cells and the production of antibodies continue unchecked. It is likely that feedback inhibition by antibody operates to resolve the response to both B and T lymphocytes. *Immunological enhancement* is the term used to describe prolongation of allograft survival or promotion of tumor growth, often achieved by experimental curtailment of B and T cell functions with specific antibody. Similar observations have been made regarding antibody inhibition of T cell function in some human cancer patients.[100] Whether the antibody is of a certain class or whether it works alone or in conjunction with antigen in the form of soluble antigen-antibody complexes has not been resolved. Nor has the site of effect been ascertained, since evidence exists to implicate the afferent (recognition), central (sensitization), and efferent (mediator production) phases of the immune response under given conditions. Once the offending antigen population is eliminated, the body must shut off lymphocytes already sensitized and functioning as well as inhibit noncommitted cells from responding to degraded but antigenic remnants that may still exist. This ultimate central control is exquisite and must surely extend to the genome of lymphocytes, for memory cells are thought to remain dormant, ready to be triggered by a secondary challenge.

DISORDERS OF IMMUNE SYSTEM

The differentiation and maturation of lymphocyte precursor stem cells from the bone marrow normally produce cells capable of recognizing and responding to foreign but not self-antigens. Genetic or somatic disturbances during the many critical steps involved in this process can result in an inability to cope with foreignness and a propensity to form self-reactive lymphocytes. Thus immunodeficiency states and autoimmunity are thought to be interrelated and may result from the same etiological events during ontogeny.[83] More than twenty immunodeficiency states have been recognized[87] and are characterized by the component of the immune system that appears defective[166] (Fig. 11-3).

Immunodeficiencies

Hypogammaglobulinemia and agammaglobulinemia. Abnormalities in the B cell system can result in an altered ability to produce antibodies. People so affected gen-

erally suffer from repeated bacterial infections often manifested in and about the oral cavity. The Bruton-type agammaglobulinemia is one example of this type of deficiency. It is due to a genetic defect in B cells at some stage of differentiation after the T-B cell dichotomy. The T cell system appears intact, since a normal thymus is found and the affected children can express delayed hypersensitivity. It is inherited as an X-linked recessive trait, and affected males have low or undetectable levels of one or several classes of immunoglobulins.[90] These children often succumb to overwhelming bacterial infections after the protective maternal antibodies are depleted during the first year after birth. Unfortunately these children also suffer an unusually high incidence of rheumatoid arthritis and other autoimmune diseases.

IgA deficiency. Other genetic defects affect the B lymphocytes in such a way that only particular classes of immunoglobulins are affected. A selective IgA deficiency is such a case and occurs with a frequency estimated between 1:700[92] and 1:3000.[193] Like other immunodeficiencies it is often manifested as a sex-linked recessive in males. A chromosomal aberration has been cited,[79, 92, 210] but the evidence is inconclusive. IgA is the major immunoglobulin of the external secretions, and individuals deficient in this antibody suffer repeated infections of the mouth, sinuses, and respiratory tree, and gastrointestinal disturbances like celiac disease.[192] Gingivitis is also a frequent finding among these people,[14] and the incidence of dental caries may be increased.[188]

In this selective immunological disorder both the serum and secretory forms of IgA are deficient or absent altogether, although the number of IgA-B lymphocytes may be found within normal limits.[84] The levels of IgG and IgM in saliva are markedly increased[32, 192] from the normally low concentrations. IgG is thought to gain access to the external fluids by passive diffusion, but IgM appears to be actively transported.[32] In fact, secretory piece, thought to be essential for the transport of dimeric IgA from the tissues, is usually found only with IgA. However, it is

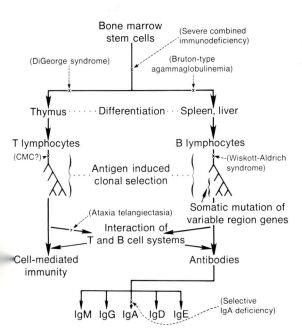

Fig. 11-3. Stem cells from bone marrow proceed through definitive maturation steps in central lymphoid organs, thymus, spleen, and liver. After contact with antigen, reactive clones of lymphocytes complete their differentiation by induced genetic mutation processes during cellular proliferation. Gene defects at any of these critical stages result in aberrant immunological responsiveness. Broken lines indicate the probable site that gene defects occur for a variety of immunological disorders.

found with the IgM in IgA-deficient people.[52] Unlike sIgA, neither IgG nor IgM is stable in the oral fluids, and they are not resistant to the proteases and the harsh external environment.[52] IgA-deficient patients also show autoantibodies to their own IgA and IgM.[4, 228] IgE may be elevated,[192] but it is probably not protective.[55]

People suffering from an IgA deficiency also frequently have an associated autoimmune state such as rheumatoid arthritis, lupus erythematosus, allergic rhinitis, or autoimmune thyroiditis.[31] IgA deficiency is frequently encountered in the combined immunodeficiency ataxia telangiectasia. In both cases thymic function may be depressed.[84]

People with IgA deficiency also have a high incidence of circulating precipitating antibodies to food substances,[193] particularly to a bovine milk protein.[39] Secretory IgA may well act as a barrier to antigen penetration of the mucosa.[1, 101] Thus without sIgA the milk proteins gain access to the local immune system through the mucosa and stimulate an immune response.

Deficiencies of cell-mediated immunity. The diGeorge syndrome is due to a deficit in the T cell system due to the abnormal development of the third and fourth pharyngeal pouches. In this case the B cell system develops normally, and the individuals make normal amounts of antibody. However, the thymus is either absent or rudimentary, so that the thymic-dependent areas of lymph nodes are absent, and a lymphopenic state usually exists. The associated parathyroids are usually affected, resulting in a calcium imbalance. These people do not express any delayed hypersensitivity. Consequently they usually suffer from repeated and severe viral and fungal infection and from small bowel disease[109] and cannot reject foreign tissue grafts. The incidence of cancer among these individuals would no doubt be high should they survive into adulthood. The genetic basis for this developmental anomaly is not known.

Chronic mucocutaneous candidiasis

Chronic mucocutaneous candidiasis (CMC) is characterized by a generalized cutaneous anergy manifested by a persistent, therapy-resistant superficial infection of the cutaneous and mucosal surfaces by *Candida albicans*. The epithelium may be hyperplastic with infiltration by hyphae, lymphocytes, and plasma cells. Recurring respiratory tract infections and endocrine disorders are often associated with this disease.[89, 135, 206] CMC is the result of an immunological defect in the T cell system.[40] Specifically, lymphocytes from people with this abnormality display a decreased transformation to mitogens like phytohemagglutinin (PHA),[36] a decreased production of lymphokines,[135] and decreased chemotactic factor.[205] In addition, lymphocytes are less able to kill appropriately labeled target cells and fail to respond to skin tests.[135] Moreover, many patients have lower than normal levels of serum immunoglobulins. Although some evidence suggests that these patients also have an altered capacity to form antibodies against *C. albicans* antigens,[48, 135] this is not always the case, since some can indeed form antibodies to one or more of the many *C. albicans* antigens.[10] Serum antibodies may have a detrimental effect in an indirect way, since it has been reported that the plasma from patients with CMC inhibits lymphocyte transformation in vitro to a variety of antigens.[44, 176] A deficiency of sIgA seems to heighten the severity of the disease.[135]

Although precipitating antibodies to *Candida* antigens are found,[10] this proposed genetic defect is likely to involve either a selective clone of lymphocytes that specifically reacts to *C albicans,* or a mutant Ir gene. Ir gene function is often associated with T cell funciton, and a T cell defect has been postulated in CMC.[40] In any case, the defect appears to be well defined and limited to these particular antigens.

Combined immunodeficiencies. There also exist several states that are due to abnormalities in both the T and B cell systems.[57, 91] In these cases the genetic defect occurs before the branching of T-B cell differentiation among the bone marrow stem cells. For example, the Swiss-type severe combined immunodeficiency can be inherited as a sex-linked or autosomal recessive and is characterized by severe bacterial, viral, and fungal infections. These children have neither delayed hypersensitivity nor antibody formation.

Ataxia telangiectasia is inherited as an autosomal recessive trait and appears to be a defect primarily of the T cell system, since patients with this disease usually have only a vestigial thymus and little or no delayed hypersensitivity, predisposing them to viral and fungal infections. Most immunoglobulins appear in normal amounts. However, many people fail to form IgG, and a great number have small amounts of IgA or IgE.

The Wiskott-Aldrich syndrome is another severe combined immunodeficiency and is inherited as an X-linked recessive trait. The genetic defect leaves the individual with a general inability to process antigen and with low or negligible amounts of IgA, IgM, and IgE, although IgG may be normal in amount. These people also suffer severe, recurrent infections. A tendency for chromosomal breaks and an unusually high association with leukemia are additional general characteristics of this disorder.

Autoimmunity

The immune system of an individual does not normally react against self components or tissue, but when it does, the phenomenon is called *autoimmunity*. In some cases self-antigens can be made foreign by chemical alteration, but most autoimmune states are the result of a deficient immune system. This is made strikingly clear by the observation that the incidence of autoimmune phenomena and cancer increases with advancing age as the immune system deteriorates.[93, 220, 225] Moreover, an unusually high incidence of autoimmune diseases is found associated with many immunodeficiency states. Although certain families seem to have a propensity for autoimmune phenomena, just as others do for cancer, allergies and other diseases, no proof exists yet to identify a genetic cause for autoimmune diseases.

Several diseases are recognized as autoimmune states. In each case, one or more parts of the body are the target of its own immune system. In Hashimoto's thyroiditis, for example, antibodies are made against indigenous thyroglobulin. Moreover, sensitized T lymphocytes are also found.[41] In rheumatoid arthritis there are circulating antibodies against self-immunoglobulins. The complexes formed in the tissues contribute significantly to the pathogenesis of the disease.

Lupus erythematosus is another autoimmune disease characterized by degeneration of the connective tissue and manifested as lesions of the skin and other tissues and organs. It occurs as a chronic discoid type and as an acute systemic, fatal form. Oral lesions are found and take on the appearance of leukoplakia with time.[104, 151] Salivary gland involvement is not uncommon.[120] Antinuclear antibodies are found, but their role in the cause of the disease is not clear. In fact, they may be the result of the widespread cellular damage and the altered immune system.

Sjögren's syndrome. Sjögren's syndrome is an autoimmune disease that manifests itself primarily in the mouth.[3] The clinical diagnosis is made if two or more of the following triad is present: keratoconjunctivitis sicca, xerostomia, and one of the several connective tissue diseases, including rheumatoid arthritis, lupus erythematosus, systemic sclerosis, polyarteritis nodosa, polymyositis, or dermatomyositis. Clinically, Sjögren's syndrome may resemble Behcet's syndrome, Reiter's syndrome, and scleroderma. It is found most often in women after the age of 40 years.[59, 133, 212] Histologically the salivary glands are heavily infiltrated by lymphocytes. The acinar tissue is replaced by these cells, eventually leading to fibrosis and glandular ectasia.

The infiltrating lymphocytes synthesize large amounts of IgG and IgM locally.[6, 213] Some antibody-forming lymphocytes have multiple H chain types on their surface, which is atypical.[224] The multiple classes of Ig associated with the cells may be due to immune complexes or autoantibodies, since the infiltrating cells do make anti-immunoglobulins, including rheumatoid factor.[6]

The salivary ducts appear to be the target for a unique organ-specific autoantibody (ASD). This antibody may be protective, since when it is present in measurable amounts, there is less infiltration and glandular damage.[7] The ASD appears in serum but not in saliva.[23]

There also appears to be a defect in the T cell system, since peripheral blood lymphocytes from people with Sjögren's syndrome have a decreased response to stimulation by mitogens and decreased delayed hypersensitivity reactivity.[21, 140] However, lymphocytes from patients with Sjögren's syndrome do react to parotid gland extract as if they were sensitized.[21]

It can be seen that Sjögren's syndrome presents the typical picture for an autoimmune disease. It is almost always found in conjunction with an impaired immune system, and self-reactive lymphocytes are the destructive agents. The target appears to be the ducts of the salivary glands. The destruction is probably mediated by T cells, since they react to antigen in vitro as if they were sensitized, but the role of antibody cannot be excluded. The B cell system appears aberrant, since an unusually high concentration of IgG and IgM but not IgA appears locally. Other unusual states of immunoglobulin synthesis are also reported, including IgM macroglobulinemia and anti-IgG. The T cell defect, if it exists, appears low grade but general as defined by common tests for delayed hypersensitivity, such as DNCB.

Oral ulceration. Another oral disease that may have an autoimmune etiology is that of recurrent oral ulcerations.[134, 136] The principle of autoimmunity to epidermal tissues is certainly not unusual, since pemphigus results from autoallergy to mucus membranes and skin.[183, 196] The concept of autoimmunity in oral ulceration is not new.[199] Circulating antibodies that react specifically with cells from epithelium and mucosa are found in people suffering from this affliction,[136] and antibodies against nuclear material can also be demonstrated.[2] Furthermore, T lymphocytes may also be involved in the pathogenesis of aphthous stomatitis.[72, 173]

Lymphoid cancer

A third type of immunological disorder is lymphoid neoplasia. Whereas the immuno-

deficiency diseases and autoimmunity involve altered states of competence, the neoplastic disorders are due to uncontrolled and excessive cellular proliferation (leukemia, lymphoma) or protein synthesis (myeloma).

Leukemia. The leukemias are debilitating, usually fatal diseases of unknown cause.[181] The gene-controlled maturation of affected cells is thought to be defective, so that the proliferation of lymphocytes, monocytes, or stem cells (myelogenous leukemia) is uncontrolled. The result is abnormally high numbers of the cells and their precursors in the peripheral blood and in cellular infiltrations of the spleen, liver, bone marrow, and lymph nodes.[229] In some cases the leukemic cells express new, nonself surface antigens.[77] Acute lymphocytic leukemia occurs most frequently in the first decade of life, whereas acute monocytic and myelocytic leukemias may occur at any age. In general the chronic forms are more frequent after the age of 30.[26, 103, 181]

Spontaneous bleeding of the gingiva, petechiae and ecchymoses, pallor, and ulceration are among the most frequently reported oral findings.[61, 103] Gingival hypertrophy is found in the chronic forms,[180] especially in the monocytic types,[103] but is rare in children.[61] Oral pain is a common complaint,[121, 229] often including the joints.[102, 103] The gingivitis that often accompanies this disease can some times be ameliorated by instituting appropriate oral hygiene measures.[141] The cervical and submandibular nodes are often palpable.[26, 229] Involvement of the lacrimal and salivary glands can lead to dysfunction.[26]

The acute leukemias are often associated with agranulocytopenia,[26] which makes these individuals more susceptible to bacterial infections.[229] Necrosis of the mucosa[103] and secondary bacterial infections are not uncommon.[102, 103]

Radiographic signs of leukemia have also been reported,[61, 62] particularly in the chronic forms.[103] Cellular infiltration of alveolar bone can lead to resorption, displaced and loose erupted teeth, and in some cases to displacement of developing teeth.

Myeloma. The hypergammaglobulinopathies are another form of lymphoid neoplasia. The primary characteristic is excessive production and secretion of antibody molecules and their heavy and light chain components. Although more than one type of antibody may be formed as in multiple myeloma, usually the disease is limited to a selective abnormality of one type: IgG, IgM, or IgA.

Each heavy and light chain pair, whether incorporated into an intact molecule or alone (as in Bence Jones proteins of IgM macroglobulinemia, which are light chains in the urine) are identical for each individual as regards amino acid sequence. In addition, chromosomal abnormalities are regularly observed.[106] Thus affected individuals may suffer a defect in the regulation of protein synthesis involving a unique set of antibody structural genes. The fact that oligomeric serum myeloma IgA molecules combine with secretory piece and are secreted like sIgA[51] emphasizes the normal quality albeit abnormal quantity of the antibodies.

The clinical signs and symptoms of the myelomas are similar to those of the leukemias. Surface petechiae and ecchymoses, bleeding tendencies, bone and joint pains, ulceration, and lymphadenopathy often involving the oral and facial structures are reported.[94, 201] Moreover, radiographic lesions of cancellous bone have also been observed.

The incidence of hypergammaglobulinemia is much greater in men than in women[197] and tends to increase with age,[201] as do most diseases that involve the immune system.[93, 225]

Myeloma is thought to have a genetic basis,[197] and abnormal chromosomes have been reported.[94] Hypercalcemia is frequently associated, as is primary amyloidosis.[201]

Immunotherapy. The treatment of patients with aberrant immune systems often entails heroic efforts designed to eliminate environmental insults,[27, 71] such as sequestration in a germ-free environment. Immunotherapy may be instituted to reconstitute the immunological system.[91, 154, 159] When chemicals are used to suppress already abnormal lymphoid systems as in leukemias and lymphomas (such as Hodgkin's disease), infections of many

sorts are a predictable and extremely dangerous consequence.[8] Bacterial,[189] fungal,[17] viral,[209] and protozoan[182] infections are common problems. In these cases the side effects of therapy may be as debilitating as the disease.

Immune complex disease

The nonspecific chemical mediators unleashed by the interaction of antigen with antibody and T lymphocytes are insensitive to the genetic origin of the biological material in the immediate area. Ordinarily, the antigen bears the brunt of the attack, and any incidental damage to the host tissue is quickly repaired. However, when the battle front persists in the same locale for extended periods, the accumulative insult to the host can be destructive. Such is the case for periodontal disease.

Periodontal disease begins with an accumulation of bacteria and debris about the teeth, which elicits a gingivitis. Bacteria growing in the plaque release soluble substances such as hyaluronidase,[87] which increase the permeability of the gingiva[74] and enhance further antigen uptake.[158] The bacterial products that permeate the gingiva maintain the inflammatory state and contribute to the stimulation of the immune system.[19] Although many bacterial substances can play a direct role in the pathogenesis of periodontitis,[87, 99] the accumulation of immunological mediators[19, 138] within the gingiva also contributes to the severe damage characteristic of the disease.

The lack of a good experimental model has precluded the definitive experiments that would firmly establish and define the influence of sensitized T lymphocytes in periodontal disease. Nevertheless, enough evidence exists to confidently predict a major pathogenic role for cell-mediated immunity,[54, 112, 135, 139, 148] although contradictory evidence does exist.[167, 168] Peripheral blood lymphocytes from people with periodontal disease are stimulated to divide and are transformed into blast cells in vitro when cultured with plaque. Moreover, the antigens necessary for stimulation of these presumptively sensitized lymphocytes are also found in a soluble form in saliva,[110, 205] although the validity of this technique has been questioned.[122]

Lymphocytes from nondiseased people are not transformed by plaque, but sensitization can occur in as few as 7 days after cessation of normal hygiene.[139] Lymphocytes taken from patients with periodontal disease and stimulated in vitro release lymphotoxin, which can kill cultured fibroblasts[111, 195] and MIF, which inhibits motile cells from leaving the area of its influence.[117] In addition to these and other well characterized lymphocyte-derived mediators that are thought to contribute to the tissue destruction, plaque-stimulated lymphocytes also release a factor that directly causes resorption of bone in vitro.[113]

Plaque regularly stimulates transformation and chemical mediator formation when the lymphocytes are taken from people with mild to moderate periodontal disease. However, lymphocytes from patients suffering severe periodontitis are not usually so affected by plaque.[116] This is somewhat surprising in view of the fact that these same lymphocytes are able to display a strong chemical mediator response.[117] A possible explanation for this discrepancy might be related to the observation that in these people serum factors, presumably antibodies, can be shown to be inhibitory for lymphocyte transformation, not only for autologous cells but also for cells from different donors.[115] In these cases the blocking antibodies are correlated with the severity of the disease. In other cases, antibodies have been shown to enhance cell-mediated immunity. Thus it appears that humoral immunity also plays a significant role in the pathogenesis of periodontal disease.[88]

Antibodies specific for oral bacteria and antibody-producing cells are found within the gingiva and in the peripheral lymphoid tissues of people with periodontal disease.[86, 153] By combining with soluble and particulate antigen in the gingiva, antibodies no doubt protect the host against disseminated bacterial infections and toxic reactions. Nevertheless, the very act of containment results in tissue damage. Both immune complexes and endotoxins activate the complement system,[205]

which can also be found within diseased gingiva.[87] Some of the activated complement components, including C5a or chemotactic factor, enhance inflammation by attracting polymorphonuclear leukocytes (PMNs), increasing the permeability of small blood vessels and causing smooth muscle contraction.[205] The lysosome enzymes released by the PMNs increase tissue damage. In addition, the activation of the complement system leads to factors that cause the degranulation of mast cells, liberating histamine and heparin. The number of mast cells has been inversely correlated with the severity of periodontal disease.[87, 164]

IgE, the cytophilic antibody that contributes to atopy, has also been associated with periodontal disease. IgE and IgE-producing cells can be found in diseased gingiva[86] and are thought to combine specifically with bacteria present in the tissue.[165] The proposed effect of IgE is strengthened by the finding of a significant positive correlation between immediate hypersensitivity to actinomyces from dental plaque and periodontal disease.[164]

IgA and IgA-containing cells are reported to be in higher concentrations relative to IgG in the gingiva of diseased patients.[87] Serum IgA is also known to rise in concentration in proportion to the severity of the disease,[164] although correlations of precipitating serum antibodies with oral bacteria are tenuous at best.[86] Secretory IgA from parotid saliva appears to be unrelated to periodontal disease,[47] but IgA in whole saliva has been found to be higher in periodontal disease,[143] probably due to leakage of serum IgA from crevicular fluids.

TRANSPLANTATION GENETICS
Histocompatibility system

Tissues grafted from one person to another nonidentical individual will be rejected because the immune system of the latter recognizes cell-associated antigens of the former as foreign. This seemingly simple and straightforward phenomenon is the basis for one of the most complex and fascinating fields of scientific endeavor, histocompatibility genetics.[155] From its modest beginnings in blood group serology,[203] this facet of immunogenetics has blossomed to include such diverse fields as transplantation, cancer, and phylogeny (the reader is referred to the excellent text by Hildemann[106] for an in-depth approach to immunogenetics).

Cells possess molecularly distinct[215] surface components, many of which are glycoproteins, which serve to distinguish the individual from the rest of the universe. Recent evidence suggests that these antigens may share a common structural unit.[119] They are necessarily antigenic when exposed to another host, and transplantation was the means by which they were discovered. These histocompatibility antigens, their genes, and the genes and gene products associated with them are the objects of intense investigation by the immunological community.[214]

The histocompatibility genes of mice,[126, 127] rabbits,[53, 219] rhesus monkeys,[13] and man[218] are concentrated in a polygenic region called the major histocompatibility complex

(MHC). The murine system has been studied the most, and although differences are thought to exist, each species shares the overall design. Included in the complex are genes that determine immunological individuality, the histocompatibility (H) genes, those which control immunological responsiveness, the Ir genes, and those which provoke lymphocyte proliferation, the MLR (mixed lymphocyte reaction) genes. Included in the murine system are the Ss, Slp genes, which encode serum β-globulins, which influence complement levels.[69]

The MHC of mice and man are compared in Fig. 11-4. In mice, many H genes have been defined, but the ones that provoke the strongest rejection episodes are called H-2 genes and are found within the MHC. The rest of the murine H genes are distributed throughout the genome in a manner that may well prove to be analogous to the well-known MHC of chromosome 17.[106] In man, the corresponding strong antigens are called HL-A

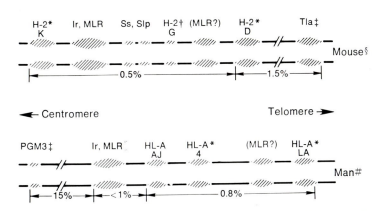

Fig. 11-4. Diagram exemplifies major histocompatibility complex (MHC) of all mammalian species studied to date. Each pair of double lines represents diploid chromosomes of mouse and man, respectively. Relative positions for known genetic loci of each set are represented by shaded areas, and map distances, expressed as recombination frequencies, are given below chromosome sets. H-2 and HL-A gene products are characterized using cytotoxic antisera, whereas MLR gene products are detected by in vitro lymphocyte transformation. Ir genes are characterized by innate responsiveness of experimental animals to defined antigens. *Murine H-2D and H-2K specificities are thought to correspond to human HL-A (LA) and HL-A (4) specificities, but otherwise no comparisons are intended between the two species as regards gene positions or loci size. †From Snell, G. D., Cherry, M., and Demant, P.: Transplant. Rev. 15:3, 1973. ‡PGM3 and Tla are nonimmune genetic loci on same chromosome but unrelated to MHC of man and mouse, respectively. §Modified from Klein, J., Bach, F. H., and Festenstein, F.: Immunogenetics 1:184, 1974. ‖From Blumenthal, M. N., et al.: Science 184:130, 1974. #Modified from Thorsby, E.: Transplant. Rev. 18:51, 1974.

(for human leukocyte antigens), and the MHC resides on chromosome 6.[133a, 218]

The histocompatibility antigens elicit the formation of antibodies and are characterized by serological techniques, primarily lympho-cytotoxicity (SD antigens). Although the H-2 antigens were originally discovered using erythrocytes, they do not carry all the specific-ities, whereas nucleated cells do. It must be noted that the ABO blood group antigens of erythrocytes are also antigenic and act as transplantation antigens.

As shown in Fig. 11-4, the H-antigen genes are located in two regions called *loci,* al-though more than one gene may be responsi-ble for a given H-specificity.[63] In man, a third locus has been described,[218] which may be analogous to the proposed third H-2 locus described by Snell.[204] The first two loci are thought to be separated by a distance cor-responding to a recombination frequency of about 0.5%. The alleles at each locus are mutually exclusive so that in the diploid cell there may be as many as four or as few as two different H genes. Each is codominant, and the gene products are expressed as dis-tinct units on the cell membrane.

The H genes are highly polymorphic.[125] That is, more than one heritable gene form exists for each locus. At least fifteen alleles have been defined for the first locus and twenty for the second in man.[68] Moreover, there is some speculation that H genes may mutate at an unexpectedly high rate.[200] What, then, is the biological function of this diverse genetic system? Three major hypotheses have been advanced. In brief, the first[118] proposes that the H genes acting through a process of clonal selection and random mutation generate lymphocytes, particularly B cells, capable of responding to any antigen except endogenous H antigens (self-tolerance). This necessarily implies simultaneous genetic evo-lution of H genes and antibody V genes, even though the two systems are not known to be so linked. The second theory[28] emphasizes the potential role of H antigens in cellular differ-entiation and cell-to-cell recognition, genetic polymorphism being a requirement for the integrity of the animal. The third hypothesis[38]

suggests that the polymorphic H system evolved to protect the host against the possi-bility of contamination by cells from an-other individual, particularly cancer cells. Whatever the evolutionary drive, the H sys-tem provides sufficient diversity through heterozygosity to ensure uniqueness and vigor of the individual.[68] This, of course, is of para-mount importance for immunological surveil-lance and the detection of aberrant, neo-plastic cells, viruses, and other foreign material.

The second group of genes located within and near the MHC are called MLR (mixed lymphocyte reaction) genes. Their gene prod-ucts do not stimulate antibodies like the SD antigens but will cause genetically disparate lymphocytes to proliferate in vitro, hence their designation as lymphocyte-defined (LD) antigens. In most species there appear to be at least two such loci, at least one of which is within the MHC. That one is closely as-sociated with one of the SD loci (Fig. 11-4) but is not always inherited with it, producing a linkage disequilibrium. The recombination frequency between the second HL-A locus and the major MLR of man is estimated to be about 0.1%.[218] Other genetic loci have been described that also contribute to in vitro lymphocyte activation but are outside the MHC, such as the M locus.[78]

LD antigens stimulate proliferation in non-sensitized cells, whereas SD antigens can only stimulate blastogenesis among sensitized lymphocytes.[218] The LD antigens are con-sidered by many to represent T cell antigen receptors. Thus in vitro blastogenesis may duplicate primary antigen recognition and the proliferation of some antigen-reactive cell clones.

Current evidence links these LD antigens (MLR loci gene products) with the third major component of the MHC, immune response (Ir) genes.[97] They were originally described in guinea pigs and defined on the basis of responsiveness to synthetic poly-nucleotide antigens. Responder strains ex-pressed a primary IgM response as well as secondary IgG and memory. Nonresponders produced only the initial IgM antibody.

Many Ir genes are now thought to be expressed on both T and B lymphocytes, although the gene products could represent antigen receptors for T cells, amplifying T and B cell functions, and perhaps are involved in the regulation of cellular tolerance.[149]

Like the LD antigens, Ir gene products were thought not to evoke antibodies in a genetically dissimilar host, but recent evidence with mice is to the contrary.[67, 98] The Ir genes are involved in a variety of immunological phenomena, including antibody responsiveness to several defined synthetic antigens as well as naturally occurring proteins,[66] susceptibility and resistance of laboratory animals to cancer viruses, and graft versus host (GVH) disease.[98] The MLR genes correlate most closely with the proposed chromosomal locations of the Ir genes and may be one and the same.

T cell function may also be controlled genetically. Recent evidence[222] suggests that recessive genes, in concert with the sex-linked recessive immunodeficiency states, may influence the level of responsiveness to defined antigens.

Histocompatibility (HL-A) antigens have been linked to the incidence of a number of diseases in humans.[64, 73] Hodgkin's disease,[76] celiac disease,[144] acute lymphatic leukemia, systemic lupus erythematosus, ankylosing spondylitis, and others have been cited.[76, 218] Recent studies link sensitivity to ragweed antigens E[24, 142] and RA-5[150] to HL-A SD antigens and suggest the presence of Ir genes in man.[36] As in other species, the Ir genes of man are placed outboard of the second SD locus in the MHC in concert with current dogma. Certain other HL-A antigens of the second locus have also been correlated with the incidence of some immunological diseases.[156]

The discovery of the importance of MHC antigens in transplantation has led to many efforts to match donor and recipients for SD and LD antigens to circumvent rejection. The results are encouraging[65, 217] but are by no means as good as was expected.[5, 96] Tissue grafted between related humans who are SD identical and LD negative (no stimulation in MLR) is the best combination[217] but is rare.[63] In general, transplants between human siblings do better than between unrelated people, and the more alike the individuals are as regards MHC genes, the better the grafts will do.[208] Paradoxically, selective mismatches may also contribute to prolonged graft survival,[33] perhaps because of an immunoblocking mechanism or an undetected LD antigen identity.

The ABO blood group antigens must also be considered when searching for prospective donors of organs, since they certainly do influence the survival of transplanted tissue.[147]

As regards kidney transplantation in humans, organs from cadavers can be used successfully, provided the donor and recipient can be properly matched for HL-A (SD) antigens.[216] In these cases MLR typing is not always possible. Kidneys are the most successfully grafted organs, with a predicted survival rate of from 60% to 90%.[208] The factors influencing the survival of kidneys include HL-A haplotype differences (the H genes inherited on each chromosome of the diploid pair), unresponsiveness to HL-A antigens, and presensitization (many transplant candidates have received transfusions of whole blood and thus have been exposed to HL-A antigens on the cells). Cadaver donor transplants are influenced by the preceding factors to a lesser extent than they are by the production of HL-A antibodies after transplantation.[172]

Transplantation is not without hazard. Certainly, the host is expected to become sensitized to donor antigens should they differ from his own. In fact, the onset of cytotoxic antibodies against HL-A antigens is considered to herald the clinical demise of the graft.[172] Preexisting HL-A antibodies as in multiparous women and in patients who have had many transfusions make for a guarded prognosis, although preexisting anti–HL-A lymphocytotoxic antibodies have little effect on kidney allograft survival as long as they are not specific for donor antigens.[43] Diseases of many sorts may also be transferred with the graft, so that precautions must be taken in screening potential donors. Cancer itself can be transmitted with the tissue or may arise de novo as a result of immunosuppressive drugs that are frequently administered to prevent rejection.[81] Nevertheless, these are infrequent occurrences; in the majority of cases, the transplant prolongs a useful life.

Tooth transplantation

Transplantation techniques and theory are of particular interest to the dental community because of their potential applicability to prosthetic, endodontic, and periodontal surgery. Teeth, bone, and mucosa have been transplanted in the past, even among humans, with scant regard for immunological processes. Modern dental scientists are now re-examining these techniques with great expectations.

Numerous reviews of tooth transplantation have appeared in the past decade.[49, 163, 198, 227] All emphasize the fact that teeth and tooth germs, like other tissues, are usually rejected when grafted to a genetically different host. This has been demonstrated in a variety of species, utilizing not only orthotopic graft sites but also an array of heterotopic transplant locations. Primary grafts of teeth sensitize a host to subsequent transplants of donor-type tissue, resulting in accelerated rejection of the second-set graft. The converse is also true, indicating that both mature teeth and tooth buds express the histocompatibility antigens.

Although antibodies are formed against tooth transplants,[184, 185] rejection of teeth, like other tissues, is mediated to a large extent by T lymphocytes.[184, 187] Without a thymus, animals cannot reject teeth.[145, 174] That the antigens of the histocompatibility gene complex are responsible for and are the targets of the rejection episodes is amply confirmed by experiments utilizing genetically defined laboratory animals.

Tooth buds are rejected within 7 to 10 days when transplanted heterotopically[128] or orthotopically[186] among mice who differ at the major, H-2, histocompatibility loci. H-2 compatibility with multiple non–H-2 loci differences also leads to prompt graft rejection.[187] On the basis of histological tech-

niques,[186, 187] the events leading to tooth rejection are similar to those observed for other tissue. Within 4 or 5 days after transplantation, the grafts are revascularized in the host. Shortly thereafter, lymphocytes begin to accumulate about the apices of the teeth and within the pulp cavities about the blood vessels. As the density of the infiltrating cells increases, graft cell damage becomes apparent. The cytolysis begins within the coronal portion of the pulp and proceeds toward the apex, so that by the second week after transplantation, most of the pulp tissue has been destroyed. The cemental surfaces are attacked later than the pulp tissue, and resorption of the cementum and dentin occurs over a period of several weeks. Thus radiographical and clinical examination of transplanted teeth are unreliable parameters of graft rejection.

However, when only single non–H-2 gene loci differences exist, teeth are permanently accepted,[123] whereas skin grafts among the same combinations are eventually rejected. When two non–H-2 loci differ between donor and recipient, another factor, allelic direction, becomes critical.[186] Allelic direction identifies the influence of those genes not serologically defined but which contribute to host responsiveness. For example, mouse strain B10.129 (21M) skin grafts[45] and tooth grafts[186] on B10.129 (10M) recipients result in moderately prompt rejection; skin is rejected within 22 to 30 days and teeth within 9 to 13 days. The speed is also dependent on graft size, the smaller the faster. The events differ when grafts are exchanged in the opposite direction. 10M skin grafts are rejected by 21M host within 60 days, but tooth germs, although they experience a transient immunological crisis, do survive.[186] Thus the antigens of the donor and the ability of the host to recognize and respond to them influence graft survival. The influence of MLR genes has not been determined.

To avoid the rejection phenomena altogether and to take advantage of the biostatic character of avital teeth, a variety of techniques have been employed to condition teeth and increase their usefulness. Cryopreservation and tissue culture,[15, 50, 58, 179, 202] irradiation,[80, 169] and fluoride treatment[85] have all been tried with equivocal results. In humans, teeth from mismatched donors are rejected and eventually resorbed. Even isogeneic or autogeneic mature donor teeth are usually resorbed to some degree.[29] Endodontic treatment before storage in the cold for short periods may increase the transplantability of teeth.[162]

Bone transplantation

The restoration of bony defects induced by trauma or disease is a major concern of dental surgeons, especially oral surgeons and periodontists. The use of bone and bonelike substances to fill the defects and stimulate bone formation to effect the repair is the most popular form of treatment. However, bone grafts must not only survive transplantation but must also actively contribute to the reestablishment of normal contours. Incompatible grafts of bone are rejected unless the organic antigenic components are first removed. The product of such treatment is a biostatic material lacking osteogenic capacity, which, like cartilage, is useful only for space filling.[29] Attempts to transplant genetically disparate bone capable of osteogenic activity have been generally unsuccessful, although some favorable results have been reported.[75] The use of autogenous bone and marrow circumvents the problem of histoincompatibility.[30]

Periodontal defects can usually be repaired using autogenous alveolar bone,[22] with or without an immunologically inert scaffolding material.[129] However, larger facial defects require more substantial grafts. Notwithstanding the problems encountered when incompatible tissue is used, the restoration of large defects involves the undesirable consequences of mobility, resorption, and fibrous unions of free bony grafts.[30] Furthermore, the use of autogenous tissue necessitates at least one additional operation site to procure the required mass of graft material, thus imposing further stress and trauma on the patient. Another approach is to use tissue from a source other than the patient, preferably from another human to avoid strong interspecies antigens.

Surprisingly little effort has been expended to explore the usefulness of bone transplantation among humans. However, the excellent studies by Hiatt and Schallhorn[105, 194] have laid the groundwork for further studies toward that end. They found that allogeneic bone from donors matched for HL-A and ABO antigens with recipients could be transplanted with results comparable to other more conventional methods. This approach would offer an unlimited supply of physiologically favorable donor tissue. However, tissue typing facilities are not universally available to the dental clinician. Moreover, the genetic parameters that would define acceptable donor-recipient matches have yet to be elucidated. It must also be emphasized that allogenic transplantation is not without hazard,[105] as discussed previously (see Transplantation section). Nevertheless, with the surge of immunological research in the field of transplantation biology, these problems should be overcome soon.

SUMMARY

Animals at almost every level of phylogenetic development have evolved cellular defense mechanisms with some resemblance to the mammalian immune system. At the heart of the immune system are the lymphocytes. The phenotype of these cells is determined during ontogeny, and their single most important characteristic is the ability to distinguish between self and nonself. Reactive clones selectively reproduce when stimulated immunologically, generating functionally active lymphocytes, which react specifically with the inciting antigen.

Each animal inherits a unique but finite array of genes, which determine its immunological stature. Although some await definition, many have been characterized. The histocompatibility genes are expressed on virtually every cell and serve as markers of self. The immune response genes and MLR genes are essential for and may, in fact, govern the initiation of immune responsiveness. Other genes encode the structure of immunological mediators and regulate their synthesis.

Perturbances within the genome can lead to alterations of the functional capacity of the immune system and, consequently, to a decreased ability of the animal to survive. Immunodeficiency diseases are due to defective maturation of one or more of the components of the immune system. The stage of development at which the genetic disturbance occurs dictates the scope of involvement and the severity of the disease. Immune responsiveness to self-antigens is likewise a sign of an immunological disturbance. This lack of discrimination, autoimmunity, may be due to acquired alterations or to genetic defects within the recognition mechanism. Lymphoid cancer, characterized by either the uncontrolled proliferation of cells (leukemia) or by the unregulated synthesis of immunoglobulins (myeloma), is yet another immunological disorder. The infrequent occurrence of these diseases emphasizes the genetic stability and essential nature of the immune system.

The immune system may play a critical role in the pathogenesis, if not the cause, of periodontal disease. Certainly a substantial body of evidence has accumulated implicating both T and B cell mediators as the causative factors of much of the characteristic tissue destruction and bone resorption. Recurrent oral ulceration may also have an immunological basis. In both cases, a protective immune response may lead to incidental host tissue destruction because of repeated, chronic insults to the tissue.

Advances in understanding of the immune system have led to new concepts in medical therapy. In particular, the transplantation of tissues and organs from one individual to another after matching for the genes of the major histocompatibility gene complex has led to prolonged graft and host survival. These successes have promoted interest in applying transplantation techniques to surgical and prosthetic problems within the dental profession. In particular, the transplantation of teeth and bone hold great promise as alternatives to conventional dental surgery techniques.

Although the emphasis of this chapter has been on disorders of the immune system, it must be recalled to the reader that for the vast majority of living creatures the immune system, to whatever extent it has evolved, permits the continued existence of life in what can only be considered a most inhospitable environment. The higher life forms are surrounded by a sea of microorganisms and inundated by harsh chemicals and energy emissions. That life persists at all is in no small way due to the extraordinarily efficient immune system.

REFERENCES

1. Adams, D.: The effect of saliva on the penetration of fluorescent dyes into the oral mucosa of the rat and rabbit, Arch. Oral Biol. 19:505, 1974.
2. Addy, M., and Dolby, A. E.: Aphthous ulceration: the antinuclear factor, J. Dent. Res. 51:1594, 1972.
3. Akin, R. K., Kreller, A. J., III, Walters, P. J., and Trapani, J. S.: Sjögren's syndrome, J. Oral Surg. 33:27, 1975.
4. Ammann, A. J., and Hong, R.: Selective IgA deficiency and autoimmunity, Clin. Exp. Immunol. 7:833, 1970.
5. Amos, D. B., and Yunis, E. J.: Histocompatibility matching and donor selection. In Yunis, E. J., Gatti, R. A., and Amos, D. B., editors: Tissue typing and organ transplantation, New York, 1973, Academic Press, Inc., p. 117.
6. Anderson, L. G., Cummings, N. A., and Asofsky, R.: Salivary gland immunoglobulin and rheumatoid factor synthesis in Sjögren's syndrome, Am. J. Med. 53:456, 1972.
7. Anderson, L. G., Tarpley, T. M., Talal, N., et al.: Cellular-versus-humoral autoimmune responses to salivary gland in Sjögren's syndrome, Clin. Exp. Immunol. 13:335, 1973.
8. Armstrong, D.: Infectious complications in cancer patients treated with chemical immunosuppressive agents, Transplant. Proc. 5:1245, 1973.
9. Aster, R. H., Miskovich, B. H., and Rodey, G. E.: Histocompatibility antigens of human plasma: localization to the HLD-e lipoprotein fraction, Transplantation 16:205, 1973.
10. Axelsen, N. H., Kirkpatrick, C. H., and Buckley, R. H.: Precipitins to *Candida albicans* in chronic mucocutaneous candidiasis studied by crossed immunoelectrophoresis with intermediate gel, Clin. Exp. Immunol. 17:385, 1974.

11. Bach, M. L., and Bach, F. H.: The genetics of histocompatibility. In McKusick, V. A., and Claiborne, R., editors: Medical genetics, New York, 1973, Hospital Practice Publishing Co., p. 183.

12. Bach, M. L., Huang, S. W., Hong, R., and Poulik, M. D.: β_2-Microglobulin: association with lymphocyte receptors, Science 182:1350, 1973.

13. Balner, H.: Current knowledge of the histocompatibility complex of rhesus monkeys, Transplant. Rev. 15:50, 1973.

14. Barrickman, R. W., Callerame, M. C., and Condemi, J. J.: Gingivitis in hypogammaglobulinemia, J. Periodontol. 44:171, 1973.

15. Bartlett, P. F.: Cryopreservation of tooth germs, J. Dent. Res. 51:830, 1972.

16. Bartlett, P. F., and Reade, P. C.: Cryopreservation of developing teeth, Cryobiology 9:205, 1972.

17. Bennett, J. E.: Diagnosis and therapy of systemic mycoses in the immunosuppressed host, Transplant. Proc. 5:1255, 1973.

18. Berg, K.: Compositional relatedness between histocompatibility antigens and human serum lipoproteins, Science 172:1136, 1971.

19. Berglund, S. E.: Introduction to conference, J. Periodontol. 41:195, 1970.

20. Berkel, A. I.: Developmental aspects of delayed hypersensitivity, Boll. Ist. Sieroter. Milan. 53:147, 1974.

21. Berry, H., Bacon, P. A., and Davis, J. D.: Cell-mediated immunity in Sjögren's syndrome, Ann. Rheum. Dis. 31:298, 1972.

22. Bierly, J. A., and Sottosanti, J. S.: Osseous filtration: an improved technique for bone implantation, J. Periodontol. 45:414, 1974.

23. Bluestone, R., et al.: Salivary immunoglobulins in Sjögren's syndrome, Int. Arch. Allergy 42:686, 1972.

24. Blumenthal, M. N., et al.: Genetic mapping of Ir locus in man: linkage to second locus of HL-A, Science 184:1301, 1974.

25. Boackle, R. J., Pruitt, K. M., and Mestecky, J.: The interactions of human complement with interfacially aggregated preparations of human secretory IgA, Immunochemistry 11:543, 1974.

26. Bodey, G. P.: Oral complications of myeloproliferative disease, Postgrad. Med. 49:115, 1971.

27. Bodey, G. P.: Patient isolation units for cancer patients treated with chemical immunosuppressive agents, Transplant. Proc. 5:1279, 1973.

28. Bodmer, W. F.: Evolutionary significance of the HL-A system, Nature 237:139, 1972.

29. Boyne, P. J.: Transplantation, implantation and grafts, Dent. Clin. North Am. 15:433, 1971.

30. Boyne, P. J.: Osseous grafts and implants in the restoration of large oral defects, J. Periodontol. 45:378, 1974.

31. Brandtzaeg, P.: Human secretory immunoglobulin. II. Salivary secretions from individuals with selectively excessive or defective synthesis of serum immunoglobulins, Clin. Exp. Immunol. 8:69, 1971.

32. Brandtzaeg, P., Fjellanger, I., and Gjeruldsen, S. T.: Human secretory immunoglobulins. I. Salivary secretions from individuals with normal or low levels of serum immunoglobulins, Scand. J. Haematol. (Suppl.) 12:3, 1970.

33. Braun, W. E., Straffon, R. A., and Nakamoto, S.: Mismatched HL-A haplotypes with antigens HL-A1, 3, and 11 associated with excellent renal allograft function, Transplantation 15:86, 1973.

34. Bretscher, P. A.: Hypothesis: on the control between cell-mediated, IgM and IgG immunity, Cellular Immunol. 13:171, 1974.

35. Buckley, C. E., III, Dorsey, F. C., and Corley, R. B.: HL-A linked human immune response genes, Proc. Natl. Acad. Sci. U.S.A. 70:2157, 1973.

36. Buckley, R. H., et al.: Defective cellular immunity associated with chronic mucocutaneous moniliasis and recurrent staphylococcal botryomycosis: immunological reconstitution by allogeneic bone marrow, Clin. Exp. Immunol. 3:153, 1968.

37. Burnet, F. M.: The clonal selection theory of acquired immunity, New York, 1959, Cambridge University Press.

38. Burnet, F. M.: Multiple polymorphism in relation to histocompatibility antigens, Nature 245:359, 1973.

39. Butler, J. E., and Oskvig, R.: Cancer, autoimmunity and IgA-deficiency related by a common antigen-antibody system, Nature 249:830, 1974.

40. Cahill, L. T., Ainbender, E., and Glade, P. R.: Chronic mucocutaneous candidiasis: T-cell deficiency associated with B cell dysfunction in man, Cell. Immunol. 14:215, 1974.

41. Calder, E. A., Penhale, W. J., McLeman, D., et al.: Lymphocyte-dependent antibody-mediated cytotoxicity in Hashimoto thyroiditis, Clin. Exp. Immunol. 14:153, 1973.

42. Calder, E. A., et al.: Characterization of human lymphoid cell-mediated antibody-dependent cytotoxicity (LDAC), Clin. Exp. Immunol. 18:579, 1974.

43. Callender, C. O., et al.: Anti-HL-A antibodies: failure to correlate with renal allograft rejection, Surgery 76:573, 1974.

44. Canales, L., et al.: Immunological observations in chronic mucocutaneous candidiasis, Lancet 2:567, 1969.

45. Cantrell, J. L., and Hildemann, W. H.: Characteristics of disparate histocompatibility barriers in congenic strains of mice. I. Graft-versus-host reactions, Transplantation 14:761, 1972.

46. Capra, J. D., and Kindt, T. J.: Antibody diversity: can more than one gene encode each variable region?, Immunogenetics 1:417, 1975.

47. Chandler, D. C., et al.: Human parotid IgA and periodontal disease, Arch. Oral Biol. 19: 733, 1974.

48. Chilgren, R. A., et al.: Chronic mucocutaneous candidiasis, deficiency of delayed hypersensitivity, a selective local antibody defect, Lancet 2:688, 1967.

49. Coburn, R. J.: Bibliography of tooth transplantation, Transplantation 5:1553, 1967.

50. Coburn, R. J., Henriques, B. L., and Francis, L.: The development of an experimental tooth bank using deep freeze and tissue culture techniques, J. Oral Ther. Pharm. 2:445, 1966.

51. Coelho, I. A., Pereira, . T., and Virella, G.: Analytical study of salivary immunoglobulins in multiple myeloma, Clin. Exp. Immunol. 17:417, 1974.

52. Coelho, I. A., et al.: Salivary immunoglobulins in a patient with IgA deficiency, Clin. Exp. Immunol. 18:685, 1974.

53. Cohen, C., and Tissot, R. G.: Specialized research applications. II. Serological genetics. In Weisbroth, S. H., Flatt, R. E., and Krans, A. L., editors: The biology of the laboratory rabbit, New York, 1974, Academic Press, Inc., pp. 167-177.

54. Cohen, S., and Winkler, S.: Cellular immunity and the inflammatory response, J. Periodontol. 45:348, 1974.

55. Collins-Williams, C., Chiu, A. W., and Varga, E. A.: The relationship of atopic disease and immunoglobulin levels with special reference to selective IgA deficiency, Clin. Allergy 1:381, 1971.

56. Colten, H. R.: Synthesis and metabolism of complement proteins, Transplant. Proc. 6:33, 1974.

57. Cooper, M. D., and Lawton, A. R., III: The development of the immune system, Sci. Am. 231:59, 1974.

58. Costich, E. R., et al.: Freezing and *in vitro* culture of hamster teeth before replantation and transplantation, J. Oral Surg. 24:500, 1966.

59. Cummings, N. A.: Oral manifestations of connective tissue disease, Postgrad. Med. 49: 134, 1971.

60. Cunningham, A. J., and Fordham, S. A.: Antibody daughter cells can produce antibody of different specificities, Nature 250:669, 1974.

61. Curtis, A. B.: Childhood leukemias: osseous changes in jaws on panoramic dental radiographies, J. Am. Dent. Assoc. 83:844, 1971.

62. Curtis, A. B.: Childhood leukemias: initial oral manifestations, J. Am. Dent. Assoc. 83: 159, 1971.

63. Dausset, J.: The genetics of transplantation antigens, Transplant. Proc. 3:8, 1971.

64. Dausset, J., Dejos, L., and Hors, J.: The association of the HL-A antigens with disease, Clin. Immunol. 3:127, 1974.

65. Dausset, J., and Hors, J.: HL-A and kidney transplantation, Nature (New Biol.) 238:150, 1972.

66. David, C. S., Freilinger, J. A., and Scheffler, D. C.: New lymphocyte antigens controlled by the Ir-IgG region of the H-2 gene complex, Transplantation 17:122, 1974.

67. David, C. S., and Shreffler, D. C.: I region-associated antigen system (Ia) of the mouse H-2 gene complex, Transplantation 18:313, 1974.

68. Degos, L., et al.: Selective pressure on HL-A polymorphism, Nature 249:62, 1974.

69. Demant, P., et al.: The role of the H-2 linked Ss, Slp region in the control of mouse complement, Proc. Natl. Acad. Sci. U.S.A. 70:863, 1973.

70. Diener, E.: Evolutionary aspects of immunity and lymphoid organs in vertebrates, Transplant. Proc. 2:309, 1970.

71. Dietrich, M., and Fliedner, T. M.: Gnotobiotic care of patients with immunologic deficiency diseases, Transplant. Proc. 5:1271, 1973.

72. Dolby, A. E.: Recurrent aphthous ulceration, Immunology 17:709, 1969.

73. Edwards, J. H.: HL-A and disease: the detection of associations, J. Immunogen. 1: 249, 1974.

74. Ellison, S. A.: Oral bacteria and periodontal disease, J. Dent. Res. 49:198, 1970.

75. Emmings, F. G.: Chemically modified osseous material for the restoration of bone defects, J. Periodontol. 45:385, 1974.

76. Falk, J. A., and Osoba, D.: The association of the human histocompatibility system with Hodgkin's disease, J. Immunogen. 1:53, 1974.

77. Fefer, A., Michelson, E., and Thomas, E. D.: Leukemia antigens: mixed leukocyte culture tests on twelve leukaemic patients with identical twins, Clin. Exp. Immunol. 18:237, 1974.

78. Festenstein, H., Abbasi, K., and Demant, P.: The genetic basis of the generation of effector capacity for cell mediated lympholysis in mice, J. Immunogenetics 1:47, 1974.

79. Finley, S. C., et al.: Immunological profile in a chromosome 18 deletion syndrome with IgA deficiency, J. Med. Genet. 6:388, 1969.

80. Fong, C., and Berger, J.: Tissue response to x-irradiated tooth transplants, Oral Surg. 29: 275, 1970.

81. Fortner, J. G., and Shiu, M. H.: Organ transplantation and cancer, Surg. Clin. North Am. 54:871, 1974.

82. Friedlaender, M. H., and Baer, H.: Human X chromosome carriers quantitative genes for immunoglobulin M, Science 176:311, 1972.

83. Fudenberg, H. H.: Are autoimmune diseases immunologic deficiency states? In Good, R. A., and Fisher, D. W., editors: Immuno-biology, Stamford, Conn., 1971, Sinauer Associates, Inc., p. 175.

84. Gatti, R. A., and Seligmann, M.: The primary immunodeficiency diseases: classification, pathogenesis and treatment, Turk. J. Pediatr. 15:195, 1973.

85. Gedalia, I., Shulman, L. B., and Goldhaber, P.: Fluoride uptake by root surfaces of teeth, J. Dent. Res. 48:1148, 1969.

86. Genco, R. J.: Immunoglobulins and periodontal disease, J. Periodontol. 41:196, 1970.

87. Genco, R. J., et al.: Antibody-mediated effects in the periodontium, J. Periodontol. 45:330, 1974.

88. Gilmour, M. N., and Nisengard, R. J.: Interactions between serum titres to filamentous bacteria and their relationship to human periodontal disease, Arch. Oral Biol. 19:959, 1974.

89. Goldberg, L. S., et al.: Studies on lymphocyte and monocyte function in chronic mucocutaneous candidiasis, Clin. Exp. Immunol. 8: 37, 1971.

90. Goldblum, R. M., et al.: X-linked B lymphocyte deficiency. I. Panhypo-γ-globulinemia and dys-γ-globulinemia in siblings, J. Pediatr. 85:188, 1974.

91. Good, R. A.: Disorders of the immune system. In Good, R. A., and Fisher, D. W., editors: Immunobiology, Stamford, Conn., 1971, Sinauer Associates, Inc., p. 3.

92. Good, R. A., and Rodey, G. E.: IgA deficiency, antigenic barriers and autoimmunity, Cell. Immunol. 1:147, 1970.

93. Good, R. A., and Yunis, E.: Association of autoimmunity and immunodeficiency and aging in man, rabbits, and mice, Fed. Proc. 33:2040, 1974.

94. Gorlin, R. J., and Pindborg, J. J.: Macroglobulinemia of Waldenström. In Syn-

dromes of the head and neck, New York, 1964, McGraw-Hill Book Co., pp. 339-344.

95. Gotze, O., and Muller-Eberhard, H. J.: The C3 activator system: an alternate pathway of complement activation, J. Exp. Med. 134: 905, 1971.

96. Graham, A. F., et al.: Heart transplantation: current indications and long term results, Transplant. Proc. (Supp. 1) 6:17, 1974.

97. Green, I.: Genetic control of immune responses, Immunogenetics 1:4, 1974.

98. Hauptfeld, V., Klein, D., and Klein, J.: Serological identification of an Ir-region product, Science 181:167, 1973.

99. Hausmann, E.: Potential pathways for bone resorption in human periodontal disease, J. Periodontol. 45:338, 1974.

100. Hellstrom, K. E., and Hellstrom, I.: Immunologic defenses against cancer. In Good, R. A., and Fisher, D. W., editors: Immunobiology, Stamford, Conn., 1971, Sinauer Associates, Inc., p. 209.

101. Heremans, J. F., Crabbe, P. A., and Masson, P. L.: Biological significance of exocrine gamma-A-immunoglobulin, Acta Med. Scand. (Supp. 445) 179:84, 1966.

102. Herschfus, L.: Blood dyscrasias as seen in the oral cavity, J. Mich. Dent. Assoc. 52:260, 1970.

103. Herschfus, L.: Oral manifestations of blood disorders, J. Oral Med. 25:56, 1970.

104. Herschfus, L.: Lupus erythematosus, J. Oral Med. 27:12, 1972.

105. Hiatt, W. H., and Schallhorn, R. G.: Human allografts of iliac cancellous bone and marrow in periodontal osseous defects. I. Rationale and methodology, J. Periodontol. 42: 642, 1971.

106. Hildemann, W. H.: Immunogenetics, San Francisco, 1970, Holden-Day, Inc.

107. Hildemann, W. H.: Some new concepts in immunological phylogeny, Nature 250:116, 1974.

108. Hildemann, W. H.: Phylogeny of immune responsiveness in invertebrates, Life Sci. 14: 605, 1974.

109. Horowitz, S., et al.: Small intestinal disease in T cell deficiency, J. Pediatr. 85:457, 1974.

110. Horton, J. E., Leikin, S., and Oppenheim, J. J.: Human lymphoproliferative reaction to saliva and dental plaque-deposits: an *in vitro* correlation with periodontal disease, J. Periodontol. 43:522, 1973.

111. Horton, J. E., Oppenheim, J. J., and Mergenhagen, S. E.: Elaboration of lymphotoxin by cultured human peripheral blood leucocytes stimulated with dental plaque deposits, Clin. Exp. Immunol. 13:383, 1973.

112. Horton, J. E., Oppenheim, J. J., and Mer-

genhagen, S. E.: A role for cell-mediated immunity in the pathogenesis of periodontal disease, J. Periodontol. 45:351, 1974.

113. Horton, J. E., Raisz, L. G., Simmons, H. A., et al.: Bone resorbing activity in supernatant fluid from cultured human peripheral blood leukocytes, Science 117:793, 1972.

114. Ishizaka, T., Sian, C. M., and Ishizaka, K.: Complement fixation by aggregated IgE through alternate pathway, J. Immunol. 108: 848, 1972.

115. Ivanyi, L., Challacombe, S. J., and Lehner, T.: The specificity of serum factors in lymphocyte transformation in periodontal disease, Clin. Exp. Immunol. 14:491, 1973.

116. Ivanyi, L., and Lehner, T.: Lymphocyte transformation by sonicates of dental plaque in human periodontal disease, Arch. Oral Biol. 16:1117, 1971.

117. Ivanyi, L., Wilton, J. M. A., and Lehner, T.: Cell-mediated immunity in periodontal disease; cytotoxicity, migration inhibition and lymphocyte transformation studies, Immunology 22:141, 1972.

118. Jerne, N. K.: The somatic generation of immune recognition, Eur. J. Immunol. 1:1, 1971.

119. Katagiri, M., et al.: Common antigenic structures of HL-A antigens. III. An HL-A common antigenic marker closely associated with HL-A alloantigenic activity and detected by use of rabbit anti-rhesus monkey cell membrane antibodies, Immunology 27:487, 1974.

120. Katz, W. A., and Ehrlich, G. E.: Acute salivary gland inflammation associated with systemic lupus erythematosus, Ann. Rheum. Dis. 31:384, 1972.

121. Keene, J. J., Jr., Hussman, L., and Bruner, G.: Terminal oral manifestations of acute lymphoblastic leukemia, J. Oral Med. 27: 117, 1972.

122. Kiger, R. D., Wright, W. H., and Creamer, H. R.: The significance of lymphocyte transformation responses to various microbial stimulants, J. Periodontol. 45:780, 1974.

123. Klein, J.: Tooth transplantation in the mouse. III. The role of minor (Non-H-2) histocompatibility loci in tooth germ transplantation, Transplantation 12:500, 1971.

124. Klein, J.: H-2 system in wild mice. I. Identification of 5 new H-2 chromosomes, Transplantation 13:291, 1972.

125. Klein, J.: Genetic polymorphism of the histocompatibility-2 loci of the mouse, Ann. Rev. Gen. 8:63, 1974.

126. Klein, J., Bach, F. H., and Festenstein, F.: Genetic nomenclature for the H-2 complex of the mouse, Immunogenetics 1:184, 1974.

127. Klein, J., and Schuffler, D. C.: The H-2

model for the major histocompatibility systems, Transplant. Rev. 6:3, 1971.

128. Klein, J., and Secosky, W. R.: Tooth transplantation in the mouse. II. The role of the histocompatibility-2 (H-2) system in tooth germ transplantation, Oral Surg. 32:513, 1971.

129. Klingsberg, J.: Periodontal scleral grafts and combined grafts of sclera and bone: two year appraisal, J. Periodontol. 45:262, 1974.

130. Kohler, H., Kaplan, D. R., and Strayer, D. S.: Clonal depletion in neonatal tolerance, Science 186:643, 1974.

131. Kohler, H., Shimizu, A., Paul, C., et al.: Three variable-gene pools immune to IgM, IgG, and IgA immunoglobulins, Nature 227: 1318, 1970.

132. Kolata, G. B.: Antibody diversity: how many antibody genes?, Science 186:432, 1974.

133. Krolls, S. O.: Salivary gland diseases, J. Oral Med. 27:96, 1972.

133a. Lamm, L. U., Friedrich, U., Peterson, G. B., et al.: Assignment of the major histocompatibility complex to chromosome no. 6 in a family with pericentric inversion, Hum. Hered. 24:273, 1974.

134. Lehner, T.: Autoimmunity and breach of the blood-epithelial barrier, J. Dent. Res. (Supp.) 48:685, 1969.

135. Lehner, T.: Cell-mediated immune responses in oral disease: a review, J. Oral Path. 1:39, 1972.

136. Lehner, T.: Immunologic aspects of recurrent oral ulcers, Oral Surg. 33:380, 1972.

137. Lehner, T., Wilton, J. M. A., and Ivanyi, L.: Immunodeficiencies in chronic mucocutaneous candidiasis, Immunology 22:775, 1972.

138. Lehner, T., Wilton, J. M. A., Ivanyi, L., et al.: Immunological aspects of juvenile periodontitis (periodontosis), J. Periodont. Res. 9:261, 1974.

139. Lehner, T., et al.: Sequential cell-mediated immune responses in experimental gingivitis in man, Clin. Exp. Immunol. 16:481, 1974.

140. Leventhal, B. G., Waldorf, D. S., and Talal, N.: Impaired lymphocyte transformation and delayed hypersensitivity in Sjögren's syndrome, J. Clin. Invest. 46:1338, 1967.

141. Levin, S. M., and Kennedy, J. E.: Relationship of plaque and gingivitis in patients with leukemia, Va. Dent. J. 50:22, 1973.

142. Levine, B. B., Stember, R. H., and Fotino, M.: Ragweed hayfever: genetic control and linkage to HL-A haplotypes, Science 178: 1201, 1972.

143. Lindstrom, F. D., and Folke, L. E. A.: Salivary IgA in periodontal disease, J. Odontol. Scand. 31:31, 1973.

144. Ludwig, H., Granditsch, G., and Polymenidis, Z.: HL-A8 and haplotype HL-A 1-8 in coeliac disease, J. Immunogen. 1:91, 1974.

145. Macedo-Sobrinho, B., and Iranpour, B.: The effect of thymectomy on tooth germ allografts in rats, Arch. Oral Biol. 16:1215, 1971.

146. Mackay, J. R., Rampton, V. N., and Fyles, J. G.: Autosensitization of lymphocytes against thymus reticulum cells, Science 176:1324, 1972.

147. Mackintosh, P.: ABO matching in kidney graft survival, Nature 250:351, 1974.

148. Mackler, B. F., et al.: Blastogenesis and lymphokine synthesis by T and B lymphocytes from patients with periodontal disease, Infect. Immun. 10:844, 1974.

149. Marchalonis, J. J., Morris, P. J., and Harris, A. W.: Speculations on the function of immune response genes, J. Immunogenetics 1:63, 1974.

150. Marsh, D. G., Bias, W. B., and Hsu, S. H.: Association of the HL-A7 cross-reacting group with a specific reaginic antibody response in allergic man, Science 179:691, 1973.

151. Martin, D. W.: Lupus erythematosus—its oral manifestations, Oral Surg. 29:846, 1970.

152. Mayer, M. M.: The complement system, Sci. Am. 229:54, 1973.

153. Mayron, L. W., and Loiselle, R. J.: Bacterial antigens and antibodies in human periodontal tissue, J. Periodontol. 44:164, 1973.

154. McCredie, K. B., et al.: Leukocyte transfusions therapy for patients with host-defense failure, Transplant. Proc. 5:1285, 1973.

155. McDevitt, H. O.: Immunogenetics. In McKusick, V. A., and Claiborne, R., editors: Medical genetics, New York, 1973, Hospital Practice Publishing Co., p. 169.

156. McDevitt, H. O., and Bodner, W. F.: Protein clinical manifestations of primary tumors of the heart, Am. J. Med. 52:1, 1972.

157. McKearn, T. J.: Antireceptor antiserum causes specific inhibition of reactivity to rat histocompatibility antigens, Science 183:94, 1974.

158. Mergenhagen, S. E., Tempel, T. R., and Snyderman, R.: Immunologic reactions and periodontal inflammation, J. Dent. Res. 49:256, 1970.

159. Meuwissen, H. J.: Bone marrow transplantation in immunosuppressed or congenitally immune deficient patients, Transplant. Proc. 5:1291, 1973.

160. Moller, G., and Swehag, S. E.: Specificity of lymphocyte-mediated cytotoxicity induced by in vitro antibody-coated target cells, Cell. Immunol. 4:1, 1972.

161. Mozes, E., and Fuchs, S.: Linkage between immune response potential to DNA and X chromosome, Nature 249:167, 1974.

162. Nasjleti, C. E., Castelli, W. A., and Blakenship, J. R.: The storage of teeth before reimplantation in monkeys, Oral Surg. 39:20, 1975.

163. Natiella, J. R., Armitage, J. E., and Greene, G. W.: The replantation and transplantation of teeth, Oral Surg. 29:397, 1970.

164. Nisengard, R.: Immediate hypersensitivity and periodontal disease, J. Periodontol. 45:344, 1974.

165. Nisengard, R. J., and Beutner, E. H.: Relation of immediate hypersensitivity to periodontitis in animals and man, J. Periodontol. 41:223, 1970.

166. Nisonoff, A.: Molecules of immunity. In Good, R. A., and Fisher, D. W., editors: Immunobiology, Stamford, Conn., 1971, Sinauer Associates, Inc., p. 65.

167. Nobreus, N., Attstrom, R., and Egelberg, J.: Effect of anti-thymocyte serum on chronic gingival inflammation in dogs, J. Periodont. Res. 9:236, 1974.

168. Nobreus, N., Attstrom, R., and Egelberg, J.: Effect of anti-thymocyte serum on development of gingivitis in dogs, J. Periodont. Res. 9:227, 1974.

169. Nordenram, A., and Gergman, G.: Allogeneic transplants using cobalt-60 irradiated teeth in monkeys, Oral Surg. 29:944, 1970.

170. Norman, M. E., and South, M. A.: Evaluation of children for immunologic deficiency diseases, Clin. Ped. 13:644, 1974.

171. O'Neill, P. A., and Romsdahl, M. M.: IgA as a blocking factor in human malignant melanoma, Immunol. Commun. 3:427, 1974.

172. Opelz, G., Mickey, M. R., and Terasaki, P. I.: HL-A and kidney transplants: reexamination, Transplantation 17:371, 1974.

173. Oppenheim, J. J., and Francis, T. C.: The role of delayed hypersensitivity in immunological processes and its relationship to aphthous stomatitis, J. Periodontol. 41:205, 1970.

174. Oprisin, C., Doroga, H., and Serban, A.: Homografts of tooth buds in thymectomized rats, J. Dent. Res. 43:498, 1968.

175. Owen, J. J. T., Cooper, M. D., and Raff, M. C.: *In vitro* generation of B lymphocytes in mouse foetal liver, a mammalian "bursa" equivalent, Nature 249:361, 1974.

176. Patterson, P. Y., et al.: Mucocutaneous candidiasis, anergy and a plasma inhibitor of cellular immunity; reversal after amphotericin B therapy, Clin. Exp. Immunol. 9:595, 1971.

177. Porter, R. R.: Structural studies of immunoglobulins, Science 180:713, 1973.

178. Poulik, M. D., et al.: Aggregation of HL-A antigens at the lymphocyte surface induced by antiserum to β_2-microglobulin, Science **182:**1352, 1973.

179. Pourtouis, M., and Porta, G.: Culture of tooth buds in defined chemical environments, Bull. Group Int. Rech. Sci. Stomatol. **15:**71, 1972.

180. Presant, C. A., Jafdar, S. H., and Cherrick, H.: Gingival leukemic infiltration in chronic lymphocytic leukemia, Oral Surg. **36:**672, 1973.

181. Reichart, P.: Leukemia—the dental aspects, J. Dent. Assoc. Thai. **22:**165, 1972.

182. Remington, J. S., and Anderson, S. E., Jr.: Diagnosis and treatment of pneumocystosis and toxoplasmosis in the immunosuppressed host, Transplant. Proc. **5:**1263, 1973.

183. Rickles, N. H.: Allergy in surface lesions of the oral mucosa, Oral Surg. **33:**744, 1972.

184. Riviere, G. R.: Cytotoxic antibodies and lymphocytes induced by orthoptic tooth bud allografts in mice, J. Immunol. **112:**776, 1974.

185. Riviere, G. R., and Hansen, R. W.: Allo-antibodies induced in histoincompatible rats by single pulp and tooth grafts, J. Dent. Res. **52:**1186, 1973.

186. Riviere, G. R., and Hildemann, W. H.: Orthotopic transplantation of tooth buds among histoincompatible mice, Transplantation **16:**655, 1973.

187. Riviere, G. R., Sabet, T. Y., and Hoffman, R. L.: Transplantation of tooth buds across a multiple non-H-2 barrier, Transplantation **12:**271, 1971.

188. Robertson, P. B., and Cooper, M. D.: Oral manifestations of IgA deficiency, Adv. Exp. Med. Biol. **45:**497, 1974.

189. Rodrigues, V., and Bodey, G. P.: Bacterial infections in immunosuppressed patients: diagnosis and management, Transplant. Proc. **5:**1249, 1973.

190. Rowley, D. A., et al.: Specific suppression of immune responses, Science **181:**1133, 1973.

191. Ruddy, S.: Chemistry and biologic activity of the complement system, Transplant. Proc. **6:**1, 1974.

192. Savilahti, E.: IgA deficiency in children, Clin. Exp. Immunol. **13:**395, 1973.

193. Savilahti, E., Pelkonen, P., and Visakorpi, J. K.: IgA deficiency in children, Arch. Dis. Child. **46:**665, 1971.

194. Schallhorn, R. G., and Hiatt, W. H.: Human allografts of iliac cancellous bone and marrow in periodontal osseous defects. II. Clinical observations, J. Periodontol. **43:**67, 1972.

195. Schroeder, H. E., and Page, R.: Lymphocyte-fibroblast interaction in the pathogenesis of inflammatory gingival disease, Experimentia **28:**1228, 1972.

196. Scopp, I. W.: Immune response and oral disease, J. Oral Med. **27:**26, 1972.

197. Shawkat, A. H., and Phillips, J. D.: Multiple myelomas, Oral Surg. **37:**969, 1974.

198. Shulman, L. B.: The current status of allogeneic tooth transplantation. In Hard tissue growth, repair, and remineralization, Ciba Foundation Symposium 11, Amsterdam, 1973, North-Holland Publishing Co., p. 91.

199. Shulman, L. D.: Recent concepts of autoimmunity in oral disease—with emphasis on recurrent oral ulceration, Diastema **3:**47, 1971.

200. Silvers, W. K., and Gasser, D. L.: The genetic divergence of sublines as assessed by histocompatibility testing, Genetics **75:**671, 1973.

201. Sippel, H. W., Natiella, J. R., and Greene, G. W., Jr.: A case of multiple myeloma with oral manifestations, Trans. Congr. Int. Assoc. Oral Surg. **4:**132, 1971.

202. Soder, P. O., and Lundquist, G.: Autotransplantation of teeth with use of cell cultivation technique, Int. Dent. J. **22:**327, 1972.

203. Snell, G. D.: Immunogenetics: retrospect and prospect, Immunogenetics **1:**1, 1974.

204. Snell, G. D., Cherry, M., and Demant, P.: H-2: its stucture and similarity to HL-A, Transplant. Rev. **15:**3, 1973.

205. Snyderman, R.: The role of the immune response in the development of periodontal disease, Int. Dent. J. **23:**310, 1973.

206. Snyderman, R., et al.: Defective mononuclear leukocyte chemotaxis; a previously unrecognized immune dysfunction, Ann. Int. Med. **78:**509, 1973.

207. Spiers, R. S.: Multiple cellular and subcellular responses to antigen: literature review and hypothesis of immunization, Immunochemistry **8:**665, 1971.

208. Stenzel, K. H., Whitsell, J. C., and Stubenbord, W. T.: Kidney transplantation: improvement in patient and graft survival, Ann. Surg. **180:**29, 1974.

209. Stevens, D. A.: Immunosuppression and virus infections, Transplant. Proc. **5:**1259, 1973.

210. Stewart, J. M., et al.: Absent IgA in deletion of chromosome 18, J. Med. Genet. **1:**11, 1970.

211. Strayer, D. S., et al.: Neonatal tolerance induced by antibody against antigen-specific receptor, Science **186:**640, 1974.

212. Sussman, R. N., et al.: Sjögren's syndrome: an autoimmune disease, J. Oral Surg. **30:**23, 1972.

213. Talal, N., Asofsky, R., and Lightbody, P.: Immunoglobulin synthesis by salivary gland

lymphoid cells in Sjögren's syndrome, J. Clin. Invest. **49**:49, 1970.

214. Tanigaki, N., and Pressman, D.: The basic structure and the antigenic characteristics of HL-A antigens, Transplant. Rev. **21**:15, 1974.

215. Thieme, T. R., Raley, R. A., and Fahey, J. L.: Demonstration of molecular individuality of HL-A antigens, J. Immunol. **113**: 323, 1974.

216. Thompson, J. S., Bonney, W. W., Lawton, R. L., et al.: Effect of HL-A haplotype matching on renal transplantation, Transplantation **17**:438, 1974.

217. Thompson, J. S., Flink, R. J., Caldwell, J. L., et al.: Relationship of mixed lymphocyte culture response, HL-A histocompatibility antigens, and renal transplantation, Transplant. Proc. **5**:1763, 1973.

218. Thorsby, E.: The human major histocompatibility system, Transplant. Rev. **18**:51, 1974.

219. Tissot, R. G., and Cohen, C.: Histocompatibility in the rabbit, Transplantation **18**:142, 1974.

220. Toh, B. H., et al.: Depression of cell-mediated immunity in old age and the immunopathic diseases, lupus erythematosus, chronic hepatitis and rheumatoid arthritis, Clin. Exp. Immunol. **14**:193, 1973.

221. Tomasi, T. B.: The gamma A globulins: first line of defense. In Good, R. A., and Fisher, D. W., editors: Immunobiology, Stamford, Conn., 1971, Sinauer Associates, Inc., p. 76.

222. Vacheck, H., and Kolsch, E.: The genetic control of T cell-mediated immunity. I. Characterization of a mouse strain whose low responsiveness is inherited as a recessive trait, Immunology **27**:507, 1974.

223. van Boxel, J. A., and Buell, D. N.: IgD on cell membranes of human lymphoid cell lines with multiple immunoglobulin classes, Nature **251**:443, 1974.

224. van Boxel, J. A., et al.: Multiple heavy-chain determinants on individual B lymphocytes in the peripheral blood of patients with Sjögren's syndrome, N. Engl. J. Med. **289**:823, 1973.

225. Walford, R. L.: Immunologic theory of aging: current status, Fed. Proc. **33**:2020, 1974.

226. Wang, A. C., and Fudenberg, H. H.: IgA and evolution of immunoglobulins, J. Immunogenetics **1**:3, 1974.

227. Weinreb, M. M., and Sharav, Y.: The immunobiology of tooth transplantations, Int. Dent. J. **21**:488, 1971.

228. Wells, J. V., Bleumers, J. F., and Fudenberg, H. H.: Human anti-IgM isoantibodies in subjects with selective IgA deficiency, Clin. Exp. Immunol. **12**:305, 1972.

229. White, G. E.: Oral manifestations of leukemia in children, Oral Surg. **29**:420, 1970.

230. Zighelboim, J., et al.: A sensitive in vitro microassay for detecting antibody-dependent cellular cytotoxicity, Transplantation **18**:27, 1974.

12

Heritable mucocutaneous disorders

ROBERT J. GORLIN

In a book of this degree of specialization it might be expected that all known genetic mucocutaneous disorders would be discussed. Yet, even this is impossible, since several new disorders are recognized each year, and many more are not fully defined or limned.

The disorders I have chosen represent a wide spectrum, the only common denominator being involvement of the mucocutaneous surfaces. Although some attempt has been made to group the entities in a gesture toward nosology, one should not draw any conclusion concerning a commonality in causes. A white mucosa is usually a thickened mucosa, but there must be numerous mechanisms involving the shedding of cells. No studies have been carried out that have shed significant light on the anomaly in any one of the disorders discussed. This is the work of future generations of investigators. It is my sincere hope that this brief dissertation shall serve a heuristic role.

DYSKERATOSIS CONGENITA (ZINSSER-ENGMAN-COLE SYNDROME)

Zinsser[16] reported the first example of a syndrome comprising reticular atrophy of the skin with pigmentation, dystrophy of nails, and oral leukoplakia. His report went unrecognized, and 20 years later, the same syndrome was reported under almost the same title by Engman.[6] Various authors developed the syndrome, noting the association of aplas-

tic anemia and hypersplenism. Wilgram and Weinstock[15] pointed out that the oral lesions are characterized by a decreased number of keratinosomes associated with a decreased epithelial cell turnover. Thus the disorder is not really a dyskeratosis.

Heredity

The hereditary pattern of the disorder is not clear. Although most patients are male and there is clearly X-linked inheritance in one report,[4] a few fully expressed examples of the condition have been described in females. There have been several affected male sibs, and in two cases a brother and sister have been affected.[1, 9, 13] This variability probably is due to genetic heterogeneity, there being X-linked and autosomal recessive forms of the disorder. About thirty-five cases have been published.

Systemic manifestations

There is generalized growth retardation and frailty.

Skin and skin appendages. The most prominent skin changes closely resemble those seen in poikiloderma atrophicans vasculare, involving especially the face, neck, and chest and appearing approximately at puberty. A prominent reticulated hyperpigmentation of skin, usually described as gunmetal in color, involves the same areas. Microscopically, one notes atrophy of the epidermis and subcutaneous tissues accompanied by capillary hyperplasia. Melanin pigment is heavily deposited, especially near blood vessels. Characteristically, there is no inflammatory exudate.

Hyperhidrosis of the palms and soles and generalized hypohidrosis elsewhere have been noted in over half the cases. In most cases the fingernails and toenails become dystrophic at about puberty (Fig. 12-1).

Eyes and ears. Chronic blepharitis, ectropion, and profuse tearing due to keratinization with obstruction of the lacrimal punctae have been noted (Fig. 12-2).

Central nervous system. Mental retarda-tion and/or schizophrenia has been reported in about 30% of patients.

Blood. Several investigators have noted an associated aplastic anemia and hypersplen-ism.[1-4, 7, 14]

Other findings. Small testes have been described in about 15%.

Oral manifestations. Crops of vesicles and bullae appear on the oral mucosa, most frequently during the 5- to 7-year-old period or, in some cases, earlier. These flaccid bullae are recurrent and essentially painless. Because of moisture and maceration, they rupture early,

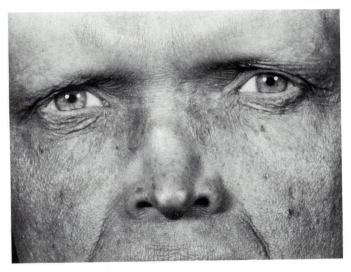

Fig. 12-1. Dystrophy of nails. (Courtesy H. Reich, Münster, Germany.)

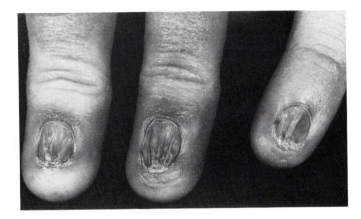

Fig. 12-2. Absence of eyebrows and eyelashes. Note crinkly, atrophic skin. (Courtesy H. Reich, Münster, Germany.)

leaving ulcerated areas with epithelial tags along the margin. After several attacks, the mucosa becomes atrophic, and the tongue loses its papillae and becomes smooth (Fig. 12-3). Under ultraviolet light, the normal orange fluorescence of the tongue is missing.

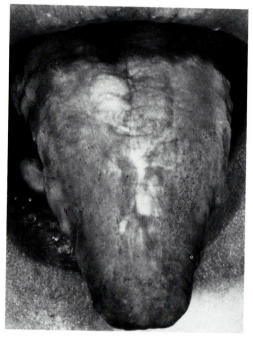

Fig. 12-3. Atrophy of tongue mucosa with premalignant dyskeratosis. (Courtesy H. Reich, Münster, Germany.)

Eventually the mucosa becomes thickened, fissured, and white. About 20% complain of dysphagia; esophageal diverticula have been noted with increased frequency. Several studies[1, 5, 10, 13] have reported large verrucous carcinomatous lesions on the buccal and cervical mucosa of patients with this syndrome. Microscopically, dyskeratotic changes are seen, clearly branding the lesion as true leukoplakia.

Laboratory aids

Demonstration of pancytopenia may aid in the diagnosis.

Steier and associates,[14] and many other authors have pointed out similarities and differences between dyskeratosis congenita and Fanconi's anemia. More prominent in dyskeratosis congenita are cutaneous telangiectatic erythema and atrophy, ungual dysplasia, mucosal leukoplakia and carcinomatosis, and esophageal diverticula. Prominent in Fanconi's anemia but absent in dyskeratosis congenita are renal and skeletal anomalies.

EHLERS-DANLOS SYNDROMES

Within the past decade, seven or more types of Ehlers-Danlos syndrome have been defined. Within the compass of this chapter, my discussion must necessarily be brief.

Ehlers[24] described the association of hyper-

Table 12-1. Characteristics of seven variants of the Ehlers-Danlos syndrome*

Type of Ehlers-Danlos syndrome	Skin hyperextensibility	Joint hypermobility	Skin fragility	Bruising
Severe (type I)	Marked	Marked	Marked	Moderate
Mild (type II)	Moderate	Moderate	Moderate	Moderate
Benign hypermobile (type III)	Variable; usually marked	Marked	Minimal	Minimal
Ecchymotic (type IV)	Minimal	Limited to digits	Marked	Marked
X-linked (type V)	Marked	Limited to digits	Minimal	Minimal
Ocular variety (type VI)	Marked	Marked	Minimal	Minimal
Procollagen peptidase deficiency (type VII)	Moderate	Marked	Moderate	Moderate

*Modified from McKusick, V. A.: Editorial: multiple forms of the Ehlers-Danlos syndrome, Arch. Surg. 1

elastic skin, skin hemorrhages, and loose jointedness. Danlos[23] added cutaneous pseudotumors and fragility. Several of those affected had jobs as human pretzels and India rubber men at circus sideshows. Comprehensive surveys are those of McKusick[27] and Beighton and co-workers.[20, 22]

There are at least seven variants of the syndrome, three of which exhibit autosomal dominant inheritance. A fourth type is X-linked, and three forms are autosomal recessive. The interested reader is also referred to the classification of Barabas.[17]

The basic defect is not known for types I-III, but a defect in elastin has been suggested, a view that I do not share. In the ecchymotic form (type IV), a type 3 collagen deficiency has been demonstrated. In type V, there is a deficiency of lysyl oxidase. In a recessive form (type VI), the collagen has been shown to be hydroxylysine deficient.[29] In another recessive form (type VII), procollagen peptidase is deficient (Table 12-1).

Systemic manifestations

Prematurity is frequently observed in the severe form (type I) due to early rupture of fetal membranes. Death in youth or early adult life may occur in the ecchymotic type (type IV). Friable tissues and operative difficulties due to abnormal bleeding have been seen in both the severe and ecchymotic forms.

Facies. Scars on the forehead and chin are present in about half the cases (Fig. 12-4). The ears may project outward and somewhat downward (lop ears). Epicanthal folds are

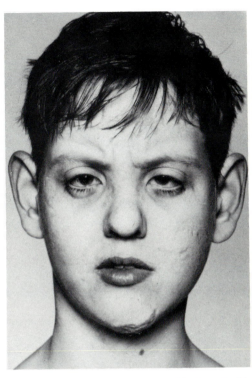

Fig. 12-4. Scars of chin. (From Barabas, G. M., and Barabas, A. P.: Br. Dent. J. **123**:472, 1967.)

Major complications	Inheritance	Basic defect
Musculoskeletal deformities common; varicose veins, prematurity due to ruptured membranes	Autosomal dominant	Unknown
	Autosomal dominant	Unknown
	Autosomal dominant	Unknown
Death from arterial rupture, aortic dissection, intestinal perforation; musculoskeletal abnormalities absent	Autosomal dominant	Type III collagen deficiency
Musculoskeletal disorders common	X-linked	Lysyloxidase deficiency
Fragility of cornea and sclera; musculoskeletal disorders common	Autosomal recessive	Hydroxylysine deficiency
Marked short stature and multiple joint dislocations	Autosomal recessive	Procollagen peptidase deficiency

frequent, causing the nasal bridge to appear wide.

Skin. The skin has a velvety or doughy feel and is hyperplastic, especially over the major joints (Fig. 12-5). After being stretched, it returns to its normal position. The hyperextensible skin fold in the X-linked form is thicker than that in the severe variety.

The skin is fragile, and minimal trauma produces gaping wounds. After healing, papyraceous scars result. These can usually be detected over the forehead, knees, shins, or elbows (Fig. 12-6). Bruising in the severe form is variable in degree but is particularly marked in the ecchymotic type.

Molluscoid or raisin-like pseudotumors over the heels and major joints are not uncommon, and there is often redundancy of the skin of the hands and feet. Calcified structures, 2 to 10 mm in diameter, may be found subcutaneously, especially over bony prominences of the forearms and shins, in about 30% of cases.

Musculoskeletal system. Hyperextensibility of joints (Fig. 12-7), a weak hand clasp, and pes planus are usually present in the severe form of the syndrome. Genu recurvatum has been noted in about 25% of cases, and there may be recurrent joint dislocations.

Other findings. Various gastrointestinal complications have been observed, including hiatus hernia, intestinal diverticula, diaphragmatic eventration, and rectal prolapse during infancy. Occasionally there is spontaneous perforation of the intestines, massive gastrointestinal hemorrhage, or arterial rupture, especially in the ecchymotic form.

Oral manifestations. The oral mucosa is excessively fragile and easily bruised. The oral mucosa does not hold sutures satisfactorily. Healing may be slightly retarded, since the edges of the wound draw apart, but there is no evidence of excessive scar formation in the mouth. The gingiva is said to be more liable to injury, and periodontal disease occurs at an early age. In addition, severe bleeding has been noted after tooth extraction. Recurrrent subluxation of the temporomandibular joint has been reported.[25, 31]

Barabas and Barabas[19] found that premolar

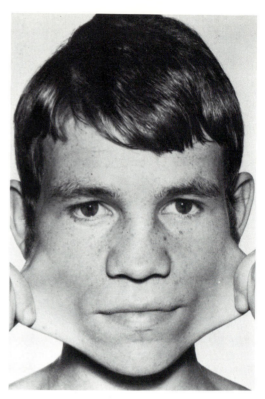

Fig. 12-5. Hyperstretchability of skin. (Courtesy P. Beighton, Baltimore, Md.)

and molar teeth had high cusps and deep occlusal fissures. Radiographically, the teeth may have stunted and deformed roots and large pulp stones in the coronal part of the pulp chamber. This observation was first made by Selliseth[30] and later confirmed by Barabas and Barabas[19] and Pindborg.[28] Barabas[18] found hypoplastic areas in the enamel, irregularities of amelodentinal and cementodentinal junctions, formation of pathological dentin, occurring more often in the root than in the crown and containing vascular inclusions, dentinal tubules following abnormal courses, and many denticles. The finding of abnormalities in the dentin, which has no significant elastic tissue content, indicates that collagenous tissue is affected regardless of whether elastic tissue is present.

Gorlin and Pindborg[26] observed that at least 50% of patients with the Ehlers-Danlos syndrome have the ability to touch the nose with the tongue, an ability manifest by only

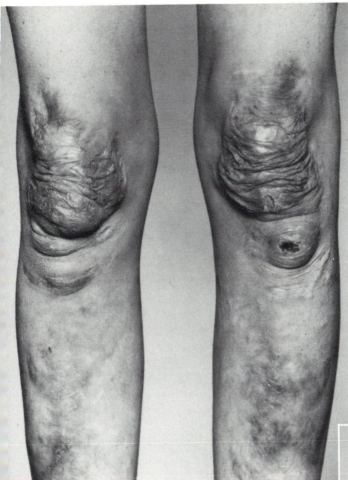

Fig. 12-6. Cigarette-paper scars of knees and shins. (From Barabas, G. M., and Barabas, A. P.: Br. Dent. J. **123**:472, 1967.)

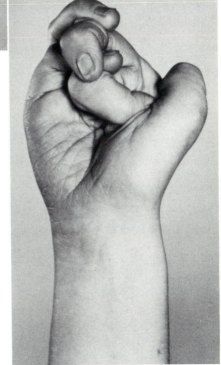

Fig. 12-7. Hypermobility of joints. (From Barabas, G. M., and Barabas, A. P.: Br. Dent. J. **123**:472, 1967.)

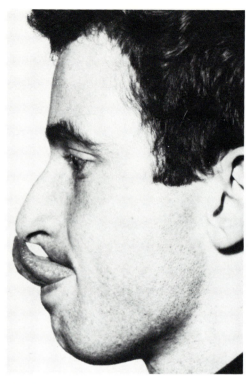

Fig. 12-8. Ability to touch nose with tongue tip seen in 50% of patients with Ehlers-Danlos syndrome. (Courtesy P. Beighton, Baltimore, Md.)

about 8% to 10% of ostensibly normal persons (Fig. 12-8).

Laboratory aids

Joint mobility and skin elasticity may be estimated by standard methods.[22, 27]

ENDOCRINE CANDIDOSIS SYNDROME (ADDISON'S DISEASE, IDIOPATHIC JUVENILE HYPOPARATHYROIDISM, AND SUPERFICIAL CANDIDOSIS)

The association of candidosis with idiopathic hypoparathyroidism and Addison's disease has been known for several decades. In some patients, one or more of the following disorders may be present: a celiac-like condition with malabsorption, chronic liver disease, achlorhydria, pernicious anemia, malfunction of the thyroid gland (Hashimoto's disease), and pulmonary infiltrates of undetermined cause. It should be emphasized

that not all of the cardinal elements of the syndrome need be present in the same individual or in a single family.

Defective delayed hypersensitivity to *Candida albicans* has been demonstrated in patients with the syndrome. Congenital abnormalities of the thymus may also be associated with mucocutaneous candidosis. Defective lymphocyte function has been demonstrated in vitro. Excellent reviews are those of Gass,[35] Hermans and Ritts,[37] and Kirkpatrick and associates.[38]

Heredity

The syndrome exhibits autosomal recessive inheritance.

Systemic manifestations

Not all components of the syndrome appear simultaneously. The candidosis is nearly always the first component to appear, usually during the first 6 years of life. It is followed from 3 months to 13 years later by the other components. The hypoparathyroidism and hypoadrenal corticism become manifest most frequently during the prepubescent period, the former usually preceding the latter.

Endocrine system. The hypoparathyroidism is usually manifested by tetany. The serum calcium level is reduced and the serum phosphorus level elevated in the absence of significant disease of the genitourinary and gastrointestinal systems. Furthermore, parathyroid hormone injection results in an increase in the level of serum calcium and in elevated urinary phosphorus excretion. At necropsy, absence of the parathyroid glands or their replacement with fat has been noted.

Addison's disease becomes manifest soon after the appearance of the hypoparathyroidism. Lassitude, anorexia, progressive weakness, hypotension, and progressive pigmentation of the skin and mucous membranes signal its onset, and laboratory findings confirm the low serum sodium and high potassium levels. Death from adrenal crisis is a common outcome, and necropsy shows adrenocortical atrophy of the cytotoxic type.

The relation of the candidosis to the endocrine glands is not known. Necropsy does not

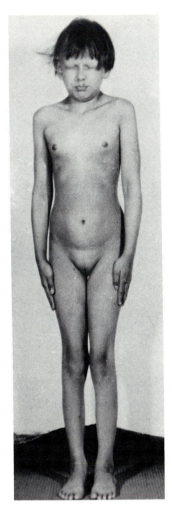

Fig. 12-9. Note increased skin pigmentation and photophobia. (From Gass, J. D.: Am. J. Ophthalmol. **54:**660-674, 1962.)

suggest mycotic involvement of these organs, nor does the fungus elaborate a toxin that is capable of producing changes. It has been suggested that the candidosis is a superficial expression of undetermined abnormalities already present in the host that favor the development of the infection as well as the endocrinopathies.[33, 34]

Skin and skin appendages. The skin is dry, and the body and scalp hair are usually brittle and diminished. The eyebrows and axillary and pubic hair are remarkably sparse (Fig. 12-9). Total alopecia may develop, most notably after therapy with dihydrotachysterol. The fingernails and toenails are frequently thin, ridged, and brittle and are often the site of infection by *Candida* organisms. If infected, they become brown, irregular, and thickened, with a crumbled outer edge[32] (Fig. 12-10).

Oral manifestations. The candidosis may be superficial or deepseated and may involve the lips, tongue, buccal mucosa, palate, and larynx with thick creamy-white plaques. The mucosa between the plaques is often hyperemic, and the tongue may be smooth and devoid of papillae. Perleche, or angular stomatitis, may extend over a considerable portion of the perioral skin. Similar involvement of the anal and vaginal mucosae has been described.

With the advent of Addison's disease, areas of splotchy melanin pigment are seen in the

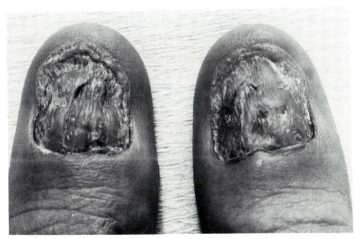

Fig. 12-10. Moniliasis of nails. Also note increased skin pigmentation. (Courtesy K. H. Sjöberg, Sandviken, Sweden.)

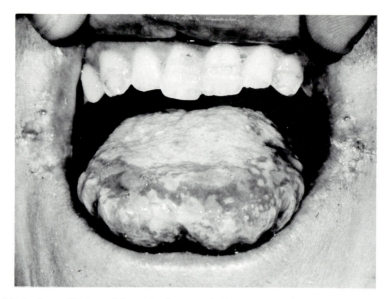

Fig. 12-11. Oral moniliasis and hypoplastic enamel. One can see that hypoparathyroidism was treated by normal enamel near cervices of teeth.

mouth, especially on the buccal mucosa and palate.

The teeth are chalky, with the crowns pitted or exhibiting transverse grooves of enamel hypoplasia (Fig. 12-11).

Laboratory aids

Serum levels of calcium, phosphorus, potassium, and chloride are indicated. Thyroid function studies should also be carried out.

EPIDERMOLYSIS BULLOSA

Epidermolysis bullosa includes several hereditary vesicular disorders that involve skin and often oral and other mucosas. The vesicles usually arise at points of trauma. For some types, however, heat may be the precipitating factor, or the blisters may arise spontaneously.

The interested reader is referred to the work of Gedde-Dahl[46] for a detailed historical review.

Epidermolysis bullosa is classified into autosomal dominant and recessive forms, each of which may be divided into two or more types. These will be considered separately.

Dominant simplex form

Systemic manifestations. Sites of friction or trauma are most frequently involved. Nails are affected in about 20% of cases. Scarring and/or pigmentation does not result after healing. The disorder usually appears neonatally or during infancy when the child begins to crawl and principally involves the feet, hands, and neck, rarely the ankles, knees, trunk, and elbows. After the third year of life, usually only the hands and feet are affected. The nails are normal. Generally, the condition improves markedly at puberty.

Oral manifestations. The frequency of oral bullae is not sufficiently documented. Tilsley and Beard[50] and Davidson,[46] for example, found no oral involvement. Gedde-Dahl[47] noted lingual and/or palatal lesions in several patients.

Histopathological study reveals cleavage through the basal layer, that is, above the PAS-positive basement membrane.

Dominant dystrophic (hypertrophic) form

Systemic manifestations. The dominant dystrophic form of epidermolysis bullosa is characterized in decreasing order of frequency by flat, pink, scar-producing bullae of the ankles, knees, hands, elbows, and feet.[47] Milia are common but less numerous than in the recessive dysplastic type. The nails are usually (80%) thick and dystrophic. In contrast to the recessive dystrophic cases, the conjunctiva and cornea are never involved. About 20% of cases show changes before the age of 1 year. Improvement seems to occur with age.

Oral manifestations. About 20% of cases manifest oral bullae.[51] Oral milia were noted by Andreasen and associates.[42] These milia are not retention cysts but epidermoid cysts, which originate from detached islands of epithelium in areas of earlier bulla formation.

Recessive dystrophic type

Systemic manifestations. The extensive studies of Gedde-Dahl[47] suggest that this disorder is genetically heterogeneous. The reader is referred to his text for a discussion of the many subtypes.

Bullae are usually manifested at or shortly after birth, arising at sites of pressure or trauma or appearing spontaneously. In infants, the most commonly affected areas are the feet, buttocks, scapulas, elbows, fingers, and occiput. In older children, the hands, feet, knees, and elbows are most often involved (Fig. 12-12). When a bulla ruptures or the roof peels off, a raw, painful surface is evident. The fluid contained in the bulla is at first sterile but may become secondarily infected and bloody. On healing, the bullae often are followed by keloidal scars, causing contraction, and by various degrees of pigmentation or depigmentation. They are frequently associated with milium-like cysts. The scars may lead to loss of bony structures or to interference with growth and resultant dwarfism (Fig. 12-13, *A*). Formation of claw-hand and the enclosure of the hand in a glovelike epidermal sac have been noted frequently (Fig. 12-13, *B*). Nikolsky's sign is often present. The nails may be extremely involved, often being dystrophic or absent (Fig. 12-13, *B*).

Changes are essentially limited to the hands, feet, and esophagus. The esophagus may become segmentally stenotic (most often the upper half) in childhood with consequent dysphagia.[45] The metacarpals become slender and overconstricted, and the distal phalanges become pointed and clawlike.

Oral manifestations. Although a considerable number of authors have remarked on the teeth having hypoplastic enamel with

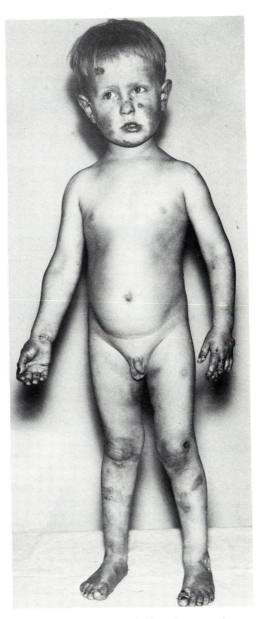

Fig. 12-12. Epidermolysis bullosa (autosomal recessive dystrophic). Note blisters on face and extremities. (Courtesy A. Lodin, Stockholm, Sweden.)

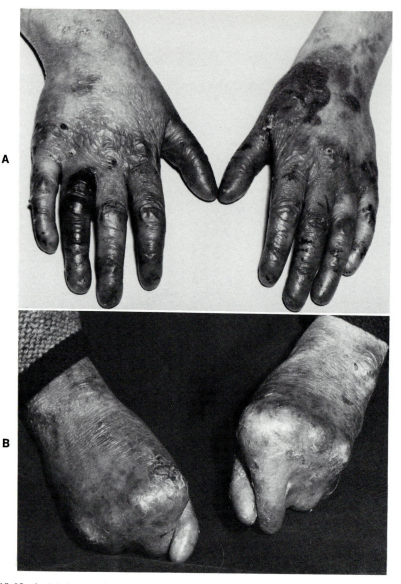

Fig. 12-13. A, Moderate destruction of hands. Note blisters and nail dystrophy. **B,** Advanced destruction of hands. (**A** courtesy D. Winstock, London. **B** from Rocke, H.: Hautarzt **7:**463, 1956.)

great susceptibility to dental caries, delayed eruption, and frequent retention, there is little documentation concerning frequency. I share with Rodermund[48] the belief that there is no correlation between the degree of cutaneous and dental involvement. Pock-marked alteration of the enamel has been handsomely illustrated by Rodermund[48] (Fig. 12-14). Excellent histological studies of unerupted teeth

have been published by Arwill and co-workers,[44] who noted hypoplasia of enamel with absence of prismatic structure. The dentin is probably not significantly affected.

Oral mucosal involvement occurs soon after birth, vesicles apparently forming from the negative pressure involved in the sucking reflex. Although oral bullae are said to occur in at least 15%, our impression is that it is

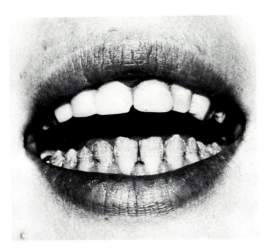

Fig. 12-14. Pitted enamel. (From Rodermund, O. E.: Dermatol. Wochenschr. **153:**350, 1967.)

much higher. The lingual mucosa appears thick, gray, and smooth and may become bound down. The sulci may become obliterated, with much scarring, microstomia, and immobility of the lips. Even routine dental management may cause the eruption of bullae on the lips and oral mucosa. The slightest abrasion from normal toothbrushing may cause serious sequelae. Other oral changes, the frequencies of which have not been established, are atrophy of the maxilla with resultant relative mandibular prognathism, increased mandibular angle, and oral carcinoma.

Histopathological changes in the oral mucosa were well demonstrated by Arwill and associates.[43] The bullae occur below the PAS-positive basement membrane.

Epidermolysis bullosa letalis

Systemic manifestations. The criteria for diagnosis of the Herlitz lethal type are (1) neonatal onset, (2) death within the first 3 months of life, and (3) absence of milia, pigmentary changes, and scarring. Many authors view the lethal type as a severe form of the dystrophic recessive disorder. At the present time, we have only clinical criteria, such as early death and absence of scarring, pigmentation and/or milia to separate the two forms.

Usually the vesicles, often hemorrhagic, are

noted at the base of the fingernails within the first few hours of life. The nails soon become loose and are shed. This is followed by involvement of the trunk, umbilicus, face, scalp, and extremities. The palms and soles are never affected. There seems to be an absence of reaction to traumatic provocation.

Light-microscopic examination demonstrates epidermal-dermal cleavage that follows the rete ridge contour.

Oral manifestations. Bullae that are remarkably fragile and hemorrhagic are found in nearly all patients, especially at the junction of the hard and soft palates. Histological study reveals cleavage between the epithelium and connective tissue or within the epithelium between the basal layer and the stratum spinosum. The cells of the basal layer seem palisaded as a result of extracellular vacuolization.

Arwill and co-workers[43] investigated skin as well as oral mucosa ultrastructurally in four cases of the letalis form. They found that the gingiva and skin exhibited less hemidesmosomes and tonofilaments. Although the desmosomes remained intact, minute vesicles were found between the basement membrane and the basal cell membrane in the intermediate zone.

FABRY'S SYNDROME (ANGIOKERATOMA CORPORIS DIFFUSUM UNIVERSALE)

The clinical syndrome was described independently by Anderson[52] in England and Fabry[55] in Germany. The disorder is characterized by the systemic accumulation of the glycosphingolipid, trihexosyl ceramide, particularly in the cardiovascular-renal system. The primary metabolic defect is the deficient activity of ceramide trihexosidase, which normally catabolizes the accumulated glycosphingolipid.[53]

Heredity

Opitz and associates[57] documented the X-linked transmission with complete penetrance and variable expressivity of this disease in hemizygous males. Heterozygous females may be asymptomatic or may manifest many of the same symptoms as the hemizygous males in attenuated form. Skin lesions and corneal opacities are present in the majority of carriers. Studies[56, 57] have demonstrated that the loci for Xg and Fabry's disease are linked.

Systemic manifestations

Skin. The cutaneous, vascular lesions (angiokeratoma corporis diffusum) are telangiectases; they do not blanch with pressure and usually appear as clusters of individual macular to papular, punctate, dark-red angiectases in the superficial layers of the skin. There may be moderate keratosis over these lesions. They usually appear during childhood and progressively increase in size and number with age. Characteristically, they are most dense over the iliosacral area, scrotum, posterior thorax, thighs, buttocks, and umbilicus (Fig. 12-15).

Eye. Ocular manifestations include aneurysmal dilation and tortuosity of conjunctival and retinal vessels with corneal opacities in hemizygous males. The opacities are characterized by diffuse haziness or whorled streaks in the corneal epithelium, resembling changes seen in chloroquine intoxication, and must be observed by slit lamp microscopy. These lesions do not impair vision.

Cardiovascular-renal system. With increasing age, the major symptoms result from involvement of the cardiovascular-renal system. Early in the disease, casts, red cells, and lipid inclusions with characteristic birefringent Maltese crosses appear in the urinary sediment. Proteinuria, isosthenuria, and gradual deterioration of renal function and development of azotemia occur in the second to fourth decades of life. Cardiovascular findings in late maturity may include hypertension, left ventricular hypertrophy, myocardial ischemia or infarction, and cerebral vascular disease. Death most often results from uremia or vascular disease of the heart or brain during the fourth decade of life.

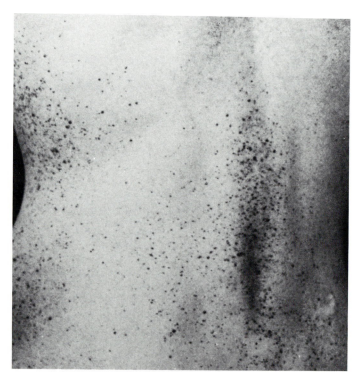

Fig. 12-15. Numerous angiokeratomas over trunk. (Courtesy M. Ruiten, Gröningen, The Netherlands.)

Nervous system. Onset of the disease in hemizygous males usually occurs during childhood or adolescence and is characterized by periodic, excruciating acroparesthesias, which may become more frequent and severe with age. These painful episodes may last several days and are associated with low-grade fever and elevation of the erythrocyte sedimentation rate. During the second and third decades of life, these recurrent episodes become progressively more painful and may occur weekly, usually lasting 12 to 24 hours, but occasionally persisting for 1 or 2 weeks. Affected individuals may be incapacitated for prolonged periods of time.

Oral manifestations. The majority of patients have symmetrical, pinpoint, macular, purplish spots on the lips, especially on the lower lip near the skin-mucosal junction, on either side of the midline. The lesions are smaller than those on the skin (Fig. 12-16). The buccal mucosa appears to be involved to a lesser degree. Only rarely are other oral tissues—gingiva, soft palate, and uvula—involved. The tongue is not affected. The nasal mucosa has been involved, with resultant epistaxis. Glycosphingolipid accumulation has been demonstrated in dental pulp from hemizygous males.[54]

Laboratory aids

Birefringent lipid inclusions can be observed histologically in biopsied tissues (including dental pulp), bone marrow macrophages, or urinary sediment.[54] All cases should be confirmed biochemically by the demonstration of increased levels of trihexosyl ceramide in urinary sediment, plasma, or cultured fibroblasts, or by deficient activity of the specific enzyme, ceramide trihexosidase, or nonspecific α-galactosidase in plasma, leukocytes, biopsied tissue, or cultured fibroblasts. Prenatal detection can be accomplished by the demonstration of deficient α-galactosidase in cultured amniotic cells obtained by amniocentesis.

FAMILIAL DYSAUTONOMIA (RILEY-DAY SYNDROME)

A syndrome consisting of absence of overflow tears, vasomotor instability, hypoactive deep tendon reflexes, relative indifference to pain, feeding difficulties, and absence of lingual fungiform papillae was first described by Riley and associates.[65] Subsequently, Riley[64]

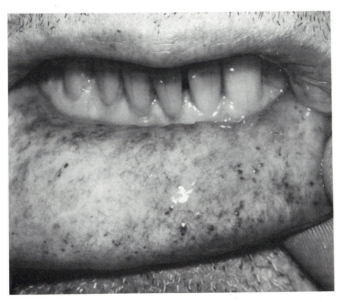

Fig. 12-16. Labial involvement. Note that angiokeratomas are smaller than lesions of hereditary hemorrhagic telangiectasia.

and Riley and Moore[66] presented thorough reviews of the clinical picture in this syndrome.

Heredity

Genetic studies have shown autosomal recessive inheritance. Virtually all parents had Ashkenazic Jewish ancestry, the great majority stemming from eastern Europe (Galicia, the Ukraine, or Romania). About one American Jew in 10,000 to 20,000 has familial dysautonomia. The frequency is similar among Israeli Jews of Ashkenazic extraction. Parental consanguinity has been noted in at least 5% of cases.[62]

Systemic manifestations

Stature is small, and intellectual development is delayed. About 25% of these patients die of pulmonary infection by the age of 10 years. Recurrent bronchopneumonia is common, probably because food is frequently aspirated.

Facies. A frightened, fixed expression with a slitlike mouth and a peculiar "working" of the tongue is typical. The face is thin, with a pale to grayish color except during excitement. External strabismus is common.

Nervous system. Difficulties in swallowing and regurgitation appear soon after birth, and the infant fails to produce overflow tears with usual stimuli.[65] Other frequent signs are absent to hyporeactive deep tendon reflexes, poor motor coordination, breath-holding spells, scanning nasal speech, postural hypotension, paroxysmal hypertension, emotional lability, and relative indifference to pain. On the other hand, many of these children do not like their feet or scalp to be touched (dysesthesia). The indifference to pain may result in Charcot joints as the child grows older. Skin blotching, abnormal sweating, erratic temperature control, and episodic vomiting are frequently seen. About 80% of patients exhibit growth retardation, and about 55% have severe progressive scoliosis, which appears around the eighth or ninth year of life. Intelligence is normal. Speech is often monotonous and slurred with an unusual nasal quality.[62]

Eyes. Constant features are decreased tearing, absent corneal reflex, and absent pupillary constriction in response to subconjunctival instillation of methacholine.[66] Neuroparalytic keratitis, mild keratitis sicca, or corneal ulceration have been noted in at least 30% of cases.

Oral manifestations. Characteristically the

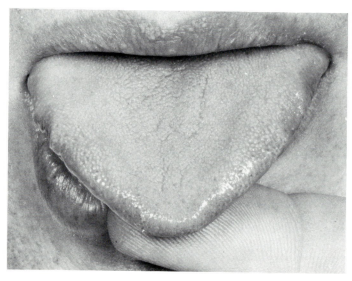

Fig. 12-17. Absence of fungiform papillae.

mouth is transversely elongated into a horizontal slit. Smith and co-workers[67] reported absence of fungiform papillae on the tongue (Fig. 12-17). Henkin and Kopin[60] reported that circumvallate papillae were also absent or greatly diminished in number. Sensitivity to sweet and bitter taste is reduced in these patients and usually provides the first anatomical evidence of a peripheral sensory defect in the disease. There is excessive drooling and diminished gag reflex or swallowing disturbance in about 80% of the patients. Dental caries is infrequent, perhaps due to the reduced taste sensibility and consequent lowered desire for sweets. However, periodontal disease, malocclusion, and dental arch crowding are common.[63]

HEREDITARY HEMORRHAGIC TELANGIECTASIA (OSLER-RENDU-WEBER SYNDROME)

Hereditary hemorrhagic telangiectasia is characterized by multiple capillary and venous dilations of the skin and mucous membranes.

Heredity

The mode of transmission is autosomal dominant.[68, 74] The so-called lethal homozygotic state[71] we cannot accept as a valid example.

Systemic manifestations

The telangiectasia observed in the syndrome may vary in appearance from pinpoint to spider-like to nodular. The lesions are bright red, violaceous, or purple. When a glass slab is pressed on them, they blanch. Often the patients are pale and may have a history of fatigue and weakness caused by bleeding from the telangiectases with resultant anemia. The hemorrhage, often nontraumatic, is the most severe complication and becomes more frequent with advancing age.

Skin. Telangiectases are observed on the facial skin, especially on the cheeks, ears, and nasal orifices in about 60% of patients.[72] They may also occur on the fingers, toes, and nail beds in about 30% of cases. They usually appear in the second to third decades of life and increase in number and size with age. The lesions may be purpuric. In elderly persons, spider-like configurations may be seen.

Nasal mucosa. Telangiectasia of the nasal mucosa is common and in 80% to 90% results in recurrent epistaxis, which tends to become more severe with time. As a rule, epistaxis precedes the appearance of telangiectasia on the skin, often appearing in childhood. Bleeding from the nose may be oozing, sometimes persisting continuously for several days, or there may be profuse hemorrhage initiated by sneezing or coughing. Hemorrhagic death has resulted in 2% to 4%.

Other mucous membranes. The gastric mucosa is often involved, resulting in melena and hematemesis, which increase with age in about 20% of the cases.[68] Other areas of the gastrointestinal tract (pharynx, esophagus, jejunum, sigmoid colon) or the conjunctiva may be the seat of telangiectasia. When located in the bladder, vagina, or uterus, the telangiectases may lead to genitourinary bleeding.[70]

Other findings. Almost any organ may be affected by angiodysplasias: liver, brain, spinal cord, and lungs.[70]

Oral manifestations. The lips and tongue (frequently the dorsum and tip) are sites of telangiectasia in about 60% of cases (Fig. 12-18). The palate, gingiva, buccal mucosa and mucocutaneous junctions may be similarly affected in about 20% of cases. Bleeding from the mouth is second in frequency to epistaxis, having been noted in about 20% of cases. Hemorrhage from the gingiva and buccal mucosa occurs less frequently than from the lips and tongue. Labial lesions are more common (about 85%) in those with gastrointestinal bleeding.

Laboratory aids

The hemoglobin and erythrocyte counts may be lowered because of hemorrhage. When telangiectases are suspected in the gastrointestinal tract, gastroscopy and sigmoidoscopy may be carried out.

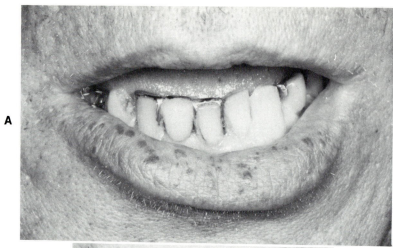

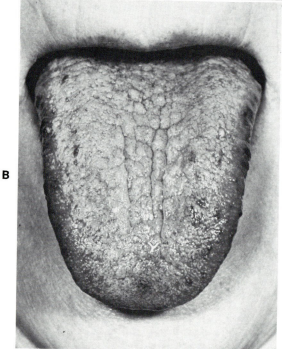

Fig. 12-18. **A,** Telangiectasia of lower lip. **B,** Telangiectasia of tongue. (Courtesy J. J. Pindborg, Copenhagen, Denmark.)

ACRODERMATITIS ENTEROPATHICA (DANBOLT-CLOSS SYNDROME)

Acrodermatitis enteropathica is a rare childhood disorder characterized by skin lesions, hair loss, nail changes, and gastrointestinal disturbances, which was completely delineated in 1943 by Danbolt and Closs. The reader is referred to the review of Wells and Winkelmann.[78] Over 200 cases have been reported.

Heredity

In 65% of reported cases, there has been a history of familial occurrence.[78] A recessive mode of transmission appears evident. The disease is evenly distributed all over the

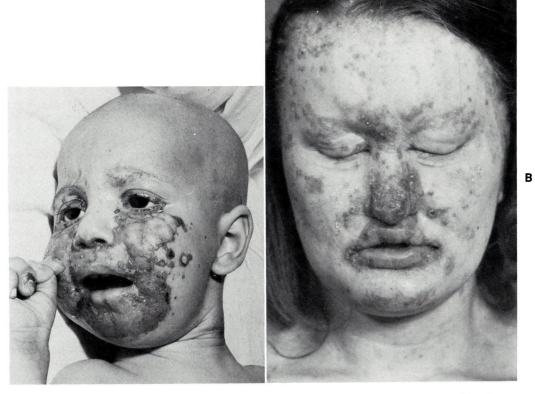

Fig. 12-19, **A**, Acrodermatitis enteropathica in an infant. **B**, Acrodermatitis enteropathica in postpubescent girl. (**A** courtesy Dr. S. Freier, Jerusalem, Israel; **B** courtesy N. Danbolt, Oslo, Norway.)

world. Although the exact mechanism is not known, the syndrome is related to a low serum zinc level.[77]

Systemic manifestations

Acrodermatitis begins early in life, usually between the ages of 3 weeks and 10 years, with an average age at onset of 9 months. Occasionally, the syndrome has been reported in adults[79] (Fig. 12-19). The disorder seems to improve by puberty. The onset is insidious and follows an intermittent course, often with spontaneous, partial remissions, succeeded by increasingly severe exacerbations. The majority of cases ended fatally before the use of zinc dietary supplements.[76]

Body growth is retarded in 80% of the patients, and 40% present mental changes, often in the form of schizophrenic behavior associated with the exacerbations of the disease.

Facies. Children suffering from acrodermatitis enteropathica exhibit a striking uniformity of appearance, mainly because of the alopecia and the orificial location of lesions.

Skin. The syndrome usually starts with small erythematous, moist skin eruptions localized around the natural orifices and symmetrically on the buttocks, elbows, knees, hands, and feet, especially between the fingers and toes and around the nails. The trunk is only slightly affected. The rash in most cases is of vesiculobullous type, but vesicles or bullae are not always present. After a short period of time, the vesicular lesions begin to dry and crust, subsequently turning into sharply marginated lesions, sometimes with psoriasiform appearance.[78] When the lesions heal, they leave no scars.

Gastrointestinal tract. Gastrointestinal disturbances consist of bouts of diarrhea with increased excretion of fat.

Oral manifestations. A large number of children with the syndrome suffer from thrush. The buccal mucosa, less often the palate, gingiva, and tonsils, presents red and white spots or edema with erosions, ulcerations, and desquamation. The white coating of the oral mucosa is reported to be rather firmly attached to underlying structures. On the buccal mucosa and borders of the tongue, there may be numerous small papillomas with a whitish, thickened epithelial covering. Severe halitosis is often present.

Laboratory aids

Serum zinc levels should be determined.

MULTIPLE MUCOSAL NEUROMAS, PHEOCHROMOCYTOMA, MEDULLARY CARCINOMA OF THE THYROID, AND MARFANOID BODY BUILD WITH MUSCLE WASTING

Initially described in part about fifty years ago, the syndrome of (1) multiple mucosal neuromas, (2) pheochromocytoma, (3) medullary carcinoma of the thyroid, and (4) Marfanoid build with muscle wasting of the extremities had its description enlarged by Williams and Pollock,[85] Gorlin and associates,[81, 82] Schimke and co-workers,[84] Levy and associates,[83] and Carney et al.[80]

Heredity

The syndrome is inherited as an autosomal dominant trait. An analysis of forty-four cases was carried out by Gorlin and Mirkin.[81] Most aspects of the syndrome can be explained by hyperplasia and/or neoplasia of neural crest derivatives.

Systemic manifestations

Facies. A distinct facies has been noted, which is characterized by large nodular lips and thickening and often eversion of upper eyelids.

Mucosal neuromas

Oral neuromas. The mucosal neuromas principally involve the lips and tongue, although buccal, gingival, palatal, pharyngeal, nasal, conjunctival, and other mucosae can be the site of these lesions. Both lips are extensively and nodularly enlarged. The lingual lesions are largely limited to the anterior dorsal surface of the tongue and appear as pink pedunculated nodules (Fig. 12-20). Oral and labial involvement is the first component of the syndrome to appear, almost invariably before the eighth year of life. Microscopically, the mucosal nodules are plexiform neuromas, that is, unencapsulated masses of convoluted myelinated and unmyelinated nerves (Fig. 12-21). An occasional ganglion cell is noted.

Eyes. The eyelid margins are thickened and often everted. Pedunculated nodules, up to 6 mm in diameter, are present on the palpebral conjunctiva in nearly all patients. The cornea is the site of white medullated nerve fibers, which can easily be seen under slit-lamp examination using low power with a broad beam of light. They extend into the pupillary area, where they anastomose.

Other sites of involvement. Nasal and laryngeal mucosa may also be the site of neuromas. In addition to hyperplasia of neurenteric ganglion cells throughout the entire gastrointestinal tract wall, similar changes have been observed in the bronchi, bladder, or spinal nerve roots.

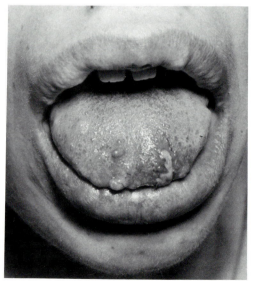

Fig. 12-20. Bumpy lips and nodular tongue due to mucosal neuromas.

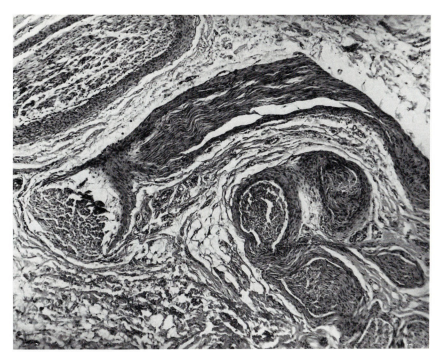

Fig. 12-21. Microscopic appearance of mucosal neuroma.

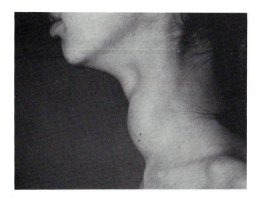

Fig. 12-22. Medullary carcinoma of thyroid.

Pheochromocytoma. The presence of pheochromocytoma is often heralded by weakness, flushing, pounding headache, nausea, hypertension, dyspnea, palpation, flatulence, paresthesia, blanching of the extremities, profuse sweating, and intractable diarrhea.

Pheochromocytoma, commonly bilateral, has been diagnosed in about 50% of cases, most becoming evident during the second and third decades of life.

Medullary carcinoma of the thyroid. Medullary carcinoma of the thyroid has been diagnosed in over 65% of patients with the syndrome. Most have been between 18 and 25 years of age at the time of the tumor's initial appearance. In no case has the tumor become manifest before the twelfth year of life (Fig. 12-22).

Musculoskeletal alterations. The majority of patients have exhibited an asthenic or somewhat Marfanoid build with severe muscle wasting, especially of the extremities, simulating a myopathic state (Fig. 12-23). A host of skeletal alterations have been noted: pes cavus, severe lordosis, aseptic necrosis of lumbar spine, kyphosis, scoliosis, and increased mobility of joints. These have been reviewed by Gorlin and Mirkin.[80]

Laboratory aids

Serum calcitonin levels should be ascertained to monitor the presence of medullary carcinoma of the thyroid. Intracutaneous injection of 1:1000 histamine produces a wheal but no flare. Vanilmandelic acid or

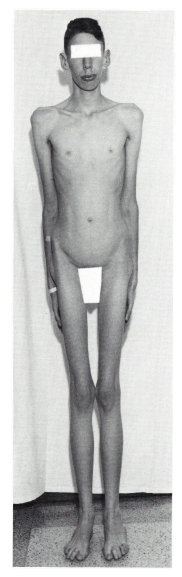

Fig. 12-23. Asthenic body build with muscle wasting.

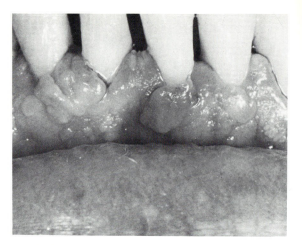

Fig. 12-24. Numerous fibrous growths of gingiva. (From Rosenbluth, M.: Periodontics **1**:81-83, 1963.)

other catecholamine levels should be employed to monitor the presence of pheochromocytoma.

MULTIPLE HAMARTOMA AND NEOPLASIA SYNDROME (COWDEN SYNDROME)

This syndrome was first described by Lloyd and Dennis.[89] Weary and associates[91] published five examples of the syndrome, emphasizing its hamartomatous character and sug-

gesting that it principally involved the skin, gastrointestinal tract, breasts, and thyroid. Gentry and co-workers[87] reported additional cases.

Heredity

The syndrome is inherited in an autosomal dominant manner.[87]

Systemic manifestations

Breasts. Fibroadenomatosis, virginal hypertrophy, and breast carcinoma have been described.

Thyroid. Thyroid alteration has included fetal adenoma, follicular adenocarcinoma, and so-called goiter.

Other tumors. A wide variety of neoplasms has been noted: ovarian cysts, colonic polyposis and/or diverticulosis, ganglioneuromatosis of the colon, meningioma of ear canal, angiomatous lesions of soft and hard tissues, and lipomas, both subcutaneous and retroperitoneal. Angiomyomas have been described in the extremities.

Skin. The pinnae, the lateral neck, the nasal, periorbital, glabellar, perioral areas, and the dorsum of hands and forearms are the most frequently involved sites of lichenoid and papillomatous lesions. Histological examination suggests that they are hamartomas of hair follicle origin similar to inverted follicular keratoses. The palms may exhibit waxy punctate keratoderma.[90]

Other findings. Hydronephrosis has been described. However, in one case,[88] it was thought to be secondary to a huge retroperitoneal lipoma.

Oral manifestations. Papular lesions of the lips and gingiva and, to a lesser extent, the palate, as well as papillomatous lesions of the buccal, faucial, and oropharyngeal mucosa have been noted in most patients. The tongue is pebbly and fissured (Fig. 12-24).

Laboratory aids

No laboratory aids are known.

PEUTZ-JEGHERS SYNDROME (MUCOCUTANEOUS MELANOTIC PIGMENTATION AND GASTROINTESTINAL POLYPOSIS)

The syndrome of mucocutaneous melanotic pigmentation associated with intestinal polyposis received its eponym from Peutz,[98] a Dutch physician who described the syndrome in three generations, and from Jeghers and associates,[95] who published a comprehensive account of ten cases. Since that time, nearly 350 cases have been recorded. The surveys of Dormandy[93] and Klosterman[96] furnished added knowledge of the syndrome.

Heredity

The syndrome is transmitted as an autosomal dominant disorder with virtually complete penetrance.

Systemic manifestations

Gastrointestinal system. Polyposis of the gastrointestinal tract is the clinically more important component of the syndrome. The polyps are hamartomatous in origin. The following sites are involved with the approximate frequency: jejunum, 65%; ileum, 55%; large bowel and rectum, 35% each; stomach, 25%; duodenum, 15%; appendix, 5%.

Thus the polyps may be found anywhere in the mucus-secreting portion of the gastrointestinal tract and may make themselves apparent by producing intussusception. Often

the intussusception is self-resolving but may lead to serious intestinal obstruction and death. Onset of symptoms varies widely, from a few weeks to old age. However, about 70% of patients experience some type of gastrointestinal symptoms—intermittent colicky pain (85%) and melena or rectal bleeding (35%)—before diagnosis.

The polyps are usually described as benign adenomatous tumors varying in size from 0.5 to 7 cm in diameter. Dormandy[93] suggested that these growths are hamartomatous, arising from primitive adenomatous vesicles embedded in the bowel wall. Although several authors have described malignant degeneration of a polyp, Dozois and co-workers[94] reviewed these cases and found no parallelism between location of the malignant tumor and the general location of polyps in this syndrome; that is, the most common sites for the adenocarcinomas (stomach and colon) are least likely to be sites of polyps.

Microscopically, the polyps represent focal overgrowths, in improper proportions, of tissues indigenous to that part of the gastrointestinal tract. A branching-tree arrangement of smooth muscle may be seen scattered throughout the growths. Frequent mitotic figures are also characteristic. The growths may extend to the serosal surface.

Skin. In about 50% of affected persons, numerous, usually discrete, brown to bluish-black macules are present on the skin, especially about the facial orifices—perioral, perinasal, periorbital (Fig. 12-25). Although some patients exhibit only a few pigmented macules, others are markedly pigmented. In addition, pigmented spots occur on the extremities in about a third of affected individuals.

Ovarian cysts and tumors. Ovarian neoplasms, most often granulosa cell tumors, have been found in about 10% of women with Peutz-Jeghers syndrome.[92, 99]

Oral manifestations. On the lips, especially the lower lip, and on the oral mucosa, round, oval, or irregular, rarely confluent macules of bluish gray pigment of variable intensity may be seen. They vary in size from 1 to 12 mm, usually somewhat larger than those on the cutaneous surface. About 98% of 117 patients

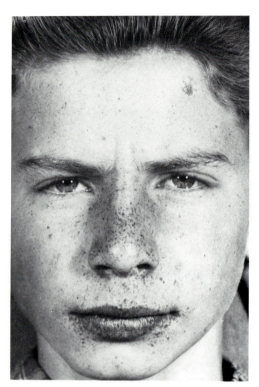

Fig. 12-25. Perioroficial melanotic macules.

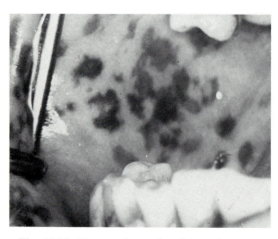

Fig. 12-26. Pigmented macules of buccal mucosa. (From Klosterman, G. F.: Arch. Klin. Exp. Dermatol. **226:**182-189, 1966.)

had pigmentation of the lips, and 88% had involvement of the buccal mucosa[97] (Fig. 12-26).

WHITE SPONGE NEVUS

White sponge nevus, better called *white folded dysplasia of mucous membrane,* was first reported by Cannon.[101]

Heredity

White sponge nevus is inherited as an autosomal dominant disorder.

Mucous membranes

White folded dysplasia may be congenital or may appear by puberty. The white spongy plaques may occur on any part of the oral mucosa, with variable involvement of the esophageal, anal, vulval, and vaginal mucosa[102] (Fig. 12-27).

The histological appearance is similar to that seen in pachyonychia congenita.[100, 103, 104, 106, 107] The epithelium is thickened with hyperkeratosis. The cells of the stratum spinosum manifest intracellular edema with pyknotic nuclei. Parakeratinized plugs extend deep toward the basal layer. Whitten's[105] ultrastructural studies showed virtually total absence of differentiation of epithelial cells beyond the parabasal level. He thought that the basic defect may reside in abnormal storage of fibrous protein in the epithelial cells and in increased production of extracellular cementing substances produced by the membrane-producing granules, which prevents normal desquamation and hence clinical thickening.

HEREDITARY BENIGN INTRAEPITHELIAL DYSKERATOSIS (WITKOP–VON SALLMANN SYNDROME)

The syndrome of hereditary benign intraepithelial dyskeratosis was described in a North Carolina triracial isolate (Caucasian-Negro-Indian) in 1960 by Witkop and associates and by von Sallmann and Paton. The chief components are plaques of the bulbar conjunctiva and oral mucosal thickenings clinically similar to white sponge nevus of Cannon.

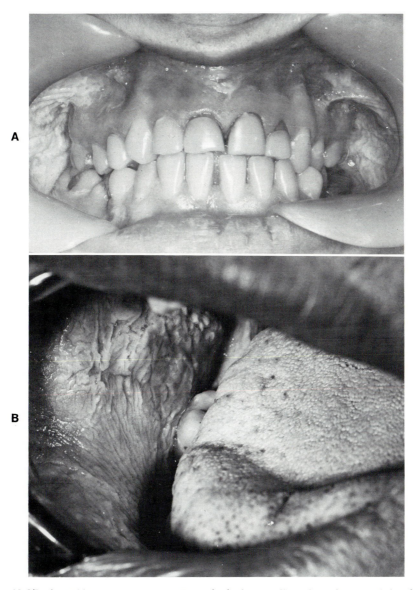

Fig. 12-27. A, White sponge nevus. Note gingival as well as buccal mucosal involvement. **B,** Marked rugosity of buccal mucosa. (**A** courtesy W. G. Browne, Inverness, Scotland; **B** courtesy C. J. Witkop., Jr., Minneapolis, Minn.)

Heredity

The syndrome exhibits autosomal dominant inheritance with a high degree of penetrance.[110] Attempts to link this disorder with several blood groups have met with negative results.[108]

Systemic manifestations

Eyes. About the limbus, both nasally and temporally, there are foamy gelatinous plaques, more superficial than pterygia, on a hyperemic bulbar conjunctiva (Fig. 12-28). The eye lesion is usually noted within the first year of life.[109]

The dyskeratotic process may involve the cornea, producing blindness from shedding and resultant vascularization of this structure. Photophobia, especially in children, is common.

Oral manifestations. The oral mucosal thickenings are asymptomatic. They appear as soft white folds and plaques, resembling white sponge nevus (Fig. 12-29). Although the thickenings appear at birth, they are mild, increasing in severity to about 15 years of age. There does not appear to be a tendency for the plaques to undergo malignant degeneration.

Tissue sections or Papanicolaou-stained smears of buccal mucosal or conjunctival scrapings are characteristic. Acanthosis, vacuolization of the stratum spinosum, and intraepithelial dyskeratosis characterized by waxy eosinophilic cells called *tobacco cells,* and a cell-within-a-cell pattern are noted. These latter changes are especially evident in Papanicolaou-stained smears (Fig. 12-30).

Witkop and Gorlin[110] found similarities in oral smears from hereditary benign intraepithelial dyskeratosis and keratosis follicularis (Darier-White disease). The grains of the latter resemble the so-called tobacco cells of the former, and the corps ronds of the latter resemble the cell-within-a-cell body seen in the syndrome under discussion. However, the cell-within-a-cell is far more common in oral smears of hereditary benign intraepithelial dyskeratosis, and, in addition, one rarely sees the small blue parabasilar cells so often seen in keratosis follicularis. Patients receiving methotrexate also exhibit the cell-within-a-cell phenomenon in exfoliated buccal cells.

Laboratory aids

Papanicolaou-stained smear or biopsy as just noted may be used.

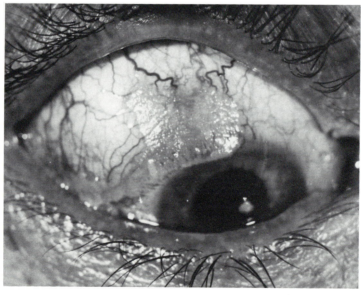

Fig. 12-28. Gelatinous plaques and vascularity of bulbar conjunctiva. (Courtesy C. J. Witkop, Jr., Minneapolis, Minn.)

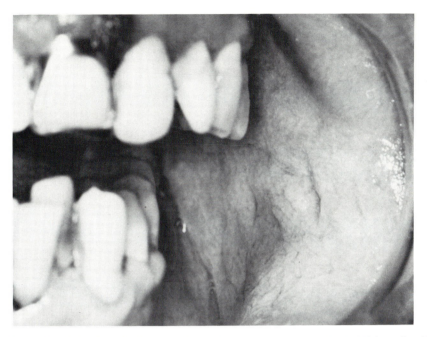

Fig. 12-29. Marked white thickening of buccal mucosa. (Courtesy C. J. Witkop, Jr., Minneapolis, Minn.)

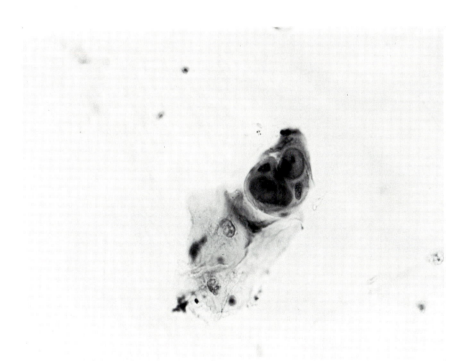

Fig. 12-30. Cell-within-cell dyskeratosis. (Courtesy C. J. Witkop, Jr., Minneapolis, Minn.)

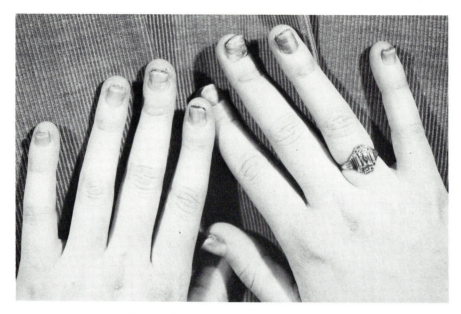

Fig. 12-31. Nails are thickened from birth.

PACHYONYCHIA CONGENITA (JADASSOHN-LEWANDOWSKI SYNDROME)

Pachyonychia congenita is genetically heterogeneous, two distinct syndromes being subsumed under the term. Although both syndromes exhibit some similarities, their differences are never observed within the same pedigree. I will limit my discussion to the one having oral mucosal involvement.

Jadassohn and Lewandowski[114] described the syndrome of pachyonychia congenita, palmoplantar keratosis and hyperhidrosis, follicular keratosis, and oral leukokeratosis.

Heredity

The syndrome follows an autosomal dominant mode of transmission.

Systemic manifestations

Skin and skin appendages. In most cases, at birth or soon thereafter, the fingernails and toenails become thickened, tubular, and hard, the undersurface being filled with a horny, yellowish-brown material. This substance causes the nail to project upward from the nail bed at the free edge (Fig. 12-31).

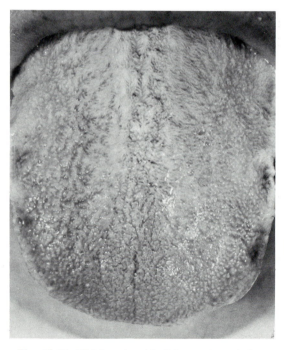

Fig. 12-32. Thickened epithelial covering of dorsum of tongue. (From Gorlin, R. J., and Chaudhry, A. P.: Oral Surg. **11**:541-544, 1958.)

Palmar and plantar hyperkeratoses are noted in 40% to 65% of the cases during the first few years of life. During warm weather, bullae appear on the feet, especially on the plantar surface of the toes and heels along the sides. They burst, become infected, and are extremely painful, often making walking an extremely difficult task. Hyperhidrosis of the palms and soles nearly always occurs, the rest of the skin being dry.

During the first few years of life, pinhead-sized follicular papules appear over the elbows, knees, popliteal areas, and buttocks in over 50% of the cases.[115]

Oral manifestations. The dorsum of the tongue is thickened, presenting a white or grayish white appearance (Fig. 12-32). Less commonly involved is the buccal mucosa at the interdental lines. Oral aphthae are frequent.

The oral mucosa is thickened by a uniform acanthosis. There is marked intracellular vacuolization. The microscopic picture greatly resembles that seen in white sponge nevus.[113]

Laboratory aids

No laboratory aids are known.

DARIER'S DISEASE

Darier's disease (keratosis folliculosis) is manifest as cutaneous hyperkeratotic papules usually first appearing in childhood. Not un-

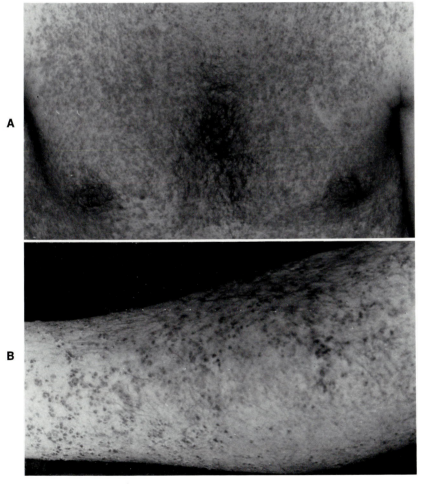

Fig. 12-33. Darier's disease. **A,** Confluent papular lesions of trunk. **B,** Similar involvement of leg. (From Spouge, J. D., Trott, J. R., and Chesko, G.: Oral Surg. **21:**441-457, 1966.)

commonly, the mucous membranes of the oral cavity, pharynx, larynx, vagina, and rectum are similarly involved.

Heredity

The disorder exhibits autosomal dominant inheritance.

Systemic manifestations

Skin. In the early stage, the cutaneous lesions are small (2 or 3 mm), firm pruritic papules that appear initially at the orifices of hair follicles. Gradually they enlarge and change from skin color to grayish-brown and become encrusted with greasy keratin. Often they are initially noted in the scalp or on the face and extend over the extremities, chest, and genital region (Fig. 12-33). Papillomatous masses may form in the axillae, groin, or retroauricular areas, which produce an offensive, rancid odor. Subungual hyperkeratoses are also common.

Microscopically, the cutaneous and mucosal lesions present a diagnostic picture. There are hyperkeratosis, acanthosis, dyskeratosis, and formation of cleftlike intraepithelial lacunae, usually suprabasilar in location. Two variants of dyskeratotic cells are identifiable: (1) intensely basophilic-staining, small, elongated grains and (2) corps ronds (Fig. 12-34), which are cells with homogeneous eosinophilic material surrounding a basophilic pyknotic nucleus. Caulfield and Wilgram[117] suggested that the cause is an error in synthesis, organization, or maturation of the tonofilament-desmosomic complex.

Oral manifestations. The oral lesions are 1 to 3 mm papules somewhat resembling cobblestones.[119, 120] They principally involve the hard and soft palates[118] (Fig. 12-35).

Laboratory aids

Biopsy of skin or oral mucosal lesions may be useful.

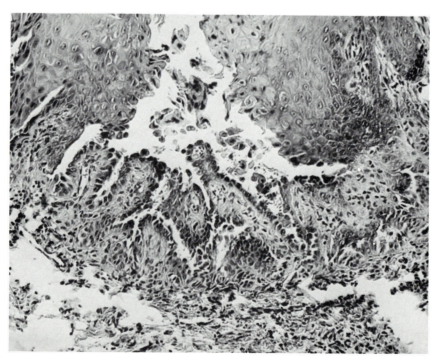

Fig. 12-34. Characteristic microscopic picture showing cleftlike intraepithelial lacunae, suprabasilar in position. Note elongated grains and corps ronds.

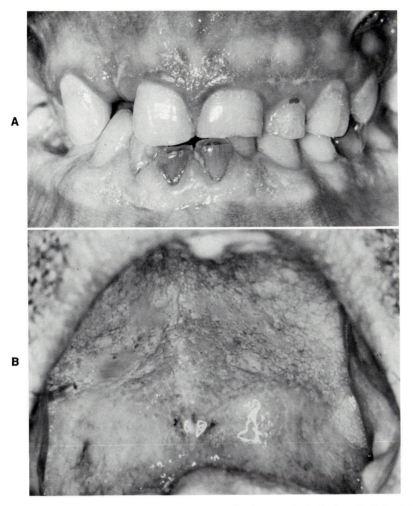

Fig. 12-35. A, Early lesions of maxillary and mandibular attached gingiva. **B,** Palatal involvement. (**A** from Spouge, J. D., Trott, J. R., and Chesko, G.: Oral Surg. 21:441-457, 1966; **B** courtesy J. Payne, Northwood, Middlesex, England.)

PALMOPLANTAR HYPERKERATOSIS AND ATTACHED GINGIVAL HYPERKERATOSIS

Raphael and associates[112] reported the combination of palmoplantar hyperkeratosis and attached gingival hyperkeratosis in a kindred involving several generations. In 1974, while visiting Athens, Greece, I had the opportunity to see another family with the same disorder, and, in 1975, I examined a large kindred in Minneapolis. An isolated example was reported by Fred and co-workers.[121]

Heredity

Autosomal dominant inheritance is indicated by transmission of the disorder through several generations. There was male-to-male transmission in all kindreds.

Systemic manifestations

Cutaneous findings. Focal hyperkeratosis of the soles was more marked over the weight-bearing areas, the heels, toe pads, and metatarsal heads. Hyperkeratosis of the palms also seemed trauma related. Hyperhidrosis was noted in the hyperkeratotic areas (Fig. 12-36).

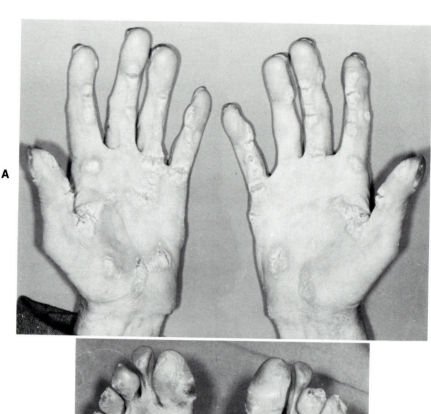

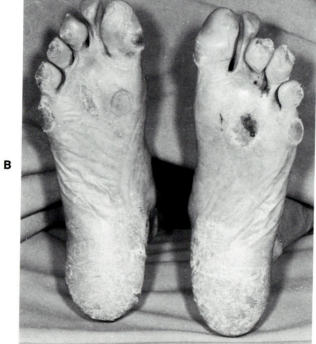

Fig. 12-36. Hyperkeratosis of **A,** palms and **B,** soles.

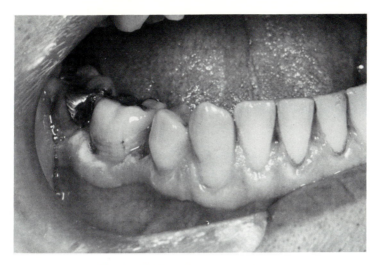

Fig. 12-37. Hyperkeratosis of gingiva.

The hyperkeratotic areas appeared around puberty in most patients.

Involvement of the distal portion of the finger and toe nails with keratin deposits first involved the toes at 4 or 5 years of age followed by fingernail changes at 8 or 9 years of age.

Oral findings. Sharply marginated hyperkeratosis involved the labial and lingual attached gingiva (Fig. 12-37). The hyperkeratotic area appeared in early childhood and increased in severity with age.

Laboratory aids

Biopsy is of no value in establishing the diagnosis.

HYPERKERATOSIS PALMOPLANTARIS AND PERIODONTOCLASIA IN CHILDHOOD (PAPILLON-LEFÈVRE SYNDROME)

Papillon and Lefèvre[126] described a syndrome consisting of hyperkeratosis of palms and soles and destruction of the supporting tissues of both primary and permanent dentitions.

Heredity

The syndrome is inherited in an autosomal recessive manner.[125]

Systemic manifestations

Skin. At approximately the same time that periodontal involvement first occurs, sometime between the second and fourth years of life, or on rare occasions even earlier, the palms and soles become red and scaly (Fig. 12-38). The hyperkeratotic involvement of the palms is usually well demarcated, extending to the edges and over the thenar eminences. The soles are usually more severely involved, the process frequently spilling over the edges, where it may be most marked, extending to the Achilles tendon. Occasionally, the external malleoli, tibial tuberosities, and dorsal finger and toe joints may exhibit a scaly redness.[124, 127]

Oral manifestations. The development and eruption of the deciduous teeth proceeds normally, but almost simultaneously with the appearance of palmar and plantar hyperkeratosis, the gingiva swell and become boggy, and marked halitosis develops. Destruction of the periodontium almost immediately follows eruption of the last primary molar tooth (Fig. 12-39). The teeth are involved in roughly the same order in which they erupt. One observes deep periodontal pocket formation followed by exfoliation of the teeth. By the age of 4 years, nearly all primary teeth have been lost. With exfoliation of the teeth, the inflamma-

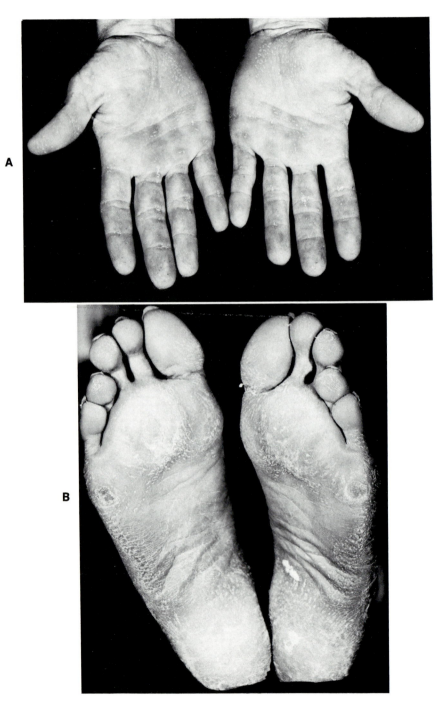

Fig. 12-38. Hyperkeratosis of **A,** palms and **B,** soles. (From Gorlin, R. J., Sedano, H., and Anderson, V. E.: J. Pediatr. **65:**895-908, 1964.)

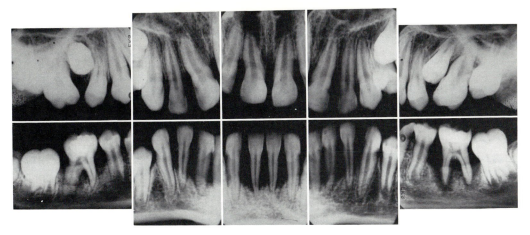

Fig. 12-39. Premature destruction of periodontium. (From Dekker, G., and Jansen, L. H.: J. Periodontol. **29:**266, 1958.)

tion subsides, and the gingiva resumes its normal appearance. The mouth then appears normal until the permanent dentition erupts, when the process is repeated in essentially the same manner. Only the wisdom teeth do not exfoliate. Bony destruction is usually severe, and the alveolar process is often completely destroyed. Even during the stage of active periodontal breakdown, the rest of the oral tissues appear entirely normal.

Laboratory aids

No laboratory aids are known.

ACATALASIA

Acatalasia as described by Takahara[135, 136] is characterized by progressive oral gangrene.

Heredity

Normal parents of affected sibs and increased parental consanguinity indicate autosomal recessive inheritance. Heterozygotes have shown blood catalase activities intermediate between normal controls and homozygote acatalasemic individuals. In Japan, carriers vary in different communities from 0.09% to 1.4% of the population.[130, 131]

Asymptomatic acatalasia has been found in Koreans, Swiss, and Israelis.[128, 134] Heterozygotes have been found in the United States and Sweden. There is suggestive evidence that there is genetic heterogeneity in acatalasia.[130, 137]

Systemic manifestations

Lesions in this disorder are limited to the mouth. There is remarkable range of severity, cases ranging from asymptomatic to those with severe oral lesions. Among families with acatalasia, approximately 25% of those exhibiting the enzyme defect have no oral lesions. About 60% develop oral lesions before the age of 10 years.

The mildest and most common form of the disorder consists of small, painful crater-like ulcerations situated on the free gingiva, which spontaneously heal. They first appear after the eruption of the primary teeth. In moderately severe cases, the entire free gingiva is involved followed by progressive bone loss. With extension of the gangrenous process, there is loosening and exfoliation of teeth followed by spontaneous healing. A few patients have had osteomyelitis with bony sequestration and/or invasion of the maxillary sinus or nasal cavity.

The pathogenesis as postulated by Takahara[136] involves the invasion of the gingival tissue by normally present hydrogen peroxide–producing organisms. In homozygotes, hydrogen peroxide accumulates and destroys hemoglobin, thus depriving the tissues of oxygen with resultant necrosis. The necrotic tissue, in turn, favors additional growth of bacteria.

Laboratory aids

Blood catalase levels should be determined in carriers and affecteds.

POROKERATOSIS

Porokeratosis (Mibelli's disease) reveals cutaneous and/or mucosal lesions characterized by patches with atrophic centers surrounded by a raised keratotic wall.

Heredity

The disorder is inherited as an autosomal dominant trait. However, it has been reported in about twice as many males as females.

Systemic manifestations

Skin. The cutaneous lesion is a chronic, slowly growing, well-defined ringlike formation. Initially, there is a keratinous papule that slowly enlarges, leaving a cleared, flattened atrophic center with a peripheral, open circular wall of keratin. It appears early in life and persists for years. The hands and feet most often are affected.

Oral manifestations. Possibly 50% of the patients have been reported to have lesions on the mucous membranes.[138, 140] The upper lip is rather frequently involved.[139] The microscopic picture is diagnostic. The central atrophic area reveals dermal fibrosis and atrophy of the prickle layer with overlying hyperkeratosis, whereas the wall shows acanthosis and a deep central groove filled with parakeratotic epithelium (cornoid lamella).

Laboratory aids

Biopsy as just noted may be useful.

PSEUDOXANTHOMA ELASTICUM (GRÖNBLAD-STRANDBERG SYNDROME)

The syndrome of alterations of the skin, recurrent severe gastrointestinal hemorrhages, weak peripheral pulses, and failing vision was identified and named by Darier in 1896.[144] Angioid streaks were added to the syndrome by Grönblad and Strandberg in 1929.[146,149]

Heredity

Pseudoxanthoma elasticum appears to be genetically heterogeneous. Most examples are inherited in an autosomal recessive manner. Consanguinity has been found in at least 20% of the cases. A dominant form may also exist.[117]

Systemic manifestations

Skin. The primary alteration in pseudoxanthoma elasticum is calcification of elastic fibers. The skin becomes thickened and the markings accentuated by raised, yellowish, flat papules (Fig. 12-40), especially about the mouth, neck, axilla, elbows, and groin. These changes are usually recognized after the second decade, although they may appear as early as the third or fourth year of life. The thickened, yellowish skin becomes redundant, resembling pig skin, especially on the neck and axilla.

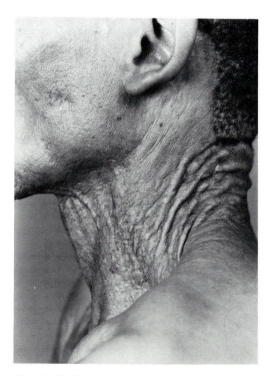

Fig. 12-40. Skin becomes thickened with markings accentuated by yellowish papules. (From Heyl, T.: Arch. Dermatol. 96:528, 1967. Copyright 1967, American Medical Association.)

Eyes. Visual disturbances have been noted in almost 30% of cases. Fundoscopic examination has demonstrated brownish or gray streaking (angioid streaks) of the fundus in over 85% of patients. The streaks resemble vessels in the way that they course over the fundus but actually represent involvement of Bruch's membrane. Retinal hemorrhage, followed by organization, results in loss of vision.[142]

Cardiovascular system. By the third decade, there may be weakness or absence of the pulses in the arms and legs, accompanied by variable degrees of intermittent claudication in about 20% of cases. Radiographic examination has revealed calcification of peripheral arteries, especially those of the lower extremities in about 15% of cases. Hypertension has been noted in about 20% of cases. Angina of effort is seen in at least half the patients.

Hemorrhage, especially gastrointestinal, occurs in 15% of cases because of involvement of small blood vessels. Bleeding may also occur in the retina, kidney, uterus, or bladder.[143, 145, 148]

Oral manifestations. The skin about the mouth may become redundant. The mucosal surfaces of the lip, especially the lower lip, may exhibit yellowish intramucosal nodules in about 10% of the cases. The buccal mucosal, soft palate, and tonsillar areas may be similarly affected (Fig. 12-41).

Laboratory aids

Both skin and mucous membrane exhibit similar histopathological alterations. The connective tissue fibers are thickened, fragmented, curled, granulated, and basophilic. They exhibit the staining qualities of elastic fibers. Calcium can be demonstrated within the degenerated fibers.

HYALINOSIS CUTIS ET MUCOSAE (URBACH-WIETHE SYNDROME, LIPOID PROTEINOSIS)

The syndrome consists of yellowish nodular infiltration of skin and mucous membranes and hoarseness. Wiethe[158] and Urbach[157] defined the condition and applied the terms "lipoidosis cutis et mucosae" and "lipoid proteinosis." Over 200 cases have been described to date.[152, 155]

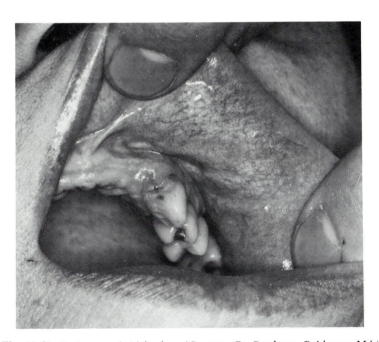

Fig. 12-41. Oral mucosal thickening. (Courtesy R. Goodman, Baltimore, Md.)

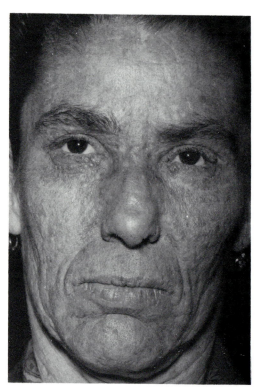

Fig. 12-42. Infiltration of skin. (Courtesy A. Wiedemann, Vienna, Austria.)

Heredity

The syndrome is transmitted in an autosomal recessive manner. It has appeared in sibs, and in about 20% of the cases there has been parental consanguinity. Many have been of Dutch, German, or Swedish extraction.[155]

Systemic manifestations

Skin and skin appendages. Discrete or confluent yellowish-ivory or waxy nodules, from pinhead to matchhead in size, usually occur on the face, neck, axillae, and hands early in life (Fig. 12-42). On the margin of the eyelids, beadlike excrescences appear in about 50% of cases, followed by loss of cilia. Brownish-yellow, wartlike hyperkeratotic lesions appear on the knees, elbows, and proximal interarticular surfaces of the fingers.

Central nervous system. Intracranial calcification has been found in at least 70% of reported cases, located above the pituitary fossa in the hippocampus, falx cerebri, or temporal lobes, and may be more often seen in individuals over the age of 10 years. Rarely there is associated epilepsy.[153]

Larynx and other mucosal involvement. The voice may be hoarse from birth or within the first few years of life. The inability to cry at birth in the majority of the cases testifies to early laryngeal involvement. Laryngoscopic examination reveals yellowish-white plaques

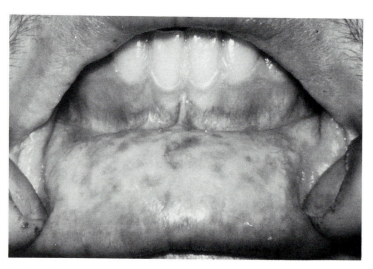

Fig. 12-43. Infiltration of lower lip. (Courtesy J. A. Keipert, Melbourne, Australia.)

on the epiglottis, aryepiglottic folds, and interarytenoid region. The cords are thickened and nodular, and closure is insufficient. Dyspnea may be severe, and laryngectomy may be necessary.

Other mucosal surfaces, such as the vulva, rectum, esophagus, stomach, and nostril mucosa are rarely affected.

Oral manifestations. The mouth is the most extensively involved area. Nearly all oral tissues become infiltrated with yellowish-white, elevated, pea-sized plaques, which appear most frequently before puberty and gradually increase in severity. The lower lip, usually more severely affected, assumes a cobblestone appearance (Fig. 12-43). Radiating fissures may appear at the angles of the mouth.

The tongue becomes firm or woody, thick, large, and bound to the floor of the mouth (Fig. 12-44), with marked infiltration of the frenum and sublingual and fimbriated plicae, which become inelastic cords. The dorsum loses its papillae. Ulcers may develop.

With infiltration of the buccal mucosa, the opening of the parotid duct may become stenosed, with ensuing retrograde parotitis. Extension of the infiltration to the pharynx may result in dysphagia. The uvula is infiltrated and usually retracted. The tonsils may be extensively infiltrated.

Teeth may fail to develop or may be hypoplastic, especially the upper lateral incisors, canines, and upper or lower premolar teeth, or the enamel may be severely hypoplastic.

Microscopically, one notes hyalinosis of the upper layers of the corium or dermis, beginning about the small arterioles. Histochemical study has revealed the presence of a carbohydrate but few or no lipids. The hyaline material stains intensely with the PAS procedure, thus appearing to be a glycoprotein either free or loosely bound to collagen.[151] Ultrastructural studies have been carried out on the hyaline material, suggesting that it represents an altered collagen.[154, 156]

TANGIER DISEASE (FAMILIAL HIGH-DENSITY LIPOPROTEIN DEFICIENCY)

Tangier disease, a disorder deriving its name from a small island in the lower Chesapeake Bay, was first described by Fredrickson.[162] It is characterized by almost complete absence of plasma high-density lipoproteins, abnormal composition of low-density lipoproteins, plasma cholesterol values below 120 mg/dl, reduced phospholipids, and nor-

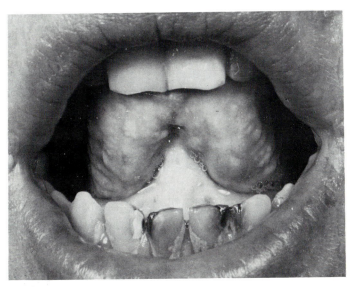

Fig. 12-44. Infiltration of undersurfaces of tongue and oral floor. (Courtesy A. Jensen, Oslo, Norway.)

mal-to-elevated triglycerides. Cholesterol esters are stored in large amounts in foam cells, particularly in reticuloendothelial cells.

Heredity

The disorder is inherited as an autosomal recessive trait.[160] Other kindreds have been described in Missouri, Kentucky, England, and Germany.[162, 164]

Tissue storage of cholesterol esters has not been observed in heterozygotes. Heterozygotes, however, have lower than normal values of high-density lipoproteins than control subjects.

Systemic manifestations

Patients present with characteristic enlargement of the tonsils and an orange to yellowish-gray color of the tonsillar, pharyngeal, and rectal mucosa which results from deposition of cholesterol esters in these tissues. In addition, there may be enlargement of lymph nodes, thymus, spleen, and liver and, less often, a finely granular corneal infiltration and maculopapular skin rash.

Histologically, the involved tissues exhibit collections of foam cells. Peripheral nerves manifest a loss of myelin sheaths. These areas of degenerated peripheral nerves are surrounded by cells that contain lipid. On chemical analysis, the lipid has been demonstrated to be cholesterol esters.[159, 163]

Nervous system. There may be loss of pain and temperature sense and progressive muscle wasting and weakness. Eyelid closing may be difficult.[165]

XANTHOMATOSIS

Xanthomatosis of the oral mucosa, especially that of the hard palate, occurs in combination with eruptive, often transient, cutaneous xanthomas, episodic abdominal pain, and hepatosplenomegaly in *familial hyperchylomicronemia* (familial fat-induced, type I hyperlipemia; Bürger-Grütz disease).[167, 168, 171] The disorder is inherited as an autosomal recessive trait. Oral xanthomatosis also may be seen in so-called *type V familial hyperlipoproteinemia,* which is hyperchylomicronemia with hyperprebeta-lipoproteinemia. α-lipoproteins and β-lipoproteins are normal or low. In addition to the clinical findings mentioned, often there is an associated abnormal glucose tolerance or diabetes mellitus that presents in adult life.[172] Similar cases were described by Braun-Falco and Braun-Falco[166] and by Schirren.[173]

Infants with severely elevated cholesterol and phospholipid levels may manifest oral, especially gingival, xanthomatosis. Oral xanthomas were seen in a child with cholangitic transient icterus of unknown cause by Svendsen.[174] Eruptive xanthomatosis results from sufficiently prolonged marked elevation of blood fat levels from whatever cause[169, 170] (Figs. 12-45 to 12-47).

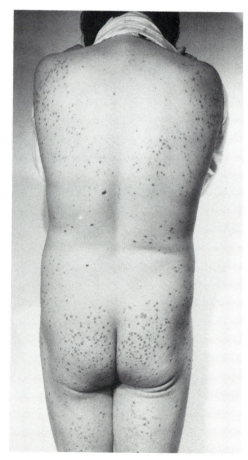

Fig. 12-45. Eruptive xanthomas of back, buttocks, and legs.

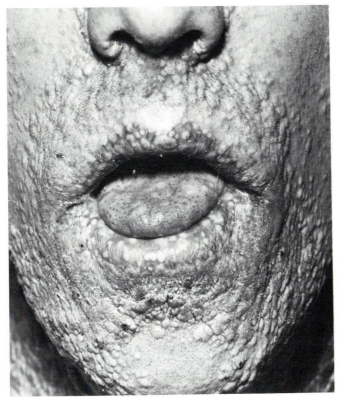

Fig. 12-46. Disseminated xanthomas of skin and mucosa. Patient had biliary cirrhosis and diabetes insipidus. (Courtesy R. K. Winkelmann, Rochester, Minn.)

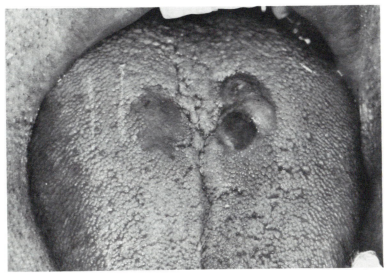

Fig. 12-47. Xanthomas of dorsum of tongue in diabetic patient. (From Raffle, E. J., and Hall, D. C.: Br. Dent. J. **125**:62-66, 1968.)

MULTICENTRIC RETICULOHISTIOCYTOSIS

Multicentric reticulohistiocytosis is a systemic disease characterized by weight loss, frequent bouts of pyrexia, arthritis, and deposits of large histiocytic cells in numerous organs such as skin, lymph nodes, bone marrow, and endocardium.

Heredity

The patients are usually in the middle to older age group, and there appears to be a predilection for women. The condition is probably inherited as an autosomal recessive trait.

Systemic manifestations

Skin. The eruption consists of numerous firm, red, brown, yellow, or flesh-colored papules. Common sites of involvement are the hands, arms, scalp, face, ears, neck, and upper trunk. Individual lesions may disappear and recur, and the total eruption may eventually fade.

Joints. The frequently deforming, usually symmetrical polyarthritis mimics rheumatoid arthritis involving the knees, hands, wrists, shoulders, ankles, hips, feet, vertebrae, and jaw. Stiffness followed by tenderness and pain, redness, and swelling with consequent limitation of movement is the usual course. In about 20% of cases the arthritis becomes mutilating.

Oral manifestations. The oral mucosa appears to be involved in about half the patients. Papules are present most frequently in the lips and tongue. Less often involved are the buccal mucosa, gingiva, pharynx, sclera, and larynx.[175-179] A strongly positive PAS reactive material is found in histiocytes and giant cells, indicating that the material is a sort of mucin, mucoprotein, or glycoprotein.

REFERENCES
Dyskeratosis congenita (Zinsser-Engman-Cole syndrome)

1. Addison, M., and Rice, M. S.: The association of dyskeratosis congenita and Fanconi's anemia, Med. J. Aust. 1:797-799, 1965.
2. Bazex, A., and Dupré, A.: Dyskératose congénitale (type Zinsser-Cole-Engman) associée à une myelopathie constitutionelle (purpura thrombopenique et neutropenie), Ann. Dermatol. Syphiligr. (Paris) 84:497-513, 1957.
3. Bodalski, J., Defecinska, E., Judkiewicz, L., and Pacanowska, M.: Fanconi's anemia and dyskeratosis congenita as a syndrome, Dermatologica 127:330-342, 1963.
4. Bryan, H. G., and Nixon, R. K.: Dyskeratosis congenita and familial pancytopenia, J.A.M.A. 192:203-208, 1965.
5. Cannell, H.: Dyskeratosis congenita, Br. J. Oral Surg. 9:8-20, 1971.
6. Engman, M. F., Sr.: A unique case of reticular pigmentation of the skin with atrophy, Arch. Dermatol. Syph. 13:685-687, 1926.
7. Inoue, S., Mekanik, G., Mahallati, M., and Zuelzer, W. W.: Dyskeratosis congenita with pancytopenia, Am. J. Dis. Child. 126:389-396, 1973.
8. Koszewski, B. J., and Hubbard, T. F.: Congenital anemia in hereditary ectodermal dysplasia, Arch. Dermatol. 74:159-166, 1956.
9. Marshall, J., and van der Meulen, H.: Dyskeratosis congenita—its occurrence in the female, Br. J. Dermatol. 77:162, 1965.
10. Milgrom, H., Stoll, H. L., and Crissey, J. T.: Dykeratosis congenita, Arch. Dermatol. 89:345-349, 1964.
11. Orfanos, C., and Gartmann, H.: Leukoplakien, Pigmentverschiebungen und Nageldystrophie, Med. Welt. 17:2589-2594, 1966.
12. Ortega, J. A., Swanson, V. L., Landing, B. H., and Hammond, G. D.: Congenital dyskeratosis, Am. J. Dis. Child. 124:701-705, 1972.
13. Sorrow, J. M., and Hitch, J. M.: Dyskeratosis congenita, Arch. Dermatol. 88:340-347, 1963.
14. Steier, W., van Voolen, G. A., and Selmanowitz, V. J.: Dyskeratosis congenita: relationship to Fanconi's anemia, Blood 39:510-521, 1972.
15. Wilgram, G. F., and Weinstock, A.: Advances in genetic dermatology, Arch. Dermatol. 94:456-479, 1966.
16. Zinsser, F.: Atrophica cutis reticularis cum pigmentatione, dystrophia unguium et leukoplakia oris, Ikonograph Derm. Kioto, 1906, pp. 219-223.

Ehlers-Danlos syndrome

17. Barabas, A. P.: Heterogeneity of the Ehlers-Danlos syndrome: description of three clinical types and a hypothesis to explain the basic defects, Br. Med. J. 21:612-613, 1967.
18. Barabas, G. M.: The Ehlers-Danlos syndrome: abnormalities of the enamel, dentine, cementum and the dental pulp: a histological

examination of 13 teeth from 6 patients, Br. Dent. J. **126**:509-515, 1969.

19. Barabas, G. M., and Barabas, A. P.: The Ehlers-Danlos syndrome: a report of the oral and haematological findings in nine cases, Br. Dent. J. **123**:472-479, 1967.

20. Beighton, P.: The Ehlers-Danlos syndrome, Springfield, Ill., 1972, Charles C Thomas, Publisher.

21. Beighton, P., and Horan, F.: Orthopaedic aspects of the Ehlers-Danlos syndrome, J. Bone Joint Surg. (Br.) **51**:444-453, 1969.

22. Beighton, P., Price, A., Lord, J., and Dickson, E.: Variants of the Ehlers-Danlos syndrome: clinical, biochemical, haematological, and chromosomal features of 100 patients, Ann. Rheum. Dis. **28**:228-245, 1969.

23. Danlos, H.: Un cas de cutis laxa avec tumeurs par contusion chronique des coudes et des genoux, Bull. Soc. Franç. Derm. Syph. **19**:70-72, 1908.

24. Ehlers, E.: Cutus laxa, Neigung zu Hemorrhagien in der Haut, Lockerung mehrerer Artikulationen, Derm. Z. **8**:173-174, 1901.

25. Goodman, R. M., and Allison, M. L.: Chronic temporomandibular joint subluxation in Ehlers-Danlos syndrome, J. Oral Surg. **27**:659-661, 1969.

26. Gorlin, R. J., and Pindborg, J. J.: Syndromes of the head and neck, New York, 1964, McGraw-Hill Book Co.

27. McKusick, V. A.: Heritable disorders of connective tissue, ed. 4, St. Louis, 1972, The C. V. Mosby Co.

28. Pindborg, J. J.: Pathology of the dental hard tissues, Philadelphia, 1970, W. B. Saunders Co.

29. Pinnell, S. R., Krane, S. M., Kenzora, J. E., and Glimcher, M. J.: A heritable disorder of connective tissue: hydroxylysine-deficient collagen disease, N. Engl. J. Med. **286**:1013-1021, 1972.

30. Selliseth, N. E.: Odontologische Befunde bei einer Patientin mit Ehlers-Danlos Syndrom, Acta Odontol. Scand. **23**:91-101, 1965.

31. Thexton, A.: A case of Ehlers-Danlos syndrome presenting with recurrent dislocation of the temporomandibular joint, Br. J. Oral Surg. **2**:190-193, 1965.

Endocrine candidosis syndrome

32. Blizzard, R. M., and Gibbs, J. H.: Candidiasis: studies pertaining to its association with endocrinopathies and pernicious anemia, Pediatrics **42**:231-237, 1968.

33. Castello, S., Fikrig, S., Inamdar, S., and Orti, E.: Familial moniliasis, defective delayed hypersensitivity and adrenocortico-tropic hormone deficiency, J. Pediatr. **79**: 72-79, 1971.

34. Chilgren, R. A., Meuwissen, H. J., Quie, P. G., et al.: Chronic mucocutaneous candidosis, deficiency of delayed hypersensitivity and selective local antibody defect, Lancet **2**:688-693, 1967.

35. Gass, J. D.: The syndrome of keratoconjunctivitis, superficial moniliasis, idiopathic hypoparathyroidism and Addison's disease, Am. J. Ophthalmol. **54**:660-674, 1962.

36. Greenberg, M. S., Brightman, V. J., Lynch, M. A., and Ship, I. I.: Idiopathic hypoparathyroidism, chronic candidosis and dental hypoplasia, Oral Surg. **28**:42-53, 1969.

37. Hermans, P. E., and Ritts, R. E.: Chronic mucocutaneous candidiasis: its association with immunologic and endocrine abnormalities, Minn. Med. **53**:75-80, 1970.

38. Kirkpatrick, C. H., Rich, R. R., and Bennett, J. E.: Chronic mucocutaneous candidiasis: model-building in cellular immunity, Ann. Intern. Med. **74**:955-978, 1971.

39. Spinner, M. W., Blizzard, R. M., and Childs, B.: Clinical and heterogeneity in idiopathic Addison's disease and hypoparathyroidism, J. Clin. Endocrinol. **28**:795-804, 1968.

40. Wells, R. S.: Chronic oral candidiasis (autosomal recessive inheritance), Proc. R. Soc. Med. **63**:10-11, 1970.

41. Wuepper, K. D., and Fudenberg, H. H.: Moniliasis, "autoimmune" polyendocrinopathy, an immunologic family study, Clin. Exp. Immunol. **2**:71-82, 1967.

Epidermolysis bullosa

42. Andreasen, J. O., Hjørting-Hansen, E., Ulmansky, M., and Pindborg, J. J.: Milia formation in oral lesions in epidermolysis bullosa, Acta Pathol. Microbiol. Scand. **63**: 37-41, 1965.

43. Arwill, T., Bergenholtz, A., and Olsson, O.: Epidermolysis bullosa hereditaria. IV. Histologic changes of the oral mucosa in the polydysplastic dystrophic and the letalis forms, Odontol. Rev. **16**:101-111, 1965.

44. Arwill, T., Olsson, O., and Bergenholtz, A.: Epidermolysis bullosa hereditaria. III. A histologic study of changes in teeth in the polydysplastic dystrophic and lethal forms, Oral Surg. **19**:723-744, 1965.

45. Becker, M. H., and Swinyard, C. A.: Epidermolysis bullosa dystrophica in children; radiologic manifestations, Radiology **90**:124-128, 1968.

46. Davidson, B. C. C.: Epidermolysis bullosa, J. Med. Genet. **2**:233-242, 1965.

47. Gedde-Dahl, T., Jr.: Epidermolysis bullosa; a clinical, genetic, and epidemiologic study,

Baltimore, 1971, The Johns Hopkins University Press.

48. Rodermund, O. E.: Zahnveränderungen bei Epidermolysis bullosa, Dermatol. Wochenschr. **153:**350-357, 1967.

49. Schnyder, U. W., and Eichhoff, D.: Zur Klinik und Genetik der dominant dystrophische Epidermolysis bullosa hereditaria, Arch. Klin. Exp. Derm. **218:**62-90, 1964.

50. Tilsley, D. A., and Beard, T. C.: Epidermolysis bullosa simplex in Tasmania, Lancet **2:** 905-907, 1963.

51. Touraine, A.: Classification des épidermolyses bulleuses, Ann. Dermatol. Syphiligr. (Paris) **2:**309-312, 1942.

Fabry's disease

52. Anderson, W.: A case of "angiokeratoma," Br. J. Dermatol. **10:**113-117, 1898.

53. Brady, R. O., Gal, A. E., Bradley, R. M., et al.: Enzymatic defect in Fabry's disease: ceramide trihexosidase deficiency, N. Engl. J. Med. **275:**1163-1167, 1967.

54. Desnick, S. J., Witkop, C. J., Jr., Krivit, W., Theis, J. K., and Desnick, R. J.: Fabry's disease (ceramide trihexosidase deficiency), diagnostic confirmation by analysis of dental pulp, Arch. Oral Biol. **17:**1473-1479, 1972.

55. Fabry, J.: Ein Beitrag zur Kenntnis der Purpura haemorrhagica nodularis (Purpura papulosa haemorrhagica Hebrae), Arch. Derm. Syph. (Berl.) **43:**187-200, 1898.

56. Johnston, A. W., Frost, P., Spaeth, G. L., and Renwick, J. H.: Linkage relationships of the angiokeratoma (Fabry) locus, Ann. Hum. Genet. **32:**369-374, 1969.

57. Opitz, J. M., Stiles, F. C., Wise, D., Race, R. R., et al.: The genetics of angiokeratoma corporis diffusum (Fabry's disease), and its linkage with Xg(a) locus, Am. J. Hum. Genet. **17:**325-342, 1965.

58. Wise, D., Wallace, H. J., and Jellinek, E. H.: Angiokeratoma corporis diffusum: a clinical study of eight affected families, Q. J. Med. **31:**177-206, 1962.

Familial dysautonomia (Riley-Day syndrome)

59. Brunt, P. W., and McKusick, V. A.: Familial dysautonomia: a report of genetic and clinical studies with a review of the literature, Medicine **49:**343-374, 1970.

60. Henkin, R., and Kopin, I.: Abnormalities of taste and smell thresholds in familial dysautonomia: improvement with methacholine, Life Sci. **3:**1319-1325, 1964.

61. Mahloudji, M., Brunt, P. W., and McKusick, V. A.: Clinical neurological aspects of familial dysautonomia, J. Neurol. Sci. **11:**383-395, 1970.

62. McKusick, V. A., Norum, R. A., Farkas, H. J., et al.: The Riley-Day syndrome—observations on genetics and survivorship, Israel J. Med. Sci. **3:**372-379, 1967.

63. Reitman, A. A., Blacharsh, C., and Levy, J. M.: Clinical evaluation of the dental aspects of familial dysautonomia, J. Am. Dent. Assoc. **71:**1436-1446, 1965.

64. Riley, C. M.: Familial dysautonomia, Adv. Pediatr. **9:**157-190, 1957.

65. Riley, C. M., Day, R. L., Greeley, D. M., and Langford, W. S.: Central autonomic dysfunction with defective lacrimation, Pediatrics **3:**468-481, 1949.

66. Riley, C. M., and Moore, R. H.: Familial dysautonomia differentiated from related disorders, Pediatrics **37:**435-446, 1966.

67. Smith, A. A., Farbman, A., and Dancis, J.: Tongue in familial dysautonomia, Am. J. Dis. Child. **110:**152-154, 1965.

Hereditary hemorrhagic telangiectasia (Osler-Rendu-Weber syndrome)

68. Bird, R. M., Hammarsten, J. F., Marshall, R. A., and Robinson, R. R.: A family reunion: a study of hereditary hemorrhagic telangiectasia, N. Engl. J. Med. **257:**105-109, 1957.

69. Ecker, J. A., Doave, W. A., Dickson, D. R., et al.: Gastrointestinal bleeding in hereditary hemorrhagic telangiectasia, Am. J. Gastroenterol. **33:**411-421, 1960.

70. Quickel, K. E., and Whaley, R. J.: Subarachnoid hemorrhage in a telangiectasia, Neurology **17:**716-719, 1967.

71. Snyder, L. H., and Doan, C. A.: Studies in human inheritance: is homozygous form of multiple telangiectasia lethal? J. Lab. Clin. Med. **29:**1211-1216, 1944.

72. Stecker, R. H., and Lake, C. F.: Hereditary hemorrhagic telangiectasia, Arch. Otolaryngol. **82:**522-526, 1965.

73. Trell, E., Johansson, B. W., Linell, F., and Ripa, J.: Familial pulmonary hypertension and multiple abnormalities of large systemic arteries in Osler's disease, Am. J. Med. **53:** 50-63, 1972.

74. Tünte, W.: Klinik und Genetik der Oslerschen Krankheit, Z. Menschl. Vererb. Konstit.-Lehre **37:**221-250, 1964.

Acrodermatitis enteropathica (Danbolt-Closs syndrome)

75. Danbolt, N.: Akrodermatitis enteropathica, Acta Derm. Venereol. (Stockh.) **23:**127-169, 1943.

76. der Kaloustian, V. M., Musallam, S. S., Sanjad, S. A., et al.: Oral treatment of acro-

dermatitis enteropathica with zinc sulfate, Am. J. Dis. Child. **130**:421-423, 1976.

77. Moynahan, E. J.: Acrodermatitis enteropathica: a lethal inherited human zinc-deficiency disorder, Lancet **2**:399-400, 1974.

78. Wells, B. T., and Winkelmann, R. K.: Acrodermatitis enteropathica, Arch. Dermatol. **84**:40-52, 1961.

79. Wittels, W.: Akrodermatitis enteropathica beim Erwachsenen (Danbolt u. Closs), Derm. Wochenschr. **144**:765-772, 1961.

Multiple mucosal neuromas, pheochromocytoma, medullary carcinoma of the thyroid, and Marfanoid body build with muscle wasting

80. Carney, J. A., Sizemore, G. W., and Lovestedt, S. A.: Mucosal ganglioneuromatosis, medullary thyroid carcinoma, and pheochromocytoma: multiple endocrine neoplasia, type 2b, Oral Surg. **41**:739-752, 1976.

81. Gorlin, R. J., and Mirkin, B.: Multiple mucosal neuromas, medullary carcinoma of the thyroid, pheochromocytoma and Marfanoid body build with muscle wasting, Z. Kinderheilkd. **113**:313-325, 1972.

82. Gorlin, R. J., Sedano, H., Vickers, R., and Cervenka, J.: Multiple mucosal neuromas, pheochromocytoma and medullary carcinoma of the thyroid: a syndrome, Cancer **22**:293-299, 1968.

83. Levy, M., Habib, R., Lyon, G., Schweisguth, O., et al.: Neuromatose et epithelioma à stroma anyloide de la thyroide chez l'enfant, Arch. Fr. Pédiatr. **27**:561-583, 1970.

84. Schimke, R. N., Hartmann, W., Prout, T., and Rimoin, D.: Syndrome of bilateral pheochromocytoma, medullary thyroid carcinoma and multiple neuromas: a possible regulatory defect in the differentiation of chromaffin tissues, N. Engl. J. Med. **279**:1-7, 1968.

85. Williams, E. D., and Pollock, D. J.: Multiple mucosal neuromata with endocrine tumors—a syndrome allied to von Recklinghausen's disease, J. Pathol. **91**:71-80, 1966.

Multiple hamartoma and neoplasia syndrome (Cowden syndrome)

86. Carlier, G., Larere, L., Carlier, C., and Houcke: Sclérose tubéreuse de Bourneville avec papillomatose de la muqueuse buccale, Rev. Stomatol. (Paris) **72**:607-614, 1971.

87. Gentry, W. C., Eskritt, N. R., and Gorlin, R. J.: Multiple hamartoma syndrome (Cowden's disease), Arch. Dermatol. **109**:521-529, 1974.

88. Lattes, R. (New York, N.Y.), Gellmani, S., and Zuflacht, J. (Valley Stream, N.Y.): Personal communications, 1974.

89. Lloyd, K. M., and Dennis, M.: Cowden's disease: a possible new symptom complex with multiple system involvement, Ann. Intern. Med. **58**:136-142, 1963.

90. Rosenbluth, M.: Multiple noduli cutanei: an unusual case of multiple noduli cutanei with gingival manifestations, Periodontics **1**:81-83, 1963.

91. Weary, P. E., Gorlin, R. J., Gentry, W. C., et al.: The multiple hamartoma syndrome (Cowden's disease), Arch. Dermatol. **106**:682-690, 1972.

Peutz-Jeghers syndrome (mucocutaneous melanotic pigmentation and gastrointestinal polyposis)

92. Christian, C. D.: Ovarian tumors—an extension of the Peutz-Jeghers syndrome, Am. J. Obstet. Gynecol. **111**:529-534, 1971.

93. Dormandy, T. L.: Gastrointestinal polyposis with mucocutaneous pigmentation: Peutz-Jeghers syndrome, N. Engl. J. Med. **256**:1093-1102, 1141-1146, 1186-1190, 1956.

94. Dozois, R. R., Judd, E. S., Dahlin, D. C., and Bartholomew, L. G.: The Peutz-Jeghers syndrome, Arch. Surg. **98**:509-517, 1969.

95. Jeghers, H., McKusick, V. A., and Katz, K. H.: Generalized intestinal polyposis and melanin spots of the oral mucosa, lips, and digits, N. Engl. J. Med. **241**:993-1005, 1031-1036, 1949.

96. Klosterman, G. F.: Pigmentfleckenpolypose: Klinische, histologische und erbbiologische Studien am sogenannten Peutz-Syndrom, Stuttgart, Germany, 1960, Georg Thieme Verlag KG.

97. Klostermann, G. F.: Zur Kenntnis der Pigmentfleckenpolypose: Bemerkungen zu Diagnostik, Verlauf und Erbbiologie des sogenannten Peutz-Jeghers-Syndroms aufgrund katamnestischer Daten, Arch. Klin. Exp. Dermatol. **226**:182-189, 1966.

98. Peutz, J. L. A.: Very remarkable case of familial polyposis of mucous membrane of intestinal tract and nasopharynx accompanied by peculiar pigmentation of skin and mucous membrane, Ned. Maandschr. Geneesk. **10**:134-146, 1921.

99. Scully, R. E.: Sex cord tumor with annular tubules: a distinctive ovarian tumor of the Peutz-Jeghers syndrome, Cancer **25**:1107-1121, 1970.

White sponge nevus

100. Browne, W. G., Izatt, M. M., and Renwick, J. H.: White sponge naevus of the mucosa: clinical and linkage data, Ann. Hum. Genet. **32**:271-282, 1969.

101. Cannon, A. B.: White sponge nevus of the

mucosa (naevus spongiosus albies mucosae), Arch. Dermatol. Syph. 31:365-370, 1935.

102. Haye, K. R., and Whitehead, F. I. H.: Hereditary leukokeratosis of the mucous membranes, Br. J. Dermatol. 80:529-533, 1968.

103. Simpson, H. E.: White sponge nevus, J. Oral Surg. 24:463-466, 1966.

104. Stüttgen, G., Berres, H. H., and Will, W.: Leukoplakische, epitheliale Naevi der Mundschleimhaut und ihre Keratinisierungsform, Arch. Klin. Exp. Dermatol. 221:433-446, 1965.

105. Whitten, J. B.: The electron microscopic examination of congenital keratoses of the oral mucous membranes. I. White sponge nevus, Oral Surg. 29:69-84, 1970.

106. Witkop, C. J., Jr., and Gorlin, R. J.: Com-Dermatol. 84:762-771, 1961.

107. Zegarelli, E. V., Everett, F. G., Kutscher, parative histology and exfoliative cytology of four hereditary mucosal syndromes, Arch. A. H., Gorman, J., and Kupferberg, N.: Familial white folded dysplasia of the mucous membranes, Arch. Dermatol. 80:59-65, 1959.

Hereditary benign intraepithelial dyskeratosis (Witkop–von Sallmann syndrome)

108. Pollitzer, W. S., Menegaz-Bock, R. M., Renwick, J. H., and Witkop, C. J.: Hereditary benign intraepithelial dyskeratosis: a linkage study, Am. J. Hum. Genet. 17:104-108, 1965.

109. von Sallmann, L., and Paton, D.: Hereditary benign intraepithelial dyskeratosis. I. Ocular manifestations, Arch. Ophthalmol. 63:421-429, 1960.

110. Witkop, C. J., and Gorlin, R. J.: Four hereditary mucosal syndromes, Arch. Dermatol. 84:762-771, 1961.

111. Witkop, C. J., Shankle, C. M., Graham, J. B., et al.: Hereditary benign intraepithelial dyskeratosis. II. Oral manifestations and hereditary transmission, Arch. Pathol. 70:696-711, 1960.

112. Yanoff, M.: Hereditary benign intraepithelial dyskeratosis, Arch. Ophthalmol. 79:291-293, 1968.

Pachyonychia congenita (Jadassohn-Lewandowski syndrome)

113. Gorlin, R. J., and Chaudhry, A. P.: Oral lesions accompanying pachyonychia congenita, Oral Surg. 11:541-544, 1958.

114. Jadassohn, J., and Lewandowski, K.: In Neisser, A., and Jacobi, E.: Ikonographia Dermatologica, Berlin, 1906, Urban & Schwarzenberg, p. 29.

115. Laing, C. R., Hayes, J. R., and Scharf, G.: Pachyonychia congenita, Am. J. Dis. Child. 111:649-652, 1966.

116. Moldenhauer, E., and Ernst, K.: Das Jadassohn-Lewandowsky Syndrom, Hautarzt 19:441-447, 1968 (Case 1).

Darier's disease

117. Caulfield, J. B., and Wilgram, G. F.: An electron-microscope study of dyskeratosis and acanthosis in Darier's disease, J. Invest. Dermatol. 41:57-65, 1963.

118. Cernéa, P.: Un cas de maladie de Darier avec atteinte de la muqueuse buccale, Rev. Stomatol. (Paris) 66:699-706, 1965.

119. Gorlin, R. J., and Chaudhry, A. P.: The oral manifestations of keratosis follicularis, Oral Surg. 12:1468-1470, 1959.

120. Spouge, J. D., Trott, J. R., and Chesko, G.: Darier-White's disease: a cause of white lesions of the mucosa, Oral Surg. 21:441-457, 1966.

Palmoplantar hyperkeratosis and attached gingival hyperkeratosis

121. Fred, H. L., Gieser, R. G., Berry, W. R., and Eiband, J. M.: Keratosis palmaris et plantaris, Arch. Intern. Med. 113:866-871, 1964.

122. Raphael, A. L., Baer, P. N., and Lee, W. B.: Hyperkeratosis of gingival and plantar surfaces, Periodontics 6:118-120, 1968.

Hyperkeratosis palmoplantaris and periodontoclasia in childhood (Papillon-Lefèvre syndrome)

123. Bach, J. N., and Levan, N. E.: Papillon-Lefèvre syndrome, Arch. Dermatol. 97:154-158, 1968.

124. Brownstein, M. H., and Skolnik, P.: Papillon-Lefèvre syndrome, Arch. Dermatol. 106:533-534, 1972.

125. Gorlin, R. J., Sedano, H., and Anderson, V. E.: The syndrome of palmar-plantar hyperkeratosis and premature periodontal destruction of the teeth, J. Pediatr. 65:895-908, 1964.

126. Papillon and Lefèvre, P.: Deux cas de kératodermie palmaire et plantaire symétrique familiale (maladie de Meleda) chez le frère et la soeur: coexistence dans les deux cas d'altérations dentaires graves, Bull. Soc. Fr. Dermatol. Syph. 31:82-84, 1924.

127. Smith, P., and Rosenzweig, K. A.: Seven cases of Papillon-Lefèvre syndrome, Periodontics 5:42-46, 1967.

Acatalasia

128. Aebi, H., Heiniger, J., Bütler, R., and Hassig, A.: Two cases of acatalasia in Switzerland, Experientia 17:466-467, 1961.

129. Hamilton, H. B., and Neel, J. V.: Genetic

heterogeneity in human acatalasia, Am. J. Hum. Genet. **15:**408-419, 1963.

130. Hamilton, H. B., Neel, J. V., Kobara, T. Y., et al.: Frequency in Japan of carriers of the rare recessive gene causing acatalasemia, J. Clin. Invest. **40:**2199-2208, 1961.

131. Nishimura, E. T., Hamilton, H. B., Kobara, T. Y., et al.: Carrier state in human acatalasemia, Science **130:**333-334, 1959.

132. Paul, K. G., and Engstedt, L. M.: Normal and abnormal blood catalase activity in adults, Scand. J. Clin. Lab. Invest. **10:**26-33, 1958.

133. Richardson, M., Huddleson, E., Bethea, R., and Trustdorf, M.: Study of catalase in erythrocytes and bacteria. III. Catalase activity of erythrocytes from humans and animals in various pathological states, Arch. Biochem. **47:**338-345, 1953.

134. Szeinberg, A., deVries, A., Pinkhas, J., et al.: A dual hereditary red blood cell defect in one family; hypocatalasemia and glucose-6-phosphate dehydrogenase deficiency, Acta Genet. Med. (Roma) **12:**247-255, 1963.

135. Takahara, S.: Progressive oral gangrene probably due to lack of catalase in the blood (acatalasaemia); report of nine cases, Lancet **2:**1101-1104, 1952.

136. Takahara, S.: Progressive oral gangrene due to acatalasemia, Laryngoscope **64:**685-688, 1954.

137. Takahara, S., Hamilton, H. B., Neel, J. V., et al.: Hypocatalasemia; a new genetic carrier state, J. Clin. Invest. **39:**610-619, 1960.

Porokeratosis

138. Butterworth, T., and Strean, L. P.: Clinical genodermatology, Baltimore, 1962, The Williams & Wilkins Co.

139. Ramanathan, K., Omar-Ahmad, U. D., Kutty, M. K., et al.: Porokeratosis Mibelli, Br. Dent. J. **126:**31-32, 1969.

140. Schuermann, H., et al.: Krankheiten der Mundschleimhaut und der Lippen, ed. 3, München/Berlin, 1966, Urban & Schwarzenberg.

Pseudoxanthoma elasticum (Grönblad-Strandberg syndrome)

141. Berlyne, G. M., Bulmer, M. G., and Platt, R.: The genetics of pseudoxanthoma elasticum, Q. J. Med. **30:**201-212, 1961.

142. Carlborg, V., Ejrup, B., Grönblad, E., and Lund, F.: Vascular studies in pseudoxanthoma elasticum with a series of color photographs of the eyeground lesions, Acta Med. Scand. (Suppl.) **350:**1-84, 1959.

143. Danielsen, L., Kobayasi, T., Larsen, H. W., et al.: Pseudoxanthoma elasticum, a clinico-pathological study, Acta Derm. Venereol. (Stockh.) **50:**355-373, 1970.

144. Darier, J.: Pseudoxanthoma elasticum, Mh. Prakt. Dermatol. **23:**609-617, 1896.

145. Eddy, D. D., and Farber, E. M.: Pseudoxanthoma elasticum: internal manifestations: a report of cases and a statistical review of the literature, Arch. Dermatol. **86:**729-740, 1962.

146. Grönblad, E.: Angioid streaks—Pseudoxanthoma elasticum: Vorläufige Mitteilung, Acta Ophthalmol. (Kbh.) **7:**329, 1929.

147. McKusick, V. A.: Heritable disorders of connective tissue, ed. 4, St. Louis, 1972, The C. V. Mosby Co.

148. Nellen, M., and Jacobson, M.: Pseudoxanthoma elasticum (Grönblad-Strandberg disease) with coronary artery calcifications, S. Afr. Med. J. **32:**649-651, 1958.

149. Strandberg, J.: Pseudoxanthoma elasticum, Zbl. Haut. Geschl. Kr. **31:**689, 1929.

Hyalinosis cutis et mucosae (Urbach-Wiethe syndrome, lipoid proteinosis)

150. Caplan, R. M.: Visceral involvement in lipoid proteinosis, Arch. Dermatol. **95:**149-155, 1967.

151. Fleischmajer, R., Nederwich, A., and Ramos e Silva, J.: Hyalinosis cutis et mucosae: a histochemical staining and analytical biochemical study, J. Invest. Dermatol. **52:**495-503, 1969.

152. Gordon, H., Gordon, W., Botha, V., and Edelstein, I.: Lipoid proteinosis, Birth Defects **7:**164-177, 1972.

153. Grosfeld, J. C. M., Auping, J., and Spaans, J.: Hyalinosis cutis et mucosae (lipoid proteinosis Urbach-Wiethe), Dermatologica **130:**239-266, 1965.

154. Hashimoto, K., Klingmüller, G., and Rodermund, O. E.: Hyalinosis cutis et mucosae: an electron microscope study, Acta Derm. Venereol. **52:**179-195, 1972.

155. Hofer, P.: Urbach-Wiethe disease, Acta Derm. Venereol. **53** (suppl. 71): 1-52, 1973.

156. Rodermund, O. E., and Klingmüller, G.: Elektronenmikroskopische Befunde des Hyalins bei Hyalinosis cutis et mucosae, Arch. Klin. Exp. Derm. **236:**238-249, 1970.

157. Urbach, E.: Über eine familiäre lokale Lipoidose der Haut und der Schleimhäute auf Grundlage einer diabetischen Stoffwechselstörung, Arch. Dermatol. Syph. (Berl.) **159:**451-466, 1929.

158. Wiethe, C.: Kongenitale diffuse Hyalinablagerungen in den oberen Luftwegen familiär auftretend, Z. Hals. Nase. Ohrenheilkd. **10:**359-362, 1924.

Tangier disease

159. Fenans, V. J., and Fredrickson, D. S.: The pathology of Tangier disease, Am. J. Pathol. **78**:101-158, 1975.
160. Fredrickson, D. S.: The inheritance of high density lipoprotein deficiency (Tangier disease), J. Clin. Invest. **43**:228-236, 1964.
161. Fredrickson, D. S., Altrocchi, P. H., Arioli, L. V., et al.: Tangier disease, Ann. Intern. Med. **55**:1016-1031, 1961.
162. Fredrickson, D. S., Gotto, A. M., and Levy, R. I.: Familial lipoprotein deficiency. In Stanbury, J. B., Wyngaarden, J. B., and Fredrickson, D. S., editors: The metabolic basis of inherited disease, ed. 3, New York, 1972, McGraw-Hill Book Co., pp. 493-530.
163. Hoffman, H. N., II, and Fredrickson, D. S.: Tangier disease (familial high density lipoprotein deficiency), Am. J. Med. **39**:582-593, 1965.
164. Huth, K., Kracht, J., Schoenborn, W., et al.: Tangier-Krankheit (Hyp-α-Lipoproteinämie), Dtsch. Med. Wochenschr. **95**:2357-2361, 1970.
165. Kocen, R. S., Lloyd, J. K., Lascelles, P. T., et al.: Familial alpha-lipoprotein deficiency (Tangier disease) with neurological abnormalities, Lancet **1**:1341-1344, 1967.

Xanthomatosis

166. Braun-Falco, O., and Braun-Falco, F.: Zum Syndrome Diabetes insipidus und disseminerte Xanthome, Z. Laryngol. Rhinol. Otol. **36**:378-387, 1957.
167. Bürger, M., and Grütz, O.: Über hepatosplenomegale Lipoidose mit xanthomatösen Veränderungen in Haut und Schleimhaut, Arch. Dermatol. Syph. (Berl.) **166**:542-548, 1932.
168. Chapman, F. D., and Kinney, T. D.: Hyper-

lipemia; "idiopathic lipemia," Am. J. Dis. Child. **62**:1014-1024, 1941.
169. Fleischmajer, R.: The dyslipidoses, Springfield, Ill., 1960, Charles C Thomas, Publisher.
170. Fredrickson, D. S., and Levy, R. I.: Familial hyperlipoproteinemia. In Stanbury, J. S., Wyngaarden, J. B., and Fredrickson, D. S., editors: The metabolic basis of inherited disease, ed. 3, New York, 1972, McGraw-Hill Book Co., pp. 545-614.
171. Goodman, M., Schuman, H., and Goodman, S.: Idiopathic lipemia with secondary xanthomatosis, hepatosplenomegaly and lipemic retinalis, J. Pediatr. **16**:596-606, 1940.
172. Raffle, E. J., and Hall, D. C.: Xanthomatosis presenting with oral lesions, Br. Dent. J. **125**:62-66, 1968.
173. Schirren, C. G.: Hyperlipidämische Xanthomatosen, Hautarzt **8**:119-127, 1957.
174. Svendsen, H. M.: Icterus and xanthomatosis, Acta Paediatr. Scand. **50**:171-176, 1961.

Multicentric reticulohistiocytosis

175. Baccaredda-Boy, A.: Paraxanthomatöse (thesaurotische) System-Histiocytose, Hautarzt **11**:58-63, 1960.
176. Francois, J.: Dystrophie dermo-chondrocorneenne familiale, Ann. Oculist. (Paris) **182**:409-442, 1949.
177. Orkin, M., Goltz, R. W., Good, R. A., Michael, A., and Fisher, J.: A study of multicentric reticulohistiocytosis, Arch. Dermatol. **89**:640-654, 1964.
178. Warin, R. P., Evans, C. D., Hewitt, M., et al.: Reticulohistiocytosis (lipoid dermatoarthritis), Br. Med. J. **1**:1387-1391, 1957.
179. Wiedemann, H. R.: Zur Francoisschen Krankheit, Aerztl. Wochenschr. **13**:905-909, 1958.

13

Oral facial manifestations of inborn errors of metabolism

GERALD H. PRESCOTT

Metabolism is a series of biochemical reactions, each step of which is catalyzed by a specific enzymatic reaction. Since the structure of each enzyme is controlled by one or more genes (depending on the number of polypeptide chains contained within the particular enzyme), each biochemical reaction in any metabolic pathway is under genetic control.

An inborn error of metabolism is a genetically determined biochemical disorder in which an enzymatic protein is either not made or is so structurally altered that it cannot perform its normal metabolic role. The English physician, Sir Archibald Garrod, first postulated the concept of inborn errors of metabolism in 1902 when he began his studies on alcaptonuria, which were to culminate in his classic Croonian Lectures in 1908, and his monograph, *Inborn Errors of Metabolism,* which appeared in 1909 and again in 1923. From his work on patients with diseases such as alcaptonuria, cystinuria, albinism, and pentosuria, Garrod hypothesized that certain chronic diseases arise because an enzyme controlling a single metabolic step is reduced in activity or missing altogether. Garrod surmised that the accumulation of homogentisic acid in alcaptonuria was evidence that the substance, which is a normal metabolite in the breakdown of tyrosine, accumulates in excessive amounts due to a failure of the oxidation of homogentisic acid. Fifty years later, his hypothesis was proved by the demonstration of an absence of measurable homogentisic acid oxidase activity in the liver of a patient with alcaptonuria.

Garrod observed that many of the diseases that he studied had a familial distribution, and that although frequently one or more of the patient's siblings were similarly involved, the parents and more distant relatives were, in most cases, free of the disease. He also noted a particularly high incidence of consanguineous marriages in the parents of affected individuals, as well as the parents of other similarly affected individuals who had been reported elsewhere in the literature.

Garrod's work went unnoted by geneticists for several decades; however, consistent with his observations, work in this area in the past twenty years has shown that most inborn errors of metabolism are inherited as autosomal recessive traits, although a few are transmitted as autosomal dominant (Wilson's disease) and X-linked traits (Lesch-Nyhan syndrome).

One of the most significant concepts that has emerged in the past twenty years is that inborn errors of metabolism do not necessarily arise from a single unique mutation in the genotype, but that a whole spectrum of clinical expression occurs due to the presence of multiple alleles, presumably due to multiple mutations at a given gene locus. The molecular basis for this concept has been well documented in studies on the hemoglobin molecule. Investigators have examined the structure of the hemoglobin molecule from samples of blood derived from patients with various hemoglobin disorders and have clearly demonstrated that the degree of functional impairment of the molecule is directly related to the strategic location of specific amino acid substitutions or deletions, which arise by various mutational changes in the DNA molecule. It is now clear that the observed variability in the clinical expression and severity of many inborn errors of metabolism arises in part from the existence of allelic genes, each of which is responsible for an altered enzyme or structural protein molecule and, in some cases, for no protein at all. It is also now clear that similar minor and well-tolerated alterations in the molecular structure provide for the normal inherited variations, for example, heterozygosity among individuals and among populations.

Although this chapter will not attempt to deal with the detailed biochemical aspect of alterations in the normal metabolic pathways that result in the various inborn errors of metabolism, it is important to briefly review the various mechanisms by which gene mutations may occur and how these alterations in gene structure may affect the structure and function of a protein molecule. For a detailed discussion of the biochemistry of the various inborn errors, the reader is referred to one of several excellent works dealing directly with these aspects.[5, 25, 52, 57]

INBORN ERRORS AS ERRORS IN PROTEIN SYNTHESIS

Alterations in the base sequence of the DNA molecule may result in an altered enzyme or structural protein, which frequently impairs the function of that protein. These alterations occur by a process known as mutation. There are a number of types of mutation that have been identified and studied extensively in bacterial and eukaryotic systems.

Point mutations are due to a change in one base pair affecting one nucleotide in the DNA sequence. These changes can be due to *substitution, deletion,* or *insertion* of a base that alters the triplet codons, which code for the specific amino acids in the protein structure. A purine-for-purine or pyrimidine-for-pyrimidine base substitution is called a *transitional point mutation,* whereas a purine-for-pyrimidine or pyrimidine-for-purine substitution is called a *transversional point mutation.*

Point mutations involving the insertion or deletion of a single base in the DNA sequence lead to *frame shift mutations.* This results in a new amino acid sequence in the remainder of the polypeptide chain, which may result in a nonfunctional protein (with or without the same antigenic properties), a poorly functional protein, or no protein at all (Tables 13-1 and 13-2).

Point mutations, in terms of protein made, are of two varieties, *mis-sense* and *no-sense.* In mis-sense mutations a different amino acid is substituted or deleted at a specific site in the protein molecule. The classic example occurs in sickle cell anemia, in which single base substitution ($CTT \rightarrow CAT$), where valine (CTT codon) is substituted for the glutamine (CAT codon) in the no. 6 position of the β chain of hemoglobin, results in a hemoglobin molecule with significantly altered properties with respect to the ability of the hemoglobin to bind with oxygen. No-sense mutations create such an alteration in the codon sequence that no functional protein is formed.

Several changes in the DNA sequence may result in a no-sense mutation. Perhaps the simplest is a point mutation resulting in a no-sense codon triplet that codes for no amino acid at all. This would terminate the polypeptide chain prematurely. Any frame shift mutation could cause a no-sense codon to occur because of a loss or addition of a nucleotide. Deletions of DNA material can include many (hundreds of) nucleotides, even entire genes, resulting in no protein being made.

The immediate consequence of a gene mutation is an alteration in the quantity or quality of a specific protein. The mutation may rarely be beneficial to the organism; it

Table 13-1. Types of mutation and their effects on protein

Error	Cause	Protein aberration
Mis-sense mutation	Point mutation	Substitution of different amino acid in polypeptide
No-sense mutation	Point mutation or frame shift	No protein, incomplete protein, or non-functional protein formed
Unequal crossing over*	Meiotic aberration in which there is unequal exchange of genetic material	Many abnormalities are possible depending on segregation—shortening or lengthening at polypeptide chain
Gene duplication*	Nonhomolgous pairing, nondys-junction, or equal crossing over	Increase in quantity of gene product

*Chromosomal aberrations.

Table 13-2. Effect of mutations on gene

Mutation	Alterations	Result
Point mutation	Substitution of one nucleotide in DNA by another nucleotide	Copy errors
Control gene mutation	Control gene affects other structural genes after undergoing point mutation	Nonsense code beyond point of mutation
Suppressor mutation	A mutation in a gene that may correct abnormal phenotype originally expressed by initial mutation	Correction of effects of initial point mutation by second mutation at different site in gene or cistron
Reversion	Point mutation	Correction of point mutation by second mutation at same site as original

may be neutral and lead to no recognizable biological advantage or disadvantage; or it may be deleterious and lead to an impaired fitness of the organism.

The majority of disorders discussed in the remainder of this chapter fall into the latter category.

PATHOLOGICAL CONSEQUENCES OF METABOLIC DEFECTS

Since 1952, over a hundred inborn errors have been described (Table 13-3). Many of these diseases have oral and dental manifestations, especially those in which the metabolic products are stored in body tissues. Unfortunately, an accurate and comprehensive scientific description of the orofacial manifestations of many of these entities has not been undertaken, leaving clinicians and scientists of the future with a fertile area for research.

An inborn error may manifest in a number of ways biochemically and clinically. The clinical effects of any genetically controlled protein alteration depends on (1) necessity of the altered protein to sustain normal function, (2) severity of the change in protein synthesis, and (3) whether biological or medical mechanisms are available to compensate for the mutation.

The metabolic consequences are of two main types (modified from Thompson and Thompson, 1973)[57]:

A. Deficiency of the metabolic product
   1. The product per se may be necessary for subsequent steps that effectively interrupt and stop the metabolic sequence.
   Clinical example: The most common form of the adrenogenital syndrome is due to 21-hydroxylase deficiency. The lack of this enzyme prevents the conversion of 17-hydroxy-progesterone to deoxycorticoste-

Table 13-3. Disorders in which a deficient activity of a specific enzyme has been demonstrated in man*

Condition	Enzyme with deficient activity	Condition	Enzyme with deficient activity
Acatalasia	Catalase	Gangliosidosis, generalized	β-Galactosidase
Acid phosphatase deficiency	Acid phosphatase	Gaucher's disease	Glucocerebrosidase
Adrenal hyperplasia I	21-Hydroxylase†	G6PD deficiency (favism, primaquine sensitivity, etc.)	Glucose-6-phosphate dehydrogenase
Adrenal hyperplasia II	11-β-Hydroxylase†		
Adrenal hyperplasia III	3-β-Hydroxysteroid dehydrogenase†	Glycogen storage disease I	Glucose-6-phosphtase
Adrenal hyperplasia V	17-Hydroxylase†	Glycogen storage disease II	α-1,4-Glucosidase
Albinism	Tyrosinase		
Aldosterone synthesis, defect in	18-Hydroxylase†	Glycogen storage disease III	Amylo-1,6-glucosidase
Alcaptonuria	Homogentisic acid oxidase	Glycogen storage disease IV	Amylo-(1,4 to 1,6)-transglucosidase
Angiokeratoma, diffuse (Fabry)	Ceramide-trihexosidase	Glycogen storage disease V	Muscle phosphorylase
Apnea, drug-induced	Pseudocholinesterase	Glycogen storage disease VI	Liver phosphorylase†
Argininemia	Arginase		
Argininosuccinic aciduria	Argininosuccinase	Glycogen storage disease VII	Muscle phosphofructokinase
Aspartylglycosaminuria	Specific hydrolase (AADG-ase)	Glycogen storage disease VIII	Liver phosphorylase kinase
Carnosinemia	Carnosinase	Gout, primary (one form)	Hypoxanthine-guanine phosphoribosyl transferase
Cholesterol ester deficiency (Norum's disease)	Lecithin cholesterol acetyl transferase (LCAT)		
Citrullinemia	Arginosuccinic acid synthetase	Hemolytic anemia I	Adenosine triphosphatase
Crigler-Najjar syndrome	Glucuronyl transferase	Hemolytic anemia II	Diphosphoglycerate mutase
Cystathioninuria	Cystathionase		
Disaccharide intolerance I	Invertase	Hemolytic anemia III	Glucose-6-phosphate dehydrogenase
Disaccharide intolerance II	Invertase, maltase	Hemolytic anemia V	Glutathione reductase
		Hemolytic anemia VI	Hexokinase
Disaccharide intolerance III	Lactase	Hemolytic anemia VII	Pyruvate kinase
		Hemolytic anemia VIII	Triosephosphate isomerase
Formimino transferase deficiency	Formimino transferase		
Fructose intolerance	Fructose-1-phosphate aldolase	Hemolytic anemia IX	Hexosephosphate isomerase
		Hemolytic anemia X	Phosphoglycerate kinase
Fructosuria	Hepatic fructokinase	Histidinemia	Histidinase
Fucosidosis	Fucosidase	Homocystinuria	Cystathionine synthetase
Galactokinase deficiency	Galactokinase	Hydroxyprolinemia	Hydroxyproline oxidase
Galactosemia	Galactose-1-phosphate uridyl transferase	Hyperammonemia I	Ornithine transcarbamylase

*From McKusick, V. A.: Ann. Rev. Gen. **4:**1-46, 1970.
†Inferred from functional deficit. Specific assays not performed.

Table 13-3. Disorders in which a deficient activity of a specific enzyme has been demonstrated in man—cont'd

Condition	Enzyme with deficient activity	Condition	Enzyme with deficient activity
Hyperammonemia II	Carbamyl phosphate synthetase	Neonatal jaundice	Glutathione peroxidase
Hyperglycinemia, ketotic form	Propionate carboxyl-ase†	Niemann-Pick disease	Sphingomyelinase
		Orotic aciduria	Orotidylic pyrophos-phorylase and oroti-dylic decarboxylase
Hyperlysinemia	Lysine-ketoglutarate reductase		
Hyperoxaluria, with		Pentosuria	L-Xylulose reductase
I Glycolic aciduria	2-Oxo-glutarate-glyox-ylate carboligase	Phenylketonuria	Phenylalanine hydroxy-lase
II Glycolic aciduria	D-Glyceric dehydro-genase	Porphyria, acute inter-mittent	Uroporphyrinogen I synthetase†
Hyperprolinemia I	Proline oxidase	Porphyria, congenital erythropoietic	Uroporphyrinogen III cosynthetase
Hyperprolinemia II	δ-1-Pyrroline-5-car-boxylate dehydro-genase†	Pulmonary emphysema (one type)	α-1-Antitrypsin
Hypophosphatasia	Alkaline phosphatase	Pyridoxine-dependent infantile convulsions	Glutamic acid decar-boxylase†
Intestinal lactase deficiency (adult)	Lactase	Pyridoxine-responsive anemia	δ-Aminolevulinic acid synthetase†
Isovaleric acidemia	Isovaleric acid CoA dehydrogenase	Refsum's disease	Phytanic acid α-oxidase
Leigh's necrotizing en-cephalomyelopathy	Pyruvate carboxylase	Sulfite oxidase deficiency	Sulfite oxidase
		Tay-Sachs disease	Hexosaminidase A
Lesch-Nyhan syndrome	Hypoxanthine-guanine phosphoribosyl transferase	Testicular feminization	Δ⁴-5α-Reductase
		Thyroid hormonogenesis, defect in	Iodotyrosine dehalo-genase (deiodinase)
Lipase deficiency, con-genital	Lipase (pancreatic)	Trypsinogen deficiency disease	Trypsinogen
Lysine intolerance	L-lysine:NAD-oxido-reductase	Tyrosinemia I	Para-hydroxyphenyl-pyruvate oxidase
Mannosidosis	α-Mannosidase	Tyrosinemia II	Tyrosine transaminase
Maple sugar urine disease	Keto acid decar-boxylase	Valinemia	Valine transaminase
		Vitamin D–resistant rickets	Cholecalciferase†
Metachromatic leukodystrophy	Arylsulfatase A (sul-fatide sulfatase)	Wolman's disease	Acid lipase
Methemoglobinemia	NAD-methemoglobin reductase	Xanthinuria	Xanthine oxidase
		Xanthurenic aciduria	Kynureninase
Methylmalonic aciduria I	Methylmalonic CoA carboxymutase	Xeroderma pigmento-sum	DNA-specific endo-nuclease
Methylmalonic aciduria II	5′ Deoxyadenosylco-balamin synthe-tase†		
Myeloperoxidase defi-ciency with dissemi-nated candidiasis	Myeloperoxidase		

rone (Substance S). Substance S is necessary to make cortisol resulting in low serum and urinary levels of cortisol and the subsequent clinical effects.

2. Feedback inhibitor control of protein synthesis is impaired.

   Clinical example: Some metabolic errors, such as Hartnup disease, are due to the lack of enzymes necessary to carry substrates across membranes. In Hartnup disease the amino acid tryptophan, necessary for nicotinamide synthesis, cannot be transported across the intestinal mucosa; therefore the clinical signs of nicotinamide deficiency develop.

B. Accumulation of precursors of the blocked reaction

1. The precursor substrate may be increased and cause clinical symptoms.

   Clinical example: The lack of an enzyme can cause the buildup of the substrate immediately preceding the block. The accumulation of the precursor can lead to severe clinical effects seen in the storage diseases such as mucopolysaccharidosis type I (Hurler's syndrome). The deficient enzyme is α-L-iduronidase, causing the accumulation of gangliosides in tissues, thereby causing mental and growth retardation.

2. Alternative metabolic pathways may start to function and produce toxic levels of certain metabolites due to overproduction.

   Clinical example: Although the use of al-

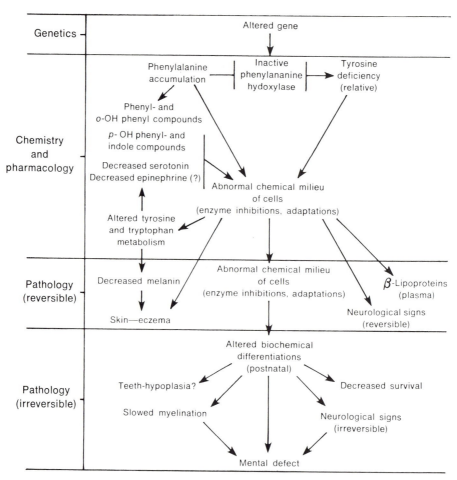

Fig. 13-1. Pathogenesis of phenylketonuria. Irreversible changes such as mental defect are considered to result from altered biochemical differentiation in developing brain. (From Stanbury, J. B., Wyngaarden, J. B., and Fredrickson, D. S., editors: The metabolic basis of inherited disease, ed. 3, New York, 1972, McGraw-Hill Book Co. Copyright 1972; used with permission of McGraw-Hill Book Co.)

ternative pathways of metabolism to circumvent a blocked reaction can be helpful to an organism, it can also lead to pathologic conditions if the products in the alternate pathways are toxic. A good example of this phenomenon is phenylketonuria, in which the severe mental retardation occurs due to the accumulation of toxic metabolites of the alternative pathway of phenylalamine metabolism (that is, phenylpyruvic acid, hydroxyphenylacetic acid, and others) (Fig. 13-1).

CLASSIFICATION

Inborn errors of metabolism have been classified in a variety of ways. One of the simplest and most common methods is by grouping these diseases into general catagories according to the metabolic pathways or cycles that are altered to produce the observed clinical abnormalities. We have chosen to categorize the inborn errors of metabolism that have as part of their clinical findings certain oral facial manifestations by the system used by Stanbury and associates in their text, *The Metabolic Basis of Inherited Disease.*

    I. Lysosomal storage diseases
    II. Disorders primarily related to abnormal lipid metabolism
    III. Disorders of amino acid metabolism
    IV. Abnormalities of carbohydrate metabolism and glycogen storage diseases
    V. Abnormalities of purine and pyrimidine metabolism
    VI. Abnormalities of mental metabolism
    VII. Miscellaneous metabolic disorders, including disorders of steroid metabolism; disorders manifesting primarily as transport disorders; deficiencies of circulating enzymes and plasma proteins, etc.

ORAL MANIFESTATIONS OF METABOLIC DISEASES
Diseases characterized by lysosomal storage and/or lipid disorders

Mucopolysaccharidoses. The mucopolysaccharidoses are characterized by abnormal deposition in soft and hard tissues and/or urinary excretion of acid mucopolysaccharides. Effects on mentation and life expectancy are variable, but dysostosis multiplex is a constant finding. The biochemical and clinical aspects of the mucopolysaccharides are discussed thoroughly by McKusick[32] and Stanbury and co-workers[52] (Table 13-4) and, with respect to their effects on the dental pulp, in Chapter 10 of this book.

Mucopolysaccharidosis I (Hurler's syndrome, MPS I). The head is large with a scaphocephalic skull due to premature closure of the sagittal and frontal sutures. Often there is a prominent ridge along the sagittal suture secondary to hyperostosis of the sutural area. Saddle nose is generally present and the facial features are coarse with large lips, expressionless facies, and hypertelorism. Corneal clouding is a consistent finding. Intraorally, the tongue is enlarged, and most cases show hypertrophy of the bony alveolar ridges as well as the gingival tissue and adenoids.[9] Radiographs of the head show enlargement of the bony structures, in general, as well as a "slipper-shaped" or "J-shaped" sella turcica and enlarged optic foramina. The inferior surface of the sphenoid bone approximates the hard palate, effectively narrowing the nasopharyngeal airway.[26]

The incisors are frequently small, peg shaped, and widely spaced.[8] Delayed root formation of the permanent teeth is common. Horrigan describes the mandibular ramus to be narrow and short and the condyle to be hypoplastic and absent in some cases.[23] The coronoid notch can be deeply grooved or cleft. Gardner,[14] in a review, reported that the body of the mandible was shorter and broader than normal, the gonions were prominent, and the intergonial distance was wide. The large mandible may account for the widely spaced teeth as well as the teeth being small.

Cawson[8] described "dentigerous cysts" in the molar region of the jaws of these patients, which appear by 3 years of age. Gorlin[21] believes that these localized areas of bone destruction are pools of chondroitin sulfate B. The margins of the lesions are smooth and well defined. The lesions that appear in the mandible are smaller and less frequent than those seen in the maxilla. These punched-out lesions are also seen in MPS IV. The pheno-

Table 13-4. The genetic mucopolysaccharidoses (as classified in 1972 by McKusick) *

	Designation	Clinical features	Genetics	Excessive urinary MPS	Substance deficient
MPS I H	Hurler's syndrome	Early clouding of cornea, grave manifestations, death usually before age 10	Homozygous for MPS I H gene	Dermatan sulfate Heparan sulfate	α-L-iduronidase (formerly called Hurler corrective factor)
MPS I S	Scheie's syndrome	Stiff joints, cloudy cornea, aortic regurgitation, normal intelligence, ?normal life span	Homozygosity for MPS I S gene	Dermatan sulfate Heparan sulfate	α-L-iduronidase
MPS I H/S	Hurler-Scheie syndrome	Phenotype intermediate between Hurler and Scheie	Genetic compound of MPS I H and I S genes	Dermatan sulfate Heparan sulfate	α-L-iduronidase
MPS II A	Hunter's syndrome, severe	No clouding of cornea, milder course than in MPS I H, but death usually before age 15 years	Hemizygous for X-linked gene	Dermatan sulfate Heparan sulfate	Iduronate sulfatase
MPS II B	Hunter's syndrome, mild	Survival to 30s to 50s, fair intelligence	Hemizygous for X-linked allele for mild form	Dermatan sulfate Heparan sulfate	
MPS III A	Sanfilippo's syndrome A	Identical phenotype:	Homozygous for Sanfilippo A gene	Heparan sulfate	Heparan sulfate sulfatase
MPS III B	Sanfilippo's syndrome B	Mild somatic, severe central nervous system effects	Homozygous for Sanfilippo B (at different locus)	Heparan sulfate	N-acetyl-α-D-glucosaminidase
MPS IV	Morquio's syndrome (probably more than one allelic form)	Severe bone changes of distinctive type, cloudy cornea, aortic regurgitation	Homozygous for Morquio gene	Keratan sulfate	Unknown
MPS V	Vacant				
MPS VI A	Maroteaux-Lamy syndrome, classic form	Severe osseous and corneal change, normal intellect	Homozygous for M-L gene	Dermatan sulfate	Arylsulfatase B
MPS VI B	Maroteaux-Lamy syndrome, mild form	Severe osseous and corneal change, normal intellect	Homozygous for allele at M-L locus	Dermatan sulfate	Arylsulfatase B
MPS VII	β-glucuronidase deficiency (more than one allelic form?)	Hepatosplenomegaly, dysostosis multiplex, white cell inclusions, mental retardation	Homozygous for mutant gene at β-glucuronidase locus	Dermatan sulfate	β-glucuronidase

...14, St. Louis, 1972, The C. V. Mosby Co.

type frequency is estimated between 1 in 40,000 to 1 in 100,000.[29]

Mucopolysaccharidosis I S (Scheie's syndrome, MPS I S). Although MPS I S shares the same biochemical defect with MPS I, the clinical features are markedly different. Mental retardation is not a hallmark, nor are the coarse facies or the intraoral findings similar to those in MPS I.

The facies is described as "broad mouthed." Corneal clouding is a complication in many cases. The phenotype frequency is estimated by Lowry and Renwick to be 1 in 500,000.[29]

Mucopolysaccharidosis I H/S (Hurler-Scheie syndrome, MPS I H/S). MPS I H/S probably represents allelism between the Hurler and Scheie genes; therefore one would predict the patient to exhibit an intermediate phenotype between the extremes of Hurler's and Scheie's syndromes. This is indeed the case in those few cases reported.[33, 34]

Craniofacial findings that have been noted include facial hemiparesis, blindness, deafness, rhinorrhea, hypertelorism, corneal clouding, enlarged tongue, saddle nose, ocular proptosis, diastemas, and an enlarged sella turcica. The frequency of the disorder is estimated to be 1 in 20,000.

Mucopolysaccharidosis II (Hunter's syndrome, MPS II). MPS II is inherited as an X-linked recessive trait and is presumed to have two allelic forms. Type A causes death before age 15, and type B allows survival to the third to fifth decades with mild to moderate impairment of intelligence. The general facial appearance is similar to Hurler's syndrome; however, corneal clouding is not a feature. Older affected patients tend to have a ruddy complexion, rosy cheeks, a saddle nose, and prominent superciliary ridges. Papilledema and optic atrophy have been described.[11]

Reports of intraoral findings frequently note tongue enlargement. No accurate description of the dentition has been noted.

The relative frequency is estimated to be 0.66 in 100,000 births,[29] which McKusick believes to be an underestimate.

Mucopolysaccharidosis III (Sanfilippo's syndrome A or MPS III A, Sanfilippo's syndrome B or MPS III B). MPS III, types A and B, are autosomal recessive in inheritance and are clinically identical but are biochemically distinguishable, since A and B have different enzyme deficiencies (Table 13-4).

The skull and orbital ridges are thickened; the sella turcica is usually normal. The cornea usually remains clear. The lips are large with flaring nostrils and a saddle nose. Mouth breathing is common. Mentation is severely impaired.

The permanent teeth are reported to erupt late and are small. O'Brien[39] had two patients, one of who had widely spaced teeth; however, an affected sib had "crowded, irregular teeth." A rough estimate of the frequency is 1 in 100,000 to 1 in 200,000.[56]

Mucopolysaccharidosis IV (Morquio's syndrome, MPS IV). MPS IV is autosomal recessive, and McKusick believes there are two allelic forms, a keratan sulfate–excreting form and a non–keratan sulfate–excreting form. Clinically, there is marked short stature, and the facies, although characteristic, are not as coarse as seen in MPS I. There is a prominent maxilla with a wide mouth. Cloudy corneas are usually found.

The teeth are widely spaced. Garn[16] reports enamel defects in the primary and permanent dentition. The enamel is thin, fractures off easily, and has a grayish opaque appearance. Sharp, pointed molar cusps are noted, as is a predisposition to caries. Gingival hypertrophy or tongue enlargement is not striking.

Intelligence is usually normal; however, progressive neurosensory hearing loss is a hallmark. The frequency is approximately 1 in 40,000.[34]

Mucopolysaccharidosis VI (Maroteaux-Lamy syndrome, MPS VI). MPS VI is inherited as an autosomal recessive trait and is characterized by severe skeletal dwarfism, normal intelligence, and corneal opacities. McKusick has tentatively chosen to call the classic Maroteaux-Lamy syndrome MPS VI, type A, and a rare, milder form he calls MPS VI, type B.

The facial features are reminiscent of but not identical to those found in MPS I (Hurler's).[49] The face is usually small with a saddle nose. Hydrocephalus may be a complication.

Radiographs demonstrate fused lambdoidal sutures, slipper-shaped sella turcica, and a ground-glass appearance of the calvarium.[34]

Worth[59] described a number of dental findings found in MPS I; however, the clinical pictures of his patients were those of MPS VI. Some of his findings were delayed eruption of permanent teeth, decreased height of the mandibular ramus, and deep position of many of the mandibular, unerupted, permanent teeth in the body of the mandible.

Mucopolysaccharidosis VII (β-glucuronidase deficiency, MPS VII). A few cases of MPS VII have been reported,[24, 27] and it is presumed to be autosomal recessive. Dental findings have not been thoroughly documented. In one case the facies were reported to be "unusual" with no corneal clouding or mental retardation,[47] whereas the other case had severe mental and growth retardation, corneal clouding, and radiographic findings similar to those seen in MPS I and II. McKusick speculates that two allelic forms of the syndrome may be present.

Mucolipidoses. Mucolipidoses are characterized by mental deterioration in general, dysostosis multiplex, and, usually, early death. Visceral storage of mucopolysaccharides, glycolipids, and/or sphingolipids is a hallmark of these diseases. Many mimic MPS I, MPS II, or MPS III clinically[50, 51] (Table 13-5).

Mucolipidosis I (lipomucopolysaccharidosis, ML I). In ML I disorder there is an accumulation of glycolipids and mucopolysaccharides causing facial features mildly reminiscent of Hurler's syndrome. The skeletal changes are similar to MPS III.

Mucolipidosis II (I-cell disease, ML II). The ML II disease also accumulates glycolipids and mucopolysaccharides, and the facial appearance is strikingly similar to Hurler's syndrome. Shortly after birth the gingiva becomes hypertrophied, and the head enlarges to become scaphocephalic. The ears may be small, firm, and somewhat fleshy. Corneal clouding is neglible. X-ray studies may show the sella turcica to be infantile (Fig. 13-2).

Mucolipidosis III (pseudo-Hurler polydystrophy, ML III). ML III exhibits a coarse facies with a broad mouth, thick lips, saddle nose, prominent supraorbital ridges, and corneal clouding.[36] The teeth have been reported to be widely spaced and "stubby."[32] The tongue and gingiva are not enlarged, and the severity of mental impairment is variable.

Mannosidosis. The patients with mannosidosis have facies very similar to Hurler's,

Table 13-5. Mucolipidoses

Name	Genetics	Life expectancy (years)	Enzyme defect	Dysostosis multiplex	Hurler-like orofacial manifestations
Mucolipidosis I	Autosomal recessive	?	?	+	+
Mucolipidosis II	Autosomal recessive	2 to 6	Multiple acid hydrolases	++	++
Mucolipidosis III	Autosomal recessive	?	?	++	+
Mannosidosis	Autosomal recessive	4.5	α-Mannosidase	+	+
Fucosidosis	Autosomal recessive	4 to 6	α-Fucosidase	±	±
GM₁ gangliosidosis I	Autosomal recessive	2.0	β-galactosidase isoenzymes A, B, C	++	++
GM₁ gangliosidosis II	Autosomal recessive	2.0	β-galactosidase isoenzymes B, C	+	±
Juvenile multiple sulfatidosis	Autosomal recessive	14	Aryl sulfatases A, B, C	+	±

although less coarse.[41] The stature of the patients is not generally dwarfed. Intraorally there is no gingival or tongue hypertrophy. Although the teeth may be widely spaced, they are of normal size (Fig. 13-3).

Fucosidosis. No significant oral or dental findings have yet to be noted in fucosidosis, a rare entity.

GM₁ gangliosidosis I (neurovisceral lipidosis, generalized gangliosidosis, pseudo-Hurler's disease). Coarse facies and severe mental and motor retardation are the clinical features of gangliosidosis I. Macroglossia may be present.

GM₁ gangliosidosis II (juvenile gangliosidosis). Gangliosidosis II is essentially the same as type I except that the onset is later

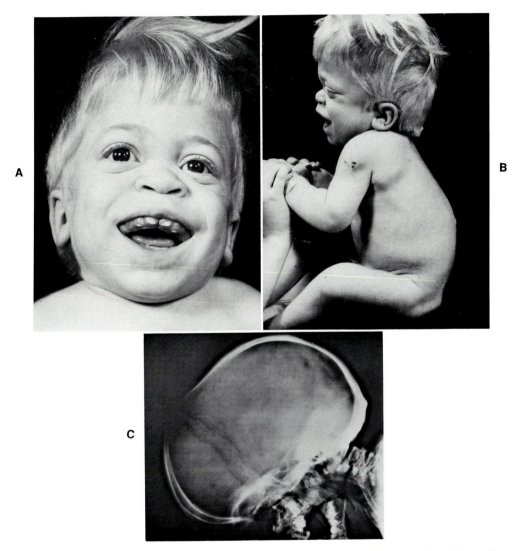

Fig. 13-2. Mucolipidosis II (I-cell disease) in C. McK., 25-month-old boy. Peculiar facies and right inguinal hernia were noted at birth. At 6 months of age, abnormal facies was again noted, as well as hypertrophied gums and triangular-shaped head. Examination at 25 months showed child with severe psychomotor retardation. Facies and skull shape are demonstrated in **A.** Note marked gum hypertrophy. Marked lumbar gibbus, **B,** and limitation of both extension and flexion in all joints were present. Ears were relatively small and were thickened and firm. Bones of limbs were thick, and wrists were particularly broad. **C,** X-ray study of skull at 25 months. (From McKusick, V. A.: Heritable disorders of connective tissue, ed. 4, St. Louis, 1972, The C. V. Mosby Co.)

Fig. 13-3. A, Mannosidosis in three brothers. Note coarse facies. **B,** Note slight to moderate hepatosplenomegaly and saddle noses.

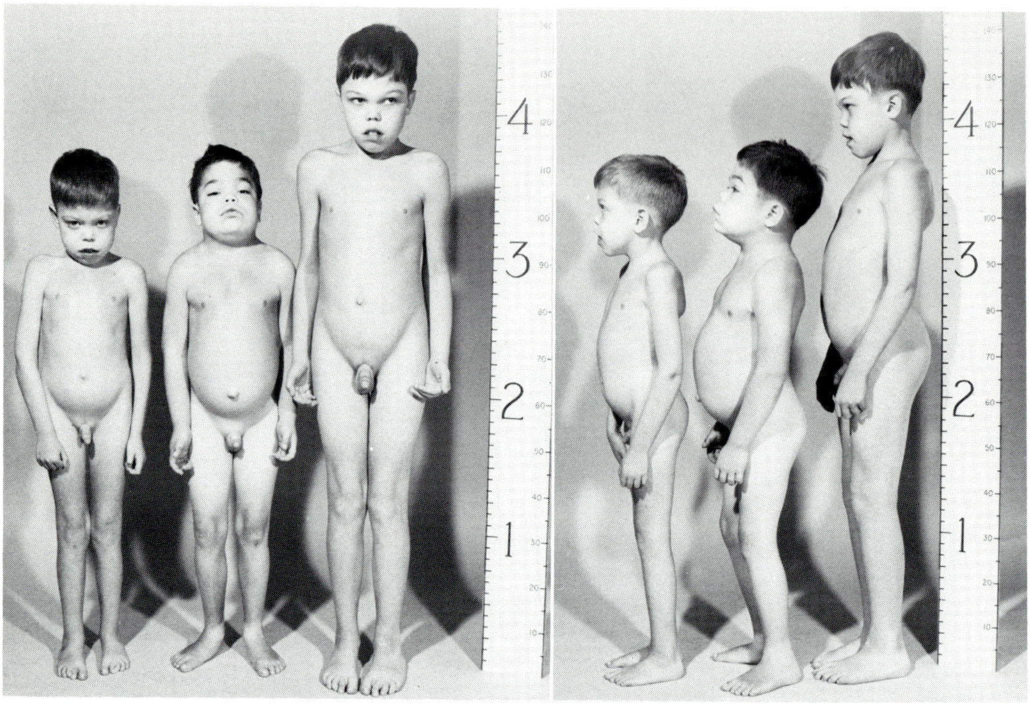

and the progression is slower.[40] There are minimal similarities to Hurler's snydrome skeletally, and no significant oral findings have been reported.

Juvenile sulfatidosis (Austin type, metachromatic leukodystrophy). Juvenile sulfatidosis, a progressive malady, impairs motor function and leads to decerebrate rigidity, blindness, deafness, and death. Szabo and associates[53] described their case as having gargoyle-like facies with an underdeveloped maxilla. The intraoral findings were not impressive.

Sphingolipidoses. The sphingolipidoses are a class of metabolic disorders in which there is mineral storage of sphingolipids and/or glycolipids. The affected patients do not have clinical features similar to the mucopolysaccharidoses or mucolipidoses, nor do they suffer from dysostosis multiplex (Table 13-6). Only those with significant oral manifestations will be discussed.

Fabry's disease (angiokeratoma corporis diffusum). Skin lesions are the hallmark of Fabry's disease, an X-linked recessive condition; however, the angiokeratomas are also seen on the lips, oral mucosa, and palate as small (<0.5 mm), diffuse, red, punctate, round lesions. The tongue is free of the lesions. The eyes can be severely involved with angiectasis of the conjunctival vessels, eyelid edema, and corneal opacities due to the glycolipid deposits. The carrier females often show cutaneous lesions, but involvement of the oral mucosa has not been reported.

Gaucher's disease. Gaucher's disease is manifest in an acute infantile form as an autosomal recessive trait and may have two chronic forms appearing later in adults and juveniles. One adult form may be inherited as an autosomal dominant trait[22] (or may be an expression of the heterozygous condition). The radiographic findings in the jaws of both adult and infantile forms are similar and feature bone marrow involvement with punched-out lesions, thinning of the cortical bone, and

Table 13-6. Sphingolipidoses

Name	Genetics	Enzyme defect	Life expectancy (years)	Oral manifestations
Fabry's disease	X-linked recessive	α-galactosyl hydrolase	30 to 60	Angiokeratomas on lip, oral mucosa, and palate
Gaucher's disease, infantile	Autosomal recessive	β-glucosidase	< 2	Dysphagia, root resorption, irregular jaw radiolucencies
Niemann-Pick disease	Autosomal recessive	Sphingomyelinase	< 3	Bluish, pigmented spots on oral mucosa
Infantile metachromatic leukodystrophy	Autosomal recessive	Aryl-sulfatase A	1 to 5	Not striking
GM$_2$ gangliosidosis I	Autosomal recessive	Hexosaminidase A	2 to 3	Not striking
GM$_2$ gangliosidosis II	Autosomal recessive	Hexosaminidase A and B	2 to 3	Not striking
GM$_2$ gangliosidosis III	Autosomal recessive	Hexosaminidase A	5 to 15	Not striking

root resorption of teeth (especially in the mandibular molar region). Tooth extraction in osteoporotic areas may result in bleeding complications.

The adult form may show yellow pigmentation of the skin, including the face and conjunctiva (pingueculae).[22, 27]

Niemann-Pick disease. According to Crocker,[10] there are at least four distinguishable forms of this sphingomyelin lipidosis: type A (acute neuronopathic form, sphingomyelinase deficient), type B (chronic form without CNS affects, sphingomyelinase deficient), type C (subacute form with CNS involvement, sphingomyelinase normal?), type D (Nova Scotia variant, sphingomyelinase normal), and type E (adult form, sphingomyelinase normal?). Type A comprises 75% of all cases and is the only type reported to have craniofacial manifestations.[52] These signs include prominence of the eyes (proptosis) and occiput, cherry red spot on the macula, and bluish, pigmented spots on the oral mucosa.

Other lipidoses. The following miscellaneous lipidoses are mentioned because they have some unique oral manifestations.

Tangier disease (familial high-density lipoprotein deficiency). Tangier disease, a rare disorder, is characterized by the absence of high-density lipoproteins in the blood plasma and the storage of cholesterol esters in the reticuloendothelial system and other tissues (gut, skin, and blood vessels).[12] The course of this autosomal recessive entity is relatively benign.

The unique yellowish-orange appearance of the tonsils is virtually pathognomonic of the disorder. The tonsils are lobulated and enlarged to the point of being obstructive and have a distinctive orange appearance overlying the normal red mucosa. This unusual symptom is due to the deposition of esters in the soft tissues.

Lipoid proteinosis (hyalinosis cutis et mucosa). Lipoid proteinosis, an autosomal recessive disorder, is featured by hyaline infiltration of the skin, oral mucosa, and larynx.[20] According to Gorlin, the lesions can be nodular, verrucous, or plaquelike and be found on the oral mucosa, larynx, esophagus, stomach, and face. Intraorally the plaques are yellowish and transparent and may be fissured. Also, the tongue may be enlarged.

Hyperlipoproteinemia, type I (familial hyperlipemia, hyperchylomicronemia). Hyperlipoproteinemia type I, a rare disease, is caused by a defect in the removal of chylomicrons from the plasma, which is probably due to an autosomal recessive trait causing a deficient lipoprotein lipase enzyme. The oral manifestations are xanthomatous, yellowish white patches on the hard palate and tonsillar areas.[52] Hyperlipoproteinemia, type IV (hyperpre-β-lipoproteinemia) may also manifest oral xanthomatosis.[21]

Other rare lipid disorders such as Wolman's disease, Refsum's syndrome, Krabbe's disease, and lactosyl ceraminidosis do not have clearly defined oral manifestations.

Disorders of amino acid metabolism

Scores of inborn errors involving amino acid metabolism are known (Table 13-3), and more are delineated each year. There are only a few that have been reported to have significant oral manifestations. Many of these disorders may have minor oral signs that have been either overlooked entirely or given imprecise or cursory attention during the evaluation. Persons with a dental background have much to offer in precisely defining the oral pathology of these disorders.

Hyperlysinemia. Hyperlysinemia, a rare autosomal recessive disorder, causes severe mental and motor retardation.[2, 18] The orofacial features are striking and include (1) protruding tongue and habitual open mouth, (2) high, arched palate, (3) no speech, (4) synophrys, with scanty amounts of hair on the lateral edges of the eyebrows, (5) a fleshy pad of tissue in the glabellar area, and (6) a "high and wide" maxilla.

Homocystinuria. Homocystinuria mimics the Marfan syndrome clinically.[7, 17] The teeth are reported to be crowded, and the palate is highly arched.

Cystinosis. Cystinosis is characterized by the deposition of cystine crystals in body tissues, growth retardation, signs resembling vitamin D–resistant rickets, and photophobia. The specific enzyme defect is not known, and there appear to be two forms, a more common, serious, nephropathic disorder, and a benign entity, both inherited as autosomal recessive traits.

Nazif and Osman[38] state that the oral findings are variable and may include stomatitis, retarded dental calcification with delayed eruption of the permanent and deciduous teeth, interdental bone loss, bell-shaped roots,

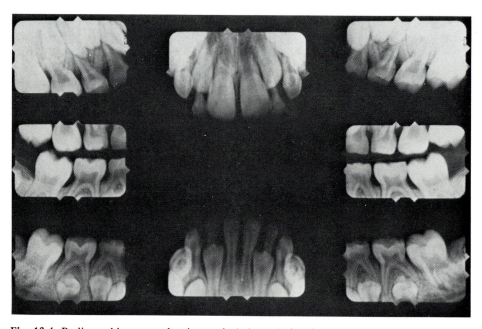

Fig. 13-4. Radiographic survey showing typical signs of vitamin D–resistant rickets. Note roots of mandibular central incisors. (From Nazif, M., and Osman, M.: Oral Surg. **35:**330-338, 1973.)

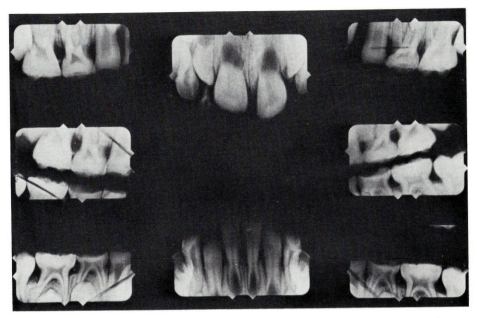

Fig. 13-5. Radiographic survey showing more pronounced signs of rickets: short roots, pronounced periapical rarefactions, and bell-shaped roots. Dental radiographs revealed absence of lamina dura, enlarged pulp chambers, periapical and interradicular rarefactions, bell-shaped roots of mandibular incisors, and severe retardation of dental calcification age. (From Nazif, M., and Osman, M.: Oral Surg. **35:**330-338, 1973.)

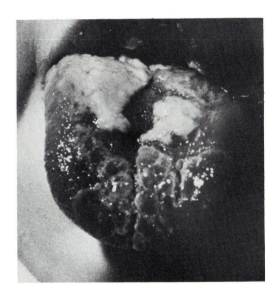

Fig. 13-6. Caucasian boy, 9 years old, diagnosed with cystinosis. Most of oral mucosa was covered with grayish tan layer, which had slightly granular surface. Tongue was more severely affected. Oral lesions involved partially labial mucosa and left corner of mouth. Teeth were free of caries. (From Nazif, M., and Osman, M.: Oral Surg. **35:**330-338, 1973.)

enlarged pulp chambers, periapical radiolucencies, and absence of the lamina dura (Figs. 13-4 and 13-5).

The stomatitis may be severe and lead to problems in eating. The oral lesions are erythematopultaceous in nature (Fig. 13-6).

Abnormalities of purine and pyrimidine metabolism

This group of diseases includes gout, xanthinuria, oroticaciduria, and the Lesch-Nyhan syndrome. Only the Lesch-Nyhan syndrome has unusual oral manifestations.

Lesch-Nyhan syndrome. This disorder is one of the few X-linked metabolic errors and is associated with nearly complete absence of hypoxanthine-guanine phosphoribosyl transferase, an enzyme in the biochemical pathway of uric acid metabolism.

The patients usually appear normal at birth, but within months vomiting, hypotonia, and mental and motor delay occur. At about a year, extrapyramidal signs appear. Soon coordinated mobility is greatly impaired, and

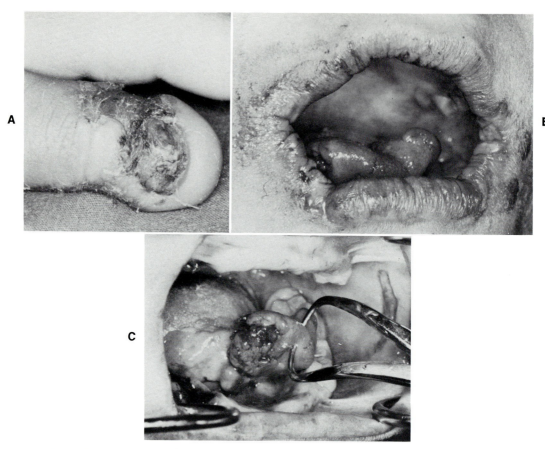

Fig. 13-7. Results of self-destructive behavior in patient with Lesch-Nyhan syndrome. Note mutilation of **A,** fingers, **B,** lips, and **C,** tongue caused by chewing of these structures. Treatment with restraints on arms led to biting of lips and tongue, which required extraction of teeth as ultimate solution of problem. (Courtesy Dr. R. Stewart, Los Angeles, Calif.)

there is marked chorioathetosis. The most striking feature of this syndrome is compulsive self-destructive behavior, which commences at 2 or 3 years of age. At this time affected children begin to bite their lips, buccal mucosa, and fingers. In many, severe mutilation can be prevented only by extracting the teeth. Restraints must often be used on the arms to prevent trauma to the fingers. This behavior is unusual because in contrast to other self-mutilation syndromes (for example, familial dysautonomia), no sensory deficits can be demonstrated.

Disorders of metal metabolism

Wilson's disease and primary hemochromatosis are the only two metabolic disorders in this category, and both have only minimal orofacial manifestations.

Wilson's disease (hepatolenticular degeneration). Wilson's disease, an autosomal recessive entity, is caused by an unknown error in copper metabolism causing brain degeneration and liver cirrhosis. Dysarthria and dysphagia are common, as is the greenish ring of copper deposition seen at the limbus of the cornea (Kayser-Fleischer ring).

Primary hemochromatosis. Primary hemochromatosis is a genetically determined aberration in iron metabolism characterized by diabetes, liver cirrhosis, and pigmentation. It is noteworthy that this iron accumulation deposited as hemosiderin in tissues causes noticeable bronzing of the face.

Abnormalities of carbohydrate metabolism

These disorders include those in which the metabolism of sugars (glucose, galactose, pentose, and fructose) and glycogen are principally involved. Few of the diseases have florid oral manifestations with the exception of uncontrolled diabetes mellitus, hence the brief comments.

Diabetes mellitus. Diabetes mellitus, a disorder of glucose metabolism, is characterized by hyperglycemia and glucosuria and results in lowered resistance of tissues to infection. The genetics of this ubiquitous disease is debatable; however, it clearly segregates in certain families, and the susceptibility is certainly conditioned by inherited factors. In controlled diabetes there are no significant oral manifestations.

In the untreated or poorly controlled patient, oral findings may include (1) fulminating periodontitis, (2) periodontal abscess formation, and (3) gingivitis with inflamed, painful and/or necrotic papillae. Russell[44-46] has reported abnormal vascular changes in the gingiva, dental pulp, and periodontal ligament. Surgical oral procedures should be undertaken with care and in collaboration with the patient's physician.

Hereditary fructose intolerance (HFI). The most common form of fructose intolerance is autosomal recessive and due to deficient fructose-1-phosphate aldolase. Because the ingestion of fructose found in sugar, sweets, and chocolate induces nausea and vomiting, these patients avoid eating these commodities and thus are extraordinarily free of dental caries.[13, 31] (See pedigree and discussion in Chapter 3.)

This striking finding substantiates the theory that a diet low in monosaccharides and disaccharides results in protection from the caries process.

Glycogen storage diseases. The glycogen storage diseases number approximately twelve and can be defined as heritable disorders of glycogen metabolism characterized by a quantitative or qualitative abnormality of the deposited glycogen (Table 13-7). The clinical effects range from death in infancy (especially the hepatomegalic forms, types I, III, VI, IX, and XII) to mild muscle problems (types VI, VII, VIII, and X). Type IV

Table 13-7. The enzymatically defined glycogenoses*

Type	Biochemical defect	Structure of glycogen	Tissue and organ involvement
0	UDPG-glycogen transferase	Normal	Liver, muscle
Ia	Glucose-6-phosphatase	Normal	Liver, kidney, GI mucosa
Ib	Glucose-6-phosphatase, functionally	Normal	Liver
IIa	Lysosomal α-1,4-glucosidase	Normal	Generalized
IIb	Lysosomal α-1,4-glucosidase	Normal	Muscle
III	Amylo-1,6-glucosidase and/or oligo-1,4 → 1,4-glucantransferase	Limit dextrin	Generalized, liver, muscle
IV	Amylo-1,4 → 1,6-transglucosylase	Amylopectin-like	Generalized
V	Muscle phosphorylase	Normal	Muscle
VI	Liver phosphorylase	Normal	Liver, leukocytes
VII	Phosphofructokinase	Normal	Muscle, erythrocytes
VIII	Phosphohexosisomerase	Normal	Muscle
IXa	Phosphorylase kinase	Normal	Liver, leukocytes
IXb	Phosphorylase kinase	Normal	Liver, muscle, leukocytes
X	Phosphorylase kinase	Normal	Muscle
XI	Phosphoglucomutase	Normal	Liver, muscle
XII	Cyclic 3',5'AMP-dependent kinase	Normal	Liver, muscle

*From Gardner, L. I.: Endocrine and genetic diseases of childhood and adolescence, ed. 2, Philadelphia, 1975, W. B. Saunders Co.

findings are those of hepatic cirrhosis and early death. Type IIa also leads to early death and primarily manifests as a muscle disorder with cardiomegaly. The symptoms of type X present in infancy; types V and VII presents in childhood to adolescence; and type VIII presents in young adulthood.[15, 52] All appear to be autosomal recessive except type VIII, which may be X-linked recessive. Only the following two types have notable oral manifestations.

Type I glycogen storage disease (von Gierke's disease, glucose-6-phosphatase deficiency). The oral problem in type I glycogen storage disease is secondary to a severe bleeding disorder. Tooth extraction or other surgical procedures may be complicated by prolonged bleeding. Also, generous fat deposits in the cheeks often may lend a cherubic appearance to these patients.

Type II glycogen storage disease (Pompe's disease, α-1,4-glucosidase deficiency, lysosomal glucosidase defect). Severe hypotonia is present in type II glycogen storage disease along with cardiomegaly. The tongue is often enlarged, presumably due to excessive accumulation of metabolites.

Miscellaneous metabolic disorders

Acatalasia (Takahara's disease, acatalasemia). Acatalasia is caused by a deficiency of the circulating enzyme catalase, which is necessary to degrade hydrogen peroxide in body tissues. In acatalasia the lesions occur exclusively in the oral cavity and may range from mild to severe, including progressive oral gangrene. Approximately 25% of the homozygous individuals are asymptomatic; however, 60% develop oral lesions before the age of 10 years. The lesions, which occur after the eruption of teeth, initially appear as small, painful ulcerations of the free gingiva that heal spontaneously. The more severe cases are characterized by lesions involving the entire gingiva. Progressive bone loss may follow, resulting in the early exfoliation of teeth. Once the teeth have been lost, most of the lesions heal spontaneously; however, a few severe cases reportedly involve bony sequestration of large portions of the maxilla

and/or mandible. The disease is inherited as an autosomal recessive trait and is more common in Japan, where it was first described by Takahara.[54, 55]

Vitamin D–resistant rickets (hypophosphatemia, phosphate diabetes, refractory rickets). Vitamin D–resistant rickets is manifested primarily as a transport defect inherited as a sex-linked dominant trait and is characterized by hypophosphatemia associated with decreased renal tubular reabsorption of inorganic phosphate, diminished gastrointestinal absorption of calcium, osteomalacia, and short stature. The oral manifestations may be striking. One of the common initial complaints of these patients is the occurrence of periapical involvement of teeth with gingival abcesses or fistulas on a tooth that appears to be free of dental caries. This phenomenon may occur in both the primary and permanent teeth. It can be explained by the fact that the teeth have large pulp chambers in which the pulp horns may extend to the dentinoenamel junction and thus be a conduit for the transmission of microorganisms to the pulp. Tracy and Campbell[58] reported decelerated maxillary and mandibular growth along with frontal and occipital bossing of the cranial vault. This condition is reviewed by Gorlin and Goldman,[21] Marks and associates,[30] Archard and Witkop,[1] and Rushton.[43]

Hypophosphatasia. Hypophosphatasia is inherited as an autosomal recessive trait and is characterized by lack of serum alkaline phosphatase; there is phosphoethanolamine in the urine. Three clinical types are noted: infantile, juvenile, and adult. In the infantile type the manifestations appear shortly after birth, and approximately 60% to 70% of the individuals die in infancy. No oral manifestations are noted.

The juvenile form becomes clinically evident after 6 months of age. The initial findings may be the premature loss of primary teeth in an otherwise normal patient. The adult form is most often found in clinically normal patients, and they usually have no pertinent oral findings.

The oral findings in this condition have been reviewed by Sobel and co-workers,[48]

Bruckner and associates,[6] Baer and co-workers,[3] and Pimstone and associates.[42] The primary mandibular central and lateral incisors followed by the maxillary incisors are the most frequently prematurely exfoliated teeth. Posterior teeth are rarely involved. It is interesting to note that teeth may be lost without any evidence of inflammatory gingival or periodontal disease. X-ray studies show many teeth to have large pulp chambers and root canals but little alveolar bone loss. (See Figs. 13-8 and 13-9.)

Porphyria. The term *porphyria* has been used to characterize a group of diseases involving inborn errors of porphyrin metabolism. There are three main classes, each characterized by overproduction of uroporphyrins and related compounds. The three classes are (1) congenital erythropoietic porphyria, (2) hepatic porphyria, and (3) protoporphyria. Each class has several subgroups, but the only entity showing oral manifestation is congenital erythropoietic porphyria. In these patients the deciduous and permanent teeth show a reddish brown or pink discoloration. Although the clinical symptoms may be mild, in ultra-

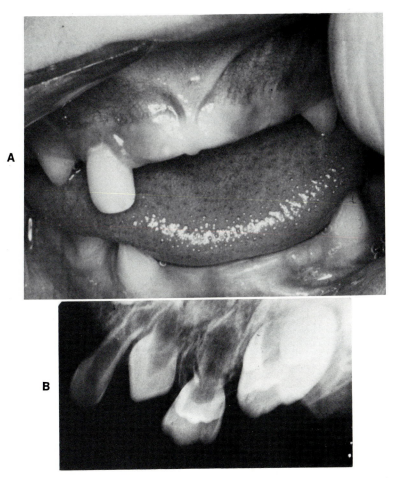

Fig. 13-8. **A,** Intraoral photograph taken at approximately 2 years of age showing loss of anterior teeth. Upper right lateral incisor has supraerupted and is abnormally mobile. Biopsy was taken from labial gingiva in this area. **B,** Radiograph of upper left quadrant taken at about 18 months of age, showing upper left lateral incisor in place. This tooth was exfoliated before patient's second birthday. (From Bruckner, R. J., Rickles, N. H., and Porter, D. R.: Oral Surg. **15:**1351-1369, 1962.)

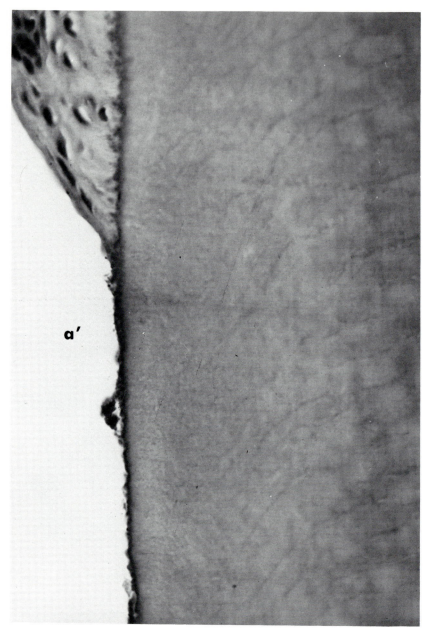

Fig. 13-9. Detail of cementum-free root surface and small portion of attached periodontal membrane fibers. (×450; reduced ⅙.) (From Bruckner, R. J., Rickles, N. H., and Porter, D. R.: Oral Surg. 15:1351-1369, 1962.)

violet light the teeth always exhibit a red fluorescence. This is due to the deposition of porphyrin in developing teeth and bones. Other systemic signs include photophobia, hypertrichosis, skin eruptions of a bullous or vesicular nature, and the excretion of red urine.

Erythroblastosis (hemolytic disease of the newborn, erythroblastosis fetalis). The most common dental finding in patients who have suffered erythroblastosis is the intrinsic staining of enamel and dentin of the deciduous teeth with or without enamel hypoplasia.[19, 28, 35, 37] This staining may be greenish in color, and the severity may be variable among the crowns of the teeth involved. Sometimes the staining can be yellowish or bluish. The enamel hypoplasia usually affects the incisal edges of the anterior teeth and the middle of the crowns of the premolars.

This disease affects families in which the mother is Rh– and the father is Rh+. Rh+ fetuses are at risk of having the mother develop antibodies against them, which results clinically in erythroblastosis.

REFERENCES

1. Archard, H. O., and Witkop, C. J., Jr.: Hereditary hypophosphatemia (vitamin D–resistant rickets) presenting primary dental manifestations, Oral Surg. **22**:184-193, 1966.
2. Armstrong, M. D., and Robinow, A. M.: A case of hyperlysinemia: chemical and clinical observations, Pediatrics **39**:546, 1967.
3. Baer, P. N., et al.: Hypophosphatasia, Periodontics **2**:209-215, 1964.
4. Beckwith, J. R., Pardee, A. B., Austrian, R., and Jacob, F.: Coordination of the synthesis of the enzymes in the pyrimidine pathway of *E. coli*, J. Mol. Biol. **5**:618, 1962.
5. Benzer, S.: The elementary units of heredity. In McElroy, W. D., and Glass, B., editors: The chemical basis of heredity, Baltimore, 1957, The Johns Hopkins University Press, p. 70.
6. Bruckner, R. J., et al.: Hypophosphatasia with premature shedding of teeth and aplasia of cementum, Oral Surg. **15**:1351-1369, 1962.
7. Carson, N. A. J., Cusworth, D. C., Dent, C. E., Field, C. M. B., Neill, D. W., and Westall, R. G.: Homocystinuria: a new inborn error of metabolism associated with mental deficiency, Arch. Dis. Child. **38**:425, 1963.
8. Cawson, R. A.: The oral changes in gargoylism, Proc. R. Soc. Med. **55**:1066-1070, 1962.
9. Craig, W. S.: Gargoylism in a twin brother and sister, Arch. Dis. Child. **29**:293, 1954.
10. Crocker, A. C.: The cerebral defect in Tay-Sachs disease and Niemann-Pick disease, J. Neurochem. **7**:69, 1961.
11. Davis, D. B., and Currier, F. P.: Morquio's disease: report of two cases, J.A.M.A. **102**:2173, 1934.
12. Fredrickson, D. S., et al.: Tangier disease, Ann. Intern. Med. **55**:1016, 1961.
13. Froesch, E. R., Wolf, H. P., Baitsch, H., Prader, A., and Labhart, A.: Hereditary fructose intolerance: an inborn defect of hepatic fructose-1-phosphate splitting aldolase, Am. J. Med. **34**:151, 1963.
14. Gardner, D. G.: The oral manifestations of Hurler's syndrome, Oral Surg. **32**:46, 1971.
15. Gardner, L. I., editor: Endocrine and genetic diseases of childhood and adolescence, ed. 2, Philadelphia, 1975, W. B. Saunders Co.
16. Garn, S. M., and Hurme, V. O.: Dental defects in three siblings afflicted with Morquio's disease, Br. Dent. J. **93**:210, 1952.
17. Gerritsen, T., and Waisman, H. A.: Homocystinuria: an error in the metabolism of methionine, Pediatrics **33**:413, 1964.
18. Ghadimi, H., Binnington, V. I., and Pecora, P.: Hyperlysinemia associated with retardation, N. Engl. J. Med. **273**:723, 1965.
19. Gibson, W. M., and Conchie, J. M.: Observation of children's teeth as a diagnostic aid. II. Developmental difficulties reflected in enamel and pigment changes in teeth, Can. Med. Assoc. J. **90**:129, 1964.
20. Gorlin, R. J.: Genetic disorders affecting mucous membranes, Oral Surg. **28**:512, 1969.
21. Gorlin, R. J., and Goldman, H. M., editors: Thoma's oral pathology, ed. 6, St. Louis, 1970, The C. V. Mosby Co.
22. Groen, J. J.: Gaucher's disease; hereditary transmission and racial distribution, Arch. Intern. Med. **113**:543-549, 1964.
23. Horrigan, W. D., and Baker, D. H.: Gargoylism; review of roentgen skull changes with description of new findings, Am. J. Roentgenol. **86**:473-477, 1961.
24. Horsch, K.: Ueber hereditäre degenerative Osteoarthropathie, Arch. Orthop. Unfallchir. **34**:536, 1934.
25. Jacob, F., and Monod, J.: Genetic regulatory mechanisms in the synthesis of proteins, J. Mol. Biol. **3**:318, 1961.
26. Lausecker, H.: Zur Symptomatologie der Dysostosis multiplex (Pfaundler-Hurler), Hautarzt **5**:538, 1954.
27. Levin, B.: Gaucher's disease; clinical and roentgenologic manifestations, Am. J. Roentgen. **85**:685-696, 1961.
28. Losch, P. K., et al.: Staining of the dental structure in jaundice of the newborn, J. Dent. Res. **19**:293, 1940.
29. Lowry, R. B., and Renwick, D. H. G.: The relative frequency of the Hurler and Hunter syndromes (letter), N. Engl. J. Med. **284**:221, 1971.
30. Marks, S. C., et al.: Dental and cephalometric findings in vitamin D–resistant rickets, J. Dent. Child. **32**:259-265, 1965.
31. Marthaler, T. M., and Froesch, E. R.: Hereditary fructose intolerance: dental status of eight patients, Br. Dent. J. **123**:597, 1967.
32. McKusick, V. A.: Heritable disorders of connective tissue, ed. 4, St. Louis, 1972, The C. V. Mosby Co.

33. McKusick, V. A., Eldridge, R., Hostetler, J. A., and Ruanguit, U.: Dwarfism in the Amish. II. Cartilage-hair hypoplasia, Bull. Hopkins Hosp. **116:**285, 1965.

34. McKusick, V. A., Kaplan, D., Wise, H., Hanley, W. B., Suddarth, S. B., Sevick, M. E., and Maumenee, A. E.: The genetic mucopolysaccharidoses, Medicine **44:**445, 1965.

35. McMillan, R. S., and Kashgarian, M.: Relation of human abnormalities of structure and function to abnormalities of the dentition. III. Relation of enamel hypoplasia to epilepsy and to diagnoses associated with Rh factor, J. Am. Dent. Assoc. **63:**38-48, 1961.

36. Melhem, R., Dorst, J. P., Scott, C. I., Jr., and McKusick, V. A.: Roentgen findings in mucolipidosis III (pseudo-Hurler polydystrophy), Radiology **106:**153, 1973.

37. Miller, J., and Forrester, R. M.: Neonatal enamel hypoplasia associated with hemolytic disease and with prematurity, Br. Dent. J. **93:** 404, 1959.

38. Nazif, M., and Osman, M.: Oral manifestations of cystinosis, Oral Surg. **35:**330, 1973.

39. O'Brien, J. S.: Sanfilippo syndrome: profound deficiency of alpha-acetylglucosaminidase activity in organs and skin fibroblasts from type B patients, Proc. Natl. Acad. Sci. U.S.A. **69:** 1720, 1972.

40. O'Brien, J. S., Stern, M. B., Landing, B. H., O'Brien, J. K., and Donnell, G. N.: Generalized gangliosidosis; another inborn error of ganglioside metabolism? (abstract), J. Pediatr. **67:**949, 1965; Am. J. Dis. Child. **109:**338, 1965.

41. Öckerman, P. A.: Diseases of glycoprotein storage, Lancet **1:**734, 1969.

42. Pimstone, B., et al.: Hypophosphatasia; genetic and dental studies, Ann. Intern. Med. **65:**722-729, 1966.

43. Rushton, M. A.: Two specimens illustrating proteolysis of dentine, Proc. R. Soc. Med. **52:** 115-117, 1959.

44. Russell, B. G.: Gingival changes in diabetes mellitus, Acta Pathol. Microbiol. Scand. **68:** 161, 1966.

45. Russell, B. G.: The dental pulp in diabetes mellitus, Acta Pathol. Microbiol. Scand. **70:** 319, 1967.

46. Russell, B. G.: The periodontal membrane in diabetes mellitus, Acta Pathol. Microbiol. Scand. **70:**318, 1967.

47. Sly, W. S., Quinton, B. A., McAlister, W. H., and Rimoin, D. L.: Beta glucuronidase deficiency: report of clinical, radiologic, and biochemical features of a new mucopolysaccharidosis, J. Pediatr. **82:**249-257, 1973.

48. Sobel, E. H., et al.: Rickets, deficiency of "alkaline" phosphatase activity and premature loss of teeth in childhood, Pediatrics **11:**309-322, 1953.

49. Spranger, J. W., Koch, F., McKusick, V. A., Natzschka, J., Wiedemann, H. R., and Zellweger, H.: Mucopolysaccharidosis VI (Maroteaux-Lamy's disease), Helv. Paediatr. Acta **25:**337, 1970.

50. Spranger, J. W., Langer, L., Jr., and Wiedemann, H. R.: Bone dysplasias: an atlas of constitutional disorders of skeletal development, ed. 1, Philadelphia, 1974, W. B. Saunders Co.

51. Spranger, J. W., and Wiedemann, H. R.: The genetic mucolipidoses; diagnosis and differential diagnosis, Humangenetik **9:**113, 1970.

52. Stanbury, J. B., Wyngaarden, J. B., and Fredrickson, D. S., editors: The metabolic basis of inherited disease, ed. 3, New York, 1972, McGraw-Hill Book Co.

53. Szabo, L. G., et al.: A Hurler's syndrome variant, Lancet **2:**1314, 1967.

54. Takahara, S.: Progressive oral gangrene probably due to lack of catalase in the blood (acatalasaemia); report of nine cases, Lancet **2:**1101-1104, 1952.

55. Takahara, S., et al.: Hypocatalasemia; a new genetic carrier state, J. Clin. Invest. **39:**610-619, 1960.

56. Terry, K., and Linker, A.: Distinction among four forms of Hurler's syndrome, Proc. Soc. Exp. Biol. Med. **115:**394, 1964.

57. Thompson, J. S., and Thompson, M. W.: Genetics in medicine, ed. 2, Philadelphia, 1973, W. B. Saunders Co.

58. Tracy, W. E., and Campbell, R. A.: Dentofacial development with vitamin D resistant rickets, J. Am. Dent. Assoc. **76:**1026-1031, 1968.

59. Worth, H. M.: The Hurler's syndrome; a study of radiologic appearances in the jaws, Oral Surg. **22:**21, 1966.

14

Oral manifestations of heritable blood disorders

RONALD J. JORGENSON

Blood is a connective tissue that differentiates from mesenchymal cells during the second through fourth week of embryonic development. During the first 2 months of development blood formation occurs primarily in the yolk sac. At 8 to 12 weeks the liver becomes the primary blood-forming organ and predominates hemopoiesis until the seventh month. Although the liver is no longer the primary hemopoietic tissue after 7 months, it continues its hemopoietic activity until birth. The spleen is actively hemopoietic during the same period, but its total contribution to formed blood is less. Bone marrow begins to elaborate elements of blood during the third embryonic month, increases its relative contribution during the second trimester, and by the seventh month is the major site of hemopoiesis. Marrow continues to produce blood after birth. The marrow elaborates erythrocytes, granulocytes, and thrombocytes, whereas lymphocytes and monocytes are formed primarily by the spleen, lymph nodes, and other lymphoid tissues. Marrow that is actively hemopoietic is red. Red marrow occupies the majority of marrow spaces in children, but it is gradually replaced by yellow, nonhemopoietic marrow with increasing age. In adults the majority of marrow spaces are filled with yellow marrow. The sternum, ribs, vertebrae, cranium,

and pelvis contain most of the red marrow in adults, and even these become filled with yellow marrow in old age. When children are challenged to produce more blood elements than the marrow is producing, the liver, spleen, and lymph nodes resume their hemopoietic activity. A similar challenge in adults is met by increased hemopoiesis of yellow marrow.

Although blood is a connective tissue, it does not have the regular structure of other connective tissues; it consists of freely mobile cells in a fluid, intracellular substrate. The identifiable structural elements of blood are the erythrocytes (red blood cells), the leukocytes (white blood cells), the thrombocytes (platelets), and the plasma.

The erythrocytes are biconcave, disclike cells that in their mature form lack nuclei. The sequence of maturation of the red blood cell and that of other blood elements is shown in Table 14-1. Red cells are elastic and can be deformed into any number of shapes. They tend to adhere to one another (at least in vitro) with their concave surfaces in contact. Red blood cells have the same capacity as other cells to synthesize certain metabolites but lack the capacity of mitotic division due to the absence of nuclei. Red cells alone have the capacity to synthesize hemoglobin, which is the principal protein

Table 14-1. Origin and relationship of blood cells*

Stem cell →

- Megakaryoblast → Promegakaryocyte → Megakaryocyte → Thrombocyte
- Myeloblast → Progranulocyte → E. myelocyte → Eosinophil
  - → N. myelocyte → N. metamyelocyte → Band cell → Neutrophil segmented
  - → B. myelocyte → Basophil
- Monoblast → Promonocyte → Monocyte
- Lymphoblast → Prolymphocyte → Lymphocyte
- Plasmablast → Proplasmacyte → Plasmacyte
- Pronormoblast (rubriblast) → Basophilic normoblast (prorubricyte) → Polychromatic normoblast (rubricyte) → Orthochromatic normoblast (metarubricyte) → Reticulocyte → Erythrocyte
- Promegaloblast → Basophilic megaloblast → Polychromatic megaloblast → Orthochromatic megaloblast → Reticulocyte → Erythrocyte

*From Leavell, B. S., and Thorup, O. A.: Fundamentals of clinical hematology, ed. 3, Philadelphia, 1971, W. B. Saunders Co.

of erythrocytes and the element that makes possible the transfer of oxygen and carbon dioxide by blood. The hemoglobin molecule consists of four globin polypeptides and four heme groups (iron-rich protoporphyrin rings). In the adult there are two alpha globin chains and two beta globin chains in a hemoglobin molecule. In the fetus the two alpha chains are combined with two gamma chains. Gamma chains differ from beta chains at thirty-eight amino acid sites and have a higher affinity for oxygen than do beta chains. Production of gamma chains usually ceases after parturition but may persist into adult life. More than eighty variants of adult hemoglobin have been described based on variation in the amino acids sequence of the alpha and beta chains.

Certain pathological conditions alter the number, size, shape, and hemoglobin content of the red blood cells. There may be a normal number of cells with a reduced content of hemoglobin (secondary anemia), a reduced number of cells that are larger than normal so that the concentration of hemoglobin is nearly normal (macrocytic anemia), or a reduction of the number and size of cells and hemoglobin content (microcytic anemia). The normal values for several red cell indices are shown in Table 14-2.

The leukocytes contain no hemoglobin, are nucleated, and are capable for the most part of ameboid movements. There are far fewer leukocytes than erythrocytes in the blood, the total number of leukocytes being equal to 1% to 2% of that of erythrocytes. The leukocytes may be divided into granular forms (neutrophils, eosinophils, and basophils) and agranular forms (lymphocytes and monocytes). The granulocytes are highly differentiated cells that lack the ability to reproduce mitotically. They develop from common progenitors, the myeloblasts. At a specific stage of maturation (the myelocyte stage) the progenitors develop the characteristic granules that are the basis for differentiating among the mature cells. The neutrophilic granulocytes are the most numerous

Table 14-2. Normal values for red corpuscles at various ages*

| Age | Red cell count (millions/ mm³) | Hemoglobin (gm/dl) | Vol. packed RBC (ml/dl) | Corpuscular values | | | |
				MCV (cμ)	MCH (γγ)	MCHC (%)	MCD (μ)
First day	5.1 ± 1.0	19.5 ± 5.0	54.0 ± 10.0	106	38	36	8.6
2 to 3 days	5.1	19.0	53.5	105	37	35	
4 to 8 days	5.1	18.3 ± 4.0	52.5	103	36	35	
9 to 13 days	5.0	16.5	49.0	98	33	34	
14 to 60 days	4.7 ± 0.9	14.0 ± 3.3	42.0 ± 7.0	90	30	33	8.1
3 to 5 months	4.5 ± 0.7	12.2 ± 2.3	36.0	80	27	34	7.7
6 to 11 months	4.6	11.8	35.5 ± 5.0	77	26	33	7.4
1 year	4.5	11.2	35.0	78	25	32	7.3
2 years	4.6	11.5	35.5	77	25	32	
3 years	4.5	12.5	36.0	80	27	35	7.4
4 years	4.6 ± 0.6	12.6	37.0	80	27	34	
5 years	4.6	12.6	37.0	80	27	34	
6 to 10 years	4.7	12.9	37.5	80	27	34	7.4
11 to 15 years	4.8	13.4	39.0	82	28	34	
Adults: Women	4.8 ± 0.6	14.0 ± 2.0	42.0 ± 5.0	87 ± 5	29 ± 2	34 ± 2	7.5 ± 0.3
Men	5.4 ± 0.8	16.0 ± 2.0	47.0 ± 5.0	87 ± 5	29 ± 2	34 ± 2	7.5 ± 0.3

*From Wintrobe, M. M.: Clinical hematology, ed. 6, Philadelphia, 1967, Lea & Febiger.
MCV, mean corpuscular volume; MCH, mean corpuscular hemoglobin; MCHC, mean corpuscular hemoglobin concentration; MCD, mean corpuscular diameter.

of the white blood cells, comprising 60% to 70% of the total. Their nuclei are highly polymorphic and usually consist of three to five chromatin masses joined by fine threads. The nuclear segmentation is thought to increase as the cell matures. Therefore an increase in the relative proportion of non-segmented cells, a shift to the left, is thought to indicate a larger proportion of young cells due to an increased demand by the body for white blood cells. An increase in the proportion of segmented cells, a shift to the right, is thought to indicate a reduction of the body's demand for white blood cells. The neutrophils elaborate proteolytic enzymes that allow them to digest bacteria and other foreign substances they phagocytose. The eosinophilic granulocytes comprise 2% to 4% of white blood cells. They also have polymorphic nuclei, although the number of lobes is not as great as in neutrophils. The function of eosinophils is also phagocytosis, but they are less active and phagocytose fewer elements than do neutrophils. Eosinophils are present in high concentrations in some of the connective tissues and in some disease processes. The basophilic granulocytes comprise 0.5% to 1.0% of white blood cells. They are relatively immobile cells and lack the clear nuclear segmentation of the other granulocytes. Basophils are only mildly phagocytic; they are associated with the release of heparin and histamine into circulating blood. Few pathological conditions affect the relative proportion of basophils in the total white cell population.

The agranulocytes are relatively undifferentiated when compared with the granulocytes. They reproduce readily by mitosis in the blood forming organs and in various connective tissues. The lymphocytic agranulocytes comprise 20% to 25% of white blood cells. Lymphocytes have a large, basophilic nucleus that is rich in ribonucleic acid (RNA). Normal circulating blood contains a small proportion of lymphocytes that are much larger than usual. These are thought to be immature lymphocytes and are more abundant than usual in certain pathological conditions. The lymphocytes migrate through capillary walls to adjacent connective tissues where their primary function is to mediate immune responses such as antibody formation and delayed hypersensitivity. They also may act as precursors of monocytes and plasma cells. Monocytic agranulocytes comprise 3% to 8% of white blood cells. Their nuclei are more irregular in shape than those of the lymphocyte and contain less RNA. Monocytes are highly phagocytic and are especially active against the tuberculus bacillus. The normal values for several commonly

Table 14-3. Relative and absolute values for leukocyte counts in 105 medical students based on differential counts on 400 cells each*

Type of cell	Percent		Absolute number	
	Mean†	95% range	Mean†	95% range
Total leukocytes			7780 ± 1460	4860-10,700
Juvenile and "band" neutrophils‡	7.9 ± 4.7	0-17.3	630 ± 410	0-1450
Segmented neutrophils	47.0 ± 9.0	25-69	3670 ± 1110	1450-5890
Total neutrophils	55 ± 8	38-70	4300 ± 1214	1870-6730
Eosinophils‡	3.0 ± 2.1	0-7.2	230 ± 170	0-570
Basophils‡	0.56 ± 0.52	0-1.6	40 ± 40	0-124
Lymphocytes	35.0 ± 7.0	21-49	2710 ± 610	1490-3930
Monocytes	6.5 ± 2.0	2.5-10.5	500 ± 180	140-860

*From Wintrobe, M. M.: Clinical hematology, ed. 6, Philadelphia, 1967, Lea & Febiger.
† ± One standard deviation.
‡These distributions are truncated at zero. For that reason the range is listed with zero as a lower limit and the mean plus two standard deviations as the upper limit.

measured white cell indices are shown in Table 14-3.

Blood platelets (thrombocytes) are minute, round elements that are produced in bone marrow by disruption of precursor cells, the megakaryocytes. Platelets appear relatively structureless in routinely stained preparations, but each is an autonomous metabolic unit rich in mitochondria, microtubules, enzymes, and glycogen. Platelets are associated with coagulation of the blood, phagocytosis, and the integrity of blood vessel walls. Coagulation factors have been identified in platelets. In addition, the platelets provide a phospholipid environment for interaction of several other coagulation factors and supply energy to the system. Platelets phagocytose numerous bacteria, spores, and particulate matter. The mechanism by which platelets contribute to the integrity of the walls of blood vessels is not clearly understood. They adhere to subendothelial tissue at the site of a break and to other platelets in the area to form a plug primarily under the influence of adenine diphosphatase (ADP).

The number and relative proportion of formed elements in the blood remain remarkably constant in healthy subjects. A closely monitored system must be responsible for the maintenance of this equilibrium. Although many aspects of the system are not fully understood, it is known that erythropoiesis, leukopoiesis, and thrombopoiesis are controlled by sensitive feedback mechanisms. The oxygen content of the blood seems to regulate erythropoiesis through the humoral factor, erythropoietin. The humoral factor, thrombopoietin, regulates the production of thrombocytes by a separate feedback mechanism. The postulated feedback mechanism of leukopoiesis is not well understood. The endocrine glands and spleen exert a secondary control on hemopoiesis, although the role of the spleen will be seen as significant in specific blood disorders discussed below. Disruption of any of the regulatory mechanisms results in clinically recognized disease. The oral manifestations of these diseases and others that are due to altered enzyme systems

or structural composition of the hemopoietic cells are the topic of this chapter. The disorders discussed here do not include all of the inherited blood disorders; only those with oral manifestations are included.

DISORDERS OF ERYTHROCYTES
Anemia

The anemias are conditions in which there is a decrease in the amount of hemoglobin in a designated quantity of blood. The term *anemia* is not etiological but is descriptive of the physiological state of the oxygen transport system.

The anemias may be classified on the basis of the cause of the alteration in the erythrocytic system into primary and secondary categories. Primary anemias are caused by a defect in erythropoiesis, a decrease in the number of erythrocytes, a decrease in the volume of the erythrocytes, or a decrease in the hemoglobin content alone. Secondary anemias are caused by excessive loss of erythrocytes from the circulating blood. Clinical signs and symptoms of anemia depend on the severity of hemoglobin reduction and on the disorder causing hemoglobin deficiency in the secondary anemias. Most clinical findings are common to all the anemias; a few are characteristic of a particular anemia. In general, the anemias are characterized by pallor of the skin, nail beds, mucous membranes, and conjunctivae, by heart palpitations and murmurs, by fatty degeneration of the heart and liver, by irregular menstruation, by small areas of hemorrhage, and by dyspnea and fatigability. Changes in erythrocyte size, shape, and staining properties are common and may serve to differentiate the types of anemia.

Iron deficiency anemia. Iron deficiency anemia is the most common form of anemia, especially in children and middle-aged women. It results from a depletion of the iron stored for hemoglobin synthesis because of a negative iron balance of the body. The common causes of iron imbalance are blood loss, pregnancy, nutritional deficiencies, and defective iron metabolism. In Western societies nutritional deficiencies are the least common of these causes, except for cases of food faddism. Heredity usually plays no role in the cause of iron deficiency anemia, but at least one Mendelian condition, hereditary hemorrhagic telangiectasia, which is discussed later in this chapter, is associated with depletion of iron because of gastrointestinal hemorrhage. The inclusion of iron deficiency anemia in this chapter is justified by its frequency and by its importance in differential diagnosis.

The clinical features of iron deficiency anemia are those of anemia in general with weakness, fatigue, dyspnea, cardiac palpitations, excessive menstruation, and pallor being most common. Changes in the epithelium occur in chronic states of iron deficiency. The nails, hair, oral mucosa, and tongue may be affected. The nails and hair are dry and brittle. The oral mucosa may be reddened, and occasionally leukoplakia or angular cheilitis are present. The papillae of the tongue may atrophy, leaving pale, smooth, irregular areas on the lateral borders or dorsum. Although a number of subjects report mild burning sensations, this form of glossitis is usually painless and is clearly different from the scarlet red, atrophic glossitis seen in the vitamin B–deficient disorders. Oral manifestations have been reported in a third of the cases of iron deficiency anemia,[11] with the severity of clinical findings being more closely correlated with the level of erythrocyte glutamic pyruvate transaminase than with the severity of the anemia. Biopsy studies of the glossal epithelium confirm the absence of fully formed filiform papillae in the denuded areas and demonstrate the absence of keratohyalin granules in these areas.

The anemia that develops from iron deficiency is at first normochromic and normocytic. As the deficiency persists, the level of hemoglobin in the erythrocytes falls, and the anemia becomes hypochromic and microcytic. Variation in the size and shape of the erythrocytes is common with elliptical and elongated cells predominating. Target cells are present in moderate numbers. Erythrocyte osmotic fragility and life span may be lower than usual. The leukocytes and platelets are usually normal in character, proportion, and absolute number.

Treatment of iron deficiency anemia consists of iron replacement and correction of the basic pathologic condition. Within 2 weeks of initiation of therapy, the atrophic filiform papillae begin to regenerate. Shortly after this, keratinization of the tongue surface can be seen. The associated angular cheilitis is slower to react to therapy and may be present several months after the papillae have rejuvenated.

Sideroblastic anemias. The common feature of the sideroblastic anemias is defective heme synthesis. The name derives from the presence in the blood of sideroblasts, cells with iron granules arranged in rings around the nucleus in the circulating blood. The rings in the sideroblast are conjugations of ferritin attached to the perinuclear mitochondria. The ferritin bound in the rings is unavailable for use in hemoglobin synthesis. Although sideroblasts are common in circulating blood and in bone marrow, the concentration of iron in the marrow is excessive in the sideroblastic anemias. Paradoxically, there are variable numbers of hypochromic cells in the circulating blood. There are two heritable forms of sideroblastic anemia.

Hereditary sideroblastic anemia (hypochromic anemia). Hereditary sideroblastic anemia has been reported in numerous families as an X-linked recessive trait.[17, 74, 102] The anemia is often detected in childhood and may be congenital, but in some cases it is not manifest until middle adult life. Clinical manifestations other than anemia include short stature, pallor of the mucosa, recurrent upper respiratory tract infections, hemic cardiac murmurs, hepatosplenomegaly, and diabetes mellitus. Occasionally the skin may be pigmented. The clinical findings may resemble those of thalassemia (p. 426). Hereditary sideroblastic anemia is differentiated from thalassemia by the absence of dermatitis, neuropathy, and glossitis. Also, levels of fetal hemoglobin and hemoglobin A_2 are normal in sideroblastic anemia. The anemia is microcytic and hypochromic. There is a pronounced poikilocytosis in some cases and a recurrent polycythemia without a rise in hemoglobin concentrations. More than 50% of the erythrocytes may be elliptical, and many are described as "signet ring" cells. Serum iron levels are raised, as is the iron clearance time. Mean survival time of the erythrocytes is normal, but their osmotic fragility may be slightly decreased. Two morphologically distinct cell lines have been grown from erythrocytes of obligate heterozygotes[95]; cells in one line are relatively normal, whereas cells in the other are microcytic and hypochromic.

An enzyme deficiency in the biosynthetic pathway of protoporphyrin has been suggested as a primary defect in sideroblastic anemia. This suggestion is based on the observation of reduced levels of free protoporphyrin in affected erythrocytes. The defect is probably at or before the synthetic step during which Δ-amino-levulinic acid is synthesized, since subsequent metabolic processes have been shown to function normally. It is possible that the increased stores of iron in affected erythrocytes bind peroxidase, preventing its metabolism to pyroxidal-5-phosphate, a coenzyme for Δ-amino-levulinic acid synthesis. Harris and co-workers[56] demonstrated in 1956 that hypochromic (sideroblastic) anemia was refractory to pyridoxine therapy. The response to pyridoxine is variable, and an individual patient may develop a tolerance to the drug. The variable response to pryidoxine may indicate etiological heterogeneity of sideroblastic anemia.

No treatment has proved effective to date. Splenectomy is contraindicated, since several patients have had fatal thrombotic episodes after surgery.

Hemochromatosis. Hemochromatosis is a rare disorder characterized by excessive storage of iron in erythrocytes and other tissues of the body, predominantly the liver. There appears to be an autosomal dominant and an autosomal recessive form of this condition.[16, 39] The dominant form is characterized by onset of symptoms at 40 or more years of age, by relatively slow progression of the disease, and by men being affected ten times more

frequently than women. The recessive form is characterized by onset of symptoms at approximately 20 years of age, relatively rapid progression, and by an equal male-to-female ratio of affliction.

Clinical features of the adult (dominant) form of hemochromatosis include hyperpigmentation of the skin, diabetes, cardiac disease, cirrhosis of the liver, hepato-splenomegaly, spider nevi, testicular atrophy, arthralgia, dyspnea, and fatigue.[7, 61, 96] Anemia is not a consistent feature of hemochromatosis. Skin pigmentation varies from bluish gray due to iron deposits to brown due to melanosis. The skin of the face and upper trunk may be the most heavily pigmented, although some workers contend that the skin of the forearm is the most heavily pigmented and is atrophic. There is excessive pigmentation around recently acquired scars, and patches of hyperpigmentation may be seen on the buccal mucosa. Clinical features of the juvenile (recessive) form include dyspnea, amenorrhea in females, hyperpigmentation of the skin, and hepatomegaly.

Although the nature of the metabolic error responsible for hemochromatosis is not understood, it is related to iron metabolism. The first recognizable symptom is increased iron absorption. The age of onset of the absorption defect has not been established, but it is probably present at birth. The absorption defect may go unnoticed until such a time as the total amount of iron absorbed surpasses the amount being lost through normal processes and an iron overload is detected. This overload usually occurs after cessation of growth in men and after menopause in women. Environmental factors such as alcoholism hasten the onset of iron overload by producing cirrhosis of the liver and increase the amount of iron in the diet. Physiological differences between men and women and differences in drinking habits easily account for the earlier age of onset and the predominance of the disease in men.

Histological studies indicate that iron is deposited first in the liver, then in the pancreas and salivary glands. Liver biopsy is the most definitive diagnostic test, but the levels of iron in circulating blood are useful for preliminary diagnosis. Treatment consists of repeated venesection or phlebotomy to increase the turnover of iron from tissue stores to peripheral blood.

Aplastic anemia. Aplastic anemia is a descriptive term for those disorders in which hemopoiesis involving all formed elements is defective. The circulating blood profile is characterized by pancytopenia (anemia, neutropenia, and thrombocytopenia) with normal or decreased cellularity of the bone marrow. Fetal hemoglobin levels are high, even in normal siblings of affected individuals. The bone marrow consists of fatty and fibrous tissues with small amounts of hemopoietic cells. The aplastic anemias may be divided into primary and secondary varieties. The causes of the secondary aplastic anemias are numerous and include poisoning by heavy metals, arsenicals, miscellaneous chemicals, drugs, and radiation. The secondary aplastic anemias may be acute or chronic and may occur at any age. Bleeding is an eventual sequela of these conditions and may eventually involve the gingiva. The prognosis for these conditions are variable.

The primary aplastic anemias are rarer than the secondary aplastic anemias, and their prognoses are far worse. Bone marrow is consistently hypocellular in the primary aplastic anemias and may consist of scattered areas of myeloid tissue only. Heritable forms of primary aplastic anemia are idiopathic aplastic anemia, Fanconi's syndrome, the Diamond-Blackfan syndrome, and dyserythropoietic anemia.

Idiopathic aplastic anemia. Idiopathic aplastic anemia occurs at all ages, although it is less common in infants and children than in other age groups. The onset of the condition is usually insidious with clinical findings related to anemia rather than to neutropenia or thrombocytopenia. Clinical findings include weakness, fatigability, and dyspnea due to the anemia, oral ulcers, fevers and recurrent infections due to the neutropenia, and hemorrhage, bruising, epistaxis, gingival bleeding, and menorrhagia due to the thrombocytopenia. Hepatospleno-

megaly and lymphadenopathy are not usual findings. The anemia is normocytic and normochromic early in the disease process, but becomes anisocytic and poikilocytic later. Sedimentation rate of the erythrocytes is elevated, and the reticulocyte count is low. Glucopenia is not a common feature, but when present, it is due to neutropenia alone. The reduced platelet count results in a prolonged bleeding time and poor clot retraction. Aplastic anemia is fatal with death often being due to overwhelming infection. There is no known treatment.

Fanconi's syndrome. Fanconi's syndrome is a constellation of pancytopenia, growth retardation, skeletal anomalies, and multiple chromosome defects.[43] It is inherited as an autosomal recessive trait. The most consistent associated skeletal anomaly is hypoplasia or aplasia of the radial ray elements of the upper limb (Fig. 14-1). Intense hyperpigmentation may involve most areas of the skin and may be patchy in distribution but does not usually involve the buccal mucosa. Upper respiratory tract infections are common and may be fatal. Fanconi's original case and several reported later had microcephaly and strabismus. The multiple chromosome defects reported in the blood of patients with the Fanconi syndrome are probably not causally related to the anemia but associated on some other basis. The chromosome defects include breaks, chromatid exchanges, and endoreduplication. Although the associated malformations may be present at birth, the symptoms of anemia are not manifest until 7 to 8 years of age. The anemia may be hypochromic, normochromic, or hyperchromic. The life span of the erythrocytes is usually shortened, but there is no appreciable increase in hemolysis. The concentration of fetal hemoglobin is higher than normal, and the number of white cells and platelets is lower than normal.

The Fanconi syndrome is usually fatal by the second decade of life and may predispose to leukemia. A deficiency of hexosekinase in the leukocytes and thrombocytes has been suggested as the basic defect in the syndrome,[73] but some workers have reported

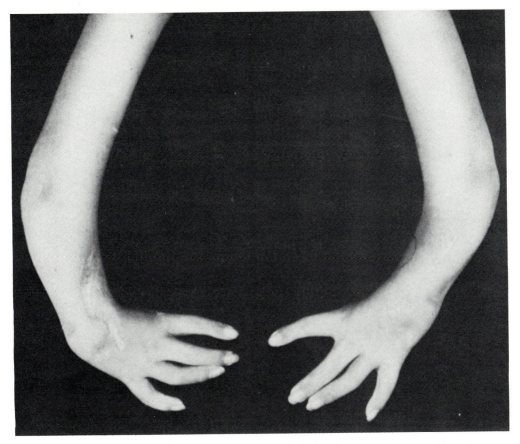

Fig. 14-1. Aplasia of radial ray elements of upper limbs in Fanconi's syndrome. (From Scott, C. I., and Haughton, P. B. T.: Birth Defects 8:191-195, 1972.)

normal levels of hexosekinase and abnormal levels of glucose-6-phosphate dehydrogenase.[21] There is no curative treatment.

Diamond-Blackfan (DB) syndrome. The DB syndrome (erythrogenesis imperfecta) is an autosomal recessive disorder of erythrocytes alone.[23, 41] It has been reported only in individuals of Caucasian ancestry. There are remarkably few clinical findings associated with the DB syndrome. The anemia of the DB syndrome is not present at birth but appears in the first few months of life. Affected individuals have been reported to be the products of premature births and to have low birth weights. In retrospect, they have been described as listless, inactive children. The onset of the anemia is particularly insidious with pallor being the first noticed and most significant finding. Anorexia and hemic murmurs may be noticed, but other findings such as hepatosplenomegaly, lymphadenopathy, growth retardation, and jaundice are absent except as complications of treatment. Pallor of the oral mucosa has been reported as the only intraoral finding, but Cathie[29] contends that the facial appearance of patients with the DB syndrome is similar from case to case (Fig. 14-2). He describes his patients as having tow-colored hair, snub noses, thick upper lips, and widely separated eyes. These facial features are similar to those in a patient reported by Robson and Sweeney,[101] who also had unilateral ptosis. The number of leukocytes and thrombocytes may be slightly decreased but not markedly so. Infections are rare in patients with the DB syndrome except as sequelae to splenectomy, which has proved to be an ill-advised form of treatment. At least one child has experienced unilateral parotitis subsequent to splenectomy.[29] The treatment of choice is repeated whole blood transfusions. Corticosteroids have produced more or less long-lasting remission in some patients but not all. Spontaneous reversal of the anemia is not uncommon. A defect in tryptophan metabolism has been suggested as the defect in this syndrome, based on the observation of excretion of anthranilic acid in the urine. This suggestion is not universally accepted.

Dyserythropoietic anemia. The term *dyserythropoietic anemia* refers in general to

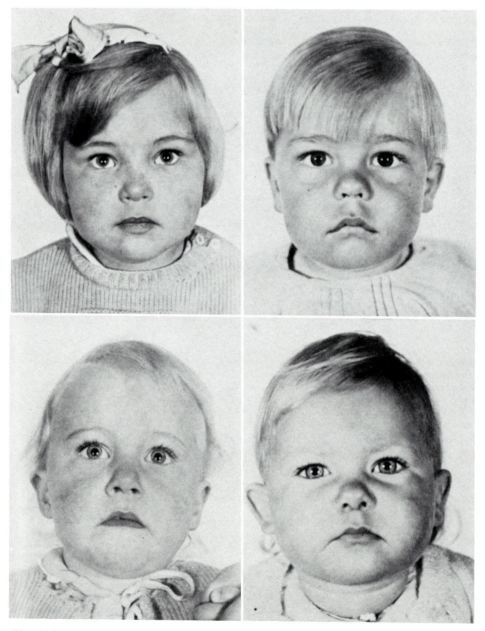

Fig. 14-2. Similar facial appearance in unrelated children with Diamond-Blackfan syndrome. (From Cathie, I. A. B.: Arch. Dis. Child. 25:313-324, 1950.)

any anemia with abnormal erythrocytes. The abnormal cells may not survive to maturation or may mature but have a short life span. Dyserythropoiesis may be due to a defect in the nucleus or in the cytoplasm; pernicious anemia is caused by a nuclear defect, a DNA-moderated enzyme deficiency in purine or pyrimidine metabolism, whereas iron deficient and sideroblastic anemias are cytoplasmic. In a more restricted sense, dyserythropoietic anemia refers to a specific autosomal recessive anemia that has been reported in two families.[114] The clinical characteristics are similar to those of thalassemia. Jaundice, pallor, splenomegaly, cardiomegaly, gallstones, and widened diploic spaces of the cranial bones have been observed in this condition. Unlike thalassemia, there is no excessive hemolysis, and the reticulate count is low. Hematological anomalies in dyserythropoietic anemia consist of hyperbilirubinemia, high serum iron levels, and low total iron binding capacity. The mechanical fragility of the erythrocytes is raised, but osmotic fragility is normal. Bone marrow studies of afflicted individuals show marked hypoplasia of erythrocyte precursors with multiple, polynucleated erythrocytes.

Megaloblastic anemia. Megaloblastic erythropoiesis is common to the anemias of vitamin B_{12} deficiency and folic acid deficiency. These anemias are characterized by abnormally large erythrocyte precursors in the marrow and abnormalities of the size and shape of mature erythrocytes. The most common abnormality of size is macrocytosis, although many red cells may be normal or smaller than normal in size. Granulocytopenia and thrombocytopenia are commonly associated with megaloblastic anemia. In addition to the common features of anemia (weakness, anorexia, weight loss, dyspnea, and fatigability) there may be associated fever, bleeding tendencies, pigmentary anomalies, and glossitis.

Addisonian pernicious anemia. The most common and one of the earliest described megaloblastic anemias is Addisonian pernicious anemia. It is a chronic disorder of middle and old age and is due to absence in gastric secretions of an intrinsic factor necessary for vitamin B_{12} absorption, which is in turn necessary for normal hemopoiesis and normal integrity of the nervous system. Defective production of the intrinsic factor has been postulated to be due to atrophy of the gastric mucosa.

The mode of inheritance of Addisonian pernicious anemia is uncertain. Between the time of Addison's treatise in 1855 and McIntyre and associates'[81] report in 1959, approximately 350 families were reported in which more than one representative had pernicious anemia. In several of these families individuals in three or more generations were affected. In others multiple siblings were affected although the parents were not. It is possible that some of these latter families represented cases of the autosomal recessive forms of pernicious anemia discussed below. Workers who have studied gastric absorption of radioactive cobalt-labeled vitamin B_{12} (Schilling test) and the production of gastric parietal cell antibodies have suggested that Addisonian pernicious anemia is an autosomal dominant trait with incomplete penetrance and variable age of onset.[81, 119] Later work has failed to substantiate these opinions.[80] There is a difference in the prevalence of Addisonian pernicious anemia among ethnic and racial groups. It occurs most frequently in people of northern European extraction and less frequently in southern Europeans and their descendants. It is rare in Asians and Africans. Certain physical features are common to patients with Addisonian pernicious anemia: fair skin, premature graying of the hair, blue eyes, broad foreheads, and short, wide chests. Pallor of the mucous membranes and a pale, smooth tongue have been described as consistent signs of Addisonian pernicious anemia. Glossitis with atrophy of the papillae occurs in about half the cases[20, 36] (Fig. 14-3). Ulcers are common and may be so painful that they interfere with eating. Leukoplakia-like changes of the tongue surface may be evident in cases of long duration. Paresthesia of the fingers and toes is not uncommon.

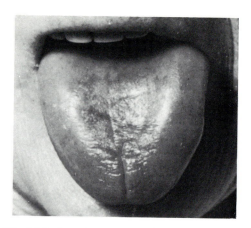

Fig. 14-3. Smooth tongue resulting from atrophy of glossal papillae in patient with Addisonian pernicious anemia. (From Gorlin, R. J., and Goldman, H. M., editors: Thoma's oral pathology, ed. 6, St. Louis, 1970, The C. V. Mosby Co.)

The initial symptoms of Addisonian pernicious anemia are usually those of anemia, although glossitis, congestive heart disease, or recurrent diarrhea may precede the anemia. If glossitis does precede the manifestations of anemia, it is frequently intermittent. The burning and soreness involve the lateral borders and the tip of the tongue and are not necessarily correlated to the severity of redness and papillary atrophy.

The anemia is variable in severity. Erythrocytes in the peripheral blood are macrocytic, anisocytic, and poikilocytic. The erythrocytes may be oval, distorted in other ways, or fragmented. There is usually an associated neutrophilic leukopenia and moderate thrombocytopenia.

Juvenile and congenital pernicious anemia. Pernicious anemia that has its onset in infants or children is due to failure of secretion of intrinsic factor by the intestinal mucosa. Two forms may be distinguished: the congenital form has normal gastric acidity and normal intestinal mucosa, whereas the juvenile form is associated with atrophy of the intestinal mucosa, achlorhydria, endocrine dysfunction, and circulating antibodies to intrinsic factor and gastric parietal cells. Each form is inherited as an autosomal recessive trait, and there is adequate evidence

that each is distinct from Addisonian pernicious anemia, not merely the homozygous state of the latter.[63, 79, 86, 118] The clinical findings are similar enough that they are discussed together. The criteria for diagnosing these conditions are onset of symptoms in the first few months of life, correction of the anemia with vitamin B_{12} or intrinsic factor therapy, malabsorption of vitamin B_{12}, objective evidence of absence of intrinsic factor in gastric juice, and exclusion of generalized malabsorption syndromes.

The clinical course of juvenile pernicious anemia is marked by neonatal onset of pallor, weakness, vomiting, and diarrhea. Somatic growth is retarded, and there may be mental retardation. Variable oral findings have been reported. Glossitis is the most common reported oral defect. Glossitis with or without depapillation and ulceration of the buccal and glossal mucosa is noted in three quarters of the cases.[71, 88] Despite significant soreness, the tongue may appear to be normal, or it may be smooth, red, and swollen.

Other clinical findings include congestive heart failure, splenomegaly, and neuropathy. Blood films are similar to those described under Addisonian pernicious anemia.

Familial vitamin B_{12} malabsorption. Megaloblastic anemia of infancy and childhood may be caused by familial vitamin B_{12} malabsorption. It is distinguished from juvenile pernicious anemia by normal intrinsic factor levels and activity and by milder clinical findings. Normal levels of intrinsic factor have been identified in some affected individuals, and lack of response of the anemia to ingested intrinsic factor has been identified in others. Normal gastric juices produce remission of the anemia, suggesting that a factor responsible for absorption of the B_{12} intrinsic factor complex is the cause of the condition. Clinical findings consist of pallor, weakness, irritability, glossitis with or without atrophy of the papillae, diarrhea, and renal malformations (variable stages of pelvis or ureter duplication). There is no interference with somatic or mental development and no associated neurologic or cardiac degeneration. The anemia is similar to that of pernicious anemia.

Megaloblastic anemia. Megaloblastic anemia is seen as an integral component of two inborn errors of metabolism, orotic aciduria and the Lesch-Nyhan syndrome. Orotic aciduria is an autosomal recessive defect of pyrimidine synthesis that presents with failure to thrive, megaloblastic anemia, and mental retardation. It is probably a regulatory gene defect giving rise to deficiencies of two consecutive enzymes in the metabolic pathway, orotidylic pyrophosphatase and orotidylic dicarboxylase. The Lesch-Nyhan syndrome is X-linked and is due to a lack of the enzyme hypoxanthine-phosphoribosyl transferase in the pathway of purine metabolism. The deficiency leads to gout, megaloblastic anemia, and self-mutilation, often of the lips and tongue.

Hemolytic anemias due to membrane defects. Excessive and premature destruction of circulating erythrocytes is a primary feature of hemolytic anemias. The anemia results from red cell hemolysis exceeding the replacement capability of the marrow. The spleen, which is the site of the erythrocyte destruction, is usually enlarged, and bilirubin levels are elevated due to the increase of heme from the destroyed cells. The hemolytic anemias may be classified according to whether the defect is intrinsic or extrinsic to the erythrocyte. Intrinsic defects for the most part are congenital and genetic, whereas extrinsic defects for the most part are acquired. The intrinsic defects may be subclassified into those which involve defects in the cell membrane and those which involve defects in the metabolism of the erythrocyte. There are at least six hereditary red cell membrane defects, five of which are associated with hemolytic anemia; hereditary permeability of the erythrocytes is not. Those with oral manifestations are spherocytosis, elliptocytosis, and acanthocytosis. Stomatocytosis is not associated with significant oral anomalies but must be mentioned because of its cause. *Stomatocyte* is the term used to describe erythrocytes that have a longitudinal mouthlike depression rather than the circular,

central concavity of normal red cells. The anemia is variable in severity, but reticulocytosis is constantly pronounced. Red cell survival is shorter than average, and osmotic fragility is increased. The most remarkable finding is an unusually high sodium ion content of the cells with concomitant reduction of potassium ion content.

Spherocytosis. An autosomal dominant form of hemolytic anemia due to a defect in the erythrocytic membrane is spherocytosis, which renders the erythrocytic membrane unusually permeable to sodium ions.[59, 60] The erythrocytes are smaller than average, stain more deeply than average, and are spherical in shape (spherocytic). The mature erythrocytes of peripheral blood are more consistently microspherocytic than the immature cells of the marrow. Spherocytes are more sensitive than the normal erythrocyte to the salinity of their environment. They tend to lyse in solutions of higher saline concentration than the normal cell. This fragility may be due in part to increased flux of sodium through the cell membrane. Spherocytes tend to accumulate in the spleen, where they are eventually lysed. Anemia results from this lysis, and consequently splenectomy usually corrects the anemia.

Spherocytosis is the most common hereditary hemolytic anemia in Northern Europeans. It affects Northern Europeans more frequently than other groups, but it has been reported in all national and racial stocks. Spherocytosis is particularly rare in Africans. The health of patients with spherocytosis is generally good. The anemia is often mild and may produce few symptoms. The majority of patients present with moderate to severe jaundice that develops in late childhood or early childhood. The jaundice may be intermittent and associated with serum bilirubin levels from 1 to 4 mg/dl. The hyperbilirubinemia leads to gallstones in approximately 50% of the cases. Mild to moderate splenomegaly is a constant finding. Persistent ulceration of the legs and growth retardation have been reported in some cases. Craniofacial involvement is not consistent but may include "tower skull," broad nasal bridge, deformities of the palate, and exophthalmos. Radiographs of the skull have been described as showing a hair-on-end appearance of the cortices (Fig. 14-4).

The anemia is spherocytic in nature. Erythrocyte osmotic fragility is raised, as are the reticulocyte count and the level of serum bilirubin. The Coombs antiglobulin test is negative. Hemoglobin levels are usually above 8 gm/dl of blood but are much lower during the frequent crises that mark the course of disease. The crises may be spontaneous or may be precipitated by an infection, in which case abnormalities of the leukocyte count may be present. Erythrocyte osmotic fragility is a certain diagnostic test for spherocytosis, although the cause of the spherocytosis is not identified by this test. Once an initial case has been identified in a family, a routine blood smear, a reticulocyte count, and determination of the level of hemoglobin and bilirubin suffice for the diagnosis in relatives.

Elliptocytosis. Elongated cells in the peripheral blood characterize elliptocytosis. There are two conditions that result in elliptical erythrocytosis. Each is inherited as an autosomal dominant trait. These conditions are distinguished on a basis of linkage with the Rh locus, the predominant shape of the erythrocytes, and clinical severity. The variety that is linked to the Rh locus is associated with oval or round cells but not with hemolytic disease.[31, 92] Cutting prefers the label *ovalcytosis* for the variety that is not linked with the Rh locus and is associated with hemolysis.[35] The clinical findings associated with ovalcytosis include pallor, weakness, jaundice, fever, cardiac disease, and splenomegaly. Darkly pigmented urine and severe bacterial stomatitis have been reported as associated findings. Although elliptocytosis that is linked to the Rh locus does not usually produce clinical disease, it may cause severe hemolytic anemia and may be fatal in the homozygous state.[92]

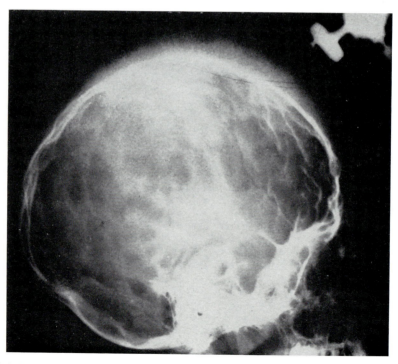

Fig. 14-4. Thick cranial vault and hair-on-end appearance of cortex in girl with spherocytosis. (From deGruchy, G. C.: Clinical haematology in medical practice, ed. 3, Oxford, England, 1970, Blackwell Scientific Publications, Ltd.)

Blood films of each form show hypochromic erythrocytes and an increased number of reticulocytes. The osmotic fragility of the erythrocytes is normal in elliptocytosis and increased in ovalcytosis. The basic defect in each may be an abnormal sodium transport system of the red cell membrane.

Acanthocytosis. An autosomal dominant disorder characterized by densely pigmented, spikelike cells in the peripheral blood is acanthocytosis. An autosomal recessive form has also been described.[30] The clinical features are predominantly neurological and have their onset in early adult life. Weakness in the lower limbs and loss of muscle control are the earliest symptoms. Uncontrolled facial grimaces and spastic tongue movement are commonly seen early in the disease process. Afflicted individuals have difficulty swallowing and talking. A particularly striking feature is self-mutilation of the tongue, lips,

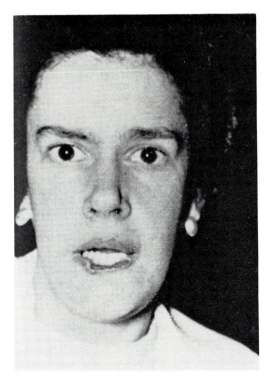

Fig. 14-5. Mutilation of lower lip in woman with acanthocytosis. (From Critchley, E. M. R., Betts, J. J., Nicholson, J. T., and Weatherall, D. J.: Postgrad. Med. J. **46:**698-701, 1970.)

and cheeks by biting[34] (Fig. 14-5). There may be drooling of oral fluids secondary to the lip mutilation, abnormal jaw jerk reflex, and tremor of the head. Acanthocytosis is differentiated from the ataxic disorder of abetalipoprotinemia and from hypobetalipoprotinemia by the association of acanthocytic erythrocytes, by neuronal rather than long-track neurological deterioration, by normal levels of β- and α-lipoproteins, and by the absence of retinitis pigmentosa. Anemia is not common in acanthocytosis, although there is a slight increase in autohemolysis of the erythrocytes. Serum enzyme studies are normal.

Hemolytic anemias due to red cell enzymopathies. A second group of hemolytic anemias is due to inborn errors of metabolism of the erythrocyte that result in energy deficiency and eventual lysis of the erythrocyte. Identification of the metabolic errors was stimulated during and after World War II by observations of severe hemolysis in persons receiving antimalarial drugs and by studies in England on relatively uncommon, heritable forms of hemolytic anemia. The several metabolic errors that have been identified can be grouped according to whether the deficiency involves glycolytic enzymes, nonglycolytic enzymes, or enzymes in the hexosemonophosphate shunt of the Krebs cycle. As a whole, the enzymatic hemolytic anemias result in a continuous destruction of red cells throughout the reticuloendothelial system. Reticulocytes are not necessarily affected in these disorders, nor is osmotic fragility of the erythrocytes. Hemoglobin structure is normal as a rule, and splenectomy does not resolve the anemia in affected persons.

Pyruvate kinase deficiency. The most common of the glycolytic enzymopathies is pyruvate kinase deficiency, which is the second most common hemolytic anemia due to inborn errors of metabolism. It is more common among Northern Europeans than other national groups, although it has been reported throughout the world. There are several alleles at the pyruvate kinase locus,[14, 123] with differences in clinical severity of the disease being the distinguishing characteristic.[40, 66] Each form of pyruvate kinase deficiency is inherited as an autosomal recessive. The age of onset of symptoms varies from infancy to adulthood. Severe cases are characterized by neonatal jaundice, recurrent upper respiratory tract infections, pigmented urine, splenomegaly, gallstones, and growth retardation. Mild cases may not be detected until the third or fourth decade of life. In retrospect, these cases are said to have had lifelong, intermittent jaundice, fatigability, and mild anemia. Severe cases appear to benefit somewhat from splenectomy, whereas no improvement is reported after splenectomy in mild cases.

Although pallor of the mucous membranes is a characteristic of mild and severe cases, other involvement of the craniofacies is more common in severe cases. Stomatitis, dysphagia, monilial infection, and a characteristic facies has been described in cases with an early age of onset. The facies have been described as mongoloid with a receding chin, wide-spaced eyes, and frontal bossing[18, 65] (Fig. 14-6). Radiographs of the skull have been reported to show thick frontal bones with a generalized widening of the diploic spaces, atrophic outer cortical plates, and a "hair-on-end" appearance of the cortices.

The basic defect in pyruvate kinase was demonstrated in 1961 by Valentine and associates[113] and stands as the first instance of an identified inborn error in the main pathway of glycolysis in humans. It is thought that erythrocytes deficient in pyruvate kinase cannot maintain normal levels of ATP, lose potassium through the cell membrane, and, as a consequence of the membrane defect, are lysed in the liver. The resultant anemia is microcytic and hypochromic. Mild leukocytosis may be present, and serum bilirubin levels may be raised. The number of thrombocytes and osmotic fragility are normal.

Hexose kinase deficiency. Hexose kinase deficiency is a glycolytic enzymopathy that has been described as an autosomal recessive trait in two families.[66, 111] The clinical findings reported in these families have been moderate anemia, pallor, intermittent jaundice, hepatosplenomegaly, and upper respiratory tract infections. Radiological findings of wide diploë of the cranial bones and alteration of trabeculation were described in one patient.[111] Since hexose kinase is involved in the first step of glucose phosphorylation and glucose concentration is extremely labile, it is impossible to assay hexose kinase activity by accumulation of glycolytic intermediates. The deficiency was demonstrated in the reported families by decreased levels of glucose-6-phosphate and by in vitro assays of hexose kinase activity. Hexose kinase activity of the leukocytes and platelets is normal.

Adenosine triphosphatase (ATPase) deficiency. ATPase deficiency is an autosomal dominant trait[54] that is characterized by susceptibility to infection, recurrent jaundice, persistent anemia, and hepatosplenomegaly.

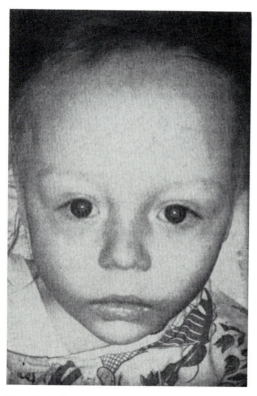

Fig. 14-6. Frontal bossing, ocular hypertelorism, and mandibular retrusion in child with pyruvate kinase deficiency. (From Bowman, H. S., and Procopio, F.: Ann. Intern. Med. **58:**567-591, 1963.)

Fever, failure to gain weight, prolonged hemorrhage, gallstones, and esophageal varices have been reported. The clinical manifestations of one case were said to be identical to those of the Banti syndrome, a disorder with significant oral facial findings (Fig. 14-7). Elevation of ATPase activity has been reported as an autosomal dominant with no recognizable sequelae on the clinical level.[19, 124]

Glucose-6-phosphate dehydrogenase (G6-PD) deficiency. G6PD deficiency is the most common of the hexosemonophosphate shunt enzymopathies that produce anemia. It has been reported in all racial and national groups, but it has its highest prevalence in people from the Mediterranean countries, West Africa, and Asia. Northern

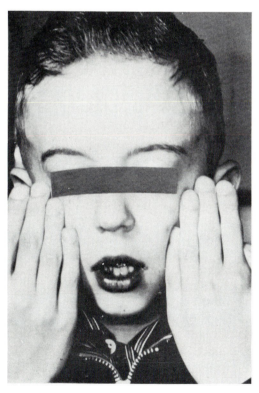

Fig. 14-7. Facies of patient with Banti syndrome. Patients with ATPase-deficient anemia reportedly have similar facies. (From Mitchell, D. F., Standish, S. M., and Fast, T. B., editors: Oral diagnosis/oral medicine, ed. 2, Philadelphia, 1971, Lea & Febiger.)

Europeans and Japanese have the lowest reported frequencies. The distribution of G6PD deficiency among the world's populations parallels that of malaria, suggesting heterozygote advantage in areas where this latter disease is endemic.

The G6PD locus is on the X chromosome and is one of the most complex and thoroughly studied multiple allele systems. Each of the many variants of G6PD is determined by a single amino acid substitution; more than a hundred variants have been more or less well documented. The variants are not randomly distributed among the world's population groups and are responsible for favism, primaquine sensitivity, other drug-induced hemolytic anemias and neonatal jaundice. Over three dozen drugs have been reported to produce hemolysis of the erythrocytes in G6PD patients.[10, 51]

Clinical features of G6PD induced hemolytic anemia appear shortly after ingestion of the responsible drug or food with the severity being related to the amount ingested. Concurrent disease, infection and hypoglycemia influence the severity of the anemia. The hemolytic process is self-limiting regardless of whether or not the causative agent continues to be ingested. Pallor, weakness, abdominal pain and dark urine are the most common findings. Individuals with G6PD deficiency may be prone to gallstones and recurrent infections. In some cases of fava bean–induced hemolytic anemia (favism, *Vicia fava* sensitivity), urticaria with itching limited to the hands and face may be the predominant feature. G6PD deficiency may also be the cause of a considerable proportion of cases of otherwise idiopathic neonatal jaundice.

The hematological profile of G6PD individuals is normal while they are not exposed to hemolytic agents. During hemolysis the red cells are anisocytic, polychromatic, and occasionally spherocytic. Erythrocyte survival time is shorter than normal, osmotic fragility is decreased, and activity of glutathione and catalase in the cells may be depressed. Reduced activity of G6PD is demonstrable in the erythrocytes of affected persons but not in the other blood elements. Intermediate levels of enzyme activity can be demonstrated in obligate heterozygote females.

Acatalasia. An autosomal recessive disorder caused by a deficiency of catalase in the erythrocytes is acatalasia. It was first described by Takahara, who noted that hydrogen peroxide did not froth normally when applied to the tissue of a patient with gangrenous stomatitis.[110, 112] In vitro investigations demonstrated that blood from individuals with acatalasia turned dark and did not froth when H_2O_2 was added, that the color faded after 20 to 30 minutes, that a yellow precipitate formed, and that the colorless supernatant contained propentdyopent, the final product of hemoglobin breakdown by H_2O_2. The acatalasia gene has been reported in 0.09% to 1.4% of the residents from different parts of Japan,[53] and for many years, acatalasia was considered to be limited to the Japanese. The gene has now been identified in several ethnic groups, although the prevalence in these groups does not approach that of its frequency in Japan.[2, 109] Based on variable levels of catalase activity in homozygotes and heterozygotes from different families and populations, it has been suggested that there are a number of alleles at the acatalasia locus.

Clinical findings of homozygosity for the acatalasia gene have been limited to the oral cavity with more than half of the documented cases having mild to severe gingivostomatitis.[110] The disease process usually begins in aseptic areas around teeth and varies from recurrent ulcers, gingivitis, and alveolar pain to generalized oral gangrene. The only treatment appears to be extraction of the teeth, debridement of the gangrenous tissue, and antibiotic therapy, although there appears to have been spontaneous regression in some cases at puberty.

Although catalase is not the most important system for reduction of H_2O_2 in the blood, the fact that its absence is associated with clinical disease attests to its significance in H_2O_2 regulation. The etiopathogenesis of oral gangrene in acatalasia may be related to repeated injury of the gingiva during mastication. The hemolytic streptococci that proliferate in the gingival wounds produce H_2O_2, which is normally reduced, but in catalase-deficient persons it initiates a cycle of oxidation of blood, anoxia, necrosis, extension of the wound, and further blood oxidation.

HEMOGLOBINOPATHIES

In the past few decades, the molecular structure of the globin moiety of hemoglobin has been delineated. Nine separate loci have been identified for the various globin polypeptide chains. The alpha and beta chains of normal adult hemoglobin are of major interest and are controlled by at least two loci. The alpha chain has been shown to consist of 141 amino acids; the beta chain consists of 146 amino acids. The precise sequence of the amino acids comprising each chain is known, and their positions are designated by number. The majority of hemoglobin variants differ from the normal at only one amino acid in the alpha or beta chain. Of the approximate 300 variants described, relatively few are associated with hemolytic anemia to varying degrees and result from the synthesis of abnormal hemoglobin chains or deficient synthesis of normal hemoglobin chains.

Stable structural variants of hemoglobin

Hemoglobin S (HbS). HbS is a major hemoglobin variant among Negroes. Its frequency is high in Western and Central Africa, in descendants of people living in these areas, and in some of the Mediterranean and Middle East countries. Its global distribution parallels that of falciparum malaria, indicating a possible selective advantage for the gene in the heterozygous state. HbS results from the substitution of valine for glutamic acid at the sixth amino acid position of the beta chain of the globin moiety. The substitution results in a molecule with reduced oxygen affinity and is associated with a myriad of erythrocyte shapes, which are collectively called *sickle cells*.

HbS is inherited as an autosomal dominant trait. It is responsible for the sickle cell trait in its heterozygous state and for sickle cell anemia in its homozygous state. Erythrocytes of heterozygotes are not overly susceptible to sickling, since a critical mass of HbS must be present for the defect to be manifest, and less than half the hemoglobin of heterozygotes is HbS. Heterozygous individuals may experience hematuria and vascular obstruction under special circumstances associated with rapid and pronounced oxygen depletion in their environment. The majority of hemoglobin in blood of homozygotes is HbS, and their erythrocytes sickle at normal, physiological levels of oxygen in the capillaries.

The symptoms of sickle cell anemia are not manifest until after the first year of life. The delay in recognition of the disease is due to the persistence of fetal hemoglobin (HbF), which has no beta chain and is, therefore, not abnormal. The level of HbS in the cell increases as the gamma chain of HbF is replaced by the defective beta chain. The most common symptoms are related to hemolysis and vascular obstruction. The hemolysis results from an increased fragility of sickled cells and produces variable degrees of anemia. Individuals with marked degrees of anemia complain of fatigue, weakness, irritability, and dyspnea, whereas those with mild anemia may have no symptoms except during a crisis. Vascular obstruction is secondary to the high viscosity of sickled cells. It results in ischemia, which in turn is responsible for the most severe symptoms of the disorders: bone and joint pain, abdominal pain, headaches, paralysis, convulsions, hematuria, hepatosplenomegaly, cardiomegaly, hypertension, persistent ulcers of the lower legs, and osteomyelitis.

Affected persons are reported to be slender and less than average in height. They are prone to respiratory tract infections and spiking fever. Frontal bossing is common. In young patients it is caused by enlargement of marrow spaces. In older patients it is caused by hyperplasia of the cortices. Hyperplasia of the marrow is most pronounced in bones normally engaged in hemopoiesis. These bones, including cranial bones, appear osteoporotic on radiographs.[85] The long bones, on the other hand, may appear on radiographs to be more dense than normal. Paranasal and frontal sinuses are reduced in size, the diploë of the skull are widened, the parietal and frontal bones are thickened, the outer cortical plate is thin, and trabeculae between the inner and outer cortices are arranged radially.[49] Trabeculation of the mandible and maxilla are more pronounced than normal and arranged in a horizontal pattern.[87, 89, 97, 100] The horizontal pattern of trabeculation is present only in alveoli where teeth are present and does not extend into edentulous areas. The lamina dura is intact, although the alveolar bone in general may be less radiodense than normal, and the mandibular cortices may appear thin.

The anemia associated with HbS homozygosity is normochromic and normocytic in nature. Leukocytosis and erythroid hyperplasia of the marrow are common. The platelet count is normal.

HbS can occur in the heterozygous state with other hemoglobin variants. The commonest occurrence of such double heterozygosity is HbS with HbC (hemoglobin SC). HbC in the homozygous state results in a mild hemolytic anemia only. However, in combination with HbS, it produces as severe a disease as sickle cell anemia. The same phenomenon has been seen with HbD and others.

Methemoglobinemia. A series of disorders that result in an excessive accumulation of methemoglobin in the erythrocytes are called, collectively, methemoglobinemia. Methemoglobin is biologically inactive due to the presence of oxidized iron rather than reduced iron in the hemoglobin complex (ferrihemoglobin rather than ferrohemoglobin). Methemoglobinemia may be congenital or acquired. Congenital forms are due to structural variants of the globin moiety, to a deficiency of nicotinamide-adenine dinucleotide (NADH)–dependent methemoglobin reductase, or to a deficiency of nicotinamide-adenine dinucleotide phosphate (NADPH)–dependent methemoglobin reductase. There are several structural variants of the globin moiety that are inherited as autosomal dominants. Individuals with these variants have variable degrees of cyanosis but no other clinical manifestations. Their cyanosis is not refactory to methylene blue therapy. The coenzyme-moderated deficiencies of methemoglobin reductase are inherited as autosomal recessive traits.[63] The primary system for reduction of methemoglobin is moderated by NADH, and consequently NADH reductase deficiency is a more common and more serious condition than NADPH reductase deficiency. In normal circumstances, NADH reductase accounts for more than 60% of methemoglobin reducing power, and NADPH reductase accounts for only 5%. Several other mechanisms account for the remainder of methemoglobin reduction.

There are several allelic forms of NADH-dependent methemoglobin reductase deficiency.[13, 121] There is no correlation between in vitro electrophoretic profiles of the several enzymes and their clinical consequences. In general, the associated methemoglobinemia is characterized by intense neonatal cyanosis, which is most pronounced in the face, lips, oral mucosa, vaginal mucosa, and nail beds. Persistent vomiting, headaches, dyspnea, fatigability, and cardiac pain are consistent symptoms. Mental retardation with strabismus, increased deep tendon reflexes, and seizures have been reported as common findings; growth retardation has been reported in some cases. In addition to cyanosis of the lips and buccal mucosa, reported oral findings have included cyanosis of the palate, gingival hypertrophy, delayed eruption of the teeth, and a highly arched palate. Cytological features of blood from affected individuals are characterized by polycythemia, variable degrees of macrocytosis, slight leukocytosis, and normal life span of the red cells.

The clinical signs and symptoms respond to treatment with methylene blue or ascorbic acid but are never completely resolved by therapy. Individuals with NADPH-dependent methemoglobin reductase deficiency have no apparent clinical disease. This disorder shows up only on routine laboratory screening with methylene blue.

Hereditary persistence of fetal hemoglobin. Hereditary persistence of fetal hemoglobin is due to an autosomal dominant hemoglobin variant, HbF. There may be a series of alleles at the HbF locus. It is probable that the reported mutations at this locus involve a deletion of a short segment of DNA. Heterozygotes for HbF are symptom free, whereas homozygotes have mild anemia with few clinical symptoms. The anemia is normochromic and microcytic with anisocytosis, poikilocytosis, numerous target cells, and occasional spherocytes. HbF produces a more morbid clinical picture when it coexists with other hemoglobin variants, including HbS, than when it is present in a homozygote state.

Thalassemias

Hemoglobinopathies that result from deficient synthesis of structurally normal hemoglobin are collectively referred to as the thalassemias. The primary defect in this group of disorders may not involve heme synthesis directly, but the amount of hemoglobin produced is certainly altered. The thalassemias are subdivided on the basis of the polypeptide chain of hemoglobin that is affected by each mutation. The most frequently described thalassemias are those which affect the beta chain, the alpha chain, or the beta and delta chain simultaneously. Deficient synthesis of the beta chain (β-thalassemia) results in a relative excess of alpha chain, and deficient synthesis of the alpha chain (α-thalassemia) results in a relative excess of the beta chain. Deficiency of the beta and delta chain simultaneously is compensated by persistent synthesis of fetal hemoglobin. The hemolytic process in the thalassemias is caused by intracellular precipitation of the chain present in excess.

Thalassemia is frequent in the Mediterranean, Middle Eastern, and Far Eastern countries. Therefore its global distribution is similar to that of G6PD deficiency, HbS, and malaria. Lately thalassemia has been reported in most racial and ethnic groups.

Thalassemia major (Cooley's anemia).
Thalassemia major results from homozygosity
for the β-thalassemia gene. Insofar as homozygosity is required to initiate the clinical
manifestations of thalassemia major, it may
be considered a recessive trait. However, the
heterozygous state may also be associated
with clinical disease (see "Thalassemia minor," p. 428), indicating dominance of the
mutant gene. However, heterozygote manifestations are much less severe than homozygote manifestations, and this may be one of
the few conditions to which we can apply
the highly abused term *incomplete autosomal
dominant.* The degree of hemolysis associated with homozygosity at the thalassemia
locus is variable, and the resultant anemia
has been categorized as severe, moderate, and
mild. Such a subjective classification serves
no useful purpose, especially since the manifestations of the disorder may vary with the
age of affected individuals.

The clinical manifestation of thalassemia
major becomes manifest sometime after birth.
Anemia is noted during the first few months
and becomes progressively severe. Failure to
thrive, poor feeding, and a protuberant abdomen usually prompt medical attention.
Affected children are short and frail and
have variable degrees of anemia, jaundice,
hepatosplenomegaly, recurrent ulcers of the
lower legs, bony abnormalities, and pigment
excretion in the stools. In children the bony
abnormalities consist of large medullary
cavities, thin cortices, and osteoporosis most
noticeable on the hands, thorax, and femurs.
The diploë of the cranial bones are dilated,
the outer cortex appears atrophied, and there
is a granular rarefaction of the trabeculae.
Similar findings are present in the spine and
pelvis. With increasing age the radiographic
picture of the hands, thorax, and femur improves while that of the skull, spine, and pelvis worsens. Medullary cavity expansion of
the facial bones is particularly prominent,
also increases with age, and may cause clinically recognized expansion of the maxilla
with resultant malalignment of the teeth
and malocclusion.[25, 55] The maxillary enlargement may be severe and may cause pro-

trusion of the middle third of the face and
tautness of the skin of the upper lip (Fig.
14-8). Ocular hypertelorism, mongoloid
orientation of the palpebral fissures, epicanthus, and, paradoxically, failure of pneumatization of the maxillary and sphenoidal sinuses have been reported in affected patients (Fig. 14-9).

The hematological profile of patients with
thalassemia major is characterized by a hypochromic and microcytic anemia. There may
be a preponderance of ovalocytes and target
cells. Levels of hemoglobin F and hemoglobin
A_2 are increased. The increase in hemoglobin
F is minimal and nondiagnostic, whereas the
increase of hemoglobin A_2 is pronounced and
is considered pathognomonic for the disorder.
The plasma bilirubin level is raised, and
there is a normoblastic hyperplasia of the
bone marrow.

The prognosis for affected individuals is
not favorable. Some cases may be fatal in

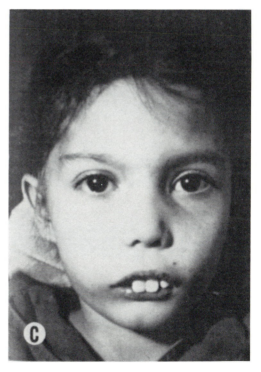

Fig. 14-8. Characteristic facies of patient with
thalassemia major. (From Caffey, J.: Am. J. Roentgenol. **78:**381-391, 1957.)

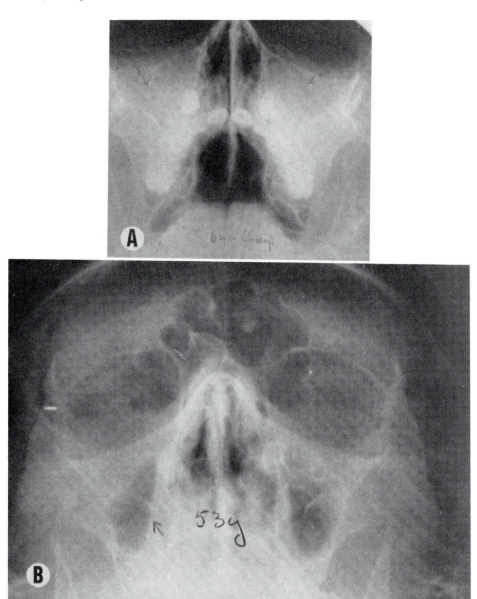

Fig. 14-9. Decreased pneumatization of maxillary sinus in adult patient with thalassemia major. (From Caffey, J.: Am. J. Roentgenol. **78:**381-391, 1957.)

early childhood, and few survive beyond 20 years of age.

Thalassemia minor. Thalassemia minor results from heterozygosity for the β-thalassemia gene. It is a relatively benign condition with few or no clinical findings. Anemia is mild to moderate, and in some cases there is erythrocytosis. Reticulocytosis is not uncommon with cells that are normoblastic and polychromic. Serum iron levels may be slightly elevated.

α-Thalassemia major and minor. α-Thalassemia major and minor are due to homozygosity and heterozygosity, respectively, for a gene causing deficient synthesis of the alpha chain of hemoglobin. The homozygous state is incompatible with life and causes hydrops fetalis and spontaneous abortion. The heterozygous state is asymptomatic and is detected during screening procedures or in families after the conception of an affected fetus.

Other forms of thalassemia have been described and are due to multiple alleles at the β-thalassemia locus or interactions of alpha or beta genes with other hemoglobin genes. The combination of β-thalassemia and HbS is most common of the latter and produces severe sickling disease.

Erythrocytosis

The term *erythrocytosis* is used here to identify disorders in which there is an increase in the absolute number of erythrocytes. When there is a concomitant increase in the number of leukocytes and thrombocytes, the term *polycythemia* is used.

Polycythemia rubra vera (PRV). PRV is a chronic disease characterized by red cell hyperplasia, leukocytosis, and thrombocytosis. The mode of inheritance of polycythemia is not clear. Pedigrees compatible with autosomal dominant and autosomal recessive inheritance have been described.[72, 91, 94] A reported higher frequency of polycythemia in Jews of Eastern European extraction and a rarity in Negroes may be due to ascertainment bias. Although cases have been reported in children, clinical symptoms first become apparent during middle age and are due to increased viscosity of the blood secondary to increased red cell mass. Some symptoms may be due to a hemorrhagic tendency of unknown cause. The earliest symptoms are usually cerebral in origin and may include headache, syncope, hearing loss, and blurred vision. Fatigability, weakness, dyspnea, hypertension, hepatosplenomegaly, varicose veins, menorrhea, weight loss, itching, burning pain in the extremities with subsequent bluish red discoloration, and gout are common. Striking features on clinical examination are ruddy cyanosis of the skin of the face and extremities and engorgement of the vessels of the mucous membranes and conjuctivae. Gingival hemorrhage has been reported as the initial symptom in some cases and a serrated, red tongue in others.[33, 72] The lips may be bluish in color, as may the gin-

giva. Facial telangiectasiae are common. Leukemia is seen commonly in patients with PRV or in their families. The nature of its association is not known, although leukemia may be the cause of death. Leukemia may also contribute to the high frequency of chromosome aneuploidies found in the blood of patients with PRV.[64] Common causes of death are thrombosis, myeloid metaplasia, and hemorrhage. Drawn blood is thick and dark. There is an increase in the number of red cells, which are normocytic and normochromic. The number of white cells, the activity of leukocyte alkaline phosphotase, and the number of thrombocytes are increased. The aim of treatment is to reduce the number of cells in the blood and thereby reduce its viscosity. Some practitioners prefer repeated phlebotomies to accomplish this, and others prefer treatment with radioactive phosphorus with or without chlornaphazin.

Erythrocytosis vera. Erythrocytosis vera may be inherited as an autosomal dominant or an autosomal recessive trait.[28, 37] The dominant variety usually has its onset later in life than the recessive variety, which is commonly seen first in children and has prompted the designation *benign, familial polycythemia of children.* However, only the erythrocyte series of blood cells is elevated in erythrocytosis, and the use of the term *polycythemia* is inappropriate.

The clinical features of the two varieties of erythrocytosis are similar. A ruddy complexion and cyanosis is noted from birth and is often severe enough to prompt the nickname of "Indian." The oral mucosa and nail beds are cyanotic. The superficial vessels, especially those of the conjuctivae, may be dilated. Involvement of the conjunctivae is often misinterpreted as pinkeye. Moderate splenomegaly is a constant finding, whereas hepatomegaly and lymphadenopathy are absent. Clubbing of the fingers and frequent headaches have been reported in some cases. Prolonged hemorrhage has been reported. In one case prolonged hemorrhage was reported after the extraction of teeth.[28] Levels of hemoglobin, red blood cells, and the hematocrit are elevated. There may be a mild erythroblastic hyperplasia of the bone marrow. Other elements of formed blood are normal in the amount.

Disorders of pigment metabolism

A group of metabolic disorders that do not ordinarily produce hemolysis and involve porphyrin metabolism are referred to as the porphyrias. There are several types of porphyria, each of which is associated with increased excretion of porphyrin or porphyrin precursors.

Congenital erythropoietic porphyria. Red urine, vesiculobullous skin lesions, erythrodontia, and hirsutism characterize congenital erythropoietic porphyria, a rare autosomal recessive disorder.[104] The clinical findings are related to excessive excretion of types I coproporphyrin and uroporphyrin.[105] The discoloration of the teeth is due to their incorporation of uroporphyrin.[118] The onset

of clinical findings is at birth or shortly thereafter; a reddish discoloration of the urine is usually the first sign. Patients with this disorder are photosensitive and develop vesiculobullous skin lesions when exposed to sunlight. The age of onset and the severity of lesions varies with the amount of light exposure. The lesions heal poorly and scar, often causing disfigurement of the face and loss of nails. Discoloration of the teeth has been reported to vary from yellow to brown with reddish brown to purple being the colors most commonly mentioned (Fig. 14-10). The teeth are discolored at the time of eruption but may darken with time. The discoloration is not uniform over the crown of affected teeth; some areas may be darkly pigmented and others almost normally white. Pigmentation has been reported as both heavier and lighter in the gingival and cervical thirds of the erupted crowns. In some cases, the crowns have been reported to be normally pigmented and only the roots discolored. The uroporphyrin that causes discoloration seems to be confined to the dentin. Discolored teeth fluoresce bright red under ultraviolet light. Size, shape, and eruption of teeth are within normal limits.

Hirsutism is most common on the trunk and extremities, although facial hirsutism may be pronounced. Marked splenomegaly is a constant finding. Erythropoietic porphyria is a debilitating disorder that causes death in early or middle adulthood. Rare cases may be fatal during childhood. It is differentiated from the other porphyrias in part by the absence of neurological deterioration, psychological disturbances, and abdominal pain. Coproporphyrin and uroporphyrin are excreted in excessive amounts in the urine and stools. Porphobilinogenuria is absent. The bone marrow of patients with erythropoietic porphyria is normoblastic and hyperplastic. Hemoglobin levels in the circulating blood are increased, as are the hematocrit and mean corpuscular volume. The normoblastic nuclei of some of the circulating erythrocytes contain conjugated porphyrins; the nuclei of other circulating erythrocytes do not contain any.

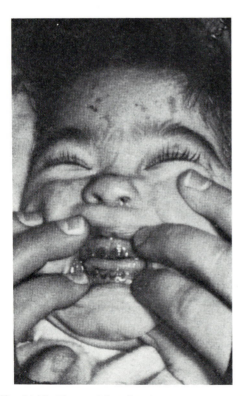

Fig. 14-10. Young child with darkly stained teeth and facial lesions caused by erythropoietic porphyria. (From Dunsky, I., Freeman, S., and Gibson, S.: Am. J. Dis. Child. **74**:305-320, 1947.)

Erythropoietic protoporphyria. Erythropoietic protoporphyria is an autosomal dominant disorder characterized by sudden onset of itching, erythema, and edema after exposure to sunlight, unlike some porphyrias, which manifest delayed onset of symptoms.[78] Itching begins after only several minutes exposure to sunlight. Erythema and edema follow within 30 minutes. Itching may be intense and may produce acute mental anguish while it persists. Vesicles rarely develop, although there may be some crusting with subsequent scarring after the edema subsides. The forehead, cheeks, and knuckles are the most severely involved areas (Fig. 14-11). In older patients the skin of these areas may appear leathery and senile. The perioral skin, especially that of the lower lip, may be fissured and cracked. Gallstones are not uncommon in affected individuals.

The age of onset of photosensitivity is in the first few years of life. Some authors report an equal male-to-female distribution of the disorder, and others report an excess of affected males.[77] Differences in life habits could account for more males than females being affected. A rather significant number of obligate carriers of the gene for erythropoietic protoporphyria are asymptomatic but do have increased levels of erythrocyte and fecal protoporphyrins and coproporphyrins. These carriers may be detected by fluorescence of their erythrocytes under ultraviolet light. The marrow is primarily responsible for excessive protoporphyrin and coproporphyrin production, although the liver may contribute to the excess.

Acute intermittent porphyria. Acute intermittent porphyria is an autosomal dominant disorder that has a higher frequency in

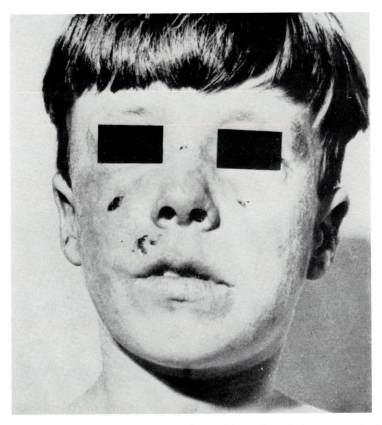

Fig. 14-11. Facial cutaneous lesions seen in patients with erythropoietic protoporphyria. (From Beattie, A. D., and Goldberg, A.: In Hardisty, R. M., and Weatherall, D. J., editors: Blood and its related disorders, Oxford, England, 1974, Blackwell Scientific Publications, Ltd.)

Sweden than elsewhere in the world.[118] The high prevalence in Sweden has led to the alternate designation of *Swedish porphyria.* Acute intermittent porphyria is characterized by profuse neurological abnormalities and gastrointestinal disturbances. Women are more frequently affected than men, and the onset of symptoms is earlier in women (during the third decade) than in men (during the fourth decade).[47] As many as half of the individuals who on the basis of family studies or on the basis of excretion of excessively high levels of porphobilinogen are obligate carriers of the gene are asymptomatic. The first symptoms noted are usually severe, intermittent, abdominal pain and weakness or paralysis of the skeletal muscles. Constipation, vomiting, and diarrhea may accompany the abdominal pain. The weakness and paralysis most frequently involve the limbs, but weakness of the facial muscles is not uncommon. There may be paralysis of the muscle supplied by the facial and trigeminal nerves, tongue weakness, and depressed gag reflex.[98] Dysphasia, dysarthria, and aphonia are not uncommon. Psychiatric disturbances and epilepsy have been reported as complicating features. Solar urticaria is rare in acute intermittent porphyria, but when present, it may manifest as vesicular eruptions over the cheeks and nasal bridge that heal with scarring and hyperpigmentation.[15]

In women, the onset of attacks often corresponds to the onset of menstruation. Barbiturates also precipitate attacks. Affected individuals usually experience two to three attacks per year. The attacks may be fatal, with the patient succumbing to infection, respiratory paralysis, and cardiovascular or cerebral complications.

Acute intermittent porphyria is distinguished from the other porphyrias on the basis of the extensive neurological involvement, the absence of photosensitivity, and the presence of porphobilinogen and Δ-aminolevulinic acid in the urine. Levels of porphyrin and porphyrin precursors in the erythrocytes are normal. The basic defect may be uroporphyrinogen 1-synthetase deficiency.[84]

Porphyria variegata. Porphyria variegata (South African porphyria), an autosomal dominant trait, is much more common in South African whites than any other population in the world.[38] This high frequency is thought to be due to founder effect; all affected individuals descend from a common ancestral couple. The clinical manifestations of porphyria variegata begin in the second to third decade and may mimic those of acute intermittent porphyria when abdominal symptoms precede those of photosensitivity. Abdominal and neurological symptoms are identical to those described for acute intermittent porphyria and are often precipitated by drugs, notably barbiturates. Photosensitive skin lesions are variable in severity, frequency, and age of onset. Rarely are they as severe as those of erythropoietic porphyria, although they are vesiculobullous and heal with scarring. The frequency and extent of skin lesions vary from patient to patient and vary with time in the same patient. Occasionally photosensitive skin lesions are the presenting sign. Porphobilinogen and Δ-aminolevulinic acid are excreted in excessive amounts in the urine during a crisis but return to normal levels during latent periods. Protoporphyrin and coproporphyrin, on the other hand, are excreted in excess in the stools during crises and remission. Erythrocyte porphyrins are normal in amount.

Porphyria variegata, like hemophilia, is one of the genetic disorders that, although rare, is of historic interest because of its occurrence in the royal houses of Europe.[76]

Coproporphyria. Coproporphyria is an autosomal dominant disorder of porphyrin metabolism that usually remains undetected until ingestion of barbiturates, anticoagulants, or tranquilizers. Even after drug use, as many as 60% of the cases may remain asymptomatic.[48] Porphyric attacks mimic those of acute intermittent porphyria with abdominal pain, nervousness, constipation, dark urine, and peripheral neuropathy predominating. Jaundice is common. Photosensitivity has been reported in several cases but is not a constant finding. In all cases in which photosensitivity was a feature, the face was conspicuously involved.[58] A single patient was reported to have coproporphyria, rickets, and riboflavin deficiency. Delayed eruption of the first tooth, hypertelorism, fragile nails, and a red tongue devoid of papillae were probably due to the latter disorders in this child, although the author postulated a causal relationship between the three conditions.[9]

Excess coproporphyrin (Isomer III) is consistently present in the stools; excessive porphobilinogen and Δ-aminolevulinic acid are excreted intermittently in the urine.

Hepatic cutaneous porphyria. Photosensi-

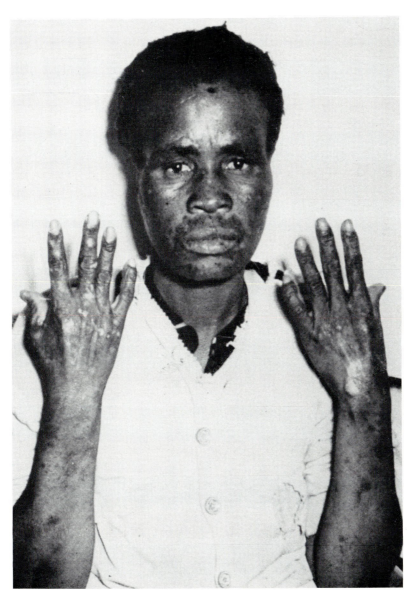

Fig. 14-12. Depigmented skin lesions with focal areas of hyperpigmentation in woman with hepatic cutaneous porphyria. (From Beattie, A. D., and Goldberg, A.: In Hardisty, R. M., and Weatherall, D. J., editors: Blood and its related disorders, Oxford, England, 1974, Blackwell Scientific Publications, Ltd.)

tivity and excessive excretion of porphyrin precursors characterize hepatic cutaneous porphyria. Clinical findings include vesiculobullous skin lesions, skin fragility, sclerodermoid skin lesions, and hirsutism. The skin lesions begin as erythema, progress to vesicles, and coalesce into bullae. The bullae bleed, crust, and heal with scarring. Skin fragility is marked and may be the only overt manifestation of the disorder. Because of scarring from the vesiculobullous lesions and fragility, sun-exposed skin develops a scleroderma-like appearance. Depigmented, shiny lesions surrounded by hyperpigmented areas are characteristic (Fig. 14-12). Females commonly complain of hirsutism of the face, arms, and hands. There are usually no reported abdominal or neurological symptoms, but a peculiar neuropathy of altered sensation over the face, scalp, and trunk has been reported in one series of patients.[5] Coproporphyrin is excreted in excess in stools and urine; uroporphyrin is excessively excreted in the urine only.

The mode of inheritance of hepatic cutaneous porphyria is not well established. Some authors describe an acquired form and a hereditary form, describing the latter as an autosomal dominant.[70, 123] Others suggest that the separation into hereditary and acquired forms is arbitrary and consider the two forms as one. Differences in clinical manifestations between the alcohol-induced disorder of middle age and the hereditary disorder of early adulthood suggest that the two are distinct entities.

DISORDERS OF LEUKOCYTES
Structural variation of granulocytes

Several conditions are associated with morphological alterations of the polymorphonuclear leukocytes. The basic defect in some of these is undoubtedly metabolic, but since each was described on the basis of morphological differences from the normal, they will be considered under this heading.

May-Hegglin anomaly. The May-Hegglin anomaly consists of inclusion bodies in the cytoplasm of neutrophils and large platelets. It is inherited as an autosomal dominant trait. The condition is usually asymptomatic, although hemorrhage and leukemia have been causally related. One subject was reported to have purpuric lesions of the oral mucosa and numerous petechiae over the cheeks. She also had severe dental caries and excess adipose tissue over the cheeks, giving her a Cushingoid appearance.[93] The cytoplasmic inclusions (Dohle bodies) in the May-Hegglin anomaly are circular or elliptical in shape, stain light blue with Wright's stain, and are usually present one to a cell. Platelets are enlarged and often rod shaped.

Chédiak-Higashi syndrome. Large granules in the leukocytes characterize the Chédiak-Higashi syndrome. The granules are single-membrane, lysosomal organelles that occur predominantly in neutrophils, although other granulocytes may be involved to variable degrees. Cells from the bone marrow, liver, adrenal cortex, and anterior pituitary contain granules also. The clinical features of this syndrome include hypopigmentation of the hair (silvery blond) and eyes, photophobia, nystagmus, lymphadenopathy, nasopharyngeal inflammation, an abnormally high susceptibility to infection, malignant lymphoma, and early death. Increased perspiration and increased thirst have been reported, although lacrimation and saliva flow are reportedly normal.

The most commonly reported orofacial findings, aside from general hypopigmentary anomalies, are a diffuse macular rash over the face, recurrent ulcers of the oral mucosa, and facial palsies late in the disease process.[69, 106] The oral ulcers have been described as shallow and patchy in distribution, resembling canker sores, and have been observed shortly after birth. Other reported oral findings have included prolonged hemorrhage after tooth extraction, excessive dental caries, "altered teeth," hemorrhagic and swollen gingivae, and premature loss of teeth.

Metabolic errors of leukocytes

Chronic granulomatous disease. Chronic granulomatous disease may be autosomal recessive or X-linked recessive in inheritance. The X-linked recessive form is the more common of the two. Clinical manifestations of this disorder include increased susceptibility to staphylococcus infection, chronic suppurative lymphadenitis, eczematoid dermatitis, chronic pulmonary disease, hepatosplenomegaly, and early death. Dermatitis may begin as a pustular rash and has been reported on the skull, face, lips, and neck. Five of the thirteen patients in one survey and another reported case have experienced recurrent ulcerative stomatitis.[27, 42, 62] The latter case also had recurrent draining abscesses of the cervical lymph nodes. His mother had firm, reddish brown plaques over the skin of her neck.

Leukocytes of affected individuals phagocytose staphylococcus organisms normally but are limited in their bactericidal activity. Failure of dissolution of bacteria ingested by the leukocytes has been documented through in vitro observations. Abnormal activity of reduced nicotinamide-adenine dinucleotide oxidase may account for the inability to digest normally phagocytosed bacteria.

A defect in leukocyte oxidase activity results in the inability to reduce nitroblue tetrazolium and is the basis for the diagnostic test for this disorder.

Leukopenia

A decrease in the number of circulating leukocytes below the normally accepted low of 4000/ml constitutes leukopenia. The neutrophils and eosinophils are involved in the hereditary leukopenias. A reduction below the normal range of the number of neutrophils and of eosinophils constitutes neutropenia and eosinophilia, respectively.

Neutropenia. Neutropenia may be caused by infection, disorders of the bone marrow, megaloblastic anemias, hypersplenism, drugs, and genetic factors. Drug-induced neutropenia is not central to the topic of this chapter but is of interest because of significant involvement of the oral cavity. Neutropenia may be associated with the ingestion of a large number of drugs, including analgesics, antihistamines, tranquilizers, anticoagulants, antimalarials, and diuretics. The early stages of drug-induced neutropenia are characterized by a reddening of the oral mucosa. Other mucosal surfaces and the skin may be involved. In more advanced cases, the oral findings include recurrent soreness of the throat, oral sepsis, ulceration and softening of the mucous membranes, and associated fever. The superficial mucosa of the gingiva, palate, tongue, and eyes may appear grayish brown and undergo necrotic changes. If the necrosis extends to the periodontium, the teeth may be excessively mobile. This condition is less common now that the role of drugs as a cause has been recognized, but it should be suspected in patients with the listed oral findings, especially in middle-aged women.

Chronic familial neutropenia. Chronic familial neutropenia is inherited as an autosomal dominant trait. Cases reported in the literature have described clinical manifestations as ranging from absent to relatively severe. It is possible that this is a heterogeneous category with asymptomatic cases being examples of benign, chronic neutropenia and more severely affected cases being examples of chronic, hypoplastic neutropenia as discussed by Spaet and Dameshek.[107] When clinical manifestations are present, the oral involvement is significant. Recurrent osteomyelitis of the maxilla, recurrent abscesses on the floor of the mouth, granulomatous lesions of the tongue, ulcerations of the gingival and buccal mucosa, hemorrhagic enlargement of the gingiva and early loss of the teeth with loss of alveolar bone have been reported as causally related to the neutropenia.[1] Afflicted individuals are unusually susceptible to infections, and extraction of teeth has precipitated severe infections in several cases. Other reported oral manifestations include pustules over the skin of the face and skull, preauricular abscesses, paranasal sinusitis, swollen salivary glands, desquamation of the palatal mucosa, discolored teeth, and persistent rhinopharyngitis. Lymphadenopathy, delayed healing of wounds, persistent infections after minor trauma and insect bites, otitis media, and lung abscesses are other common findings.

Authors who contend that there is more

than one form of chronic neutropenia state there is a relative lymphocytosis and relative monocytosis with minimal changes in eosinophils and abnormal platelets in the benign variety and an absolute lymphocytosis, an absolute monocytosis with normal eosinophils, and slight decrease in platelets in the symptomatic variety.

Cyclic neutropenia. The most frequently reported manifestations of cyclic neutropenia, another autosomal dominant trait, are fever, oral ulcers, and skin infections. Oral ulceration has been the presenting symptom in a large percentage of the cases reported and may involve the tongue, gingivae, or buccal mucosa.[8, 50] The ulcers may heal with scarring and develop before the absolute drop in neutrophil count. Multiple dental abscesses have been reported as associated findings. Teeth may be prematurely lost secondary to early destruction of alveolar bone (Fig. 14-13).

The onset of signs and symptoms of cyclic neutropenia varies from a few months of age to late adulthood. However, the majority of cases develop symptoms by the end of the first decade of life. Pharyngitis, abdominal pain, arthralgia, and infections correspond to the cyclic appearance of neutropenia and the earlier-mentioned manifestations. The periodicity of neutropenic episodes is usually reported as 3 weeks, with some cycles being as short as 15 days and others as long as 35 days. During remission the neutrophil count returns to normal or near-normal levels. Monocytosis may accompany the neutropenia. The basis for the cyclic nature of the disorder is not known. It is accentuated by pregnancy in afflicted women, but it is unrelated to their menstrual cycles.

Lethal, congenital neutropenia with eosinophilia; infantile agranulocytosis. Similar clinical courses are shown by the autosomal recessive traits of lethal, congenital neutropenia with eosinophilia and infantile agranulocytosis.[4, 68] The onset of symptoms in each is within the first few weeks to the first few months of life. Septic ulcers of the skin predominate clinical findings. These are especially common on the scalp, face, and neck. Otitis, mastoiditis, and elevated fever commonly appear with the skin lesions. Blister-like lesions and white plaques have been described on the tongue and oral mucosa. Less specific oroseptic necrosis has also been reported. One patient was reported to have

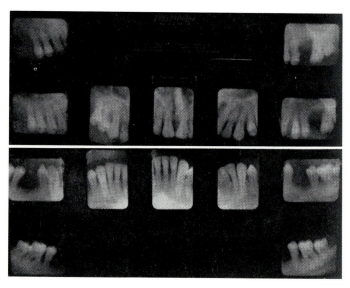

Fig. 14-13. Loss of alveolar bone in patient with cyclic neutropenia. (From Smith, J. F.: Oral Surg. 18:312-320, 1964.)

a dry mouth and enlarged gingivae by 15 months of age and another to have discolored teeth and enlarged gingivae at 11 years of age. Each of these rare recessive traits is fatal with only a few cases surviving beyond early childhood.

Andrews and co-workers[4] differentiate between the two conditions on the basis of hypoplastic marrow, monocytosis, and lack of eosinophilia in the latter.

MYELOPROLIFERATIVE DISORDERS
Leukemia

The leukemias are characterized by neoplastic proliferation of the leukoblastic tissue. The basic defect involves a failure of this tissue to respond to the factors that ordinarily regulate its growth and maturation. As a result the leukemic cells proliferate to the extent that they replace hemopoietic cells and cause bone marrow dysfunction. The white cells that consequently predominate the circulating blood are immature and abnormal in form.

Many of the essential processes of leukemia are not well understood. Epidemiological studies have shown that the frequency of leukemia has increased dramatically during the last several decades.[55] This increase in frequency cannot be explained solely on the basis of improved diagnosis and other such factors. Certain external agents and genetic factors are suspected to have contributed to the increase. Ionizing radiation has been shown to be the cause of leukemia in animal models and man. A number of cases of possible drug-induced leukemia have been reported. The drugs include benzene and melphalan.[46] Infections are known to be associated with the onset of acute leukemia of childhood. Whether the infection is the cause or effect of leukemia has not been adequately determined. The association suggests that leukemia may be transmitted by a virus, and virus-like particles have been found in the blood of patients with some forms of leukemia. In addition, the clustering of cases of leukemia in some communities suggests an infectious agent. A genetic basis for leukemia is supported by evidence that leukemia is more common in Jews than in non-Jews and more common in whites than in blacks. Cases of leukemia in more than one member of the family are not conclusive proof of a genetic basis because of the possibility of an unidentified agent in the environment shared by relatives. However, the different types of leukemia do occur in families with different frequencies. Most familial leukemia is the chronic lymphocytic variety, whereas the chronic granulocytic variety is rarely seen in families, and in most reported instances of leukemia in twins the same variety is diagnosed. The association of the Philadelphia chromosome with chronic myelocytic leukemia should not be viewed as proof that leukemia is caused by a defective G-group chromosome or that it is caused by a mutant gene on that chromosome. The chromosome defect in all probability is an acquired abnormality. However, leukemia is twenty times more common in individuals with trisomy 21 (Down's syndrome) than in the general population.[108] Based on the above and other observations, the following groups seem to be at high risk for developing leukemia: twins of children with leukemia, patients with Down's, Bloom's, or Fanconi's syndromes, patients undergoing radiation treatment, health professionals in radiology, and survivors of atomic explosions.

The leukemias are classified on the basis of the type of leukocyte predominantly involved in the proliferative process. Each type may be further categorized as acute or chronic.

Acute leukemias are more severe disorders than the chronic leukemias. It is difficult to identify the type of acute leukemia on the basis of clinical findings alone, and even laboratory studies may be inconclusive. The clinical manifestations of acute leukemias vary widely and depend more on the organ systems that are involved than on the proliferating cell types. The onset of acute leukemia may be manifested as listlessness, pallor, arthralgia, pathological fractures, fever, malaise, prostration, gingival hemorrhage, petechiae, or a generalized hemorrhagic tendency (Fig. 14-14). In general, the oral

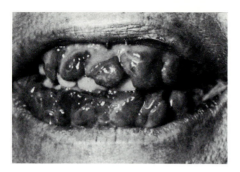

Fig. 14-14. Enlarged gingivae in patient with acute monocytic leukemia. (From Williamson, J. J.: Blood dyscrasias. In Gorlin, R. J., and Goldman, H. M., editors: Thoma's oral pathology, ed. 6, St. Louis, 1970, The C. V. Mosby Co.)

involvement of acute leukemia is more consistent and more pronounced than that in chronic leukemia.[67, 75] Oral findings have been reported in 25% to 75% of acute leukemia cases. Hemorrhage of the gingivae is the most commonly reported finding, with oral ulcers being the second most common and petechiae of the oral mucosa the third. Hemorrhaging may be intracranial and lead to headache, convulsion, sensory disturbances, papilledema, and cranial nerve palsies. The mucous membranes may appear pale because of a secondary anemia. Chloromas (myeloblast tumor masses) occur occasionally and involve the bones of the face and head. Radiographic examination of the jaws has demonstrated osseous changes in two thirds of the cases. These changes consist of alveolar bone resorption, loss of lamina dura, thick periodontal membrane spaces, resorption of the roots of teeth, and unexplained periapical radiolucencies.

Acute leukemia is consistently fatal. Some drugs have been successfully used to control acute lymphoblastic leukemia but are of no value in treating the other varieties.

Acute monocytic leukemia. A more unified clinical picture is presented by acute monocytic leukemia than by the other leukemias. It affects men more often than women and has an average onset at 45 years. Clinical features include weakness, fatigue, fever, multiple organism septicemia, hemorrhagic

tendencies, pallor, lymphadenopathy, splenomegaly, hepatomegaly, rectal and vaginal ulcers, and enlargement of the gingiva. The gingivae are swollen and pale early in the disease and ulcerated and necrotic late in the disease. Infective lesions in the oropharynx are common. These lesions may vary from small necrotic ulcers to large areas of swelling and necrosis. In contrast to acute lymphocytic leukemia, which rarely has gingival lesions, as many as half of the cases of monocytic leukemia have been described as having gingival and oropharyngeal lesions. Paralysis of muscles supplied by the facial nerve is not uncommon. A number of cases have been diagnosed on referral from dental practitioners for evaluation of these oral manifestations or for therapeutic consideration of complications after dental extractions. In one survey oral manifestations led the diagnosis equally as often as extraoral manifestations.[83]

Acute monocytic leukemia is fatal, causing death 2 to 6 months after diagnosis. Normocytic anemia, monocytosis with juvenile cells predominating, nucleation of the erythrocytes, and thrombocytopenia invariably accompany the leukemia.

Chronic leukemia

Chronic lymphocytic leukemia. The variety most commonly reported in families is chronic lymphocytic leukemia. Although it is inherited as an autosomal dominant trait,[32] men are affected more than twice as frequently as women. The onset of clinical symptoms is late in adult life. The onset is particularly insidious and may be marked by mild, nontender lymphadenopathy, moderate leukocytosis, and relative lymphocytosis. Enlargement of the superficial lymph nodes is particularly striking. The initial symptom may be enlargement of the lacrimal and salivary glands. This latter association is referred to as Mikulicz's syndrome.[32] Other clinical findings are fatigability, petechiae, gastrointestinal hemorrhage, gingival hemorrhage, hyperpigmentation of the skin, exfoliative dermatitis, hepatosplenomegaly, and susceptibility to infection. This latter finding may be related to secondary hypogammaglobulinemia.

Some patients experience recurrent episodes of herpes zoster, and others experience intense itching of the skin. Occasional spontaneous hemorrhage from the mucous membranes and gingiva are seen, but these are usually late in the disease process. Discrete, circular areas of radiolucency are commonly seen in the maxilla and mandible of advanced cases.

The prognosis for patients with chronic lymphocytic leukemia is variable. In some patients the course of disease is more rapid than in others. However, even in those with relatively static clinical findings, the disease is progressive and fatal. Since the age of onset is late in life, many patients die of causes related to senility rather than leukemia. Anemia is common in chronic lymphocytic leukemia but may not be marked. When present, it is normocytic and normochromic in nature. Moderate anisocytosis and poikilocytosis are present. The striking feature of the blood film is, of course, raised lymphocyte count.

Chronic myelocytic anemia (granulocytic leukemia). Chronic myelocytic anemia has an earlier age of onset than lymphocytic leukemia, and the sex distribution is closer to a 1:1 ratio. Like the lymphocytic variety, the onset of myelocytic leukemia is gradual and insidious. The most common early clinical findings are abdominal pain, weight loss, fevers, or nocturnal hyperhidrosis. Some patients present first with gastrointestinal hemorrhage, splenic infarction, hemorrhages of the skin, and anemia. Marked splenomegaly is a constant finding and is more pronounced than the splenomegaly in lymphocytic leukemia, the spleen tip being not uncommonly palpable below the level of the umbilicus. The liver is less consistently enlarged. Lymphadenopathy may be seen but is much less common than in the lymphocytic leukemias. The veins of the retinae are commonly engorged and may hemorrhage. The mucous membranes are pale and may be covered with petechiae. Bruising after minimal trauma and bleeding from the gingiva are common symptoms that worsen as the disease progresses. Areas of radiolucency may be seen on radiographs of the skeleton. The ends of the long bones are especially prone to osteolysis and may show alternate radiodense and radiolucent bands. The disease is invariably fatal with a mean survival time from the recognition of symptoms of only a few years.

Anemia is frequently seen in association with myelocytic leukemia. It is normocytic and normochromic and may be due in part to bleeding and in part to decreased erythropoiesis. Anisocytosis is present and poikilocytosis is not. The leukocyte count is elevated markedly with the greatest increase being in the segmented neutrophils, myelocytes, and band cells. There is also an associated thrombocytosis. The Philadelphia chromosome is seen in a large percentage of patients with myelocytic leukemia as is a low level of leukocyte alkaline phosphatase.

Erythroleukemia. Erythroleukemia is a myeloproliferative disorder that involves red cells and white cells (granulocytes). Some workers contend that the disorder begins as erythrocytic proliferation that later becomes myelocytic proliferation; others consider the disorder a single entity with variable degrees of erythrocytic or myelocytic proliferation. This is a disorder of middle age that is characterized by weakness, fatigue, dyspnea, weight loss, and hemorrhagic tendencies of the skin, mucosa, and gastrointestinal tract. Furunculosis of the scalp and face have been reported as have necrotic sores of the lips, mouth, gingivae, and petechiae of the oral mucosa. Oral petechiae are not a constant finding but when present involve the palatal mucosa. In one reported case, palatal petechiae were the only clinical sign of the disorder.[57]

Although there is no evidence that erythroleukemia is hereditary, it has been reported to be associated with multiple chromosomal abnormalities in half the cases.[57] These chromosome abnormalities include aneuploidies, increased chromosome breaks, and small fragments resembling the Philadelphia chromosome.

Multiple myeloma (myelomatosis). Multiple myeloma has been reported in numerous siblings and may represent an autosomal recessive trait.[3] One pedigree compatible with autosomal dominant inheritance has been reported.[90] Multiple myeloma is characterized by malignant proliferation of the plasma cells in the marrow. The condition affects males more frequently than females and may occur at any age, but is more common in patients over 50 years old. Clinical manifestation is variable but usually involves bone pain. The pain is aggravated by movement and may be associated with swelling. Anemia and its clinical features are not uncommon but should be considered secondary complications. Bleeding from the nose and gingiva is frequently seen. Renal failure is a common fatal complication, although it is rarely a presenting sign. Susceptibility to infection is common.

Oral findings can be particularly striking. The gingivae may be enlarged and hemorrhagic. The enlargement is due in part to amyloid deposits in the gingival tissue; the bleeding is due to gingivitis and associated thrombocytopenia. The tongue may be also enlarged secondary to amyloid deposits and may cause flaring of the teeth[22] (Fig. 14-15).

Osteoporotic lesions of the skeleton may be

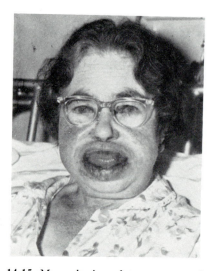

Fig. 14-15. Macroglossia and tongue protrusion in female patient with multiple myeloma. (From Buchanan, J., Frew, I. D. O., Gibson, I. J. M., Gibson, T., and Russell, A. R.: Br. J. Plast. Surg. 22:157-160, 1969.)

the only overt sign of the disease. These often are first detected by skeletal radiographs as part of a diagnostic work-up for idiopathic bone pain. The radiographic picture is one of diffuse decalcification of the skeleton with multiple small discrete radiolucencies. These lesions are common in the flat bones of the skeleton and are best seen in the skull. Occasionally the typical skeletal lesions are noted first in the jaws.[26] The mandible is more frequently involved than the maxilla; the gonial angle is the most frequently involved site of the mandible. Several cases of solitary myeloma of the jaws have been reported.[122]

Diagnosis of multiple myelomas is confirmed by the presence of abnormal plasma proteins and Bence Jones proteinuria.

HEMORRHAGIC DISORDERS

Disorders of hemostasis can be divided into three groups: disorders of the vessels, disorders of the platelets, and disorders of coagulation. It is relatively easy to identify the hemorrhagic disorders in which the platelet and coagulation mechanisms are intact, but the bleeding occurs because of fragility or other defects of the vasculature. It is harder to separate the platelet disorders from the coagulation disorders. This is because some coagulation factors are secreted by the platelets, and others must function with the platelets to produce hemostasis.

Disorders of the blood vessels

Knowledge of the role of the vessels in hemorrhagic disorders is scanty. Nonetheless there are several well-defined disorders of the blood vessels that produce a bleeding tendency. These disorders may be primary, heritable defects in the vessel, or they may be caused by environmental factors (for example, scurvy or drugs).

Hereditary hemorrhagic telangiectasia (Rendu-Osler-Weber syndrome). Hereditary hemorrhagic telangiectasia is an autosomal dominant disorder.[45] The primary defect is not known, but it is characterized by dilatations of thin-walled capillaries and arteries that do not contract normally and cause rupturing of the vessel wall. The dilatations are visible as telangiectases of the tongue tip, labial mucosa, face, conjunctivae, ears, fingers, nasal mucosa, gastrointestinal tract, and bladder. They differ from spider nevi in size, shape, and distribution. The tip of the tongue and labial mucosa are the most frequently involved sites (Fig. 14-16). The telangiectases may bleed spontaneously or with little trauma. The lesions vary in size from barely discernible to 0.5 cm in diameter and in color from red to blue. They are not usually seen in childhood but become increasingly apparent with age and are one of the triad of signs necessary for diagnosis of the condition. The other signs are spontaneous hemorrhage and positive family history as described. Cirrhosis of the liver is not uncommon in patients with this condition.

The anemia most commonly associated with hereditary hemorrhagic telangiectasia is the hypochromic, microcytic anemia of iron deficiency. Aside from anemia the blood profile is within normal limits. Treatment consists of local measures in response to epistasis, estrogen therapy, and supplemental iron to relieve the anemia that develops secondary to blood loss.

von Willebrand's disease. An autosomal dominant trait characterized by prolonged bleeding time and factor VIII deficiency is von Willebrand's disease. There is some controversy as to whether the primary defect in von Willebrand's disease is in capillary wall or in the platelets.[12] It most likely involves each. In favor of the vascular defect is the fact that the terminal capillary loops are more irregular and tortuous than normal, do not contract normally when injured, and are more fragile than normal. Favoring a platelet defect is the fact that the platelets are less adhesive than normal, presumably because of deficiency of factor VIII. The factor VIII deficiency of von Willebrand's disease is different than that of classic hemophilia, and clinical findings are milder. Cross-correcting experiments have suggested that there are two loci responsible for factor VIII deficiency. The first is on one of the autosomes and causes von Willebrand's disease; the second is on the X chromosome and is responsible for hemophilia.

The onset of hemorrhagic diathesis is early in life in von Willebrand's disease and may involve spontaneous bleeding or prolonged bleeding secondary to mild trauma. Spontaneous nosebleeds and spontaneous gingival hemorrhage are the most common symptoms.[118] Females seem to have a greater predilection for gingival hemorrhage than males and experience such bleedings most commonly at night. Gastrointestinal bleeding and menorrhagia are common. Hemarthroses are rare. The most frequent complication of medical treatment for patients with von Willebrand's disease is postextraction hemorrhage.[99]

Disorders of platelet number

Hemorrhagic conditions caused by abnormalities of the number of platelets may be caused by an excess of platelets or by a deficiency of platelets.

Thrombocythemia. Thrombocythemia is defined as a condition in which there is an increased number of platelets alone. Many of the excessive platelets are abnormal in structure, and they may be excessively adhesive. The mechanism by which thrombocythemia causes hemorrhage is not known. A concomitant deficiency of factor III has been suggested as the cause. Anemia and leuko-

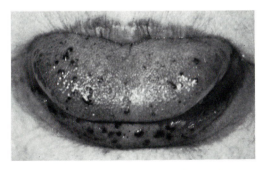

Fig. 14-16. Telangiectasiae of vermilion and tongue tip in patient with hereditary hemorrhagic telangiectasia. (From Mescon, H., Grots, I. A., and Gorlin, R. J.: Mucocutaneous disorders. In Gorlin, R. J., and Goldman, H. M., editors: Thoma's oral pathology, ed. 6, St. Louis, 1970, The C. V. Mosby Co.)

cytosis are commonly associated with the thrombocythemia and in fact may explain the bleeding tendency. Besides hemorrhaging, particularly in the gastrointestinal system, clinical findings include thromboses and splenic infarctions. Bleeding is less common from the skin and upper respiratory tract, including the oral cavity. Thrombocythemia is not known to be hereditary.

Thrombocytopenia. Thrombocytopenia is usually defined as a condition in which the platelet count is less than the normally accepted lower limit of 100,000 cells per milliliter. Thrombocytopenia may be caused by environmental agents (drugs, viruses, injuries), may be secondary to systemic conditions (hypersplenism, kidney disease, giant congenital hemangiomas, diffuse marrow disorders, Aldrich's syndrome), or may have a hereditary basis. There are autosomal dominant, autosomal recessive, and X-linked forms of thrombocytopenia.

The autosomal dominant form of thrombocytopenia has been described by numerous authors.[6] Hydronephrosis, hematuria, hemorrhagic diathesis, and aplasia of ribs have been reported in affected individuals. Aside from prolonged bleeding after tooth extraction, no particular oral involvement has been noted. A short life span of the platelet was demonstrated to be present in reported cases, although no morphological or biochemical abnormalities were discovered.

There have been convincing reports of autosomal recessive and X-linked thrombocytopenia.[103, 116] The autosomal recessive disorder is characterized by severe hemorrhagic diathesis with death in infancy being common. Spontaneous bleeding may occur simultaneously from all the mucous membranes. Hematomas of the scalp are common. X-linked thrombocytopenia may be an isolated trait, or it may be one manifestation of the Aldrich syndrome. Few families have been described in which there are no anomalies associated with the thrombocytopenia. Eczema of variable severity is the most frequently reported extrasanguine finding. The eczema is pronounced over the scalp and face and produces a dry, red, itching skin

surface. Prolonged postextraction hemorrhage is common.

It is difficult to separate these latter cases from cases of the Aldrich syndrome, a syndrome of thrombocytopenia, eczema, proneness to infection, and bloody diarrhea. This is especially true because elevated levels of IgA and decreased levels of isohemagglutinin have been reported in families with and without associated clinical anomalies.

Thrombocytopenia-absent radius (TAR) syndrome. TAR syndrome is an autosomal recessive association of thrombocytopenia and specific skeletal anomalies. This condition differs from Fanconi's syndrome described earlier by the lack of characteristic thumb abnormality, the lack of chromosomal breaks, and lack of pigmentary anomalies. Thrombocytopenia in the TAR syndrome is evident early in life but is transient. Clinical findings include petechiae of the skin and mucous membranes, bilateral absence of the radius with ulnar reduction, normal fingers and thumbs, congenital heart defects, and variable degrees of anemia. Hypoplastic mandibles and maxillae have been reported in some cases.[52]

The blood profile is one of thrombocytopenia with severe reduction in the number of marrow megakaryocytes and associated leukocytosis. The anemia is secondary to blood loss and is of the iron-deficient type.

Disorders of platelet metabolism

Relatively few conditions have been described in which a hemorrhagic diathesis is due to abnormal platelet function. Abnormal bleeding secondary to uremia is due in part to an acquired platelet defect. Several drugs also induce a qualitative change in the platelet and result in prolonged bleeding times. The most commonly used of these drugs is aspirin.

Thrombasthenia of Glanzmann and Naegeli. Thrombasthenia has been reported as an autosomal dominant[24] and autosomal recessive[44] trait. The majority of cases reported have been recessive in nature. Abnormal levels of several platelet enzymes have been reported in apparently dominant cases, whereas an unknown factor associated with platelet adhesiveness has been postulated to be causally related to the recessive form of the condition. In the recessive variety, platelets do not aggregate normally in response to extrinsic ADP. Platelet counts may be normal or slightly elevated. Platelet shape may be abnormal with round cells predominating. Bleeding time appears to be prolonged in the dominant forms but less abnormal in the recessive form. The platelets may be abnormally fragile. Severe anemia, prolonged bleeding after injury, and spontaneous bleeding from the mucous membranes have been reported in cases of thrombasthemia. Bleeding at the time of exfoliation of the primary teeth and after tooth extraction has been reported. Spontaneous bleeding from the gingiva and bleeding from the gingiva after injury and after toothbrushing have been reported.

Disorders of coagulation

The process of coagulation is complex and not entirely understood. However, a series of inherent factors associated with abnormal coagulation has been identified. These factors may be referred to by number or commonly used names. They are factors I (fibrinogen), II (prothrombin), III (tissue thromboplastin), IV (calcium), V (labile factor), VII (stabile factor), VIII (antihemophilic globulin), IX (Christmas factor), X (Stuart-Prower factor), XI (plasma thromboplastic antecedent), XII (Hageman factor), and XIII (fibrin-stabilizing factor). There is no factor VI. Inherited coagulation disorders usually involve only one factor, and it is convenient to segregate and discuss the heritable bleeding disorders according to the factors involved. Inherited abnormalities of factors I, II, V, VII, VIII, IX, X, XI, XII, and XIII have been identified.

There are no oral characteristics that serve to distinguish these disorders from one another. For the most part they share the feature of persistent, postextraction hemorrhage. The bleeding is usually of an oozing nature and may persist for several days. Oozing blood may dissect the fascial planes of the orofacial musculature and cause infraoral hematomas. This is especially true in pronounced cases of hemophilia. Physiological exfoliation of primary teeth is not associated with prolonged bleeding in these disorders, and spontaneous gingival hemorrhage is rare.

REFERENCES

1. Adams, E. B., and Witts, L. J.: Chronic agranulocytosis, Q. J. Med. **18:**173-185, 1949.
2. Aebi, H., Jeunet, F., Richterich, R., Suter, H., Butler, R., Frei, J., and Marti, H. R.: Observations in two Swiss families with acatalasia, Enzym. Biol. Clin. **2:**1-22, 1962.
3. Alexander, L. L., and Benninghoff, D. L.: Familial multiple myeloma, J. Natl. Med. Assoc. **57:**471-475, 1965.
4. Andrews, J. P., McClellan, J. T., and Scott, C. H.: Lethal congenital neutropenia with eosinophilia occurring in two siblings, Am. J. Med. **29:**358-362, 1960.
5. Asmal, A. C., Vinik, A. I., and Joubert, S. M.: A neurological disorder in porphyria cutanea tarda, S. Afr. Med. J. **44:**781-784, 1970.
6. Ata, M., Fisher, O. D., and Holman, C. A.: Inherited thrombocytopenia, Lancet **1:**119-123, 1965.
7. Balcerzak, S. P., Westerman, M. P., Lee, R. E., and Doyle, A. P.: Idiopathic hemochromatosis: a study of three families, Am. J. Med. **40:**857-873, 1966.
8. Becker, F. T., et al.: Recurrent oral and cutaneous infections associated with cyclic neutropenia, Arch. Dermatol. **80:**731-741, 1959.
9. Berger, H., and Goldberg, A.: Hereditary coproporphyria, Br. Med. J. **2:**85-88, 1955.
10. Beutler, E.: Drug-induced hemolytic anemia, Pharmacol. Rev. **21:**73-103, 1969.
11. Beveridge, B. R., Bannerman, R. M., Evanson, J. M., and Witts, L. J.: Hypochromic anaemia: a retrospective study and following of 378 inpatients, Q. J. Med. **34:**145-161, 1965.
12. Blackburn, E. K.: Primary capillary haemorrhage (including von Willebrand's disease), Br. J. Haematol. **7:**239-249, 1961.
13. Bloom, G. E., and Zarkowsky, H. S.: Heterogeneity of the enzyme defect in congenital methemoglobinemia, N. Engl. J. Med. **281:**919-922, 1970.
14. Blume, K. G., Busch, D., Hoffbauer, R. W., Arnold, H., and Lohr, G. W.: The polymorphism of nucleaside effect in pyruvate kinase deficiency, Humangenetik **9:**257-259, 1970.

15. Bolgert, M., and Cavinet, J.: Cutaneous porphyria in the adult, Br. J. Dermatol. 66:312-317, 1954.

16. Bothwell, T. H., Cohen, I., Abrahams, O. L., and Perold, S. M.: A familial study in idiopathic hemochromatosis, Am. J. Med. 27:730-738, 1959.

17. Bourne, M. S., Elves, M. W., and Israels, M. C. G.: Pyridoxine responsive anaemia, Br. J. Haematol. 11:1-10, 1965.

18. Bowman, H. S., and Procopio, F.: Hereditary non-spherocytic hemolytic anemia of the pryruvate-kinase deficient type, Ann. Intern. Med. 58:567-591, 1963.

19. Brewer, G. J.: A new inherited abnormality of human erythrocyte—elevated erythrocyte adenosine triphosphate, Biochem. Biophys. Res. Commun. 18:430-434, 1965.

20. Brown, A.: Pernicious anaemia: a clinical study of 78 cases, Glasgow Med. J. 27:313-344, 1946.

21. Brunetti, P., Neuci, G. G., Vaccaro, R., Pexeddu, A., and Migliorini, E.: Fanconi's anaemia, Lancet 2:1194-1195, 1966.

22. Buchanen, J., Frew, I. D. O., Gibson, I. I. J. M., Gibson, T., and Russell, A. R.: Macroglossia in myelomatosis, Br. J. Plast. Surg. 22:157-160, 1969.

23. Burgert, E. O., Jr., Kennedy, R. L. J., and Pease, G. L.: Congenital hypoplastic anemia, Pediatrics 13:218-226, 1954.

24. Caen, J. P., Castaldi, P. A., Leclerc, J. C., Inceman, S., Larriere, M. J., Probst, M., and Bernard, J.: Congenital bleeding disorders with long bleeding time and normal platelet count. I. Glanzmann's thrombasthenia (report of fifteen patients), Am. J. Med. 41:11-26, 1966.

25. Caffey, J.: Cooley's anemia—a review of the roentgenographic findings in the skeleton, Am. J. Roentgenol. 78:381-391, 1957.

26. Calman, H. I.: Multiple myeloma: report of a case first observed in the maxilla, Oral Surg. 5:1302-1311, 1952.

27. Carson, M. J., Chadwick, D. L., Brubaker, C. A., Cleland, R. S., and Lauding, B. H.: Thirteen boys with progressive septic granulomatosis, Pediatrics 35:405-412, 1965.

28. Cassileth, P. A., and Hyman, G. A.: Benign familial erythrocytosis: report of three cases and a review of the literature, Am. J. Med. Sci. 251:692-697, 1966.

29. Cathie, I. A. B.: Erythrogenesis imperfecta, Arch. Dis. Child. 25:313-324, 1950.

30. Cederbaum, S., Geywood, D., Aigner, R., and Motulsky, A.: Progressive chorea, dementia and acanthocytosis, a genocopy of Huntington's chorea, Clin. Res. 19:177, 1971.

31. Chalmers, J. N. M., and Lawler, S. D.: Data on linkage in man: elliptocytosis and blood groups. I. Families 1 and 2, Ann. Eugenics 17:267, 1952.

32. Chaudry, A. P., Sabes, W. R., and Gorlin, R. J.: Unusual oral manifestations of chronic lymphatic leukemia, Oral Surg. 15:446-449, 1962.

33. Cheraskin, E.: Diagnostic stomatology—a clinical pathological approach, New York, 1961, McGraw-Hill Book Co., pp. 155-156.

34. Critchley, E. M. R., Betts, J. J., Nicholson, J. T., and Weatherall, D. J.: Acanthocytosis, normolipoproteinaemia and multiple tics, Postgrad. Med. J. 46:698-701, 1970.

35. Cutting, H. O., McHugh, W. J., Conrad, F. G., and Marlow, A. A.: Autosomal dominant hemolytic anemia characterized by ovalocytosis: a family study of seven involved members, Am. J. Med. 39:21-34, 1965.

36. Darby, W. J.: The oral manifestations of iron deficiency, J.A.M.A. 130:830-835, 1946.

37. Davey, M. G., Lawrence, J. R., Lander, H., and Robson, H. N.: Familial erythrocytosis: a report of two cases, and a review, Acta Haematol. 39:65-74, 1968.

38. Dean, G.: The porphyrias: a story of inheritance and environment, Philadelphia, 1963, J. B. Lippincott Co.

39. Debre, R., Dreyfus, J. C., Frezal, J., Lasie, D., Lamy, M., Maroteaux, P., Schapira, F., and Schapira, G.: Genetics of haemochromatosis, Ann. Hum. Genet. 23:16-30, 1958.

40. deGruchy, G. C., Santamaria, J. N., Parsons, I. C., and Crawford, H.: Nonspherocytic congenital hemolytic anemia, Blood 16:1371-1397, 1960.

41. Diamond, L. K., Allen, D. W., and Magill, F. B.: Congenital (erythroid) hypoplastic anemia: a 25 year study, Am. J. Dis. Child. 102:403-415, 1951.

42. Douglas, S. D., Davis, W. C., and Fudenberg, H. H.: Granulocytopathies: pleomorphism of neutrophil dysfunction, Am. J. Med. 46:901-909, 1969.

43. Fanconi, G.: Familial constitutional panmyelocytopathy, Fanconi's anemia (F. A.). I. Clinical aspects, Semin. Hematol. 4:233-249, 1967.

44. Friedman, L. L., Bowie, E. J. W., Thompson, J. H., Jr., Brown, A. L., Jr., and Owen, C. A., Jr.: Familial Glanzmann's thrombasthenia, Mayo Clin. Proc. 39:908-918, 1964.

45. Garland, H. G., and Anning, S. T.: Hereditary hemorrhagic talangiectasia, Br. J. Dermatol. 62:289-310, 1950.

46. Girard, R., and Reval, L.: Frequency of

exposure to benzene in serious blood diseases, Nouv. Rev. Fr. Hematol. **10**:477-483, 1970.

47. Goldberg, A.: Acute intermittent porphyria: a study of 50 cases, Q. J. Med. **28**:183-209, 1959.

48. Goldberg, A., Rimington, C., and Lochhead, A. C.: Hereditary coproporphyria, Lancet **1**: 632-636, 1967.

49. Golding, J. S. R., MacIver, J. E., and Went, L. N.: The bone changes in sickle cell anaemia and its genetic variants, J. Bone Joint Surg. **41B**:711-716, 1959.

50. Gorlin, R. J., and Chaudhry, A. P.: The oral manifestations of cyclic (periodic) neutropenia, Arch. Dermatol. **82**:344-348, 1960.

51. Grimes, A. J., and deGrouchy, G. C.: Red cell metabolism: hereditary enzymopathies. In Hardisty, R. M., and Weatherall, D. J., editors: Blood and its disorders, Oxford, England, 1974, Blackwell Scientific Publications, Ltd., p. 511.

52. Hall, J. G., Levin, J., Kuhn, J. P., Ottenheimer, E. J., van Berkum, K. A. P., and McKusick, V. A.: Thrombocytopenia with absent radius (TAR), Medicine **48**:411-439, 1969.

53. Hamilton, H. B., Neel, J. V., Kobara, T. Y., and Ozaki, K.: The frequency in Japan of carriers of the rare "recessive" gene causing acatalasemia, J. Clin. Invest. **40**:2199-2208, 1961.

54. Hanel, H. K., Cohn, J. and Harvald, B.: Adenosine-triphosphatase deficiency in a family with non-spherocytic haemolytic anaemia, Hum. Hered. **21**:313-319, 1971.

55. Hardisty, R. M., and Weatherall, D. J., editors: Blood and its disorders, Oxford, England, 1974, Blackwell Scientific Publications, Ltd.

56. Harris, J. W., Whittington, R. M., Weisman, R., Jr., and Horrigan, D. L.: Pyridoxine responsive anemia in the human adult, Proc. Soc. Exp. Biol. **91**:427-432, 1956.

57. Heath, C. W., Jr., Bennett, J. M., Whang-Perg, J., Berry, E. W., and Wiernick, P. H.: Cytogenetic findings in erythroleukemia, Blood **33**:453-467, 1969.

58. Hunter, J. A. A., Khan, S. A., Hope, E., Beattie, A. D., Beveridge, G. W., Smith, A. W. M., and Goldberg, A.: Hereditary coproporphyria, Br. J. Dermatol. **84**:301-310, 1971.

59. Jacob, H. S.: Dysfunction of the red blood cell membrane in hereditary spherocytosis, Br. Haematol. **14**:99-104, 1968.

60. Jacob, H. S., and Jandl, J. H.: Increased

cell membrane permeability in the pathogenesis of hereditary spherocytosis, J. Clin. Invest. **43**:1704-1720, 1964.

61. Johnson, G. B., Jr., and Frey, W. G., III: Familial aspects of idiopathic hemochromatosis, J.A.M.A. **179**:747-751, 1962.

62. Johnson, R. B., and McMurry, J. S.: Chronic familial granulomatosis, Am. J. Dis. Child. **114**:370-378, 1967.

63. Katz, M., Lee, S. K., and Cooper, B. A.: Vitamin B(12) malabsorption due to biologically inert intrinsic factor, N. Engl. J. Med. **287**:425-429, 1972.

64. Kay, H. E. M., Lawler, S. D., and Millard, R. E.: The chromosomes in polycythaemia vera, Br. J. Haematol. **12**:507-527, 1966.

65. Keitt, A. S.: Pyruvate kinase deficiency and related disorders of red cell glycolysis, Am. J. Med. **41**:762-785, 1966.

66. Keitt, A. S.: Hemolytic anemia with impaired hexokinase activity, J. Clin. Invest. **48**:1997-2007, 1969.

67. Kirshbaum, J. D., and Preuss, F. S.: Leukemia: a clinical and pathologic study of one hundred and twenty-three fatal cases in a series of 14,400 necropsies, Arch. Intern. Med. **71**:777-792, 1943.

68. Kostman, R.: Infantile genetic agranulocytosis, Acta Paediatr. Scand. (Suppl. 105) **45**: 1-78, 1956.

69. Kritzler, R. A., Terner, J. Y., Linderbaum, J., Magidson, J., Williams, R., Praisig, R. and Phillips, G. B.: Chédiak-Higashi syndrome: cytologic and serum lipid observations in a case and family, Am. J. Med. **36**: 583-594, 1964.

70. Kushner, J. P., Lee, G. R., and Nacht, S.: The role of iron in the pathogenesis of porphyria cutanea tarda: an in vitro model, J. Clin. Invest. **51**:3044-3051, 1972.

71. Lambert, H. P., Prankerd, T. A. J., and Smellie, J. M.: Pernicious anemia in childhood: a report of two cases in one family and their relationships to the aetiology of pernicious anemia, Q. J. Med. **30**:71-90, 1961.

72. Lawrence, J. H., and Goetsch, A. T.: Familial occurrence of polycythemia and leukemia, Calif. Med. **73**:361-364, 1950.

73. Lohr, G. W., Waller, H. D., Anschutz, F., and Knopp, A.: Biochemische defekta in den Blutzellen bei familiaerer panmyelopathie (typ Fanconi), Humangenetik **1**:383-387, 1905.

74. Losowsky, M. S., and Hall, R.: Hereditary sideroblastic anaemia, Br. J. Haematol. **11**: 70-85, 1965.

75. Lynch, M. A., and Ship, I. I.: Oral mani-

festations of leukemia; a postdiagnostic study, J. Am. Dent. Assoc. **75:**932-940, 1967.

76. MacAlpine, I., Hunter, R., and Rimington, C.: Porphyria in the royal houses of Stuart, Hanover and Prussia: a follow-up study of George III's illness, Br. Med. J. **1:**7-17, 1968.

77. Magnus, I. A.: The cutaneous porphyrias, Semin. Haematol. **5:**380, 1968.

78. Magnus, I. A., Jarrett, A., Prankerd, T. A. J., and Rimington, C.: Erythropoietic porphyria: a new protoporphyria syndrome with solar urticaria due to protoporphyrinaemia, Lancet **2:**448-451, 1961.

79. McIntyre, O. R., Sullivan, L. L., Jefries, G. H., and Silver, R. H.: Pernicious anemia in childhood, N. Engl. J. Med. **272:**981-986, 1965.

80. McIntyre, P. A.: Genetic and auto-immune features of pernicious anemia. I. Unreliability of the Schilling test in detecting genetic predisposition to the disease, Johns Hopkins Med. J. **122:**181-183, 1968.

81. McIntyre, P. A., Hahn, R., Conley, C. L., and Glass, B.: Genetic factors in predisposition to pernicious anemia, Bull. Hopkins Hosp. **104:**309-342, 1959.

82. McKusick, V. A.: Mendelian inheritance in man, ed. 4, Baltimore, 1975, The Johns Hopkins University Press.

83. McPhedran, P., Heath, C. W., Jr., and Lee, J.: Patterns of familial leukemia: ten cases of leukemia in two interrelated families, Cancer **24:**403-407, 1969.

84. Meyer, V. A., Strand, L. J., Doss, M., Rees, A. L., and Marver, H. S.: Intermittent acute porphyria—demonstration of a genetic defect in porphobilinogen metabolism, N. Engl. J. Med. **286:**1277-1282, 1972.

85. Middlemiss, J. H., and Raper, A. B.: Skeletal changes in the haemoglobinopathies, J. Bone Joint Surg. **48B:**693-702, 1966.

86. Miller, D. R., Bloom, G. E., Streiff, R. R., LoBuglio, A. F., and Diamond, L. K.: Juvenile 'congenital' pernicious anemia: clinical and immunologic studies, N. Engl. J. Med. **275:**978-983, 1966.

87. Mittelman, G., Bakke, B. F., and Scopp, I. W.: Alveolar bone changes in sickle cell anemia, J. Periodontal. **32:**74-81, 1961.

88. Mohamed, S. D., McKay, E., and Galloway, W. H.: Juvenile familial megaloblastic anaemia due to selective malabsorption of vitamin B(12): a family study and a review of the literature, Q. J. Med. **35:**433-453, 1966.

89. Morris, A. L., and Stahl, S. S.: Intra-oral roentgenographic changes in sickle cell anemia, Oral Surg. **7:**787-791, 1954.

90. Nadeau, L. A., Magalini, S. I., and Stefanini, M.: Familial multiple myeloma, Arch. Pathol. **61:**101-106, 1956.

91. Nadler, S. B., and Cohn, I.: Familial polycythemia, Am. J. Med. Sci. **198:**41-48, 1939.

92. Nielsen, J. A., and Strunk, K. W.: Homozygous hereditary elliptocytosis as the cause of haemolytic anaemia in infancy, Scand. J. Haematol. **5:**486-496, 1968.

93. Oski, F. A., Naiman, J. L., Allen, D. M., and Diamond, L. K.: Leukocytic inclusions—Dohle bodies—associated with platelet abnormality (the May-Hegglin anomaly): report of a family and review of the literature, Blood **20:**657-667, 1962.

94. Owen, T.: A case of polycythemia vera with special reference to the familial features and treatment with phenyl-hydrazin, Bull. Johns Hopkins Hosp. **35:**258-262, 1924.

95. Pinkerton, P. H.: X-linked hypochromic anemia Lancet **1:**1106-1107, 1967.

96. Pollycove, M.: Hemochromatosis. In, Stanbury, J. B., Wyngaarden, J. B., and Fredrickson, D. S., editors: The metabolic basis of inherited disease, ed. 3, New York, 1972, McGraw-Hill Book Co., pp. 1051-1084.

97. Prowler, J. R., and Smith, E. W.: Dental bone changes occurring in sickle cell disease and abnormal hemoglobin traits, Radiology **65:**762-769, 1955.

98. Ridlay, A.: The neuropathy of acute intermittent porphyria, Q. J. Med. **38:**307-333, 1969.

99. Robertson, J. H.: Hereditary bleeding disorders in Western Australia, Aust. Ann. Med. **13:**143-148, 1964.

100. Robinson, I. B., and Sarnat, B. G.: Roentgen studies of the maxillae and mandible in sickle-cell anemia, Radiology **58:**517-522, 1952.

101. Robson, T., and Sweeney, P. J.: Chronic hypoplastic anaemia arising in infancy, Arch. Dis. Child. **23:**294-296, 1948.

102. Ruddles, R. W., and Falls, H. E.: Hereditary (sex-linked) anemia, Am. J. Med. Sci. **211:**641-658, 1946.

103. Schaar, F. E.: Familial idiopathic thrombocytopenia purpura, J. Pediatr. **62:**546-551, 1963.

104. Schmid, R., Schwartz, S., and Sundberg, R. D.: Erythropoietic (congenital) porphyria: a rare abnormality of the normoblasts, Blood **10:**416-428, 1955.

105. Schmid, R., Schwartz, S., and Watson, C. J.: Porphyrin content of bone marrow and liver in the various forms of porphyria, Arch. Intern. Med. **93:**167-190, 1954.

106. Sheramata, W., Kott, H. S., and Cyr, D. P.:

The Chediak-Higashi-Steinbrinck syndrome, Arch. Neurol. 25:289-294, 1971.

107. Spaet, T. H., and Dameshek, W.: Chronic hypoplastic anemia, Am. J. Med. 13:35-45, 1952.

108. Stewart, A. M.: Aetiology of childhood malignancies, Br. Med. J. 1:452-560, 1961.

109. Szeinberg, A., deVries, A., Pinkhas, J., Djaldetti, M., and Ezra, R.: A dual hereditary red blood cell defect in one family: hypocatalasemia and glucose-6-phosphate dehydrogenase deficiency, Acta Genet. Med. Gemellol. 12:247-255, 1963.

110. Takahara, S.: Progressive oral gangrene probably due to lack of catalase in the blood (acatalasemia), Lancet 2:1101-1106, 1952.

111. Takahara, S., Hamilton, H. B., Neel, J. V., Kobara, T. Y., Ogura, Y., and Nishimura, E. T.: Hypocatalasemia: a new genetic carrier state, J. Clin. Invest. 39:610-619, 1960.

112. Takahara, S., and Miyamoto, H.: Three cases of progressive oral gangrene due to lack of catalase in the blood, J. Otorhinolaryngol. Soc. Jap. 51:163, 1948.

113. Valentine, W. N., Oski, F. A., Paglia, D. E., Baughan, M. A., Schneider, A. S., and Naiman, J. L.: Hereditary hemolytic anemia with hexokinase deficiency, N. Engl. J. Med. 276:1-11, 1967.

114. Valentine, W. N., Tanaka, K. R., and Miwa, S.: A specific erythrocyte glycolytic enzyme defect (pyruvate kinase) in three subjects with congenital non-spherocytic hemolytic anemia, Trans. Assoc. Am. Physicians 74:100-110, 1961.

115. Verwilghen, R., Verhaegen, H., Waumans, P., and Beert, J.: Ineffective erythropoiesis with morphologically abnormal erythroblasts and unconjugated hyperbilirubinaemia, Br. J. Haematol. 17:27-33, 1969.

116. Vestermark, B., and Vestermark, S.: Familial sex-linked thrombocytopenia, Acta Pediatr. 53:365-370, 1964.

117. Waldenstrom, J.: The porphyrias as inborn errors of metabolism, Am. J. Med. 22:758-773, 1957.

118. Waldenstrom, J., and Haeger-Aronsen, B.: Different patterns of human porphyria, Br. Med. J. 2:272-276, 1963.

119. Waters, A. H., and Murphy, M. E. B.: Familial juvenile pernicious anaemia: a study of the hereditary basis of pernicious anaemia, Br. J. Haematol. 9:1-12, 1963.

120. Waugel, A. G., Callender, S. T., Spray, G. H., and Wright, R.: A family study of pernicious anaemia. II. Intrinsic factor secretion, vitamin B12 absorption and genetic aspects of gastric autoimmunity, Br. J. Haematol. 14:183-204, 1968.

121. West, C. A., Gomberts, B. D., Huehns, E. R., Kessel, I., and Ashby, J. R.: Demonstration of an enzyme variant in a case of congenital methaemoglobinaemia, Br. Med. J. 4:212-214, 1967.

122. Whitlock, R. I., and Hughes, N. C.: Solitary myeloma of mandible; report of a case, Oral Surg. 13:23-32, 1960.

123. Ziprkowski, L., Krakowski, A., Crispin, M., and Szeinberg, A.: Porphyria cutaneous tarda hereditaria, Isr. J. Med. Sci. 2:338-343, 1966.

124. Zueler, W. W., Robinson, A. R., and Hsu, T. H. J.: Erythrocyte pyruvate kinase deficiency in non-spherocytic hemolytic anemia: a system of multiple genetic markers? Blood 32:33-48, 1968.

125. Zurcher, C., Loos, J. A., and Prins, H. K.: Hereditary high ATP content of human erythrocytes, Folia Haematol. 83:366-376, 1965.

15

Oral and facial manifestations of cytogenetic anomalies

JAROSLAV CERVENKA

Some of the orofacial structures are known to be among the most sensitive indicators of the effect of specific (and nonspecific) teratogenic agents and environmental insults. Several chapters in this book demonstrate that malformations of the orofacial area also frequently result from the action of one mutant gene or polygenic system. However, one anatomically and embryologically well-defined aberration, for instance, cleft of the primary palate, could represent an effect of more than one etiological factor such as one mutant gene, polygenic system with a threshold, chemical teratogen, and chromosomal aberration.

In the following review it will be demonstrated that aberration of certain chromosomes manifests itself both in a specific way, affecting the development of particular facial structures, and in alteration of the phenotype, which could not be specifically attributed to the chromosome involved. For instance, cleft palate is one of the most common characteristics in the deletion of short arm of chromosome 4; on the other hand, aberration of almost any autosomal chromosome results in clefting of the palate with higher frequency than found in the general population. Deletion of a portion of DNA or extra chromosomal DNA would result in a general disturbance of developmental homeostasis as demonstrated clearly in Down's syndrome by Shapiro.[1]

HISTORICAL REMARKS

The history of human cytogenetics as a scientific field is surprisingly short. Only two decades ago the correct diploid number of human chromosomes was established to be forty-six in the publication of Tjio and Levan.[24] These authors also noted that a number of microphotographs published before their work were more in agreement with a diploid number of forty-six than forty-eight, and they credited the work by Hansen-Melander, Melander, and Kullander, which was not submitted for publication because their consistent finding of forty-six chromosomes disagreed with the "established" number of forty-eight in somatic cell. The same year the diploid number of forty-six was confirmed by Ford and Hamerton[9] by counting bivalents in human spermatocytes I.

The events of 1959 and 1960 stimulated many biologists to enter the field of human cytogenetics because of the discoveries of the first human chromosomal aberrations: trisomy 21 (Down's syndrome) by Lejeune and associates,[15] XXY (Klinefelter's syndrome) by Jacobs and Strong,[12] 45, X (Turner's syndrome) by Ford and co-workers,[10] 47, XXX syndrome by Jacobs and associates,[11] trisomy 13 by Patau and co-workers,[18] and trisomy 18 by Edwards and associates.[8]

In the following decade further chromosomal abnormalities were described. The human karyotype was classified by chromosomal morphology and size, by autoradiographical patterns, and by number of gross chromatid coils. Studies of meiotic chromosomes were expanded, and geneticists learned to obtain mitotic spreads from cells of several different tissues. Application of human cytogenetics in clinical diagnosis, genetic counseling, prenatal diagnosis, and infertility clinics was recognized, as well as application in numerous branches of biomedical research, such as cancer research, classification of established cell lines, and transplantation experiments. Electron microscopy of chromosomes brought new information about their structure, and the methods of cell hybridization provided essential basis for mapping of human chromosomes. Computerized chromosome analysis became established.

However, until 1969 almost all aspects of human cytogenetics suffered from the simple fact that cytogeneticists were not even able to reliably identify all chromosomes of the human complement.

Therefore, in 1968 and 1969, considerable excitement arose when Casperson and co-workers[3-5] discovered that fluorescent derivatives of quinacrine will stain chromosomes unevenly in such a fashion that parts of the chromosome will be brightly fluorescent and other parts will display dull fluorescence. This pattern appeared along the chromatid as bands of different width and different intensity of fluorescence—the so-called Q-bands (Fig. 15-1).

It has been demonstrated that this band-

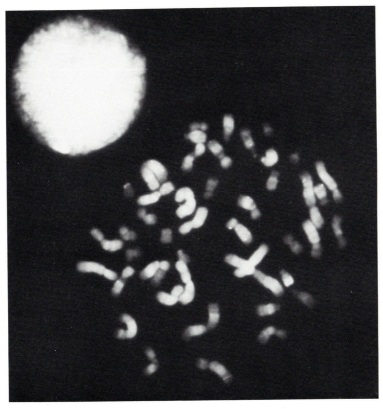

Fig. 15-1. Q-banding induced by quinacrine dihydrochloride staining and photographed under fluorescence microscope. Brightest structures are long arms of Y chromosome.

ing pattern is reproducible, consistent in chromosomes from cells of different tissues and different individuals, and characteristic for each one of the chromosomes of human complement. Thus by the method of fluorescent staining with quinacrine mustard or quinacrine dihydrochloride, all chromosomes have been identified; moreover, translocated parts and inverted, duplicated, and selected segments of sufficient length could be recognized. In a short period of time other important techniques were discovered to advance the knowledge of the human karyotype. Pardue and Gall,[17] Arrighi and Hsu,[2] and Yunis and associates[26] reported a procedure enhancing the staining of centromeric heterochromatin (C-bands) (Fig. 15-2), which became the basis for the development of the G-band, another banding technique. Specific treatment of the mitotic spreads with Giemsa stain resulted in darkly stained bands in approximately the same positions as fluorescent Q-bands. Additional techniques capable of

inducing G-bands have been reported using heat denaturation, proteolytic enzymes, and a variety of chemical agents[6, 20, 21, 23] (Fig. 15-3). The trypsin technique of Seabright[22] has been widely used, and reverse bands (R-bands) were introduced by Dutrillaux and Lejeune[7] (Fig. 15-4).

It appears certain that other avenues of cytogenetic research, such as the use of immunofluorescent studies of chromosome composition with antinucleotide antibodies[16] and the use of 5-bromodeoxyuridine (BrdU) incorporation, will provide us with important additional tools. The latter method yields a potential tool in analyzing chromosomal function and structure. It is based on the observation that BrdU is incorporated in the DNA of the chromatid biosynthetically in place of thymidine. When the bis-benzimidazole dye, such as 33258 Hoechst, is complexed with DNA, its fluorescence is partially quenched by the previously attached BrdU[14] and can be readily detected. If the cells are

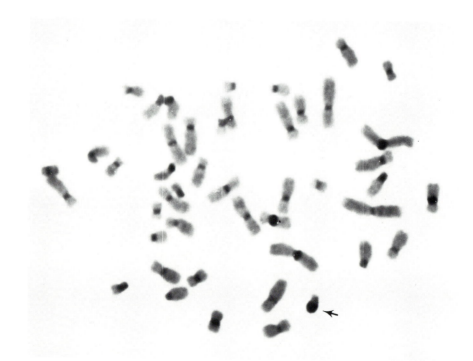

Fig. 15-2. C-banding induced by BaOH treatment and subsequent incubation in 2 × SSC. Centromeric heterochromatin and also highly repetitive DNA of Y chromosome, *arrow,* are demonstrated.

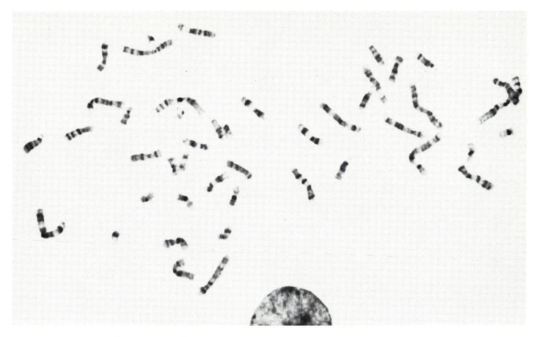

Fig. 15-3. G-banding induced by trypsin treatment. Staining by buffered Giemsa.

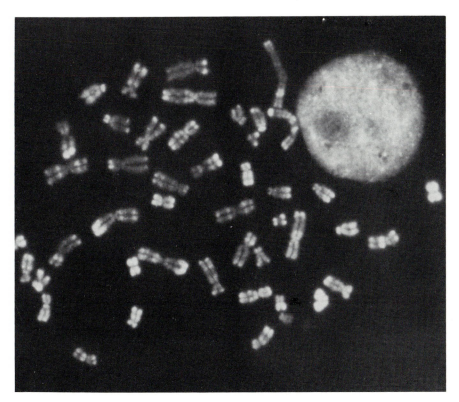

Fig. 15-4. R-banding induced by heating followed by acridine orange fluorescent stain. Chromosomal telomeres and bands reverse to G-bands are demonstrated.

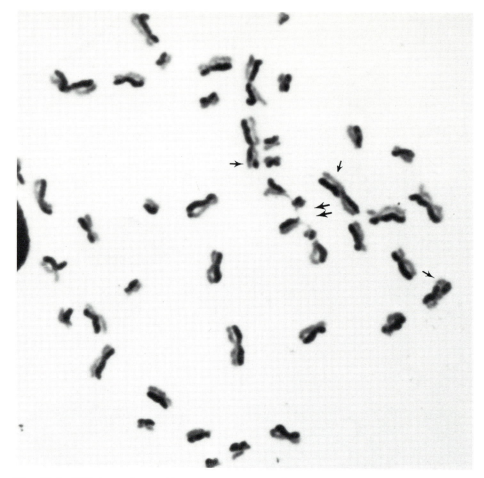

Fig. 15-5. SCE-sister chromatid exchanges, *arrows,* demonstrated by differential BrdU in-corporation and treatment of slides by heated buffer and Giemsa staining. Note satellite association of five acrocentric chromosomes, *double arrows.*

allowed to replicate in two cycles with BrdU, a lateral differentiation and exchanges between sister chromatids can be detected. Recent reports indicate that chromatid exchanges can be detected by treating the chromosomes from cells grown with BrdU by heating the slides in buffer or incubation in SSC and staining with Giemsa[13, 19, 25] (Fig. 15-5). It has been suggested that these methods provide potentially sensitive indication of chromosomal damage, since chromatid exchanges are much more frequent than gross chromatid breaks visible in metaphase chromosomes.

The most recent addition in the battery of techniques capable of differentiating classes of DNA is the method of silver staining–NOR staining (Fig. 15-6). By varying the solutions of silver nitrate and ammoniacal silver and staining conditions, it is possible to demonstrate ribosomal DNA–nucleolar organizing regions (NOR). An example of application in medical diagnosis and counseling is in patients with seemingly enlarged short arms of the D and G group chromosomes. In these cases the silver staining could reveal either harmless polymorphism of NOR or true translocation of transcriptional DNA.[10a, 10b]

The preceding paragraphs are a brief review of a few new concepts in human cytogenetics methodology, which are intended to

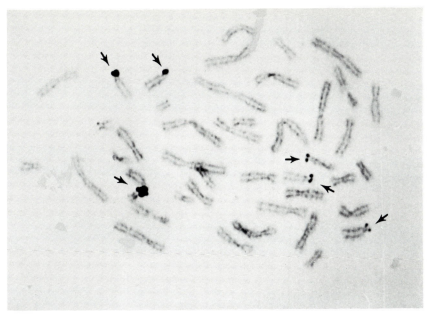

Fig. 15-6. Silver staining for nucleolus organizing regions. *Arrows,* Satellites of D and G group chromosomes.

illustrate that clinical application of cytogenetics has undergone great changes in the past 15 years. Today, not only trisomies, monosomies, and deletions and translocations are reported, but by the use of banding techniques, cytogeneticists are capable of detecting minute structural rearrangements of the chromosome and polymorphisms as well.

In the following review of orofacial expressions of chromosomal aberrations, I have chosen to review only those chromosomal syndromes which occur with a relatively high frequency, since these syndromes are most likely to be encountered in the clinic. In each instance, sufficient cases of each of the following aberrations have been described in the literature to compile meaningful clinical data.

Approximately 200 different chromosomal aberrations have been reported, and a number of texts elaborate on these in detail. In the phenotypic expression few common signs are noted, as well as few strictly specific traits for particular chromosomal defect. Thus great variability in phenotypes is probably the most common feature. This situation

forces clinicians to evaluate each patient on the basis of recognition of several characteristics, more so than on the basis of a single typical trait. The suspicion of a chromosomal defect in most cases stems from detecting a suggestive array of aberrations, including mental retardation. Only in rare examples is there one specific feature that leads clinicians to require analysis of chromosomes.

These points will hopefully be demonstrated in the following descriptions of syndromes.

TURNER'S SYNDROME

Turner's syndrome of monosomy (45,X) or partial monosomy of one of the X chromosomes, or numerous mozaicisms involving lines with 45,X constitution, is expressed as a female phenotype. It occurs in about 1 out of 5000 live births, and the frequency has been found to be extremely high in spontaneous abortions, where it has been demonstrated that about 25% of abortuses with chromosomal aberrations are due to 45,X chromosomal constitution. The most characteristic features are short stature (about 140 cm), primary amenorrhea due to streak gonads, sexual infantilism, broad, shieldlike chest with widely spaced nipples, cubitus valgus, webbing of the neck, lymphedema of extremities in newborns, occasionally coarctation of aorta, and renal anomalies. IQ is normal in the majority of patients (Fig. 15-7).

Neck

Pterygium coli, webbing of skin extending from mastoid processi to shoulders in adults

In newborns sometimes transverse folding of skin at back of the neck

Low posterior hairline recessing down into the middle of the neck

Eyes

Occasionally ptosis of upper eyelids

Epicanthi, cataracts, strabism, and corneal clouding

Ears

Protruding auricles

Sometimes longer and narrow pinna with hypoplastic helix and part of superior crus

Deafness occasionally

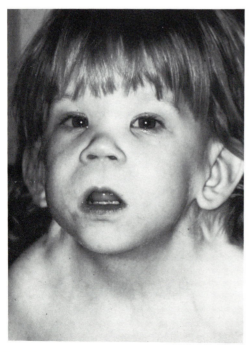

Fig. 15-7. 45,X Turner's syndrome. Note epicanthi, outstanding pinnae, and severe pterygia coli with descending hair on their ridges.

Oral cavity and jaws

Micrognathia

Crowded teeth and resulting orthodontic anomalies

Maxillary hypoplasia

Narrow, high palatal arch

Depressed mouth corners

POLY-X FEMALES

A female phenotype without severe malformations is compatible with an excess of X chromosomes. The most frequent of these conditions is triple-X female (47,XXX) or *trisomy X syndrome,* which occurs in about 1.2 per 1000 newborns and 0.73 per 1000 in the adult population. The phenotype is not characteristic: about 62% of the affected showed no abnormalities at all, and 73% have normal menstruation and breast development. Twenty-eight women of 101 surveyed by Barr and associates[29] bore sixty-seven children, most of whom were chromosomally normal. Intelligence quotients were measured in twelve XXX females by Barr and co-workers, and none exceeded an IQ of 71, the lowest value being 20. Ovarian dysfunction, sterility, and psychological and emotional disturbance of schizophreniclike expression and epilepsy were not infrequent. Delay of early motor and speech development was observed in a third of prepubertal patients by Tennes and associates.[30]

In the cases of XX/XXX mosaicism the defects occur less frequently; the number and severity of aberrations increase with the number of X chrosomes. Tetrasomies (XXXX) and pentasomies (XXXXX) are characterized by significant mental retardation as a rule.

Occasionally found abnormalities are as follows:

Eyes	**Neck**
Strabismus	Short
Hypertelorism	**Nose**
Epicanthal folds	Broad, flat
Corneal opacity	**Oral cavity and jaws**
Bilateral cataract	Relative prognathism
Nystagmus	Furrowed lips
Severe myopia	Cleft palate

KLINEFELTER'S SYNDROME

More frequent than Turner's syndrome, Klinefelter's syndrome occurs in about 1 out of 1000 liveborn infants. However, in institutions for mentally retarded the frequency is as high as 1%, which contrasts with the general finding of normal IQ in the majority of patients with Klinefelter's syndrome. Hypoplastic testes with tubular hyalinization resulting in sterility is the most constant feature. Pubertal hypogonadism associated with tall stature, gynecomastia, elevated urinary gonadotropins and low urinary 17-ketosteroids, sparse facial and axillary hair, and feminine distribution of pubic hair are frequent. In older patients crural venous stasis and crural ulcers are observed.

The typical chromosomal constitution in 80% of cases is 47,XXY (Fig. 15-8). However, great variability in number of X chromosomes and mosaicisms has been described. XXYY type of Klinefelter's syndrome is usually associated with more severe mental retardation and with a number of structural malformations that are inconsistent and vary from patient to patient (Figs. 15-9 and 15-10). Aggressiveness has been described frequently. Also, the general observation has been made that with increasing number of X chromosomes the phenotypic features of the syndrome are more severe. The 46,XX type of Klinefelter's syndrome is a rare form, associated with infertility and small testes but normal intelligence and rarely affected with structural malformations.

Skull and head
Sparse facial hair
Sometimes brachycephaly (more frequent in XXXXY)
Sometimes low nuchal hairline
In XXXXY short neck, microcephaly

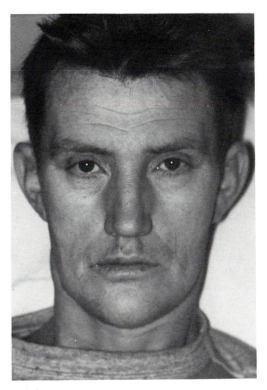

Fig. 15-8. 47,XXY Klinefelter's syndrome patient with aggressive behavior and terminal lung cancer. Only abnormal facial feature is moderate prognathism.

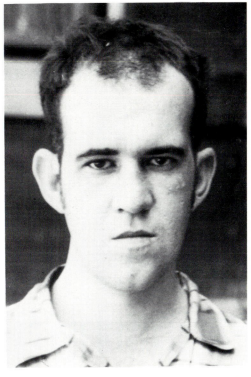

Fig. 15-9. 48,XXYY syndrome. Mentally retarded patient with prognathism and outstanding pinnae.

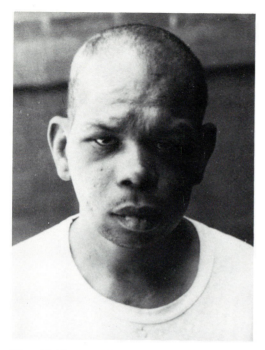

Fig. 15-10. 48,XXYY syndrome. Mentally retarded Negro patient with aggressive behavior, facial asymmetry, skeletal abnormalities, and partial indifference to pain.

Eyes
In XXXXY ocular hypertelorism (90%)
Myopia, strabismus, oblique palpebral fissures and epicanthi
Oral cavity and jaws
Mandibular prognathism in XXYY, which becomes more pronounced with increasing number of X chromosomes
15% cleft palate in XXXXY
Frequent taurodontism in XXXY and XXXXY

XYY SYNDROME

The frequency of the XYY syndrome in newborn males is about 1 in 700. However, the prevalence in penal institutions and maximum-security hospitals varies from about 1 in 10 to 1 in 200. This observation suggests psychosocial and behavioral problems with a tendency toward criminal involvement early in life. Some XYYs are of tall stature (well over 180 cm), have minor skeletal abnormalities, occasionally hypogonadism, and muscle weakness. Recent surveys and studies

indicate that a certain proportion of individuals with XYY chromosome constitution have normal behavioral patterns, intelligence, and social intercourse.

Fertility is usually unaffected, and, as a rule, children of XYYs have normal phenotypes and no chromosomal abnormality.

Abnormalities described only occasionally are as follows:

Skull and head
Mild facial asymmetry
Features of mandibulofacial dysostosis
No facial hair
Borrowing acne, neurodermatitis
Webbing of the neck
Face resembling leontiasis ossea
Eyes
Bilateral retinal detachment
Dislocated lens
Myopia
Mongoloid slanting
Strabismus
Epicanthi
Ears
Long pinnae
Prominent pinnae
One ear abnormally formed
Oral cavity and jaws
Prognathism
Glabellar mounding
Pronounced button on chin
High narrow palate
Cystic lesions in mandible
Larger mean tooth size in permanent dentition

4p–, WOLF-HIRSCHHORN SYNDROME

The Wolf-Hirschhorn syndrome occurs with lower frequency than another deletion of group B chromosomes, 5p– or cat's cry syndrome. Not more than thirty cases are described in the literature. Facial features are characteristic, and clinical diagnosis has been made frequently based on these features. The developmental impairment is generally more severe than in 5p–. Severe mental retardation with unmeasurable IQ, failure to thrive, hypotonia frequently combined with seizures, and heart defects are frequently observed. The average birth weight of 2000 gm is lower

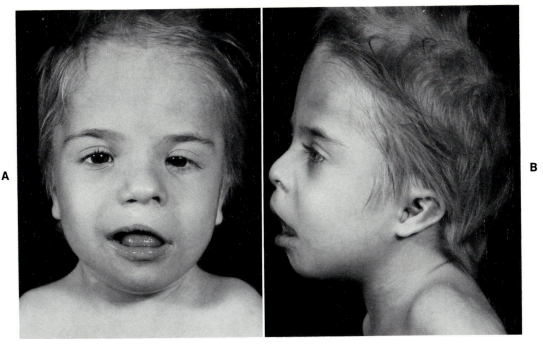

Fig. 15-11. 4p− (Wolf syndrome). **A,** Note ocular hypertelorism, convergent strabismus, repaired cleft lip, and mild facial asymmetry. **B,** Note abnormally formed pinna and low hairline. (Courtesy Dr. J. J. Yunis, University of Minnesota School of Medicine, Minneapolis, Minn.)

than that of any other chromosomal syndrome (Fig. 15-11).

Skull and head
Microcephaly is constant
Prominent glabella more than 50%
Hemangioma of the forehead
Midline scalp defects
Eyes
Marked ocular hypertelorism is constant
Strabismus in more than 50%
Ptosis of eyelids over 50%
Epicanthi
Iris coloboma
Exophthalmus
Antimongoloid slanting
Sclerocornea
Brushfield spots
Microphthalmia
Stenosis of lacrimal ducts
Nose
Beaky, broad, depressed nasal bridge
Ears
Simple formation of pinnae over 50%
Preauricular sinuses, pits

Oral cavity and jaws
Cleft palate in majority
Cleft lip less frequent
Down-turned, carplike mouth
Short, broad philtrum
Micrognathia

5p−, CRI DU CHAT SYNDROME

Cat's cry syndrome lacks typical facial features. Young patients have round faces, and older patients tend to have elongated, thin faces. Although newborns give the impression of hypertelorism, this feature becomes less obvious with increasing age.

A catlike, high-pitched, weak cry due to a hypoplastic pharynx is characteristic of almost all patients in early infancy. This cri du chat will become less pronounced and will disappear during the few months after birth. Severe psychomotor retardation with an IQ of 30 or less, low birth weight, and muscle hypotonia are fairly constant findings (Fig. 15-12).

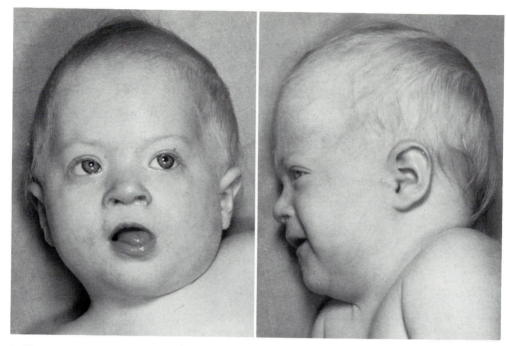

Fig. 15-12. Cri du chat syndrome. In addition to 5p−, this patient had 6q+. Hypertelorism and microcephaly are main craniofacial anomalies of this patient. (Courtesy Drs. R. C. Lewandowski and J. J. Yunis, University of Minnesota School of Medicine, Minneapolis, Minn.)

Skull and head
Microcephaly
Round facies, which later elongates
Asymmetric facies, occasionally
Premature graying of hair
Internal hydrocephalus, rarely
Short neck
Eyes
Hypertelorism, constantly
Epicanthi
Antimongoloid slanting
Strabismus, divergent
Optic atrophy, sometimes
Nose
Broad nasal bridge
Ears
Low set
Abnormalities in formation of pinna
External canals narrow, occasionally
Preauricular skin tags, occasionally
Oral cavity and jaws
Micrognathia, almost constant
Bifid uvula, cleft palate, rarely
Enlarged frontal sinuses

TRISOMY 8 SYNDROME

Trisomy 8 syndrome exists mostly (if not exclusively) in the form of mosaicism. Thirty-eight cases have been reported, which demonstrate a few consistently occurring anomalies, such as mental retardation of variable degrees, joint stiffness, vertebral anomalies, supernumerary ribs, slight muscular spasticity, long slender trunk and pelvis, and orofacial abnormalities. Deep palmar and plantar creases are pathognomonic for this syndrome (Fig. 15-13).

Skull and head
Asymmetries, almost constant
Prominent forehead, almost constant
Open mouth, occasionally
Eyes
Strabismus, about 50% cases
Nose
Abnormal shape occasionally
Ears
Low set in seventeen out of eighteen cases

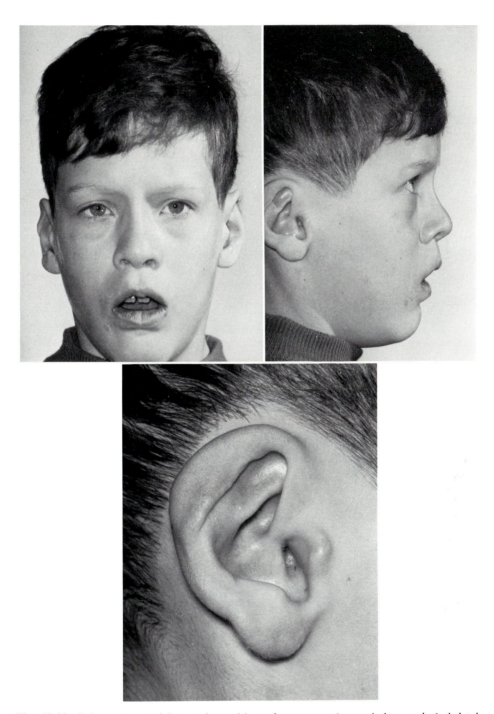

Fig. 15-13. Trisomy 8 mozaicism patient with moderate mental retardation, typical skeletal anomalies, and dermatoglyphics. Note abnormal formation of pinnae, asymmetry in central upper incisor position, and open bite.

Ears—cont'd

Malformed pinnae in twenty-six of twenty-eight cases

Oral cavity and jaws

Micrognathia, almost constant

High arched palate, almost constant

Cleft palate, five out of thirty-eight cases

TRISOMY 13, PATAU'S SYNDROME

The estimated frequency of trisomy 13 at birth is about 1 in 5000 or less; maternal age is elevated. This condition is probably the most severe chromosomal abnormality compatible with extrauterine life, which is fre-

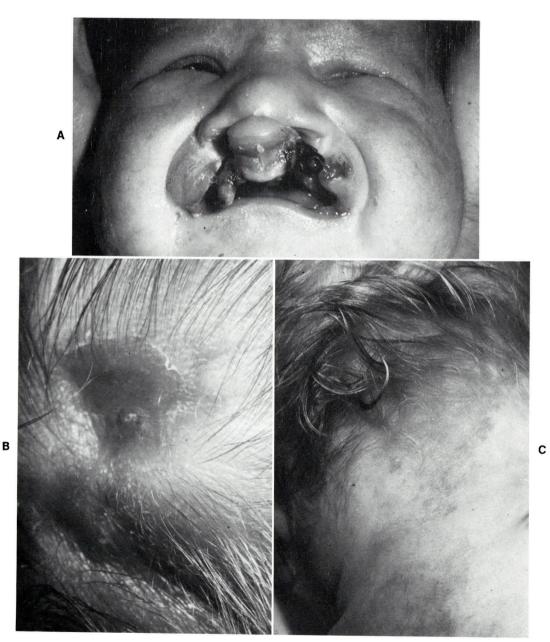

Fig. 15-14. Trisomy 13. Note bilateral cleft lip and palate, **A,** microphthalmus, scalp defect, **B,** and nuchal hemangioma, **C.**

quently of a short span. About half the new-borns with trisomy 13 will expire within several weeks after birth, and an estimated 70% will not survive to the sixth month of life. Severe psychomotor retardation, microcephaly, and a multitude of musculoskeletal malformations such as polydactyly, hyperconvex fingernails, overlapping fingers, and talipes equinovarus are consistent findings, as well as seizures, deafness, and heart defects. Diagnosis based on phenotype has frequently been possible despite the fact that over a hundred structural anomalies have been associated with the syndrome (Fig. 15-14).

Skull and head
Microcephaly, over 80%
Sloping forehead, cyclopia, ethmocephaly, cebocephaly associated with maldevelopment of the forebrain
Capillary hemangioma (mainly forehead and nuchal area)
Scalp defects (frequently midline or parieto-occipital)
Eyes
Microphthalmia (or anophthalmia unilaterally)
Hypertelorism (or hypotelorism)
Coloboma of iris
Retinal dysplasia
Epicanthal folds
Absent eyebrows
Shallow supraorbital ridges
Ears
Low set
Malformed pinna
Oral cavity and jaws
Micrognathia, 90%
Cleft lip and/or palate (up to 80%)
Occasionally cleft with agenesis of premaxilla
Narrow palate
Cleft tongue

13q– SYNDROME

A rare syndrome of deletion of long arms of chromosome 13 is characterized by low birth weight, microcephaly, micrognathia, general psychomotor retardation, undescended testes, hypospadias, imperforate anus, and wide nasal bridge. Facial asymmetry, pelvic anomalies, and webbing of the neck were described in more than half of the patients. An important feature is retinoblastoma occurring in 25% of patients.

The syndrome of 13q– has many common features with an even rarer 13 ring anomaly. Mosaicism with less pronounced malformations has been reported.

Head and skull
Microcephaly
Facial asymmetry
Trigonocephaly
Short, webbed neck
Eyes
Epicanthal folds
Hypertelorism
Ptosis
Microphthalmus
Coloboma of iris
Retinoblastoma
Glaucoma
Cataracts
Ears
Large pinna, malrotated and low set
Oral cavity and jaws
Micrognathia
Protruding upper incisors

TRISOMY 18, EDWARD'S SYNDROME

Trisomy 18, a severe anomaly, occurs with a frequency of 1 per 3000 to 1 per 6000 newborns. Over a hundred anomalies have been described as associated with this syndrome, which accounts for a high degree of variability in phenotypes. Many of these features overlap with trisomy 13, creating some confusion. However, several malformations are fairly constant (80% of patients) and characteristic, including hypertonia (preceded by neonatal hypotonia), prominent occiput, short sternum, micrognathia, small mouth, and limited hip abduction. Other important signs are failure to thrive, congenital heart defects, mainly ventricular septal defect, horseshoe kidney, rocker-bottom feet, cryptorchidism, overlapping fingers with flexion deformities, talipes equinovarus, short neck, and hernias. Females are more frequently affected than males in a ratio of 2 to 1 (Fig. 15-15).

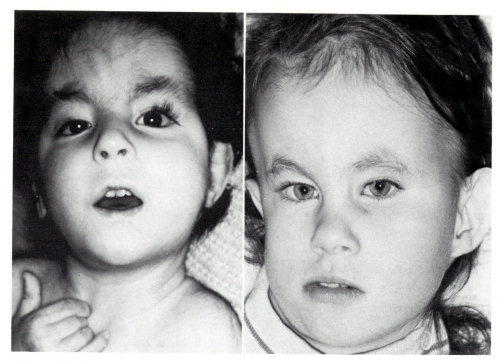

Fig. 15-15. Trisomy 18. Facial hirsutism, abnormal pinnae formation, frontal bossing, and facial asymmetry. (*Left,* courtesy Dr. M. M. Cohen, Jr., University of Washington, Seattle, Wash.)

Skull and head
Prominent occiput, constant
Microcephaly with bifrontal narrowing, 40%
Wide, open fontanels
Shallow orbital ridges
Mild hirsutism of forehead
Hypoplasia of orbital ridges
Wormian cranial bones, occasionally
Shallow, elongated sella, occasionally
Eyes
Strabismus
Short palpebral fissures, slanted
Ptosis of eyelids
Epicanthi
Hypertelorism
Colobomata iris
Corneal opacity
Microphthalmos
Cataracts, occasionally
Anisocornea, occasionally
Ears
Low set, constant
Malformed pinna, constant
Partial deafness

Oral cavity and jaws
Micrognathia, constant
Short upper lip
Small oral opening
Narrow palate
Cleft lip and/or palate in 15%
Choanal atresia
Weak, high-pitched cry

18p– SYNDROME

Although there is no characteristic clinical picture associated with the deletion of short arms of chromosome 18, several phenotypic signs are frequently observed, many of which are common to many other chromosomal observations. Mental retardation is constant but varies from severe to an IQ around 80. Other common features are low birth weight, small stature, short fingers, and webbing between the second and third toes. Characteristically, several signs of Turner's syndrome have been described, such as short stature, wide chest with laterally placed nipples,

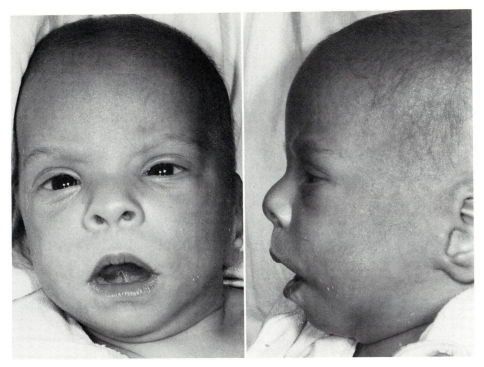

Fig. 15-16. 18p– syndrome. Note well-shaped ears, short nose with anteverted nostrils, carp-shaped mouth, no columella of upper lip, and micrognathia.

pterygium coli, and lymphedema of hands and feet at birth. Various degrees of holoprosencephaly have occasionally been observed. (See Fig. 15-16.)

Skull and head
Microcephaly
Cebocephaly occasionally
Arhinencephaly and cyclopia
Congenital alopecia

Neck
Webbing and lymphedema at birth

Eyes
Hypertelorism
Epicanthi
Ptosis of eyelids
Strabismus
Cataracts

Nose
Flattened, broad bridge

Ears
Large, low set
Poorly formed auricle

Oral cavity
Cleft lip and palate reported

Teeth, jaws
Micrognathia
Severe dental caries

18q– SYNDROME

Deletion of the long arms of chromosome 18 is characterized by typical facial dysmorphia in contrast to 18p– syndrome. Birth weight is usually below 2700 gm, and marked hypotonia is present at birth. Frequent seizures, congenital heart defects, renal anomalies, and hypoplastic genitalia occur in more than half the patients. Fingers are long, and skin dimples are observed over the knuckles as well as in subacromian and epitrochlear areas. Mental retardation has been profound in all reported cases. The phenotype is generally similar to that of the 18 ring anomaly.

Skull and head
Characteristic midfacial hypoplasia so the
  forehead and mandible relatively protrude
Mild microcephaly nearly constant
Cebocephaly was reported

Eyes

Nystagmus, constant
Deeply set
Strabismus
Optic atrophy
Tapetoretinal degeneration
Glaucoma
Hypertelorism
Epicanthi

Ears

Atresia of ear canals in over 50%
Helix well shaped but antihelix and anti-
    tragus prominent
Deep scaphoid fossae
Conductive deafness

Nose

Short but well formed
Nasal alae have triangular implantation

Oral cavity and jaws

Upper lip without columella, constant
Carp shaped in 75%
High-arched, narrow palate
Cleft lip and palate occasionally
Relative prognathism
Voice husky, broken, raw

18r– SYNDROME

Since the ring chromosome formation involves different portions of short and long
arms in different patients, the phenotypic
expression of the anomaly varies more than
do the simple 18p– or 18q– syndromes. Also,
18r– frequently exhibits features of both
18p– and 18q– syndromes.

Birth weight is low, and mental retardation, hypotonia, and microcephaly are almost
constant. Heart anomalies were reported in
about half the patients.

Skull and head

Microcephaly
Midface hypoplasia, not always observed
Pterygium coli
Low hairline

Eyes

Hypertelorism
Epicanthi
Strabismus
Antimongoloid slanting
Nystagmus
Chorioretinal atrophy

Ears

Stenosis of ear canals
Low-set pinnae, not malformed

Oral cavity and jaws

Carp-shaped mouth—most frequent
High-arched, narrow palate
Hypoplasia of enamel

TRISOMY 21, DOWN'S SYNDROME

Sometimes improperly referred to as mongoloid idiocy or mongolism, this syndrome is
the most common chromosomal abnormality
in man. The frequency is estimated to be
one per 650 live births, affecting both sexes
at about the same rate. Most of the Down's
syndrome patients have trisomy of chromosome 21 (94%), and about 3% are due to
translocation of chromosome 21 to another
chromosome of G group or D group. The
rest of the cases (3%) are the result of
chromosomal mosaicism.

The phenotype of Down's syndrome is
characteristic, although sometimes less obvious in early infancy or old age. The most
common traits are general hypotonia with
loose, hyperflexible joints; mental retardation
is always present, and pelvic bones are hypoplastic with flaring of iliac wings and shallow
acetabular angle. Characteristic are short
fingers and metacarpals, typical dermatoglyphic abnormalities with simian crease,

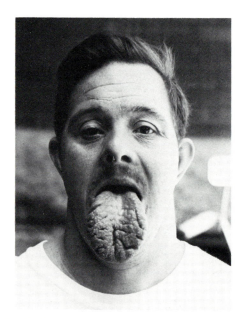

Fig. 15-17. Down's syndrome. Note marked macroglossia and fissuration of tongue.

distal placement of palmar axial triradius and frequent ulnar loops, wide space between first and second toes, excess of skin in the nuchal area, frequent cardiac abnormalities, and absent Moro's reflex. Certain minor abnormalities that occur in Down's syndrome are seen in the general population with a much lower frequency (for example, epicanthal folds, transverse palmar crease) (Figs. 15-17 to 15-19).

Skull and head

Flat profile, flat occiput, 90%
Brachycephaly, 75%
Microcephaly

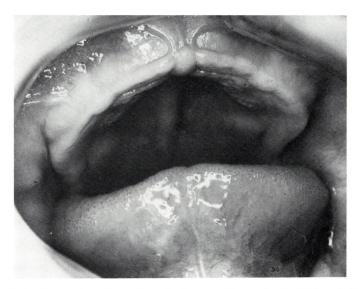

Fig. 15-18. Delayed eruption of maxillary incisors in 14-month-old child with Down's syndrome. (From Cohen, M. M., Jr., and Cohen, M. M., Sr.: Birth Defects **7:**241, 1971.)

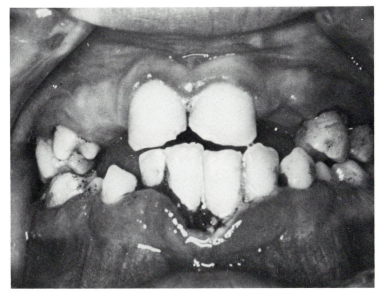

Fig. 15-19. Severe periodontal disease with necrotizing regions in 10-year-old patient with Down's syndrome. (From Cohen, M. M., Jr., and Cohen, M. M., Sr.: Birth Defects **7:**241, 1971.)

Skull and head—cont'd
Large fontanels, delayed closure
Open metopic suture past 10 years of age
Neck
Short and broad, 50%
Excess skin in nuchal area in newborn
Eyes
Oblique palpebral fissures, 80%
Epicanthi, 50%
Brushfield spots (speckled iris), 50%
Hypertelorism
Blepharitis
Convergent strabismus and nystagmus
Nose
Hypoplastic nasal bones causing depressed
    nasal bridge
Sometimes anteverted nostrils
Ears
Small earlobe, 50%
Prominent antihelix
Oral cavity and jaws
Open mouth, 70%
Narrow, markedly short palate with shelflike
    alveolar processes, 70%
Furrowed tongue, macroglossia, 50%
Broad, dry lips
Absence of frontal and sphenoid sinuses
Hypoplastic maxillary sinuses
Relative prognathism and other occlusal ab-
    normalities

Oral cavity and jaws—cont'd
Cleft lip and/or palate in 0.5%
Teeth
Delayed eruption in both dentitions
Hypodontia
Morphological abnormalities, mainly of upper
    lateral incisors
Periodontal disease frequent
Relatively low caries rate despite neglected
    oral hygiene

TRISOMY 22

Many reports have been published describing patients with a trisomy of small acrocentric chromosome of G group morphology but who do not have signs of Down's syndrome. Only recently, with the advent of banding techniques, has it been possible to recognize whether the supernumerary chromosome was actually no. 22 or just a centric fragment derived from some other than a G group chromosome.

Two syndromes of characteristic malformations appear to emerge: cat's eye syndrome or partial trisomy for long arms of chromosome 22 (22q+) and true trisomy 22.

Cat's eye syndrome (22q+) is characterized by congenital heart anomalies, genitourinary

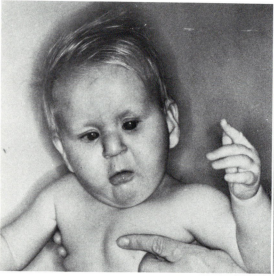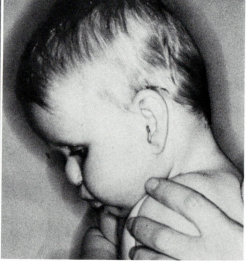

Fig. 15-20. Patient with trisomy 22. Convergent strabismus, depressed nasal bridge, and cleft of soft palate. (From Hsu, L. Y. F., Shapiro, L. R., Gertner, M., Lieber, E., and Hirschhorn, K.: J. Pediatr. **79:**12-19, 1971.)

anomalies, severe mental retardation, failure to thrive, and anal atresia.

Of the orofacial features the most striking are hypertelorism, typical iris colobomas resulting in cat's eye appearance, antimongoloid slanting of palpebral fissures, abnormally formed pinnae with preauricular skin appendages, or blind fistulas.

Considerable variability of the phenotype has been reported.

Trisomy 22 carries all the cat's eye syndrome characteristics in addition to severe hypotonia, low-placed nipples, cleft palate, microcephaly, and micrognathia. Iris coloboma has been reported in only one case of trisomy 22.

About thirty patients have been reported with these two syndromes. Authors suggest that the syndrome is compatible with a life span at least to the pubertal age. There is marked predilection for females to be affected (3:1) (Fig. 15-20).

TRIPLOIDY SYNDROME

It has been estimated that almost 20% of all chromosomal aberrations in human abortuses are triploidies, that is, they possess sixty-nine chromsomes (3n). However, in liveborn children this anomaly is exceedingly rare. Only about ten cases with true triploidy (3n) have been reported, and there have been over a dozen cases with triploid/diploid mosaicism. In these mixoploidies the lymphocytes contain primarily normal diploid karyotypes, and skin fibroblasts express the triploid chromosomal constitution.

In the true triploidy syndrome the most characteristic signs are hypospadias in boys and renal anomalies with sclerosis and hyalinization of glomeruli. Mental and physical retardation is a consistent finding.

In the cases of mosaicism, craniofacial asymmetry and delayed ossification are frequently described, as well as cleft palate, hydrocephalus, syndactyly, cryptorchidism, bifid scrotum, and, in one case, holoprosencephaly.

Orofacial malformations found both in the pure 3n and in 2n/3n mosaicism are as follows:

Head and skull
Asymmetric skull
Facial hemiatrophy
Holoprosencephaly
Hydrocephalus
Microcephaly
Eyes
Coloboma iris, most constant
Coloboma of optical papilla
Microcornea (6 × 8 mm)
Microphthalmus
Lens cataract
Mild hypertelorism
Epicanthi
Heterochromia iridis
Ears
Low set
Oral cavity and jaws
Cleft palate
Micrognathia

OTHER NEW CHROMOSOMAL SYNDROMES

The expanded potential of clinical cytogenetics brought about by banding techniques has resulted in elucidation of a large number of new chromosomal aberrations. The ability to identify all chromosomes or small segments of their arms has made possible the detection of discrete deletions, translocations, and inversions.

At present, clinical material is being evaluated in several laboratories to establish consistent pheontypic features resulting from rearrangements of particular segments of the genome. Borgankoar's catalog[70] and the article by Lewandowski and Yunis[71] include large numbers of new phenotypes, and interested readers are referred to these.

To enable an orientation in some of the important phenotypic anomalies and their association with corresponding chromosomal defects, the following list will summarize findings of Lewandowski and Yunis*:

Retardation
    Growth: 4p+, 4p–, 5p–, 9+, 10q+, 13+, 13q–, 13(q31-q32)–, 13(q32-q34)–, 14+, 18+, 18p–, 18q–, 21+, 21q–, 22+

Mental: 4p+, 4q+, 5q–, 7q+, 8+, 8q+, 9p+, 9p–, 10q⊤, 11p+, 11q+, 13+, 13q–, 13(q31-q32)–, 13(q32-q34)–, 14q+, 15q+, 18+, 18p–, 18q–, 21+, 21q–, 22q–, 22+

Psychomotor: 4p–, 4p+, 5p–, 10q+, 13+, 13q+^{d}, 13q+^{p}, 13(q21)–, 15q+, 18+, 18q–, 21+, 21q–, 22+, 22q+ (The symbol "13q+^{d}" represents partial trisomy for the distal portion of the long arm of chromosome 13. The symbol "13q+^{p}" represents partial trisomy for the proximal portion of the long arm of chromosome 13.)

Muscle tone

Hypertonia: 9p–, 18+, 21q–

Hypotonia: 4q+, 4p–, 5p–, 11p+, 15q+, 18q–, 21+, 22+, 22q–

Skull

Asymmetry: 4p–, 8+

Brachycephaly: 9p+, 21+

Fontanel closure, early: 4q+

Fontanel closure, late: 13+, 18+, 21+

Fontanel, wide: 7q+, 13+, 21+

Metopic suture: 21+

Microcephaly: 4p+, 4p–, 5p–, 9+, 9p+, 10q+, 13+, 13q–, 13q+^{d}, 13(q31-q32)–, 13(q32-q34)–, 14q+, 18q–, 21q–, 22+

Occiput, flattened: 21+

Occiput, prominent: 15q+, 18+

Sagittal sutures, wide: 13+

Sinuses, absent or hypoplastic: 21+

Trigonocephaly: 9p–, 13(q31-q32)–

Forehead

Flat: 9p+, 13q+^{d}, 15q+, 21+

Narrow: 13+, 13q+^{d}, 15q+

Prominent: 7q+, 8+, 9p–, 11p+, 13p+^{d}, 13(q32-q34)–

Sloping: 13+

Spacious: 10q+

Face

Flat and round: 5p–, 10q+, 15q+, 21+

Round: 5p–

Flat and depressed midface: 18q–

Fine and pointed midface features: 18+

Midface: midbrain septal defect: 13+, 13q+^{p}, 13q–, 18p–

Eyes

Antimongoloid: 4p+, 4p–, 5p–fi 10q+, 11p+, 15q+, 21q–, 22+, 22q+

Brushfield spots: 21+

Coloboma: 4p–, 13+, 13q–, 13q+^{p}, 22+, 22q+

Enophthalmos: 9p+, 11p+, 15q+, 18q–

Epicanthus: 4p–, 5p–, 13+, 13q–, 18p–, 21+, 22q–

Eyebrows, arched and widespread: 10q+

Eyelashes, long and incurved: 13q+^{d}

Glaucoma: 18q–

Hypertelorism: 4p+, 4p–, 5p–, 7q+, 9p+, 9p–, 13(q32-q34)–, 18p–, 22+, 22q+

Hypotelorism: 13+, 13q+, 13q–, 18p–, 21+

Lens opacity: 15q+, 21+

Microphthalmia: 4p–, 10q+, 13+, 13q–, 13q+^{p}, 14q+

Mongoloid: 9p–, 15q+, 21+

Nystagmus: 11p+, 18q–, 21+

Palpebral fissures, small: 7q+, 9+, 10q+, 18+

Palpebral fissures, horizontal: 15q+

Ptosis: 4p–, 10q+, 18p–, 22q–

Retinal dysplasia: 13+

Retinoblastoma: 13q–, 13(q21)–

Strabismus: 4p–, 5p–, 8+, 11p+, 13q+^{d}, 15q+, 18+, 18p–, 18q–, 21+

Nose

Peaked: 1q+, 4p–

Broad: 5p–, 9p–, 11q+, 22q–

Glabella, prominent: 4p–, 4p+

Nasal bridge, broad: 4p+, 4p–, 5p–, 9p–, 13q–, 21q–

Nasal bridge, depressed: 10q+, 18q–, 21+

Nasal bridge, flat: 9p–, 14q+, 18p–, 22q–

Nostrils, anteverted: 9p–

Nostrils, inverted: 9p+

Prominent: 4p+, 9+, 9p+, 21q–

Round: 4p+

Small: 7q+, 10q+, 18+, 21+

Mouth

Bow-shaped: 10q+

Dentition, abnormal: 4p+, 5p–, 13q+^{d}, 13(q32-q34)–, 15q+, 21+

Down-turned: 4p–, 9p+, 15q+, 18q–

Incisors, forward-slanting superior: 13q–, 13(q32-q34)–

Lip, lower, everted: 9p+, 15q+

Lip, lower, retracted: 11q+

Lip, upper, cleft: 4p–, 8+, 11p+, 13+, 18+, 18q–

Lip, upper, long: 9p–

Lip, upper, prominent: 10q+

Lip, upper, short: 4p–, 9p+, 15q+

Open mouth: 21+

Palate, cleft: 4p–, 7q+, 10q+, 11p+, 13+, 13q+^{p}, 14q+, 18+, 18q–, 21q–, 22+

Palate, high-arched: 8+, 9+, 10q+, 11p+, 13q+^{d}, 14q+, 21q–, 22q–

Philtrum, long: 9p–, 10q+

Philtrum, short: 4p–, 5p–

Tongue, furrowed: 21+

Tongue, large: 4p+, 7q+, 21+

Uvula, bifid: 13p–, 13(p21)–, 22q–

Jaw
  Micrognathia: 1q+, 4p–, 5p–, 7q+, 8+, 10q+, 11q+, 13+, 14q+, 18+, 18p–, 21q–, 22+
  Prominent: 4p+
Ears
  Deformed: 4p–, 4p+, 5p–, 7q+, 8+, 9+, 9p+, 9p–, 10q+, 13+, 13q+ᵈ, 13q–, 13(q32-q34)–, 14q+, 15q+, 18+, 18p–, 18q–, 21+, 21q–, 22+, 22q+
  Dimples or tags, preauricular: 4p–, 5p–, 22+, 22q+
  External canal, large: 21q–
  External canal narrow: 4p–, 18q–
  Large: 9+, 13q–, 13(q32-q34)–, 18p–, 21q–, 22+ 22q–
  Low-set: 4p–, 4p+, 5p–, 7q+, 8+, 9+, 10q+, 13+, 13q+ᵈ, 13q+ᵖ, 14q+, 15q+, 18+, 18p–, 21q–, 22+, 22q–
Neck
  Pterygium colli: 18p–, 21+
  Short: 8+, 9p+, 9p–, 10q+, 11q+, 13+, 13q–, 14q+, 15q+, 18+, 21+
Hands
  Broad: 21+
  Camptodactyly: 4p+, 8+, 10q+, 13+, 18+
  Fingers, broad: 11p+
  Fingers, long and flexed: 9+
  Fingers, long and tapering: 1q+, 18q–
  Fingers, incurved fifth: 13q+ᵖ, 13(q21)–, 21+, 22q–
  Fingers, overlapping: 10q+, 13+, 18+
  Fingers, short fifth: 8+, 15q+, 21+
  Lymphedema: 18p–
  Phalanges, hypoplastic: 8+, 9p+, 13q–, 13(q31-q32)–, 21+
  Polydactyly: 13+, 13q+ᵈ
  Short: 21+
  Syndactyly: 5p–, 22q–
  Thumbs, absent: 13q–, 13(q31-q32)–
  Thumbs, distally implanted: 18+
  Thumbs, proximally implanted: 10q+, 18q–
Feet
  Calcaneus, prominent: 13+, 18+
  Lymphedema: 18p–
  Metatarsals, delayed ossification: 4p–
  Polydactyly: 13+, 13q+ᵈ
  Rocker-bottom feet: 13+, 18+
  Short: 15q+
  Syndactyly: 10q+, 22q–
  Toes, broad: 11p+
  Toes, proximally implanted: 10q+
  Toes, wide spaces between: 10q+, 21+
Skeleton
  Articular movement, restricted: 8+, 8q+, 11q+, 15q+, 18+

Calcaneovalgus deformity: 18+, 18q–
Calcaneus, prominent: 13+, 18+
Carpal bones, delayed ossification: 4p–
Joints, hyperextensible: 15q+, 21+, 22+
Larynx hypoplasia: 5p–
Lordosis: 14q+
Hips, dislocated: 7q+, 9+, 13q–, 18+
Metacarpals, hypoplasia of first: 13q–, 13(q31-q32)–, 18q–
Metacarpals, fusion of fourth and fifth: 13q–, 13(q31-q32)–
Patella, absent: 8+
Pelvis, abnormal: 4p+, 5p–, 13+, 13q–, 18+, 21+
Pelvis, delayed ossification: 4p–
Pelvis, slender: 8+
Pes cavus: 5p–, 7q+
Ribs, abnormal: 4p+, 7q+, 8+, 8q+, 10q+, 13+, 14q+, 18q–
Sternum, short: 18+
Vertebrae, abnormal: 4p+, 5p–, 7q+, 8+, 8q+, 10q+, 13q–
Trunk
  Anal atresia: 13q–, 22+, 22q+
  Hernias: 13+, 13q+ᵈ, 18+, 21+, 21q–
  Long and slender: 8+
  Nipples, low-set: 22+
  Nipples, wide-spaced: 4p+, 18p–, 18q–
Congenital heart disease
  1q+, 4p–, 5p–, 8+, 9+, 9p–, 10q+, 11q+, 13+, 13q–, 14q+, 18+, 18q–, 21+, 22+, 22q+
Genitalia
  Ambiguous: 4q+, 4p–, 21q–
  Cryptorchidism: 4p–, 4q+, 9+, 13+, 13q–, 14q+, 15q+, 18+, 18q–, 21+, 21q–
  Hypoplastic: 18q–
  Hypospadias: 4p–, 13q–, 21q–
  Labia majora, hypoplastic: 18+, 18q–
  Ovaries, streak or hypoplastic: 4p–, 13+
  Penis, small: 9+, 15q+, 18q–, 21+
  Uterus, absent: 4p–
  Uterus, bicornuate: 13+
  Genitourinary anomalies: 4q+, 10q+, 13q–, 18+, 18q–, 22+, 22q+
Skin
  Deep furrows: 8+, 10q+
  Dimples: 4p–, 18q–
  Fingernails, hyperconvex: 4p–, 13+
  Fuzzy hair: 7q+
  Hair, premature graying: 5p–
  Hemangioma: 4p–, 13+, 13q–, 13q+ᵈ
  Nail hypoplasia: 8+, 9p+, 13+, 18+, 21q–
  Scalp defects: 4p–, 13+
Dermatoglyphics
  Arches, excess: 4p–, 18+

Flexion crease, single fifth finger: 18+, 21+

Loops, decreased ulnar: 5p–, 22q–

Loops, excess radial: 21q–

Loops, excess ulnar: 10q+, 15q+, 21+

Palmar crease, transverse: 4p–, 5p–, 7q+, 9p+, 10q+, 13+, 13q+[p], 18+, 18q–, 21+

Radial loops, thumb: 18+

Ridges, hypoplastic dermal: 4p–, 11q+, 18+

Triradius, absence of b or c: 9p+

Triradius, t' axial: 4p+, 5p–, 13+, 18+, 18q–, 21+, 21q–

Whorls, decreased: 9p+

Whorls, excess: 4p+, 5p–, 9p–, 18q–, 22q–

Miscellaneous

Birth weight, low: 4p–, 4q+, 5p–, 7q+, 11q+, 13+, 18+, 18p–, 18q–, 21q–

Hemoglobin level, persistence of elevated fetal and embryonic: 13+, 13q+[d]

Nuclear projections of neutrophils, increased: 13+, 13q+[p]

Seizures: 4p–, 13+, 14q+, 15q+, 18q–

In this list the major chromosomal syndromes (such as trisomy 21, trisomy 13, trisomy 18, and cat's cry syndrome) are included. The numbers designate the chromosome involved, p stands for short arm, q stands for long arm, + means trisomy, and – means deletion of either a total chromosome or part of it. The number following p or q designates the number of a chromosome band according to Paris conference nomenclature; for example, 13(q21)– means deletion of long arms of chromosome number 13 at the band number 21.

It appears that each of the forty-six human chromosomes has been found to be involved in translocations and other aberrations. Applying modern techniques of detailed banding also revealed high incidence of chromosomal defects and variations in as many as 0.5% to 1% of liveborn children, and it is probable that the prevalence will increase with our ability of more precise chromosomal analysis.

REFERENCES

1. Shapiro, B. L.: Amplified developmental instability in Down's syndrome, Ann. Hum. Genet. **38**:429-437, 1975.

Historical remarks

2. Arrighi, F. E., and Hsu, T. C.: Localization of heterochromatin in human chromosomes, Cytogenetics **10**:81-86, 1971.

3. Caspersson, T., Farber, S., Foley, G. E., Kudynowski, J., Modest, E. J., Simonson, E., Wagh, U., and Zech, L.: Chem. Exp. Cell. Res. **49**:219-222, 1968.

4. Caspersson, T., Zech, L., Johansson, C., and Modest, E. J.: Identification of human chromosomes by DNA reacting fluorescing agents, Chromosoma **30**:215-227, 1970.

5. Caspersson, T., Zech, L., Modest, E. J., Foley, G. E., Wagh, U., and Simonsson, E.: Chemical differentiation with fluorescent alkylating agents in *Vicia faba* metaphase chromosomes, Exp. Cell Res. **58**:128-140, 1963.

6. Drets, M. E., and Shaw, M. W.: Specific banding patterns of human chromosomes, Proc. Natl. Acad. Sci. U.S.A. **68**:2073, 1971.

7. Dutrillaux, B., and Lejeune, J.: Sur une nouvelle technique d'analyse du caryotype humain, C. R. Acad. Sci. (Paris) **272**:2638-40, 1971.

8. Edwards, J. H., Harnden, D. G., Cameron, H. H., Grosse, V. M., and Wolf, O. H.: A new trisomic syndrome, Lancet **1**:787, 1960.

9. Ford, C. E., and Hamerton, J. L.: The chromosomes of man, Nature **178**:1010, 1956.

10. Ford, C. E., Jones, K. W., Polani, P. E., deAlmeida, J. C., and Briggs, J. H.: A sex chromosome anomaly in a case of gonadal dysgenesis (Turner's syndrome), Lancet **1**:711, 1959.

10a. Goodpasture, C.: Visualization of nucleolar organizer regions in mammalian chromosomes using silver staining, Chromosoma **53**:37-50, 1975.

10b. Howell, W. M., Denton, T. E., and Diamond, J. R.: Differential staining of the satellite regions of human acrocentric chromosomes, Experientia **31**:260-262, 1975.

11. Jacobs, P. A., Baikie, A. G., Court-Brown, W. M., MacGregor, D. N., Maclean, M., and Harnden, D. G.: Evidence for the existence of the human super female, Lancet **2**:423, 1959.

12. Jacobs, P. A., and Strong, J. A.: A case of human intersexuality having a possible XXY sex determining mechanism, Nature **183**:302, 1959.

13. Korenberg, J. R., and Freedlender, F. F.: Giemsa technique for the detection of sister chromatid exchanges, Chromosoma **48**:355-360, 1974.

14. Latt, S. A.: Microfluorometric detection of deoxyribonucleic acid replication in human metaphase chromosomes, Proc. Natl. Acad. Sci. U.S.A. **70**:3395, 1973.

15. Lejeune, J., Gautier, M., and Turpin, R.: Étude des chromosomes somatique de neuf enfants mongoliens, C. R. Acad. Sci. (Paris) **248**:1721, 1959.

16. Miller, O. J., Schreck, R. R., Beiser, S. M., and Erlanger, B. F.: Immunofluorescent studies of chromosome banding with anti-nucleoside antibodies, Nobel Symposium 23, Chromosome identification, New York, 1973, Academic Press, Inc.

17. Pardue, M. L., and Gall, J. G.: Chromosomal localization of mouse satellite DNA, Science **168:**1356-1358, 1970.

18. Patau, K., Smith, D. W., Therman, E., Inhorn, S. L., and Wagner, H. P.: Multiple congenital anomaly caused by an extra autosome, Lancet **1:**790, 1960.

19. Perry, P., and Wolff, S.: New Giemsa method for the differential staining of sister chromatids, Nature **25:**156-158, 1974.

20. Patil, S. R., Merrick, S., and Lubs, H. A.: Identification of each human chromosome with a modified Giemsa stain, Science **173:**821, 1971.

21. Schnedl, W.: Analysis of the human karyotype using a reassociation technique, Chromosoma **34:**448-454, 1971.

22. Seabright, M.: A rapid banding technique for human chromosomes, Lancet **2:**971-972, 1971.

23. Sumner, A. T., Evans, H. J., and Buckland, R. A.: New technique for distinguishing between human chromosomes, Nature New Biol. **232:**31-32, 1971.

24. Tjio, J. H., and Levan, A.: The chromosome number of man, Hereditas **42:**1, 1956.

25. Wolff, S., and Perry, P.: Differential Giemsa staining of sister chromatids and the study of sister chromatid exchanges without autoradiography, Chromosoma **48:**341-353, 1974.

26. Yunis, J. J., Roldan, L., Yasmineh, W. G., and Lee, J. C.: Staining of satellite DNA in metaphase chromosomes, Nature **231:**532-533, 1971.

Turner's syndrome

27. Engel, E., and Forbes, A. P.: Cytogenetic and clinical findings in 48 patients with congenitally defective or absent ovaries, Medicine **44:**135, 1965.

28. Gordon, R. R., and O'Neill, E. M.: Turner's infantile phenotype, Br. Med. J. **1:**483, 1969.

Poly–X females

29. Barr, M. L., Sergovich, F. R., Carr, M. B., and Shaver E. L.: The Triplo-X female: an appraisal based on a study of 12 cases and a review of the literature, Can. Med. Assoc. J. **101:**247, 1969.

30. Tennes, K., Puck, M., Bryant, K., Frankenburg, W., and Robinson, A.: A developmental study of girls with trisomy X, Am. J. Hum. Genet. **27:**71-80, 1975.

Klinefelter's syndrome

31. Opitz, J.: Klinefelter syndrome. In Bergsma, D., editor: Birth defects atlas and compendium, Baltimore, 1973, The Williams & Wilkins Co. for The National Foundation–March of Dimes.

32. Zuppinger, K., Engel, E., Forbes, A. P., et al.: Klinefelter's syndrome; a clinical and cytogenetic study in 24 cases, Acta Endocrinol. (Suppl. 113) **54:**5, 1967.

XYY syndrome

33. Alvesalo, L., Osborne, R. H., and Kari, M.: The 47,XYY male, Y chromosome, and tooth size, Am. J. Hum. Genet. **27:**53, 1975.

34. Gorlin, R. J.: XYY syndrome. In Yunis, J. J., editor: Human chromosome methodology, ed. 2, New York, 1974, Academic Press, p. 222.

35. Hamerton, J. L.: Chromatin negative males with two Y chromosomes. In Hamerton, J. L.: Human cytogenetics, vol. 2, New York, 1971, Academic Press, Inc., p. 41.

4p–, Wolf-Hirschhorn syndrome

36. Guthrie, R. D., Aase, J. M., Asper, A. C., and Smith, D. W.: The 4p– syndrome, Am. J. Dis. Child. **122:**421, 1971.

37. Miller, O. J., Breg, W. R., and Warburton, D.: Partial deletion of the short arm of chromosome No. 4 (4p–): clinical studies in five unrelated patients, J. Pediatr. **77:**792, 1970.

5p–, Cri du chat syndrome

38. Breg, W. R., Steele, M. W., Miller, O. J., Warburton, D., deCapoa, A., and Allerdice, P. W.: The cri du chat syndrome in adolescents and adults: clinical findings in 13 older patients with partial deletion of the short arms of chromosome no 5 (5p–), J. Pediatr. **77:**782, 1970.

39. Howard, R. O.: Ocular abnormalities in the cri-du-chat syndrome, Am. J. Dis. Child. **73:**949, 1972.

Trisomy 8 syndrome

40. Bijlsma, J. B., Wijffels, J. C. H. M., and Tegelaers, W. H. H.: C 8 trisomy mosaicism syndrome, Helv. Paediatr. Acta **27:**281, 1972.

41. Caspersson, T., Lindsten, J., Zech, L., Buckton, K. E., and Price, W. H.: Four patients with trisomy 8 identified by the fluorescence and Giemsa banding techniques, J. Med. Genet. **9:**1, 1972.

42. Kakati, S., Nihill, M., and Sinha, A. K.: An attempt to establish trisomy 8 syndrome, Humangenetik **19:**293-300, 1973.

Trisomy 13, Patau's syndrome

43. Smith, D. W.: Autosomal abnormalities, Am. J. Obstet. Gynecol. **90:**1055, 1964.
44. Taylor, A. I.: Autosomal trisomy syndromes; a detailed study of 27 cases of Edward's syndrome and 27 cases of Patau's syndrome, J. Med. Genet. **5:**227, 1968.
45. Warkany, J., Passarge, E., and Smith, L. B.: Congenital malformations in autosomal trisomy syndromes, Am. J. Dis. Child. **112:**502, 1966.

13q–syndrome

46. Allerdice, P. W., Davis, J. G., Miller, O. J., et al.: The 13q– syndrome, Am. J. Hum. Genet. **21:**499, 1969.
47. Bloom, G. E., and Gelard, P. S.: Localization of genes on chromosome 13: analysis of two kindreds, Am. J. Hum. Genet. **20:**495, 1968.
48. Wilson, M. G., Towner, J. W., and Fujimoto, A.: Retinoblastoma and D-chromosome deletions, Am. J. Hum. Genet. **25:**57, 1973.

Trisomy 18, Edward's syndrome

49. Butler, L. J., Snodgrass, G. J., France, N. E., Sinclair, L., and Russell, A.: No. E (16-18) trisomy syndrome; analysis of 13 cases, Arch. Dis. Child. **40:**600, 1965.
50. Taylor, A. I.: Autosomal trisomy syndromes: a detailed study of 27 cases of Edward's syndrome and 27 cases of Patau's syndrome, J. Med. Genet. **5:**227, 1968.
51. Warkany, J., Passarge, E., and Smith, L. B.: Congenital malformations in autosomal trisomy syndromes, Am. J. Dis. Child. **112:** 502, 1966.

18p– Syndrome

52. de Grouchy, J.: The 18p–, 18q–, and 18r syndromes, Birth Defects **5:**74, 1969.
53. Gorlin, R. J.: Clinical manifestations of chromosome disorders. In Yunis, J. J., editor: Human chromosome methodology, New York, 1974, Academic Press, Inc.

18q– Syndrome

54. de Grouchy, J.: The 18p–, 18q–, and 18r syndromes, Birth defects: Original Article Series V, White Plains, N. Y., 1969, The National Foundation–March of Dimes, p. 74.
55. Law, E. M., and Martenson, J. G.: Familial 18q– syndromes, Ann. Genet. **12:**215, 1969.
56. Lurie, I., and Lazjerk, G.: Partial monosomies 18, Humangenetik **15:**203, 1972.

18r–Syndrome

57. Cenani, A., Pfeiffer, R., and Simon, M.: Ring chromosome 18, Humangenetik **7:**351, 1969.
58. de Grouchy, J.: The 18p–, 18q–, and 18r syndromes, Birth Defects **5:**74, 1969.
59. Kunze, J., Stephan, E., and Tolksdorf, M.: Ring-chromosom 18, Humangenetik **15:**289, 1972.

Trisomy 21, Down's syndrome

60. Cohen, M. M., Sr., and Cohen, M. M., Jr.: The oral manifestations of trisomy G_1 (Down's syndrome), Birth Defects **7:**241, 1971.
61. Mikkelsen, M., and Stene, J.: Down's syndrome: current stage of cytogenetic research, Humangenetik **12:**1, 1971.
62. Penrose, L. S., and Smith, G. I.: Down's anomaly, Boston, 1966, Little, Brown & Co.
63. Richards, B. W., Steward, A., Sylvester, P. E., and Jasiewicz, V.: Cytogenetic survey of 225 patients diagnosed clinically as mongol, J. Ment. Defic. Res. **9:**245, 1965.

Trisomy 22

64. Bass, H. N., Crandall, B. F., and Sparkes, R. S.: Probable trisomy 22 identified by fluorescent and trypsin-Giemsa banding, Ann. Genet. **16:**189, 1973.
65. Bühler, E. M., Mehes, K., Müller, H., et al.: Cat-eye syndrome, a partial trisomy 22, Humangenetik **15:**150, 1972.
66. Hirschhorn, K., Lucas, M., and Wallace, I.: Precise identification of various chromosome abnormalities, Ann. Hum. Genet. **36:**375, 1973.

Triploidy syndrome

67. Edwards, J. H., Yunchen, C., Rushton, D. I., et al.: Three cases of triploidy in man, Cytogenet. Cell Genet. **6:**81, 1967.
68. Walker, S., Andrews, J., Gregson, N. M., and Gault, W.: Three further cases of triploidy in man surviving to birth, J. Med. Genet. **10:** 135, 1973.
69. Zergollern, L., Drazancic, A., Damjanov, I., Hitrec, V., and Gorecam, V.: A liveborn infant with triploidy (69, XXX), Z. Kinderheilkd. **112:**293, 1972.

Other new chromosomal syndromes

70. Borgaonkar, D. S.: Chromosomal variation in man: a catalog of variants and anomalies, Baltimore, 1975, The Johns Hopkins University Press.
71. Lewandowski, R. C., and Yunis, J. J.: New chromosomal syndromes, Am. J. Dis. Child. **129:**515-529, 1975.

16

The genetics of cleft lip and palate

BURTON L. SHAPIRO

Facial clefts, particularly those of the lip or palate or both, are major human congenital malformations. Unquestionably these defects occurred before the written history of man. Icons with clefts dating from as early as 12 AD have been uncovered,[96] and the recorded history of surgical treatment of these debilitating conditions spans nearly 1600 years.[107] Over these years numerous etiological possibilities have been considered. The notion of "marking" or the influence on the fetus of maternal impressions such as shock or fright was a commonly held cause by the laity and persists even today in the minds of some. "Poisonous substances" such as drugs or toxins and "improper nourishment" leading to defective nutrition of the embryo have been implicated. The "mechanical influence" of pressure against the upper jaw by the embryo's knee or the mandible or tongue has been considered causative. Finally, the role of heredity factors in the production of these defects has long been recognized.[29] It is the purpose of this chapter to review current thoughts concerning the basis of clefts of the lip and of the palate.

The epidemiology of facial clefts will be considered in greater detail later. However, to place these conditions in perspective, some cursory data will be given here. Isolated cleft palate (CP) has been found in as many as 1 in 125 and as few as 1 in 5263 live births in different populations. However, the true prevalence may be as much as 60% greater because of underreporting on birth certificates.[80, 83] Cleft lip with or without cleft palate (CL ± CP) has been reported as frequently as 1 in 234 to as few as 1 in 1063 live births. Underreporting for CL ± CP has been estimated to be somewhere between 13% and 35%.[80, 83] In general CL ± CP occurs in approximately 1 in 1000 and cleft palate in 1 in 2500 live births in Caucasian populations. Prevalences are somewhat higher in populations of Oriental stock and somewhat lower in Negroes.[25]

Facial clefts account for nearly 60% of all gastrointestinal malformations.[77] Ivy[58] ranked the fifteen most common anomalies recorded on birth certificates in the state of Pennsylvania from 1956 through 1960. Facial clefts ranked second; only clubfoot was more prevalent. Accordingly, facial clefts are among the most common congenital malformations in man.

The directly associated and derived effects of facial clefts are profound and lead to important clinical consequences. The complexity of facial structures and their functions is reflected clearly in the degree and frequency of derived difficulties associated with clefts. Among the derived effects are nursing, respiratory, and swallowing difficulties. Aspiration leading to lung disease may result. Later, chewing and speech may be affected. The face is often marred by severe structural and aesthetic alterations. The dentition is often abnormal. Otitis media is frequent. Probably a greater diversity of health care specialists must interact in the habilitation of individuals with clefts of lip or palate or both than with any other congenital malformation.[100] In addition to structural and functional effects, the psychosocial effects of facial clefts are profound. Facial expression and speech provide essential means of interaction among human individuals. A defect that may affect both the facial aesthetics of an individual and his ability to speak normally suggests that facial clefts have most pervasive effects.

In any single individual the etiological basis of a congenital malformation such as a facial cleft may be (1) a teratogenic environmental factor acting on a relevant developmental pathway, (2) a single gene substitution, (3) a chromosomal anomaly, or (4) a confluence of multiple genetic and environmental factors (multifactorial). As will be discussed in much detail, the currently held explanation for most human facial clefts is based on a multifactorial model. The model suggests that when, in a developing organism, some critical number of factors (genetic and environmental) is exceeded, a cleft results. One may envision normal development as resulting from an orderly successful attainment of numerous epigenetic thresholds. Failure of a developmental pathway to overcome one or more of these developmental thresholds will lead to maldevelopment. It cannot be overemphasized that this model is no more than a generalization. Facial clefts can be associated with gross chromosomal anomalies, single gene traits, and, in experimental animals, environmental teratogens. Therefore in sporadic cases one cannot know the etiological basis except in the case of an identified single-gene syndrome. Furthermore, if the majority of cleft occurrences within a population are based on a multifactorial model, heterogeneity still exists. Within the multifactorial milieu different magnitudes of specific factors may operate in one organism in comparison with another. Human facial cleft population data is most consistent with a multifactorial threshold model. However, in any individual case a wide variety of etiological agents and pathogenetic mechanisms potentially is responsible.

Classification is prerequisite to the discussion of any malformation. Frequently traits that may not be etiologically or developmentally discontinuous are arbitrarily separated into distinct classes. Conversely, traits having diverse bases may, because of apparently similar phenotypes, be grouped together. Nevertheless, classifications are a necessary starting point. They can and must be modified. Classifications often are based on etiological concepts. Classification also influences and in some cases may inhibit understanding of pathogenesis. In recent years cleft palate has been distinguished from CL ± CP. Most modern facial cleft data are classified this way, and, for the most part, this classification will be used here. However, exceptions to the apparently sharp distinction between cleft palate on the one hand and CL ± CP on the other have occurred sufficiently frequently to warrant continued appraisal of facial cleft nosology. Moreover, the separation of conditions such as submucous clefts or clefts of the uvula from overt clefts of the palate may be arbitrary. In any case, the rigidity or flexibility of a classification system of traits has important significance for an understanding of their genetic basis.

EMBRYOLOGY

A short review of human maxillofacial development is necessary when considering a discussion of facial clefts. Genetic analysis depends on classification of cleft types, and classification is based partially on normal development. During the fourth week in utero a small maxillary and a larger mandibular process enlarge bilaterally from the first branchial arch. At about this time local ectodermal thickenings, olfactory placodes, occur at the lateral borders of the frontal prominence. By the fifth week all primordia of the lip and palate are present. Around the nasal placodes a horseshoe-like elevation arises formed by mesodermal proliferations: the medial nasal process, the lateral nasal process, and the frontonasal process. The maxillary processes enlarge intraorally as well as facially at this time. The maxillary and medial nasal processes continue to enlarge during the sixth week at the expense of the other mesodermal masses. On each side these enlargements approach one another. The basic framework of the upper lip and jaw is formed during the seventh week based on merging of the medial nasal, frontonasal, and maxillary processes on each side of the developing head. At about this time the nasal pits, which are derived from the nasal placodes, increase in depth. In part, this is due to the continued growth of processes surrounding the pits. However, the pits do tunnel internally as well, so that they soon overlie the roof of the first part of the primordial oral cavity. Mesoderm intervening between the stomodeum and the nasal pits gives way, resulting in the framework of the primary palate. The primary palate thus formed may be described as consisting of the labial, the middle, and the deep areas. The labial area forms the medial portion of the upper lip. The middle portion, which will form the premaxilla, is the incisor area of the maxillary alveolus. The deep or palatal area of the primary palate forms the small triangular plate just behind the premaxilla. This plate forms the median palatal process anterior to the future incisive foramen. Surface epithelia covering the nasal, medial, and maxillary processes abut, fuse, and break down with consequent joining of mesodermal masses of these processes. Anteriorly the two nasomedial processes lie between the nasal pits and are separated from each other along their labial surfaces by a midline furrow. This furrow is progressively smoothed out in the area of the future philtrum during the eighth week by a merging of its underlying frontal mesenchyme.

At about the time of completion of the primary palate, bilateral palatine processes enlarge intraorally from the maxillary processes. Thus at about the time of completion of the primary palate the secondary palate begins its formation. During the eighth intrauterine week the palatine shelves enlarge on both sides of the tongue, which, filling the oral cavity, maintains contact superiorly with the nasal septum. During the ninth and tenth weeks the mandibular arch enlarges, the tongue drops, and the palatal shelves are transposed horizontally. The palatal shelves fuse with each other in the midline anteriorly and with the medial palatal triangle. Fusion

between the shelves and with the nasal septum occurs in an anteroposterior direction. By 11 to 12 weeks in utero, midline contact, epithelial adhesion, cytolysis of covering epithelium, and mesenchymal coalescence of palatal shelves occur. Midline fusion is complete, except perhaps for complete formation of the posterior soft palate and uvula. Final union of the posterior secondary palate occurs, apparently, by a merging process of posterior mesenchymal pushing comparable perhaps to the mesodermal penetration that happens several weeks earlier in the anterior portion of the maxilla.[10]

Thus key events in development of the lip and palate in the human occur from about the fourth week (crown-rump length [CR] = 3.5 to 5 mm) until about 12 weeks (CR = 50 to 60 mm). Dimensional changes continue until postpuberty. However, the epigenetic events that occur in the maxillofacial region during the first trimester of development are critical. Disruption of any of these events may lead to maldevelopment of the lip or palate. The primary palate is formed by penetration and obliteration of ectodermal grooves by three mesodermal masses. Absence or deficiency of these masses or a failure of mesenchymal penetration of epithelium may result in clefts of the primary palate. Such defects occur where, during the second month of development, maxillary processes should merge with the nasomaxillary process. Since the primary palate forms the central portion of the lip, alveolus and premaxilla clefts of the primary palate can extend posteriorly as far as the incisive papilla. Clefts of the primary palate may be unilateral or bilateral. The cleft may be as slight as a notching of the lip unilaterally or so severe as to result in complete clefting of the primary palate: lip, alveolus, and premaxilla bilaterally. Rarely, the bilateral defect may be so extensive or the nasomedial process so deficient that a true midline cleft of the primary palate occurs. Clefts of the primary palate may or may not be accompanied by a cleft of the secondary palate. Here the defect is medial due to failure of the bilateral palatal shelves to unite. Such a defect results in communication between the oral and nasal cavities. The mildest manifestation of secondary palate clefting of bone would be a posterior palatal notch in the midline. Submucous cleft or cleft uvula seems to fall in the borderland between clefting and normal development and may be considered the most mild forms of cleft palate or microforms. An isolated defect of the secondary palate may extend as far forward as the incisive foramen. When associated with a cleft lip, the defects are contiguous. Since horizontal transposition is a key event, several theories of secondary palatal pathogenesis are concerned with interference with this process: a hypothetical "shelf force" may be defective, or failure of dropping of the tongue acts as a barrier to shelf movement.[134] Even if palatal shelves assume a horizontal plane, they must make midline contact. One hypothesis suggests that a cleft might result if head width is so great at the time of shelf transposition that shelves cannot contact.[97, 133] Another suggestion is that programmed epithelial cell death of covering shelf epithelium fails, thereby preventing mesenchymal coalescence.[121] Subsequent growth of the embryonic head results in rupture at the midline. Union of the soft palate and uvula probably results from posterior extension of mesenchyme through a merging process that displaces epithelium posteriorly. Mesenchymal hypoplasia in the site of the furrow where the posterior portion of the two shelves join could result in soft palate or uvula clefting.

Similar failures in development of or obliteration of seams between facial processes can account for other facial clefts, for example, various oblique and transverse facial clefts. These are exceedingly rare. Since they are not relevant to the genetic discussion that follows, they will not be considered.

CLASSIFICATION

One would think that cleft lip or cleft palate is either present or absent and that they are easily distinguished. However, for many years investigators disagreed on their classification.[63] In the last 15 years some degree of consensus has been reached about phenotypic descriptions. Clinically, all degrees of cleft lip and cleft palate may be observed from a mild notching of the vermilion border of the lip or a notched uvula to the severe bilateral complete cleft of the lip, alveolus, and entire palate. An appropriate classification of these defects is essential for pursuit of an understanding of their causes and pathogenesis as well as for clinical description. A classification is a fountainhead for further understanding, yet it may also impose a constraint. Therefore rigidity and preconceptions must be resisted. As long as causes are unclear, classifications are based on limited knowledge. One must guard against deductions to etiological conclusions from classifications based on clinical or embryological evidence.

Because of their anatomical, functional, and therapeutic relationships, cleft lip, cleft alveolus, and cleft palate must be considered together. Since a notched lip anteriorly and posteriorly a bifid uvula are perceptible anatomical gradations of the more severe defects, these phenotypes should mark the boundaries of the classification. More hypothetical, noncontiguous microforms are excluded from the classification. Excluded also from the classification are lateral and oblique facial clefts, median cleft lip, and their associated anomalies.[42]

A nomenclature committee of the American Association for Cleft Palate Rehabilitation provided a classification in 1962. The classification provides a "basis for the choice of either a simple, broadly inclusive classification or a more detailed scheme. . . . The anatomy and severity of the defect constitutes the basis for classification. The detail to which subdivision is carried depends upon the purpose of the observer in any given situation. A few broad categories may suffice for purposes of some clinical records and therapeutic measures, whereas others may require more detailed classification."[52] Major considerations were consistency, anatomical relationships, and embryological events. Early groupings considered the alveolar process as a critical boundary in the delineation of cleft subtypes. However, clinical and embryological evidence led to the general acceptance of the present classification.

Since it might be begging the etiological question to use genetic hypotheses in formulating the classification of clefts, the discussion here will consider only phenotypic considerations: embryological, anatomical, functional, and clinical.

From a functional point of view the hard palate, including the alveolus bearing the maxillary incisor teeth, and the soft palate comprise a unit. The lip represents another functional unit. However, clinically, isolated clefts of the palate occur in the midline and extend anteriorly to the incisive foramen. On the other hand, clefts of the lip may occur unilaterally (as well as bilaterally) and extend posteriorly through the alveolus to the area of the incisive foramen. To be sure, total clefts may occur, including clefts of the lip, the alveolus, and the hard and soft palate.

Embryological considerations provide the strongest basis for the current classification of clefts. Both in terms of in utero time of development and in the type of developmental processes involved, the (1) primary (prepalate) and the (2) secondary palate are distinct. The premaxilla includes the anterior portion of the hard palate: the alveolus, its four incisor teeth, and the hard palate extending posteriorly to the incisive foramen. The lip and premaxilla develop simultaneously between 4 and 7 weeks in utero. Development is essentially that of penetration by mesodermal masses of epithelial sheaths. The hard palate posterior to the incisive foramen and the soft palate develop between 7 and 12 weeks, and their development essentially involves the coalescence of two palatal shelf processes of the maxillary processes. Thus development of the primary palate and of the secondary palate are distinct.

Accordingly, a broad outline for consideration of the genetics of lip and palatal clefts is based on two major headings with two subheadings:

Prepalate
   Lip
   Alveolar process (to incisive foramen)
Palate
   Soft palate
   Hard palate (to incisive foramen)

Clefts of the prepalate may be unilateral or bilateral. Clefts of the palate are midline defects. Degrees of extent exist in each type. Clefts of the prepalate and palate may coexist.

The separation, for classification purposes, of clefts of the primary and clefts of the secondary palate is based on sound clinical and embryological bases. However, an a priori conclusion that these are etiologically distinct should be resisted. Clefts of the primary and secondary palates may coexist. Furthermore, common epigenetic events may affect development of both primary and secondary palates. The potential etiological heterogeneity of these clefts ought to counsel against strong definitive etiological assumptions. Nevertheless, this classification based on developmental derivations of the primary and secondary palates has proved extremely useful in the past twenty years and forms the basis for much of the genetic analyses.

EPIDEMIOLOGY

The inherent difficulty in estimating facial cleft incidence has been pointed out previously.[31, 55, 80, 83] Most investigators have calculated frequencies of facial clefts on the basis of birth records or hospital referrals. The inclusion of infants who die before operation will bias considerably estimates based on referral.

In terms of genetic analyses, neonatal loss is most critical. Estimates of prenatal and neonatal death of individuals with clefts vary between 17% and 25%.[25, 55, 65, 78] Clearly, a significant number of fetuses die before the time when facial clefts can be detected. Evidence exists that a disproportionate percentage of prenatal deaths are of individuals with clefts. Underreporting on birth certificates is also a critical problem in determining incidence. In several studies underreporting on birth certificates, as would be expected, varied with severity of clefts. However, even with major clefts of the lip and palate, surveys have shown that as much as a third of cases are unreported.[80] Additional difficulties arise in surveys. A subgroup may result in an unrepresentative estimate. For example, racial heterogeneity or a large kindred in which a mutant gene may be segregating could lead to an estimate not representative of the population in general. With these reservations identified we can now discuss estimates of the impact of facial clefts on human populations.

Of the total number of facial clefts, cleft lip ranges from about 20% to 30%, CL ± CP from 35% to 50%, and isolated cleft palate from 30% to 45%.[25] The incidence of all clefts of the lip and palate ranges, in different populations, from about 0.59/1000 live births to 3.63/1000 live births. The greatest contributions to these population incidence differences are due to racial differences. The average incidence of facial clefts in American Negroes is 0.59/1000,[71] in Caucasians in North America and Europe 1.78/1000,[55, 80, 83] and in individuals of Oriental stock (Japanese and North American Indians) as high as 3.27/1000.[91, 135] Incidences among different samples of similar racial ancestry have been remarkably similar. The frequency of CL ± CP is higher in Caucasians (1.34/1000 births) than in American Negroes (0.41/1000)[19] and higher in Japanese (2.13/1000)[91] than in Caucasians. In Hawaii, interracial crosses resulted in intermediate frequencies.[90] Racial differences for cleft palate do not seem to be so dramatic: American Negroes (0.41/1000), Caucasian (0.48/1000),[19] and Japanese (0.55/1000).[91] The apparent negligible differences among races for cleft palate frequency[33] are most curious in light of the highly significant racial differences for cleft uvula.[16, 54, 122] Racial differences will be analyzed in more detail when discussing etiology.

Sex differences in incidences of particular clefts exist. However, these differences are not uniform among different races, nor are the sex differences consistent when considering different degrees of cleft severity. In the literature it is usually suggested that CL ± CP occurs more frequently in males and that cleft palate occurs more frequently in females. Cleft lip appears to occur more frequently in males in Caucasian series but more frequently in female Negroes[48] with only a slight female preference in Japanese.[38, 39] CL ± CP occurs more frequently in males in Japanese

and Caucasians but, no sex difference was apparent in Negroes. Isolated cleft palate is more frequent in females in Japanese and Caucasian samples, but again, no sex difference was apparent in Negroes. Existing data suggest that more clefts occur in females in Negro samples, but male predilection occurs in Caucasian and Japanese samples. The excess of males in the latter two races appears greater with more severe clefts. That is, the excess is greater for CL ± CP than for cleft lip[31, 105] and for bilateral than unilateral clefts.[31] An explanation for sex incidence differences was suggested by Meskin and associates,[84] tested and supported by Burdi and Silvey,[11] but challenged by Janerich.[60]

A compilation of data from several series reveals that approximately 85% of cleft lip cases are unilateral, and of these more than two thirds occur on the left side.[31, 37, 80, 105] The left-side preponderance exists regardless of sex or extent of cleft. Several hypotheses concerning the basis for cleft lip sidedness have been suggested.[1, 124]

Studies that have examined a possible relationship between facial clefts and parental age,[18, 76] birth rank,[9, 25, 80] birth weight,[25, 80] and season of birth[34, 125] generally have been unrewarding in shedding light on facial cleft pathogenesis.

ETIOLOGY AND PATHOGENESIS
Heterogeneity

Successful development of the maxillofacial region requires a sequence of appropriate epigenetic events. The process involves numerous cell types that act and interact from the time of conception until late in the first trimester. Ultimately these events rest on evolved balanced genetic systems acting in a suitable milieu. Developmental pathways are channeled in such a way that there results an anatomical form that is standard for the species. Within the confines of the standard there exists a wide phenotypic variability. However, there can occur morphogenetic deviations from the standard (phenodeviants), such as facial clefts, beyond which acceptable structure and function are not attained. Standard form depends on developmental pathways, which are based on a mosaic of properly integrated elements. It should be apparent, then, that normal development does not depend on a single critical metabolic pathway or switch mechanism or cell type. Each of many elements is critical for subsequent events. Conversely, an inappropriate incident at any one or more steps can disrupt the overall pathway. Obviously no gene for normal maxillofacial development exists. Nevertheless, a single gene abnormality can disrupt its development. Products of different genes can disturb the same portion of the epigenetic course, or a product of a single gene can disrupt various steps in the pathway. Similarly, no single critical hormone or nutrient is associated with normal development. The entire system must be biochemically balanced so that as it unfolds it remains within confinements that permit subsequent development. Accordingly, appropriate development depends on a confluence of numerous factors, all of which must exist and act in concert. A grossly abnormal gene product or environmental factor can perturb the system sufficiently to displace it from its evolved direction. On the other hand, several factors individually too subtle to affect the entire system may together lead to a displacement of the overall developmental pathway to such a degree that a "normal" structure does not result. The heterogeneity just described exists in terms of the potential variety of disturbing elements in development. However, heterogeneity exists also in the relative proportion of these elements that might be meaningful in different individuals, families, or populations. Accordingly, potential agents leading to maldevelopment of the lip and palate include single gene abnormalities, gross chromosomal anomalies, teratogenic environmental factors, or combinations of these.

Environmental factors

Clefts of the lip and palate can be induced in experimental animals with a variety of teratogenic agents. Several important principles have emerged from these studies: an organism must be genetically susceptible to the agent, the agent must be suitable to produce the desired defect, and the agent must be administered by an appropriate route in a suitable dosage at a critical gestational time. The role of exogenous factors in cleft development is more difficult to discern in the human. Retrospective studies suffer from unavoidable biased reporting and lack of controls. Prospective studies require enormous numbers of individuals. Only rarely are potentially teratogenic agents present in massive or at least obvious dosages. In all likelihood subtle interactions occur that may be teratogenic. Nevertheless, the involvement of exogenous factors with susceptible genotypes is a viable hypothetical basis for clefts. Those exogenous factors that may contribute to human clefting require review.

Retrospective studies of maternal rubella infection during the first 8 weeks of gestation suggest an association with increased facial cleft incidence.[24, 56] Apparently neither maternal toxoplasmosis nor syphilis are associated with clefting.[50] A prospective study of maternal infections and subsequent clefting failed to demonstrate an association between clefts and measles, mumps, chicken pox, poliomyelitis, or influenza infections during the first trimester.[109] However, Leck[67] and Leck and co-workers[69] in a follow-up of this study did show that cleft lip risk was significantly although slightly greater in infants exposed to maternal A2 influenza infection in utero.

The ordinary use of hormones in animal studies probably has little relationship to human cleft pathogenesis. Pharmacological dosages or ablation procedures used experimentally cannot approach the subtle endocrine disbalances that may occur in human mothers. On the other hand, geographical and individual examples of human maternal hypothyroidism have consistently been associated with increased risk for clefts.[25, 50, 56, 129] In a prospective study, Pedersen and associates[99] suggested that the risk for clefting was increased in offspring of diabetic mothers. Studies on cortisone and stress in relationship to human clefts have been contradictory.[108]

Numerous isolated case histories purporting

to demonstrate some relationship between a wide variety of drugs and increased risk for facial clefts have been reviewed.[55] These reports have suffered from the usual deficiencies of retrospective studies. However, a renewed interest in the possible relationship between diphenylhydantoin (Dilantin) or its analogues and increased susceptibility to human facial clefts has occurred.[98] According to Fraser,[35] antiepileptic drugs may cause congenital malformations, particularly cleft lip, with a frequency of nearly 5%. Most recently, an association between ingestion of minor tranquilizers during pregnancy and oral clefts has been suggested.[110, 112]

In summary, clinical reports have been published in which higher frequencies of infections, endocrine disorders, or drug consumption have appeared in mothers of cleft children than in controls. It is not at all unreasonable to expect these traumatic factors to influence the apparently highly sensitive development of structures comprising the midface. Nevertheless, no factor can be selected as being of major importance. Most differences are small and often uncertain because of the retrospective methods used and absence of suitable control samples.

Racial studies

Race presupposes greater genetic similarities among individuals within a group than among different groups. At the same time, racial classifications usually include a geographical component, and, if these do not exist, cultural differences usually do. Accordingly, the bases for prevalence differences of specific conditions in different races are not always easy to identify. Nevertheless, when a racial or ethnic prevalence difference for complex traits such as facial clefts is found in populations surveyed, one has a potentially important start in discerning their basis.

The average incidence of facial clefts within essentially Caucasoid populations throughout the world is about 1.25/1000 live births. These estimates range from 0.66 in Russia[116] to 1.84 in Finland.[51] Low estimates (0.74) in essentially Caucasian populations in New York City and Tennessee[116] have been at-

tributed to a relatively large Negro proportion in these areas. Mongoloid populations have an average incidence of 1.93/1000 for all facial clefts, and incidences do not vary appreciably in estimates from China, Japan, and Malaysia.[46, 88, 91, 126] The average incidence from several surveys of American Indians was about 2.30/1000.[47, 59, 73, 86, 94] This does not differ significantly from data in the Mongoloid groups. The overall incidence of facial clefts in Negroes is about 0.46/1000.[*] Numerous studies have shown that the total frequency of facial clefts is lower in Negroes when compared with Caucasians.[†] Estimates of clefting frequency in Caucasians and Negroes even from disparate populations do not overlap. In one study the incidence of facial clefts among Mexicans was intermediate between that in Caucasians and Negroes from the same area.[75] Unquestionably the total facial cleft incidence among different racial groups is Mongoloid > Caucasian > Negro.

Following the suggestion of Fogh-Andersen that facial clefts are etiologically heterogeneous, it became the custom to survey populations in terms of cleft palate as distinct from CL ± CP. In some surveys isolated cleft lip was characterized separately from CL ± CP.

The incidence of cleft palate among Caucasian samples is about 0.32/1000.[‡] Fewer surveys of Mongoloid populations have been carried out, but the average incidence of 0.58/1000 is higher.[47, 88, 91, 126, 135] The average of 0.56/1000 in surveys among American Indians is similar to that of Orientals in Japan or China.[47, 59, 73, 94] However, estimates have varied widely (0.19 to 1.21/1000 births).[47, 94] Estimates of cleft palate incidence in Negro samples in several cities in the United States averaged approximately 0.23/1000 live births.[3, 19, 23, 47, 116] The average incidences of cleft palate in the major racial groups are Mongoloid > Caucasian > Negro. However, the differences are small and possibly not statistically significant. In the series of Chung and Myrianthopoulos,[19] for

---

*See references 3, 19, 23, 47, 72, 91, 115.
†See references 4, 23, 44, 57, 66, 72, 75, 116.
‡See references 8, 19, 21, 31, 47, 55, 130.

example, the difference between Negroes and Caucasians was not statistically significant. On the other hand the Mongoloid > Caucasian > Negro relationship for cleft palate was evident in data from several studies,[3, 91, 94] although not in others.[33] Comparisons of cleft palate incidence between Japanese and Caucasians living in Hawaii[90] and Negroes and Caucasians[19] did not reveal differences. The average incidence differences among races for CL ± CP are: Caucasian 0.98,* Mongoloid, 1.67,[47, 88, 91, 126] American Indian 1.98,[47, 73, 94] and Negro 0.36.[47, 72, 116] The average incidence differences among races for CL + CP are: Caucasian 0.54,[19, 21, 90, 94, 127] Mongoloid 1.49,[90, 91] American Indian 1.64,[59, 94, 135] and Negro 0.19.[3, 19, 94] In a few studies, data on cleft lip alone were provided: Caucasian 0.34,[21, 47, 73] Mongoloid 0.67,[47] American Indian 0.45,[47, 59, 73, 135] and Negro 0.13.[47] Clearly, incidence differences among the primary races for CL ± CP are Mongoloid (including American Indian) > Caucasian > Negro.

Morton and associates[90] showed that the frequency of CL ± CP in offspring of mixed Oriental-Caucasian parents in Hawaii was intermediate between their frequency in the parental groups. No evidence of maternal effects was noted. These findings would suggest that the involved genetic factors act additively.[90] In his review of racial findings for CL ± CP, Leck[68] found much less variation among populations of the same primary race living in different locales than between different races living in a similar area. In twenty-five series, each of which (1) included over 10,000 births, (2) was relatively homogeneous ethnically, and (3) had reasonably complete ascertainment, the statistical variance for CL ± CP among populations of different races was eight times as high as the variance within the same race in different areas. This would seem to support a meaningful genetic component in predisposition to the trait. On the other hand, Leck[68] noted that the incidence of cleft palate varies among populations of the same primary race

*See references 23, 31, 47, 72, 73, 86, 105, 116.

(except Negroes) and much less between races. He concluded that this observation coupled with the apparent association of cleft palate and maternal age and parity would suggest a relatively small genetic role in the cause of cleft palate. However, the relative degree of underreporting in different cleft types may be pertinent in this regard. In his series, Meskin[80] showed that underreporting on birth certificates was as follows: cleft palate, 53.1%; cleft lip, 35.2%; CL ± CP, 13.4%.[80, 83]

Cleft uvula (CU) will be discussed in more detail in a later section. However, racial differences in its incidence are consistent and dramatic and should be mentioned here (Table 16-10). Differences (Mongoloid > Caucasian > Negro) are highly significant.[16, 54, 122] Data are remarkably similar within racial subtypes in samples from different geographical areas. Of particular interest is the similarity of cleft uvula incidence in Orientals and populations (such as American Indians) derived from Mongoloid stock thousands of years ago.

The data presented in this section indicate that racial differences exist for facial cleft frequencies. The evidence for CL ± CP and cleft uvula is most strong. Since it is generally held that cleft uvula is a microform of cleft palate or the cleft palate component of CL ± CP, there is some question about the less strong racial difference data for cleft palate. Perhaps underreporting for cleft palate and its lower frequency account for the reported results. No evidence has been reported demonstrating cultural or environmental factors peculiar to one or another racial group that would account for the racial differences found. According to Neel,

The similarity in malformation frequencies in such diverse populations as Japanese and European thus finds an explanation in the fact that there is a malformation frequency separating the optimum balance between, on the one hand, fetal loss and physical handicap from congenital defect, and on the other hand, population gain from those very same genes which in certain combinations may someimes result in congenital defect. The differences between populations as regards the frequencies of specific defects would seem to indicate that within the framework of this optimum figure, different populations have evolved genetic systems differing significantly in their details.*

Twin studies

Despite its inclusion as a basic tool in human genetics for nearly a hundred years, criticism of the twin approach has been the subject of numerous reviews.[2] Furthermore, sampling biases must always be assumed in twin studies. In addition to biases, specific limitations in twin studies are recognized. Neither information about genotype nor identification of specific environmental factors can be obtained. Only rarely can genetic hypotheses be tested. Furthermore, inferences from twin results must usually be restricted to the population from which the sample was selected. With these caveats in mind there is a place for twin studies in human genetics. The virtual absence of any other genetic method for answering questions about the relative role of genetic and environmental factors that contribute to the development of complex traits such as facial clefts is apparent.[117] "Despite the many difficulties of twin research . . . no material but twins can provide such convincing evidence for environmental etiologic factors prior to demonstration of the factors individually."[2]

Twin studies of human facial clefts present additional specific problems. Approximately 1 in 50 live births is a twin. If we assume that a facial cleft occurs in about 1 in 600 live births, one would need to review an enormous number of newborns to obtain meaningful data. Accordingly, it is necessary to pool data from different surveys. Such pooling magnifies problems further: differences in quality of zygosity determinations by various investigators as well as different diagnostic criteria exist. It is likely that twins concordant for congenital malformations would more frequently be recorded in the literature than are discordant twin pairs.

*From Neel, J. V.: A study of major congenital defects in Japanese infants, Am. J. Hum. Genet. **10:**398-445, 1958.

Table 16-1. Twins and clefts

	MZ	DZ	h^2
CL ± CP			
Pairs	117	178	
Percentage of concordance	35.0	6.2	32.9
Cleft palate			
Pairs	43	68	
Percentage of concordance	44.2	8.8	38.8

Conversely, variation in expressivity between twins of a pair (clefts among concordant twins are seldom identical[103]) might lead to a label of discordance, resulting in an underestimate of concordance percentage. Finally, the significant underreporting that occurs in facial cleft surveys[80, 83] could affect conclusions.

In Table 16-1 data from twenty twin studies or case reports are summarized. For both CL ± CP and cleft palate, the percentage of concordance between MZ twins is greater than between DZ twins. Heritabilities (h^2) were calculated using the traditional formula:

$$h^2 = \frac{\text{\% concordant (MZ)} - \text{\% concordant (DZ)}}{100 - \text{\% concordant (DZ)}}$$

Concordance percentages agree well among the major surveys[42, 53, 85] with the exception of cleft palate in MZ twins. Metrakos and associates[85] found low concordance and Hay and Wehrung[53] found high concordance for cleft palate in MZ twins. The totals given here reflect this. Conclusions are different, however. The Metrakos and associates[85] data would support little genetic contribution for cleft palate, whereas the Hay and Wehrung[53] data suggested a relatively high genetic component. However, as Metrakos and associates noted in their study, "The number of twins in the CP group is very small and therefore unreliable."[85]

The fact that only about a third of MZ twins are concordant for facial clefts demonstrates clearly an environmental component. Concordance in DZ twins does not appear to differ significantly from sib risk estimates (p. 488). On the other hand, if the slightly greater DZ concordance in comparison with sib risk is real, it would suggest a maternal factor. The fairly consistent difference in concordance percentage between MZ and DZ twins in different series supports a genetic component in causation of facial clefts. With the exception of the Metrakos and associates[85] data, the estimates from the literature suggest that the relative contribution of environmental and hereditary factors are similar for cleft palate and for CL ± CP.

It must be emphasized that a heritability estimate (h²) based on DZ and MZ concordance of, say, $h^2 = 0.35$ does not suggest that 35% of the causative factors are hereditary. It is an estimate that 35% of the *difference* between individuals with clefts and those without may be attributable to genetic factors. Furthermore, an estimate such as this is only true for the population from which the twins were a sample. Since all the studies surveyed were essentially Caucasian inferences from the stated heritability, estimates should be to Caucasian populations only. Similarly, relative roles of environment and heredity would be expected to differ among families. In any case, heritability estimates are subject to much theoretical and practical reservation. Nevertheless, twin data reflect and confirm that which is generally accepted about the causes of facial clefts. Both genetic and environmental factors are involved. Presumably fetuses differ genetically in their susceptibility to those intrauterine environmental variables that lead to maxillofacial dysmorphology. At this writing the twin literature does not support different proportions of genetic and environmental input in clefts of the lip and palate as opposed to isolated cleft palate.

Family studies

The literature on familial analyses of facial clefts has been reviewed previously.[31, 55, 70, 115] From the earliest studies it has been recognized that facial clefts manifest familial clustering. For example, in his classical study, Fogh-Andersen[31] studied the families of 703 probands with cleft lip or cleft palate or both. If one calculates the number of relatives (first

cousins and closer) of these probands, 214 out of 24,889 had facial clefts. Since the incidence of all clefts in his population was 1.5/1000 live births, the expected number of affected relatives, if in fact no familial disposition existed, would have been thirty-seven. Clearly, the disposition to facial clefts was familial.

When one MZ twin is affected by a facial cleft, 35% of the time, on the average, the other twin will be similarly affected. This is at least 250 times the risk for the general population. Individuals who have a genotype identical to that of an individual with a cleft as well as having developed in the same uterine environment have a great chance of being equally susceptible to a facial cleft. However, DZ twins, who in general develop under conditions as similar as those of MZ twins, are concordant for facial clefts only about 6% of the time. Although this concordance percentage, too, is greater than chance, it is approximately equal to sib concordance and much lower than MZ concordance. Therefore a similar intrauterine environment is insufficient by itself to predispose to clefts. Similarly the discordance between MZ twins rules out the sufficiency of genetic factors as solitary etiological agents. On the other hand the far greater concordance between MZ twins in comparison with DZ twins supports a genetic component (p. 482). Accordingly, facial cleft susceptibility is familial with both genetic and environmental components.

For over a hundred and fifty years the hereditary basis for the familial occurrence of clefts has been supposed. However, early reports suffered from several shortcomings. They were based on hospital records, which are often incomplete; in several studies only parent-child concordance was considered hereditary, and only rarely were unaffected relatives recorded. The modern work began with a large study by Birkenfeld.[5] Between that time and the milestone work of Fogh-Andersen,[31] numerous interpretations of the data were offered. In these studies, over 25% of the cases were found to be associated with at least one affected family member in addition to the index case. Among the suggested modes of transmission offered in these studies were autosomal dominant, autosomal recessive, sex-linked recessive, "double-recessivity" (autosomal and sex-linked or partially sex-linked), "polymeric recessivity," irregular or partial autosomal dominance and "polyhybrid recessivity." von Versheur[137] believed that different hereditary dispositions could lead to clinical clefts but that "irregular dominance" was the usual form taken. He did acknowledge exogenous causes in some cases. Accordingly, theories for the genetic basis of facial clefts ranged from recessivity to irregular dominance. Despite the variety of suggested modes of transmission, it was acknowledged early that different patterns existed in different families. Failure to provide a simple explanation did not detract from the fact that positive family history, greater concordance in MZ twins in comparison with DZ twins, increased incidence in sibs, and significant differences in the frequency of clefts among inbred strains of mice indicate a meaningful genetic contribution to facial cleft predisposition.

Single gene models for the genetic component of most facial clefts are not supported by family studies.* Even if cleft palate is separated from CL ± CP as first proposed by Fogh-Andersen,[31] segregation ratios and relative risks of family members of probands with different degrees of relationship are inconsistent with a single gene model. To be sure, facial clefts are associated with specific monogenic syndromes,[43] but these comprise only a small portion of the total. An alternative explanation for the genetic component is a polygenic model in which the genetic component of facial cleft susceptibility resides in a number of genes. Under this model it is assumed that some large number of genes concerned with maxillofacial maldevelopment is distributed throughout a population. There results a continuum of genetic predispositions to the malformations. For an individual's genotype to confer susceptibility to teratogenic environmental agents, a critical combination of risk genes must occur together. For the genetic predisposition to be expressed, however, it is necessary that a sufficient number of factors, both genetic and environmental, interact so that the involved developmental pathway gets pushed over a threshold beyond which abnormalities are expressed.

The quasicontinuous model

A quasicontinuous trait is a qualitative trait in which its presence or absence or expressivity is thought to be due to variation of many genetic loci and many environmental agents. It is considered that there is an underlying normally distributed variable called *liability*.[27, 28] Manifestation of the trait depends on whether an individual's liability occurs above or below a particular threshold or thresholds.* This total phenotypic liability is multifactorial: it is the sum of two independent variables, genetic liability and environmental liability. Each of these depends on the independent action of genetic and environmental agents, each of which has small additive affects. The quasicontinuous model for facial cleft development[13, 32, 33] leads to several predictions, which can be examined in light of accumulated data.

Since it has been assumed that a large number of independent genetic variables are involved in facial cleft susceptibility, their distribution in a population will approach a normal distribution. Some individuals will possess many of these risk genes, some will possess few, and the majority of the population will possess a moderate number. Whether an organism develops a cleft will depend also on intrauterine environmental factors. Only a portion of individuals with a large number of risk genes will develop a cleft, depending on other genes and on environmental factors. However, all individuals with a cleft will possess a high proportion of the genes.

Assuming, then, that the distribution of degree of liability among individuals in the population is described by the normal or Gaussian curve of variation, the bulk of the population is concentrated in the midrange, and few individuals occur at each extreme.

---

*See references 7, 31, 55, 130, 141, 144.

*See references 13, 27, 28, 48, 49, 145.

We assume also that some critical number of so-called liability factors establishes a threshold at one end of the distribution. The liability of an individual who possesses a sufficient number of factors to predispose to a cleft is by definition beyond the threshold. Individuals who fall beneath the threshold (the majority) are not liable to the malformation. Those who do surpass the threshold are liable.

Edwards,[26] using the threshold model and several reasonable assumptions, showed that a trait with an incidence in the general population of p would be expected to have an incidence on the order of the $\sqrt{p}$ in first-degree relatives of probands. For CL ± CP,

a population frequency of $p = 0.00135$ (Table 16-2) should lead to a recurrence risk in first-degree relatives of CL ± CP subject of 0.0367. The average risk in first-degree relatives from several series was 0.0334 (Table 16-2). For isolated cleft palate, $p = 0.0004$ ($\sqrt{p} = 0.02$), and for observed affected first-degree relatives, $p = 0.0269$ (Table 16-3). Therefore, for CL ± CP and cleft palate the observed values coincide well with the expectations generated by the threshold model.

Further predictions based on the threshold model can be made and these estimates compared with data from various sources. Two assumptions are made, (1) that liabilities are

Table 16-2. Degree of relationship to CL ± CP proband and frequency of being similarly affected*

	Total number	Number affected	Percent affected	× population frequency
Population frequency	—	—	0.00135	—
First-degree relatives	6206	207	0.0334	24.7
Second-degree relatives	12,819	80	0.0062	4.6
Third-degree relatives	16,834	59	0.0035	2.6

*Modified from Carter, C. O.: The inheritance of common congenital malformations, Prog. Med. Genet. 4:59-84, 1965; Bixler, D., Fogh-Andersen, P., and Conneally, P. M.: Incidence of cleft lip and palate in the offspring of cleft parents, Clin. Genet. 2:155-159, 1971; Henriksson, T.-G.: Cleft lip and palate in Sweden; a genetic and clinical investigation, Institute for Medical Genetics, Uppsala, Sweden, 1971, University of Uppsala, pp. 1-79; Woolf, C. M.: Congenital cleft lip, J. Med. Genet. 8:65-71, 1971; and Stonova, N. S., and Messina, V. M.: A study of the family histories of patients with hare lip and cleft palate, Soviet Genet. 8:777-782, 1974.

Table 16-3. Degree of relationship to cleft palate proband and frequency of being similarly affected*

	Total number	Number affected	Percent affected	× population frequency
Population frequency	—	—	0.0004	—
First-degree relatives	2229	60	0.0269	67.3
Second-degree relatives	4173	24	0.0058	14.4
Third-degree relatives	4707	18	0.0038	9.5

*Modified from Bixler, D., Fogh-Andersen, P., and Conneally, P. M.: Incidence of cleft lip and palate in the offspring of cleft parents, Clin. Genet. 2:155-159, 1971; Henriksson, T.-G.: Cleft lip and palate in Sweden: a genetic and clinical investigation, Institute for Medical Genetics, Uppsala, Sweden, 1971, University of Uppsala, pp. 1-79; Stonova, N. S., and Messina, V. M.: A study of the family histories of patients with hare lip and cleft palate, Soviet Genet. 8:777-782, 1974; and Woolf, C. M., Woolf, R. M., and Broadbent, T. R.: A genetic study of cleft lip and palate in Utah, Am. J. Hum. Genet. 15:209-215, 1963.

distributed normally both in the general population and in relatives of probands and (2) that the variance is equal in distributions of these groups. The second assumption may be untrue but permits application of standard deviation units, which provides a basis for evaluating actual data. We can estimate liability in terms of standard deviation (S.D.) of the mean of the normal distribution.[27, 28]

We know, for example, from the properties of a normal curve, that if 2½% of the population are affected we can say that a threshold exists at + 2 S.D. above the mean. We may assume further that the mean liability of affected individuals lies someplace above +2.0 S.D., say 2.5 S.D. Therefore there is a difference *(X)* of 2.5 S.D. between the mean of the population and the mean of affected individuals. Now, first-degree relatives of probands have on the average half their genes in common, so that the mean of first-degree relatives will fall halfway between the mean of the population and the mean of the probands, or X/2. The distribution of first-degree relatives is shifted toward the threshold. The question now is, What proportion of the first-degree relatives' curve falls beyond the threshold? If the mean of this distribution lies halfway between the population mean and the proband mean, the mean of first-degree relatives occurs at 1.25 S.D. units above the mean of the general population.

Therefore the mean of first-degree relatives of probands coincides with +1.25 S.D. of the general population curve. The threshold based on population frequency was at 2.0 S.D. above the mean. Since the mean of first-degree relatives occurs at +1.25 S.D. of the general population and the threshold was at +2.0 S.D. of this distribution, the difference between the mean of first-degree relatives and the population threshold is +0.75 S.D. Therefore at +0.75 S.D. of their distribution, first-degree relatives surpass the liability threshold. If one refers to a table of areas under a normal curve, it is seen that about 77% of the first-degree relative population occurs below +0.75 S.D. of the mean—the threshold—and about 23% of first-degree relatives occur beyond the threshold. With the example used of a population frequency of 2½%, about 23% of first-degree relatives have a liability above the threshold for the trait. Second-degree relatives on the average possess a quarter of their genes in common. Therefore the mean of second-degree relatives would fall at 0.75 S.D. above the mean of the general population (X/4). Therefore the threshold for this group occurs at 1.25 S.D. (threshold [2.0 S.D.] – mean of second-degree relatives [0.75 S.D.] = 1.25 S.D.) of the distribution of the second-degree relatives. Reference to the table shows that about 8.5% of second-degree relatives surpass the thresh-

Table 16-4. Comparison of facial cleft frequencies in relatives of probands with estimates based on population frequencies using the quasicontinuous model*

	CL ± CP		Cleft palate	
	Expected	*Observed*	*Expected*	*Observed*
Population frequency	—	0.0014	—	0.0004
First-degree relatives	0.0392	0.0334	0.0582	0.0269
Second-degree relatives	0.0062	0.0062	0.0067	0.0058
Third-degree relatives	0.0019	0.0035	0.0017	0.0038

*Modified from Carter, C. O.: The inheritance of common congenital malformations, Prog. Med. Genet. 4:59-84, 1965; Bixler, D., Fogh-Andersen, P., and Conneally, P. M.: Incidence of cleft lip and palate in the offspring of cleft parents, Clin. Genet. 2:155-159, 1971; Henriksson, T.-G.: Cleft lip and palate in Sweden; a genetic and clinical investigation, Institute for Medical Genetics, Uppsala, Sweden, 1971, University of Uppsala, pp. 1-79; Woolf, C. M.: Congenital cleft lip, J. Med. Genet. 8:65-71, 1971; Stonova, N. S., and Messina, V. M.: A study of the family histories of patients with hare lip and cleft palate, Soviet Genet. 8:777-782, 1974; and Woolf, C. M., Woolf, R. M., and Broadbent, T. R.: A genetic study of cleft lip and palate in Utah, Am. J. Hum. Genet. 15:209-215, 1963.

old. Similarly about 4.5% of third-degree relatives who have an eighth of their genes in common with probands surpass the threshold.

We may apply the quasicontinuous model to actual data. In Table 16-4 estimates based on population frequencies of CL ± CP and cleft palate are compared with data obtained from several studies. As expected risk falls off sharply between first- and second-degree relatives and less sharply between second- and third-degree relatives, by the time fourth-degree relatives of probands are reached, the distinction between these individuals and the general population is slight. The data for CL ± CP and cleft palate fit these expectations reasonably well, as do data for other congenital malformations such as talipes equinovarus, congenital dislocation of the hip, and congenital pyloric stenosis.[14]

Another prediction of the quasicontinuous model is related to sex incidence differences. If sex differences exist, risks to relatives of the less frequently affected sex should be greater, since the affected individuals of the less frequently affected sex are likely to be more extreme deviants. We assume that liability exists above the threshold number of liability factors. The normal curve of the more frequently affected sex is shifted toward the threshold. Accordingly, the mean of this sex is closer to the threshold. These affected individuals do not occupy so deviant a segment of their curve as do affected individuals of the less frequently affected sex. Subjects of the sex less often affected are near the tail of the distribution and should possess more predisposing genes than do subjects of the other sex. The frequency of the trait in near relatives ought to be higher when the proband is of the less often affected sex. This prediction from the threshold model is borne out. A summary of data from several studies (Table 16-5) shows that CL ± CP occurs in nearly a 2:1 ratio of male to female. Sibs of female and male probands were similarly affected 4.71% and 3.37% of the time, respectively. Offspring of female and male probands were affected 4.30% and 3.25% of the time, respectively. Conversely, cleft palate occurs more frequently in females. Risk for cleft palate is greater in sibs of male probands and possibly greater in offspring of male cleft palate probands (Table 16-6).

Table 16-5. Sex of proband with CL ± CP and frequency of similarly affected relatives

| Sibs | Proband | | Offspring | Proband | |
	Male (514)	Female (265)		Male (472)	Female (284)
Number	1187	680	Number	749	477
Affected	40	32	Affected	23	20
Percentage	0.0337	0.0471	Percentage	0.0307	0.0419
Source	Stonova and Messina,[130] Woolf,[140] and Henriksson[55]		Source	Bixler and associates,[7] Woolf and associates,[142] Roberts,[106] and Fujino and associates[39]	

Table 16-6. Sex of proband with cleft palate and frequency of similarly affected relatives

| Sibs | Proband | | Offspring | Proband | |
	Male	Female		Male (79)	Female (106)
Number	125	256	Number	144	225
Affected	7	6	Affected	8	11
Percentage	0.0560	0.0234	Percentage	0.0556	0.0489
Source	Fraser[33] and Stonova and Messina[130]		Source	Fujino and associates[39] and Bixler and co-workers[7]	

Table 16-7. Recurrence risk for sibs according to severity of cleft in the proband*

	Number of sibs	Number affected	Percentage affected
Bilateral CL ± CP	658	37	5.62
Unilateral CL ± CP	1696	70	4.13
Unilateral cleft lip	797	21	2.63

*From Fraser, F. C.: The genetics of cleft lip and cleft palate, Am. J. Hum. Genet. **22**:336-353, 1970.

Table 16-8. Empirical recurrence risks of same type clefts*

Parents	Sibs		Percentage of CL ± CP	Percentage of cleft palate
	Affected	Normal		
Normal	1	0	4.0	3.5
	1	1	4.0	3.0
	2	0	14.0	13.0
One affected	0	0	4.0	3.5
	1	0	12.0	10.0
	1	1	10.0	9.0
	2	0	25.0	24.0
Both affected	0	0	35.0	25.0
	1	0	45.0	4.0
	1	1	40.0	35.0
	2	0	50.0	45.0

*From Tolarová, M.: Empirical recurrence risk figures for genetic counseling of clefts, Acta Chir. Plast. (Praha) **14**:234-235, 1972.

A further prediction based on the multifactorial-threshold model is that more severely affected individuals represent more extreme phenodeviants than do less severely affected ones. The state of being more or less phenodeviant with this model relates directly to distance from the population mean. A more phenodeviant individual would occur at the most tail end of the curve and would by definition possess more risk genes. Relatives of such an indivdual should be more at risk than would relatives of a less severely affected individual. Too little data exist to test this hypothesis for cleft palate. However, in Table 16-7 it is clear that if one considers unilateral cleft lip the mildest and bilateral cleft lip and palate the most severe expression of CL ± CP, the risk to sibs is indeed greatest if the proband is more severely affected. Woolf and associates[144] and Woolf[140] supported the notion that unilateral and bilateral cleft lip and palate are part of a genetic continuum in which more genes are associated with the bilateral condition. However, their data did not support the hypothesis that CL ± CP and cleft lip are part of the same continuum insofar as severity is associated with number of genes.

Empirical risks for facial clefts

Observed risks of recurrence among relatives of affected individuals provided much of the basis for the quasicontinuous explanation for facial cleft occurrence. Therefore use of these data to substantiate the model may be circular. However, empirical risk figures have utility in terms of recurrence counseling. As developed in the previous section, the multifactorial model predicts that the liability distribution of relatives of probands lies between the population distribution and that of probands. Hence a relative of an affected individual would be more at risk than a person chosen randomly from the population. Nevertheless, when one individual in a family is affected by a cleft, he or she is a sporadic case and the cleft may be due to any one of numerous factors, and risk predictions for subsequent cases in close relatives cannot be made with confidence. There is an indication that within that family there may be more predisposing factors than in families in whom no cleft occurred. When within a family more than one individual is affected and a single gene basis is ruled out, the probability increases decidedly that there exists within that family a multifactorial milieu that indeed predisposes to clefts. The expected increase in risk as the number of affected relatives increases is consistent with the multifactorial model and is of course different from expectations with single gene traits where segregation values are fixed once the mode of transmission is established. In Table 16-8 empirical risk figures for CL ± CP and cleft palate are given. These may provide a basis for counseling. However, it cannot be too strongly stated that these data are based on previous surveys. They in no way have the predictive validity of risk probabilities associated with single gene traits.

Heritability

Heritability is that portion of variance for a trait within a population attributable to genetic factors. This has been a traditional parameter with experimental species, but in man heritability usually has been derived from twin studies. With his introduction of the concept of "liability," Falconer[27, 28] developed a method for determining the heritability of liability to a multifactorial condition. He defined liability as "a graded scale of the degree of affectedness or of normal having a value above which an individual is abnormal and below which an individual is considered normal."[27] Liabilities of individuals in a population form a continuous variable and are assumed to be normally distributed. To express liability, a scale of measurement must be chosen that is also normally distributed, for example, standard deviations from the threshold. With the assumptions that liability is normally distributed and that only additive genetic variances are present, regression of relatives on index cases can be accomplished. From this regression heritability can then be determined.

Using Falconer's[27] method on data from the paper by Woolf and co-workers,[141] we have calculated heritabilities for CL ± CP (Table 16-9). Based on the regression of first-degree relatives on affected individuals it was determined that about 80% of the variability seen in liability to CL ± CP is due to additive genetic variance. This is in close agreement with heritabilities given previously.[14] It was also noted that predictions of incidence in second- and third-degree relatives within the errors of the method were in reasonably close agreement to observed incidences. The validity of these estimates is enhanced by the

Table 16-9. Estimates of heritability of liability for CL ± CP based on known frequency in general population and relatives

Calculation based on	Heritability percentage	
	Henriksson[55]	Calculated on data from Woolf and associates[141]
First-degree relatives	78	81
Second-degree relatives	88	72
Third-degree relatives	—	84

similarity of estimates based on first-, second-, and third-degree relatives.

A similar analysis was performed by Henriksson.[55] He, too, found estimates of the heritability of liability for CL ± CP about 80% (Table 16-9). The crossed-sex estimates of heritabilities for probands and relatives of unlike sex appeared to be consistent with those for probands and relatives of like sex. This finding suggested that genetic liability in the two sexes largely depends on the same genes. Furthermore, the similarity of estimates between sibs and parents suggests that the fact that sibs share a more similar environment is of no particular consequence. Similar estimates were also obtained for aunts, uncles, and grandparents indicating the same degree of genetic predisposition for these categories.

Estimates of the heritability of liability of cleft palate showed much greater variation, which could be attributed to small sample size. The heritabilities of first-degree relatives were within the expected values, but those of second-degree and particularly of third-degree relatives were unacceptably high. The presence of a major gene will increase heritability estimates made on the assumption of polygenic inheritance to over 100% for first-degree relatives and even more for second- and third-degree relatives.[26] Henriksson[55] concluded that on the basis of the evidence from his and previous investigations the genetic determinance of CL ± CP is best explained as polygenic. Evidence for a polygenic basis for cleft palate was less convincing. It was possible, based on his heritability findings, that single gene mutations are instrumental in some cases of familial occurrence of cleft palate.

It must be stressed that variance analyses as summarized by heritability are mathematical constructs that in no way reveal etiological or pathogenetic mechanisms involved in facial maldevelopment. Heritability estimates do not provide us with tools to treat or prevent the conditions under consideration. In fact calculated risk figures tell us no more than the empirical figures with which these hypotheses are compared.[30] On the other hand, the models on which these mathematical manipulations are based are of heuristic value. The complexity of underlying mechanisms is confirmed. In comparison with other models, the data can, at present, be viewed best in the context of the quasicontinuous model. This model is by no means an explanation. It provides a framework within which new questions can be asked.

Microforms

When presumed subclinical manifestations (microforms) of clinical syndromes occur more frequently in relatives of individuals with the complete syndrome than in the general population, they are likely to be associated with similar or identical genotypes.[55] Among the conditions that have been suggested as microforms of cleft lip, cleft palate, or both are malformed or missing maxillary permanent lateral incisors,[61, 64, 74] hypertelorism,[93] hypotelorism,[6] nostril asymmetry,[33] raphe or notched upper lip,[20] notching of the alveolus,[20] a high or narrow Gothic palate,[79, 126] dental abnormalities,[62] laminographically seen nasopalatine bone abnormalities,[40] submucous cleft palate,[12, 131] cleft (bifid) uvula,[82, 123] congenital palatal incompetence,[104] and facial topographical dimensions.[97] Unfortunately most speculations concerning microforms of facial clefts have not been tested rigorously. Woolf and co-workers,[143] in a well-controlled study,

ruled out missing or anomalous maxillary lateral incisors as a microform of clefting. Mills and associates[87] and Pashayan and co-workers[98] examined relatives of cleft patients and ruled out nostril asymmetry as a microform of CL(P). Laminagraphically observed nasopalatine segment abnormalities were not confirmed by Niswander.[92] In a survey of palatal dimensions of sibs and parents of CL ± CP probands, no differences were found when compared with control subjects.[119]

Of the suggested microforms of facial clefts, congenital pharyngeal incompetence (CPI), submucous cleft palate (SMCP), and cleft or bifid uvula (CU) are the most secure.

Submucous palatal clefts result from imperfect muscle union across the velum but with an intact mucosal surface. The palate is usually short and velopharyngeal closure is incompetent, resulting in hypernasal speech. SMCP is relatively uncommon. In their survey of over 10,000 randomly screened Denver school children, Stewart and co-workers[128] found SMCP in 1 in 1200. Because of its obvious anatomical relationship to cleft palate, SMCP seems to be a legitimate microform even though no family studies have been reported.

Congenital pharyngeal incompetence (CPI) is a condition in which a patient's speech is reminiscent of cleft palate speech but no morphological defect is apparent. Inability to seal the velopharyngeal opening may be due to structural or functional abnormalities of any structures contiguous with the opening, including soft palate, oral pharynx, and vertebral atlas.[102] Overt clefts of the lip and/or palate may occur with greater frequency in relatives of such individuals.[101] Furthermore, of 110 CPI subjects, 81% presented one or more of (1) bifid uvula, (2) zona pellucida of the soft palate and/or short soft palate, and (3) SMCP. These associated defects are also good candidates as microforms of facial clefts.

Cleft uvula

Replicated racial comparisons and family studies establish cleft uvula as the most secure microform of maxillofacial clefts. The uvula

Table 16-10. Cleft uvula incidence in different races of man

Racial group	Number examined	Number with cleft uvula	Number of studies	Mean frequency percentage
Japanese	4726	462	1	9.78
Chinese	191	13	1	6.81
American Indian	2508	348	3	13.87
Inuit	1868	146	2	7.82
Caucasian	29,661	440	7	1.48
Negro	4275	14	2	0.33

is a pendulous muscular mass in the midline suspended from the posterior edge of the soft palate. Fusion or merging is sometimes incomplete,[10] resulting in a cleft or bifid structure. The most complete as well as recent review of cleft uvula is that of Heathcote.[54] Surveys throughout the world confirm that the relative racial prevalence of cleft uvula is Mongoloid (10.43% [N = 9293]) > Caucasian (2.08% [N = 20,716]) > Negro (0.33% [N = 4274]) (Table 16-10). Of particular interest is the agreement among estimates made on populations of similar racial stock living in different areas of the world. These observations support strongly a genetic basis for the racial differences. Moreover, data from family studies reflect a genetic basis for this trait, which is best explained on a quasicontinuous basis.[16, 123] In an elegant test of the proposition that cleft uvula is a microform of the more severe facial clefts, Meskin and associates[82] examined relatives of probands affected by CL ± CP or by cleft palate. Cleft uvula prevalence in first-degree relations of cleft palate and CL ± CP probands was 11.2% and 17.1%, respectively. These frequencies were significantly greater than the cleft uvula prevalence of less than 1.5% in the general population from which these families were chosen. These data supported the hypothesis that cleft uvula is a microform of cleft palate and "also the cleft palate portion of the cleft lip/cleft palate complex."[82] It should be noted that the microform relationship of cleft uvula to cleft lip and cleft palate is an apparent contradiction[54] of the separate entity hypothesis implicating secondary mechanical causation of palatal clefts in embryos with cleft lip pathogenesis.[34]

The notion that cleft uvula is a microform of cleft lip or cleft palate or both has been suggested also from epidemiological data.[16, 54, 113, 122] Findings of a parallel between cleft uvula frequency and facial cleft frequency in different races strongly support this viewpoint. It is assumed that for cleft uvula to be expressed, an individual must possess a threshold number of "palatal nonfusion factors." Similarly, a threshold, but a more deviant one, exists for phenotypic expression of cleft lip or cleft palate or both. On the basis of the available epidemiological data it appears that the gene pool of some populations contains more of those genes which contribute to incomplete palatal fusion than do others. Apparently a larger number of these nonfusion genes occur in the Mongoloid race than in the Caucasian, which in turn possesses more than does the Negro population. Accordingly, one may think of the spectrum of microforms and related characteristics associated with facial clefts and the clefts themselves as comprising a family of quasicontinuous traits.[122]

Developmental instability

Fraser[33] discussed a generalized developmental instability as theoretically associated with facial cleft formation. This could account for the possible increase in other malformations associated with CL ± CP and cleft palate.[95] However, data on this point have been inconsistent.[33] Developmental instability may be viewed in another way. Whereas Fraser referred to a generalized developmental instability, one may view relative epigenetic stabilities among the many developmental pathways within an individual organism. Within a species the genotype is buffered in such a way that development is "canalized" and ordinarily proceeds along evolved developmental tracks.[138] Developmental pathways vary in their stability depending on their degree of canalization. Some are more readily displaced from the normal or standard phenotype by genetic and environmental trauma than are others.[120] Facial clefts are associated with numerous mutant single genes.[43] A large number of presumably unrelated teratogenic agents may induce clefts experimentally. All of the autosomal aneuploid states are associated with an increased risk of facial clefts. The relatively great susceptibility of lip and palatal development to such a wide variety of agents suggests that these (lip and palate) developmental pathways are indeed less stable than others in the embryonic organism.

It has been postulated that autosomal trisomy results in decreased buffering of developmental pathways and that one might expect to observe greater liability to malformation of ordinarily less stable traits.[118] Further evidence for "amplified developmental instability" in Down's syndrome (DS) was described.[120] In 21-trisomics, relatively less stable characteristics are abnormal much more frequently and more profoundly than in normal populations. If, in fact, such a pathogenetic mechanism exists in DS and if clefts represent a manifestation of developmental instability, then the frequency of clefts should be greater in DS. Recent surveys suggest that cleft lip or cleft palate or both occur in about 1 in 200 DS subjects or about ten times that in the general population.[43] Schendel and Gorlin[114] found that cleft uvula and SMCP also are about ten times more frequent in DS than in the general population. Their data supported the hypothesis of Shapiro[118] that the increase in facial cleft incidence in DS is due to the effect of trisomy on relatively unstable traits. According to a polygenic theory for the occurrence of facial clefts, thresholds for their manifestation are lowered,

and their increased frequency in DS reflects greater liability to precipitating factors. The parallel increased incidence of facial clefts and their microforms in Down's syndrome (trisomy 21) supports (1) the multifactorial basis of clefts of the uvula, palate, and lip and (2) the validity of cleft uvula and SMCP as microforms of facial clefts.

Relationship between cleft palate and CL ± CP

In much of the discussion presented in earlier sections, data on cleft palate were distinguished from those on CL ± CP. This distinction was first suggested by Fogh-Andersen,[31] in whose study sex ratios and familial clustering reflected an etiological identity of cleft lip and CL + CP, whereas these phenotypes appeared to be etiologically distinct from cleft palate. He found that the male-to-female sex ratio for cleft lip and CL + CP was about 2:1, and the ratio in cleft palate was about 1:2. First-degree relatives of cleft lip and CL + CP probands had a greater risk for cleft lip or CL + CP (0.85%) than did his general population (0.11%). However, the frequency of cleft palate in relatives of these probands was no different from the population frequency. Similarly, first-degree relatives of cleft palate probands were affected 0.73% of the time with cleft palate, which was far greater than the general population incidence (0.04%). CL ± CP occurred in only 0.05% of relatives of these cleft palate probands, which was no different from the population risk. Fogh-Andersen concluded that CL ± CP and cleft palate were distinct genetic entities. Most family studies of facial clefts since have supported this etiological distinction.* In general, cleft lip and CL + CP clustered within families, and cleft palate clustered in other families. Alternate types of clefts did not occur within the same families at frequencies any greater than that in the general population. Support for this segregation of cleft types comes from embryological evidence. In humans the lip develops between 5 and 8 weeks

---

*See references 7, 36, 38, 41, 56, 65, 111, 141.

in utero and the palate at about the ninth week. Fraser[33, 34] hypothesized that mechanical effects of cleft lip could secondarily cause cleft palate, which would account for the coincidence of the two types in families in whom cleft lip liabilities existed. On the other hand, secondary palatal maldevelopment could occur after complete formation of the primary palate. This kind of disposition would lead to cleft palate only in some families. Experiments with mice provided some evidence that such an explanation was plausible.[134]

Despite evidence for the apparent separation of cleft palate on the one hand and CL ± CP on the other, conflicting data exist that contraindicate definitive conclusions. In his major review of race and congenital malformations, Neel[91] opined that since both defects (cleft palate and CL ± CP) are, within error, increased to about the same extent from Negro to Caucasian to Mongoloid, no support is lent to the relative independence of cleft palate versus CL ± CP. Witkop[139] found that facial clefts occurred extremely frequently in Halowar Indians (CL ± CP, 1 in 125, and cleft palate, 1 in 234). He concluded also that CL ± CP and cleft palate segregate within the same families in this population. Rank and Thomson[105] examined several thousand relatives of CL ± CP and cleft palate probands in Tasmania. As expected, cleft lip and CL + CP alternated freely within families. Similarly, relatives of cleft palate probands were affected more frequently than expected by chance. However, the frequency of cleft palate in relatives of

CL ± CP probands was about five times the population risk. The frequency of CL ± CP in relatives of cleft palate probands was about 2½ times the population risk. According to these investigators, cleft palate must be produced by the same genetic system as CL ± CP in some families. Although these data supported the existence of separate genetic systems controlling the formation of CL ± CP and of cleft palate alone, the two conditions were not entirely independent in all families; some cleft palates appeared to be due to the lip-and-palate complex, and others were due to the cleft palate system. Furthermore, in an analysis of pedigrees it was found that cleft palate occurred in the same genealogy as CL ± CP in sixteen of forty-seven kindreds (34%). Drillien and co-workers[25] also observed several families in their study in whom alternate-type clefts occurred between parents and children. Woolf[140] noted that the frequency of cleft palate in all relatives of CL ± CP probands was approximately equal that in the general population. However, the frequency of cleft palate was 5.7 and 1.7 times greater in first- and second-degree relatives, respectively, than in third-degree relatives. Furthermore, the incidence in first-degree relatives was about five times that of the general population. There seemed to him to be evidence that a polygenic system can exist that affects both the palate and lip. Moreover, the distinction between CL ± CP and cleft palate apparently becomes progressively less clear as the degree of relationship to the proband decreases.[89]

The syndrome of pits of the lower lip and

Table 16-11. Type of defect found in offspring of parents with lip pits and a cleft*

| | | Offspring | | | | |
| | | Clefts with or without pits | | | | |
Parents affected with	*Pits only*	*Palate*	*Lip*	*Lip and palate*	*None*	*Total*
Pits and cleft palate	9	13	1	6	18	47
Pits and cleft lip	5	1	2	3	3	14
Pits and cleft lip and palate	13	6	0	20	32	71

*From Červenka, J., Gorlin, R. J., and Anderson, V. E.: The syndrome of pits of the lower lip and/or cleft palate, Am. J. Hum. Genet. **19:**416-433, 1967.

cleft lip and/or cleft palate (van der Woude's syndrome) was reviewed by Červenka and associates.[15] Although an association between the types of clefts in parents and their children was noted, alternate-type clefts did occur in this autosomal dominant trait (Table 16-11). This syndrome demonstrates clearly that a single etiological agent, in this case a mutant gene, can produce clefts of the lip, the lip and palate, or the palate alone. Accordingly, the genetic independence of clefts of the primary and secondary palate cannot be so complete as some authors have claimed. Moreover, the syndrome occurs too rarely to have accounted for more than a small proportion of families just cited in whom alternate-type clefting occurred. The microform cleft uvula may shed some light on this issue, also. Meskin and associates[82] examined relatives of thirty CL ± CP and twenty cleft palate probands for the presence of cleft uvula. Cleft uvula prevalence in the general population from which these families were chosen was about 1.4%.[81] Frequencies of cleft uvula in relatives of cleft probands were 8.9% in CL ± CP families and 12.6% in cleft palate families. These frequencies were significantly greater than expected by chance. The increased frequency of cleft uvula in relatives of CL ± CP probands is enigmatic. Obviously in these relatives cleft uvula is not a mechanical consequence of cleft lip. This seeming contradiction of the separate entity hypothesis is especially puzzling in view of the data[34] implicating mechanical causation of palatal clefts in embryos with cleft lip pathogenesis. The most extreme dissenting opinion concerning two genetic systems was presented by Chabora and Horowitz,[17] who analyzed selected facial cleft families from previously published series. They found that (1) the occurrence of cleft palate in families with CL ± CP probands was approximately seven times greater than expected from published population incidence figures and (2) the occurrence of CL ± CP in cleft palate pedigrees was five times greater than the frequency expected from population incidence figures. In studying alternate cleft families they found also that genetic predisposition occurred on the same side of the family too frequently to be attributed to chance. These authors concluded that a family in whom cleft palate occurs has a greater liability to CL ± CP than the general population. Similarly a family with CL ± CP has an increased liability to cleft palate. They concluded that CL ± CP and cleft palate are caused by a single genetic system.

At this time the exceptions to the dual entity assumption for clefts of the primary and secondary palates are insufficient to discount the overwhelming evidence of most family studies, which indicate their separateness. On the other hand, these exceptions point out clearly that the sharp distinction between the two groups of clefts may be too severe. In some contexts the genetical and anatomical common denominators of midfacial maldevelopment may be segregating together within families and populations. These factors could predispose to both types of clefts. The bases of facial clefts are heterogeneous. Simple explanations may be satisfying but cannot accurately reflect pathogenesis.

The lip and palate are exceedingly sensitive meters of trauma to the developing organism. Developmental pathways leading to these structures are relatively unstable and accordingly frequently develop insufficiently. Single gene abnormalities, teratogenic environmental factors, and gross chromosomal anomalies can produce clefting malformations. Nevertheless, for the bulk of facial clefts in human populations, racial, familial, and microform data fit best with a quasicontinuous model in which a critical number of genetic and environmental factors act together to predispose to these unfortunate defects.

REFERENCES

1. Adams, M. S., and Niswander, J. D.: Developmental "noise" and a congenital malformation, Genet. Res. Camb. 10:313-317, 1967.
2. Allen, G.: Twin research: problems and prospects, Prog. Med. Genet. 4:242-269, 1965.
3. Altemus, L. A., and Ferguson, A. D.: Comparative incidence of birth defects in Negro and white children, Pediatrics 36:56-61, 1965.

4. Beder, O. E., Coe, H. E., Braafladt, R. P., and Houle, J. D.: Factors associated with congenital cleft lip and cleft palate in the Pacific Northwest, Oral Surg. 9:1267-1273, 1956.

5. Birkenfeld, W.: Über die Erblichkeit der Lippenspalte und Gaumenspalte, Arch. Klin. Chir. 141:728-753, 1926.

6. Bixler, D., 1970: Cited by Fraser, F. C.: The genetics of cleft lip and cleft palate, Am. J. Hum. Genet. 22:336-353, 1970.

7. Bixler, D., Fogh-Andersen, P., and Conneally, P. M.: Incidence of cleft lip and palate in the offspring of cleft parents, Clin. Genet. 2: 155-159, 1971.

8. Böök, J. A.: The incidence of congenital diseases and defects in a South Swedish population, Acta Genet. Stat Med. 2:289-311, 1951.

9. Browne, G. A.: Birth rank and incidence of cleft lip and palate, N. Z. Dent. J. 65:176-179, 1969.

10. Burdi, A. R., and Faist, K.: Morphogenesis of the palate in normal human embryos with special emphasis on the mechanisms involved, Am. J. Anat. 120:149-160, 1967.

11. Burdi, A. R., and Silvey, R. G.: Sexual differences in closure of the human palatal shelves, Cleft Palate J. 6:1-7, 1969.

12. Calnan, J.: Submucous cleft palate, Br. J. Plast. Surg. 6:264-282, 1954.

13. Carter, C. O.: The inheritance of common congenital malformations, Prog. Med. Genet. 4:59-84, 1965.

14. Carter, C. O.: Genetics of common disorders, Br. Med. Bull. 25:52-57, 1969.

15. Červenka, J., Gorlin, R. J., and Anderson, V. E.: The syndrome of pits of the lower lip and cleft lip and/or cleft palate, Am. J. Hum. Genet. 19:416-433, 1967.

16. Červenka, J., and Shapiro, B. L.: Cleft uvula in Chippewa Indians: prevalence and genetics, Hum. Biol. 42:47-52, 1970.

17. Chabora, A. J., and Horowitz, S. L.: Cleft lip and cleft palate: one genetic system, Oral Surg. 38:181-186, 1974.

18. Chi, S., and Godfrey, K.: Cleft lip and cleft palate in New South Wales, Med. J. Aust. 2:1172-1176, 1970.

19. Chung, C. S., and Myrianthopoulus, N. C.: Racial and prenatal factors in major congenital malformations, Am. J. Hum. Genet. 20:44-60, 1968.

20. Coccia, C. T., Bixler, D., and Conneally, P. M.: Cleft lip and cleft palate: a genetic study, Cleft Palate J. 6:323-336, 1969.

21. Conway, H., and Wagner, K. J.: Incidence of clefts in New York City, Cleft Palate J. 3: 284-290, 1966.

22. Curtis, E. J., Fraser, F. C., and Warburton, D.: Congenital cleft lip and palate, Am. J. Dis. Child. 102:853-857, 1961.

23. Davis, J. S.: The incidence of congenital clefts of the lip and palate, Ann. Surg. 80: 363-374, 1924.

24. Douglas, B.: The role of environmental factors in the etiology of "so-called" congenital malformations, Plast. Reconstr. Surg. 22:214-229, 1958.

25. Drillien, C. M., Ingram, T. T. S., and Wilkinson, E. M.: The causes and natural history of cleft lip and palate, Edinburgh, 1966, Churchill Livingstone.

26. Edwards, J. H.: The simulation of mendelism, Acta Genet. 10:63-70, 1960.

27. Falconer, D. S.: The inheritance of liability to certain diseases, estimated from the incidence among relatives, Ann. Hum. Genet. 29:51-76, 1965.

28. Falconer, D. S.: The inheritance of liability to diseases with variable age of onset with particular reference to diabetes mellitus, Ann. Hum. Genet. 31:1-20, 1967.

29. Federspiel, M. N.: Harelip and cleft palate, St. Louis, 1927, The C. V. Mosby Co.

30. Feldman, M. W., and Lewontin, R. C.: The heritability hang-up, Science 190:1163-1168, 1975.

31. Fogh-Andersen, P.: Inheritance of hare lip cleft palate, Copenhagen, 1942, Munksgaard.

32. Fraser, F. C.: Hereditary disorders of the nose and mouth, Proceedings of the 2nd International Congress on Human Genetics, vol. 3, Rome, 1963, pp. 1852-1855.

33. Fraser, F. C.: The genetics of cleft lip and cleft palate, Am. J. Hum. Genet. 22:336-353, 1970.

34. Fraser, F. C.: Etiology of cleft lip and palate. In Grabb, W. C., Rosenstein, S. W., and Bzoch, K. R., editors: Cleft lip and palate, Boston, 1971, Little, Brown & Co., pp. 54-65.

35. Fraser, F. C.: Updating the genetics of cleft lip and cleft palate, Clin. Cytogenet. Genet. 10:107-111, 1974.

36. Fraser, F. C., and Baxter, H.: The familial distribution of congenital clefts of the lip and palate, Am. J. Surg. 87:656-659, 1954.

37. Fraser, G. R., and Calnan, J. S.: Cleft lip and palate: seasonal incidence, birth weight, birth rank, sex, site, associated malformations and parental age, Arch. Dis. Child. 36:420-423, 1961.

38. Fujino, H., Tanaka, K., and Sanui, Y.: Genetic study of cleft lips and cleft palates based upon 2828 Japanese cases, Kyushu J. Med. Sci. 14:317-331, 1963.

39. Fujino, H., Tashiro, Y., Sanui, Y., and Tanaka, K.: Empirical genetic risk among offspring of cleft lip and cleft palate patients, Jap. J. Hum. Genet. 12:62-68, 1967.

40. Fukuhara, T.: New method and approach to the genetics of cleft lip and cleft palate, J. Dent. Res. 44:259-268, 1965.

41. Fukuhara, T., and Saito, S.: Possible carrier status of hereditary cleft palate with cleft lip; report of cases, Bull. Tokyo Med. Dent. Univ. 10:333-341, 1963.

42. Gorlin, R. J.: Developmental anomalies of the face and oral structures. In Gorlin, R. J., and Goldman, H. M., editors: Thoma's oral pathology, St. Louis, 1970, The C. V. Mosby Co., pp. 21-95.

43. Gorlin, R. J.: Facial clefting and its syndromes, Birth Defects 7:3-49, 1971.

44. Grace, L. G.: Frequency of occurrence of cleft palates and harelips, J. Dent. Res. 22:495-497, 1943.

45. Greene, J. C.: Epidemiological research, 1964-1967, J. Am. Dent. Assoc. 76:1350-1356, 1968.

46. Greene, J. C., Vermillion, J. R., and Hay, S.: Utilization of birth certificates in epidemiologic studies of cleft lip and palate, Cleft Palate J. 2:141-156, 1965.

47. Greene, J. C., Vermillion, S. F., Gibbens, S. G., and Kerschbaum, S.: Epidemiologic study of cleft lip and cleft palate in four states, J. Am. Dent. Assoc. 68:387-404, 1964.

48. Grüneberg, H.: The genetics of a tooth defect in the mouse, Proc. R. Soc. Lond. (Biol.) 138:437-451, 1951.

49. Grüneberg, H.: Genetical studies on the skeleton of the mouse. IV. Quasi-continuous variations, J. Genet. 51:95-114, 1952.

50. Gylling, U.: Heredity of cleft lips and palates and factors influencing etiology, Excerpta Medica International Congress Series, no. 174, 1967, pp. 291-297.

51. Gylling, U., and Soivio, A. I.: Frequency, morphology and operative mortality in cleft lip and palate in Finland, Acta Chir. Scand. 123:1-5, 1962.

52. Harkins, C. S., Berlin, A., Harding, R. L., Longacre, J. J., and Snodgrasse, R. M.: A classification of cleft lip and cleft palate, Plast. Reconstr. Surg. 29:31-39, 1962.

53. Hay, S., and Wehrung, D. A.: Congenital malformations in twins, Am. J. Hum. Genet. 22:662-678, 1970.

54. Heathcote, G. M.: The prevalence of cleft uvula in an Inuit population, Am. J. Phys. Anthropol. 41:433-437, 1974.

55. Henriksson, T.-G.: Cleft lip and palate in Sweden: a genetic and clinical investigation, Institute for Medical Genetics, Uppsala, Sweden, 1971, University of Uppsala, pp. 1-79.

56. Ingalls, T. H., Taube, T. E., and Klingberg, R. A.: Cleft lip and palate: epidemiologic considerations, Plast. Reconstr. Surg. 34:1-10, 1964.

57. Ivy, R. H.: The influence of race on the incidence of certain congenital anomalies—notably cleft lip—cleft palate, Plast. Reconstr. Surg. 30:581-585, 1962.

58. Ivy, R. H.: Congenital anomalies as recorded on birth certificates in the Division of Vital Statistics of the Pennsylvania Department of Health for the period 1956-1960 inclusive, Plast. Reconstr. Surg. 32:361-367, 1963.

59. Jaffe, B. F., and Blanc, G. B.: Cleft palate, cleft lip and cleft uvula in Navajo Indians: incidence and otorhinolaryngologic problems, Cleft Palate J. 7:300-305, 1970.

60. Janerich, D. T.: Sex differences in the relative frequency of congenital oral clefts, Teratology 4:109-110, 1971.

61. John, A.: Anomalies of the lateral incisor in cases of harelip and cleft palate, Acta Odontol. Scand. 9:41-59, 1950.

62. Jordan, R., Kraus, B. C., and Neptune, C. M.: Dental abnormalities associated with cleft lip and/or palate, Cleft Palate J. 3:22-55, 1966.

63. Kernahan, D. A., and Stark, R. B.: A new classification for cleft lip and cleft palate, Plast. Reconstr. Surg. 22:435-441, 1958.

64. Kirkham, H. L. D.: Dentition in cleft palate cases, Int. J. Orthodont. 17:1076-1083, 1931.

65. Kobayoshi, Y.: A genetic study of harelip and cleft palate, Jap. J. Hum. Genet. 3:73-107, 1958.

66. Krantz, H. C., and Henderson, F. M.: Relationship between maternal ancestry and incidence of cleft palate, J. Speech Disord. 12:267-278, 1947.

67. Leck, I.: Incidence of malformations following influenza epidemics, Br. J. Prev. Soc. Med. 17:70-80, 1963.

68. Leck, I.: The etiology of human malformations: insights from epidemiology, Teratology 5:303-314, 1972.

69. Leck, I., Hay, S., Witte, J. J., and Greene, J. C.: Malformations recorded on birth certificates following A2 influenza epidemics, Public Health Rep. 84:971-979, 1969.

70. Lehmann, W., and Ritter, R.: Die Stellung der Lippen-Kiefer-Gaumenspaltenträger im Gesetz zur Verhütung erbkranken Nachwuchses, Z. Menschl. Vererb. Konstitutionslehre 23:1-16, 1939.

71. Longnecker, C. G., Ryan, R. F., and Vincent, R.: The incidence of cleft lip and cleft palate

in Charity Hospital, Plast. Reconstr. Surg. **35:**548-550, 1965.

72. Loretz, W., Westmoreland, W. W., and Richards, L. R.: A study of cleft lip and cleft palate births in California, 1955, Am. J. Public Health **51:**873-877, 1961.

73. Lowry, R. B., and Renwick, D. H. G.: Incidence of cleft lip and palate in British Columbia Indians, J. Med. Gen. **6:**67-69, 1969.

74. Lucas, R. C.: On the congenital absence of an upper lateral incisor tooth as a forerunner of harelip and cleft palate; with cases, Trans. Clin. Soc. Lond. **21:**64-66, 1888.

75. Lutz, K. R., and Moore, F. B.: A study of factors in the occurrence of cleft palate, J. Speech Hear. Disord. **20:**271-276, 1955.

76. Mackeprang, M., and Hay, S.: Cleft lip and palate mortality study, Cleft Palate J. **9:**51-63, 1972.

77. McIntosh, R., Merritt, K., Richards, M., Samuels, M. T., and Bellows, M.: The incidence of congenital malformations in a study of 5964 pregnancies, Pediatrics **14:**505-522, 1954.

78. McKeown, T., and Record, R. B.: Malformations in a population observed for five years after birth. In Wolstenholme, G. E. W., and O'Connor, C. M., editors: Ciba Foundation Symposium on Congenital Malformations, Boston, 1960, Little, Brown & Co., pp. 2-16.

79. Mengele, J.: Sippenuntersuchungen bei Lippen-Kiefer-Gaumenspalte, Z. Menschl. Vererb. Konstitutionslehre **23:**17-42, 1939.

80. Meskin, L. H.: An epidemiologic study of factors related to the extent of facial clefts, Ph.D. thesis, Minneapolis, 1966, University of Minnesota.

81. Meskin, L. H., Gorlin, R. J., and Isaacson, R. J.: Abnormal morphology of the soft palate. I. The prevalence of cleft uvula, Cleft Palate J. **1:**342-346, 1964.

82. Meskin, L. H., Gorlin, R. J., and Isaacson, R. J.: Cleft uvula—a microform of cleft palate, Acta Chir. Plast. **8:**91-96, 1966.

83. Meskin, L. H., and Pruzansky, S.: Validity of the birth certificate in the epidemiologic assessment of facial clefts, J. Dent. Res. **46:**1456-1459, 1967.

84. Meskin, L. H., Pruzansky, S., and Gullen, W. H.: An epidemiologic investigation of factors related to the extent of facial clefts. I. Sex of patient, Cleft Palate J. **5:**23-29, 1968.

85. Metrakos, J. D., Metrakos, K., and Baxter, H.: Clefts of the lip and palate in twins, Plast. Reconstr. Surg. **22:**109-122, 1958.

86. Miller, J. R.: The use of registries and vital statistics in the study of congenital malforma-

tions, Proceedings of the 2nd International Conference on Congenital Malformations, New York, 1964, International Medical Congress, Ltd., pp. 334-340.

87. Mills, L. F., Niswander, J. D., Mazaheri, M., and Brunelle, J. A.: Minor oral and facial defects in relatives of oral cleft patients, Angle Orthod. **38:**199-204, 1968.

88. Mitani, S.: Malformations of newborns, Sankato Fujinka **11:**345-356, 1943.

89. Moller, P., 1970: Unpublished data, cited by Fraser, F. C.: The genetics of cleft lip and cleft palate, Am. J. Hum. Genet. **22:**336-353, 1970.

90. Morton, N. E., Chung, C. S., and Mi, M. P.: Genetics of interracial crosses in Hawaii, Basel, Switzerland, 1967, S. Karger, A. G.

91. Neel, J. V.: A study of major congenital defects in Japanese infants, Am. J. Hum. Genet. **10:**398-445, 1958.

92. Niswander, J. D.: Laminographic X-ray studies in families with cleft lip and cleft palate, Arch. Oral Biol. **13:**1010-1022, 1968.

93. Niswander, J. D., 1970: Cited by Fraser, F. C.: The genetics of cleft lip and cleft palate, Am. J. Hum. Genet. **22:**336-353, 1970.

94. Niswander, J. D., and Adams, M. S.: Oral clefts in the American Indian, Public Health Rep. **82:**807-812, 1967.

95. Niswander, J. D., and Adams, M. S.: Major malformations in relatives of oral cleft patients, Acta Genet. **18:**229-240, 1968.

96. Ortiz-Monasterio, F., and Serrano, R. A.: Cultural aspects of cleft lip and palate. In (Grabb, W. C., Rosenstein, S. W., and Bzoch, K. R., editors: Cleft lip and palate, Boston, 1971, Little, Brown & Co., pp. 130-141.

97. Pashayan, H., and Fraser, F. C.: Facial features associated with predisposition to cleft lip, Birth Defects **7:**58-63, 1971.

98. Pashayan, H., Pruzansky, D., and Pruzansky, S.: Are anticonvulsants teratogenic? Lancet **2:**702-703, 1971.

99. Pedersen, L. M., Tygstrup, P., and Pedersen, J.: Congenital malformations in newborn infants of diabetic women, Lancet **1:**1124-1126, 1964.

100. Pruzansky, S.: Introduction. In Pruzansky, S., editor: Congenital anomalies of the face and associated structures, Springfield, Ill., 1961, Charles C Thomas, Publisher, pp. 3-10.

101. Pruzansky, S., 1970: Cited by Fraser, F. C.: The genetics of cleft lip and cleft palate, Am. J. Hum. Genet. **22:**336-353, 1970.

102. Pruzansky, S.: Personal communication, 1972.

103. Pruzansky, S., Markovic, M., and Buzdygan, D.: Twins with clefts, Acta Genet. Med. Gemellol. **19:**224-229, 1970.

104. Pruzansky, S., and Mason, R.: Family studies of congenital palatopharyngeal incompetence, 3rd International Congress on Human Genetics, Chicago, 1966, pp. 80-81.

105. Rank, B. K., and Thomson, J. A.: Cleft lip and palate in Tasmania, Med. J. Aust. 2:681-689, 1960.

106. Roberts, J. A. F.: Multifactorial inheritance and human disease, Prog. Med. Genet. 3:178-216, 1964.

107. Rogers, B. O.: History of cleft lip palate and treatment. In Grabb, W. C., Rosenstein, S. W., and Bzoch, K. R., editors: Cleft lip and palate, Boston, 1971, Little, Brown & Co., pp. 142-169.

108. Rosenzweig, S.: Psychological stress in cleft palate etiology, J. Dent. Res. 45:1585-1594, 1966.

109. Rubella and other virus infections during pregnancy, Reports on public health and medical subjects, no. 101, Ministry of Health, Great Britain, London, 1960, Her Majesty's Stationery Office.

110. Safra, M. J., and Oakley, G. P.: Association between cleft lip with or without cleft palate and prenatal exposure to diazepam, Lancet 2:478-540, 1975.

111. Sanui, Y.: Clinical statistics and genetics on the cleft-lip and cleft-palate, Jap. J. Hum. Genet. 7:194-233, 1962.

112. Saxen, I.: Associations between oral clefts and drugs taken during pregnancy, Int. J. Epidemiol. 4:37-44, 1975.

113. Schaumann, B. F., Peagler, F. D., and Gorlin, R. J.: Minor craniofacial anomalies among a Negro population, Oral Surg. 29:566-575, 1970.

114. Schendel, S., and Gorlin, R. J.: The frequency of cleft uvula and submucous cleft palate in Down's syndrome patients, J. Dent. Res. 53:840-843, 1974.

115. Schulze, C.: Anomalien, Missbildungen und Krankheiten von Zähnen. In Becker, P. E., editor: Handbuch der Humangeneti, Mund und Kiefer, vol. 11, Stuttgart, Germany, 1964, Georg Thieme, p. 344.

116. Sesgin, M. Z., and Stark, R. B.: The incidence of congenital defects, Plast. Reconstr. Surg. 27:261-267, 1961.

117. Shapiro, B. L.: A twin study of palatal dimensions—partitioning genetic and environmental contributions to variability, Angle Orthod. 39:139-151, 1969.

118. Shapiro, B. L.: Prenatal dental anomalies in mongolism: comments on the basis and implications of variability, Ann. N.Y. Acad. Sci. 171:562-577, 1970.

119. Shapiro, B. L.: Unpublished data, 1975.

120. Shapiro, B. L.: Amplified developmental instability in Down's syndrome, Ann. Hum. Genet. 38:429-437, 1975.

121. Shapiro, B. L., and Sweney, L. R.: Electron microscopic and histochemical examination of oral epithelial-mesenchymal interaction (programmed cell death), J. Dent. Res. (Suppl.) 48:652-660, 1969.

122. Shapiro, B. L., Meskin, L. H., Červenka, J., and Pruzansky, S.: Cleft uvula: a microform of facial clefts and its genetic basis, Birth Defects 7:80-82, 1971.

123. Stark, R. B.: Embryology pathogenesis and classification of cleft lip and cleft palate. In Pruzansky, S., editor: Congenital anomalies of the face and associated structures, Springfield, Ill., 1961, Charles C Thomas, Publisher, pp. 66-85.

124. Stark, R. B., editor: Congenital defects in cleft palate: a multidiscipline approach, New York, 1968, Harper & Row, Publishers.

125. Stark, R. B., Niswander, J. D., Bardanouve, V. T., and Iba, B.: Temporal-spatial clustering of oral-cleft births in Michigan and Montana, Cleft Palate J. 7:826-845, 1970.

126. Stevenson, A. C., Johnson, H. A., Golding, D. R., and Stewart, M. I. P.: A comparative study of congenital malformations, Bull. WHO 34 (supp.), Geneva, 1966.

127. Stevenson, S. S., Worcester, P. H., and Rice, R. G.: 677 congenitally malformed infants and associated gestational characteristics, Pediatrics 6:37-50, 1950.

128. Stewart, J. M., Ott, J. E., and Lagace, R.: Submucous cleft palate, Birth Defects 7:64-66, 1971.

129. Stiegler, E. J., and Berry, M. F.: A new look at the etiology of cleft palate, Plast. Reconstr. Surg. 21:52-73, 1958.

130. Stonova, N. S., and Messina, V. M.: A study of the family histories of patients with hare lip and cleft palate, Soviet Genet. 8:777-782, 1974.

131. Thaler, S., and Smith, H. W.: Submucous cleft palate, Arch. Otolaryngol. 88:184-189, 1968.

132. Tolarová, M.: Empirical recurrence risk figures for genetic counseling of clefts, Acta Chir. Plast. (Praha) 14:234-235, 1972.

133. Trasler, D. G.: Pathogenesis of cleft lip and its relation to embryonic face shape in A/J and C57BL mice, Teratology 1:33-49, 1968.

134. Trasler, D. G., and Fraser, F. C.: Role of the tongue in producing cleft palate in mice with spontaneous cleft lip, Devel. Biol. 6:45-60, 1963.

135. Tretsven, V. E.: Incidence of cleft lip and palate in Montana Indians, J. Speech Hear. Disord. 28:52-57, 1963.

136. Vaughan, H. S.: Congenital cleft lip, cleft

palate and associated nasal deformities, Philadelphia, 1940, Lea & Febiger.

137. von Versheur, O.: Über das Zusammentreffen von Lippen-Kiefer-Gaumenspalte mit Missbildungen der Gliedmassen, Erbarzt. **9:**1-11, 1941.

138. Waddington, C. H.: The canalization of development and the inheritance of acquired characteristics, Nature **150:**563-565, 1942.

139. Witkop, C.: Personal communication, 1975.

140. Woolf, C. M.: Congenital cleft lip, J. Med. Genet. **8:**65-71, 1971.

141. Woolf, C. M., Woolf, R. M., and Broadbent, T. R.: A genetic study of cleft lip and palate in Utah, Am. J. Hum. Genet. **15:**209-215, 1963.

142. Woolf, C. M., Woolf, R. M., and Broadbent, T. R.: Cleft lip and heredity, Plast. Reconstr. Surg. **34:**11-14, 1964.

143. Woolf, C. M., Woolf, R. M., and Broadbent, T. R.: Lateral incisor anomalies, microforms of cleft lip and palate? Plast. Reconstr. Surg. **35:**543-547, 1965.

144. Woolf, C. M., Woolf, R. M., and Broadbent, T. R.: Cleft lip and palate in parent and child, Plast. Reconstr. Surg. **44:**436-440, 1969.

145. Wright, S.: The results of crosses between inbred strains of guinea pigs, differing in number of digits, Genetics **19:**537-551, 1934.

17

Dysmorphic syndromes with craniofacial manifestations

M. MICHAEL COHEN, Jr.

SYNDROME DELINEATION

The word *syndrome* is derived from Greek and literally means "a running together." Minimally, a syndrome can be viewed as two or more abnormalities in the same individual. A common error in logic is made by some who readily use the term to designate a repeated pattern of abnormalities in many individuals but who refuse to apply it to a single patient with a unique pattern of abnormalities. By the same faulty reasoning, an elephant can be considered a valid concept if there are many elephants (Fig. 17-1), but if there is only one elephant in the world, then it can't be an elephant (Fig. 17-2).

The term *syndrome* can apply to a one-of-a-kind condition as well as to a many-of-a-kind condition. The importance of this becomes clear when it is considered that of the 1% of all newborns who have syndromes, only 40% of these have known, recognized entities. The other 60% represent one-of-a-kind syndromes[2] that need to be further delineated.

The significance of syndrome delineation cannot be overestimated. As an unknown syndrome becomes delineated, its phenotypic spectrum, its natural history, and its risk of recurrence become known, allowing for better patient care and family counseling. If the phenotypic spectrum is known, the clinician can search for suspected defects that may not be immediately apparent, such as a hemivertebra in the Goldenhar syndrome. If a certain complication can occur in a given disorder, such as Wilms' tumor in the Beckwith-Wiedemann syndrome, the clinician is forewarned to monitor the patient with intravenous pyelograms. Finally, if the recurrence risk is known, the parents can be counseled properly about future pregnancies. This is especially important if the risk is high and the disorder is disfiguring or has mental deficiency as one component or has a dramatically shortened life span.[1]

The delineation of syndromes discussed below is based on the work of Opitz and associates[4] and Cohen.[3] The process of delineating a syndrome can be divided into the following stages:

A. Unknown-genesis syndrome
  1. Provisionally unique-pattern syndrome
  2. Repeated-pattern syndrome
B. Known-genesis syndrome
  1. Pedigree syndrome
  2. Chromosomal syndrome
  3. Biochemical defect syndrome
  4. Environmentally induced syndrome

I am extremely grateful to Ms. Priscilla Medler for technical assistance in the preparation of this chapter.

500

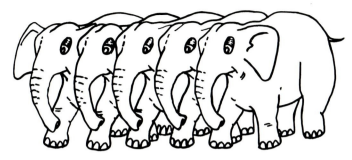

Fig. 17-1. Hey, look at all the elephants!

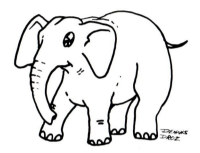

Fig. 17-2. It can't be an elephant! There's only one!

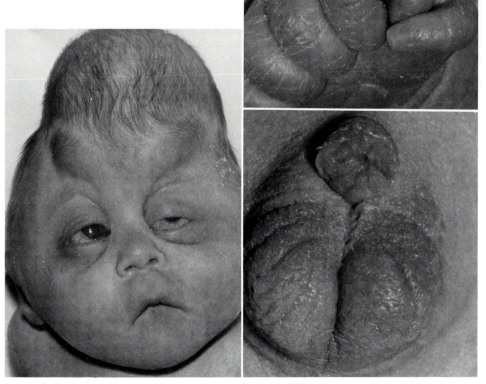

Fig. 17-3. Example of *provisionally unique-pattern syndrome* consisting of cloverleaf skull malformation, preaxial polydactyly, micropenis, cryptorchidism, and bifid scrotum. To date, no other cases are known.

In an *unknown-genesis syndrome,* the cause is simply not known. There are two types of unknown genesis syndromes. In a provisionally *unique-pattern syndrome,* two or more abnormalities are observed in the same patient such that the clinician does not recognize the overall pattern of defects from his own experience, nor from his search of the literature, nor from his consultation with the most learned colleagues in the field (Fig. 17-3). The probability that these abnormalities occur in the same patient by different causes acting independently becomes less likely the more abnormalities the patient has and the rarer these abnormalities are individually in the general population. As was indicated earlier, 60% of all newborns with two or more abnormalities represent unique-pattern syndromes. Some such syndromes are truly unique. Others seem unique at the time the initial patient is discovered but are no longer unique if a second example comes to light.

A *repeated-pattern syndrome* can be defined as a similar or identical set of abnormalities in two or more unrelated patients (Table 17-1 and Figs. 17-4 and 17-5). The same abnormalities observed in two or more patients suggest that the developmental pathogenesis in each case may be the same. In general, the validity of the defined syndrome increases the more abnormalities there are in the condition, the rarer these abnormalities are individually in the general population, and the more patients who are known to have the syndrome.

A *known-genesis syndrome* can be defined as two or more abnormalities causally related on the basis of (1) occurrence in the same family, or less conclusively, the same mode of inheritance in different families, (2) a chromosomal defect, (3) a specific defect in an enzyme or structural protein, or (4) a teratogen or environmental factor. The term *pedigree syndrome,* as used here, refers to known genesis established on the basis of pedigree evidence alone; the basic defect itself remains undefined, although it is known to represent a monogenic or possibly polygenic disorder. A *chromosomal syndrome,*

Table 17-1. Comparison of features of two patients with repeated-pattern syndrome*

	Patient 1	Patient 2
Excessive growth of prenatal onset	+++	+++
Accelerated osseous maturation	++++	++++
Performance		
Hypertonia	++	+
Hoarse low-pitched cry	++	++
Developmental delay	?	?
Excessive appetite	++	++
Craniofacial		
Large bifrontal diameter	+++	+++
Flat occiput	+	+
Large ears	+++	+++
Ocular hypertelorism	++	++
Long philtrum	++	+
Relative micrognathia	+	+
Limbs		
Hands		
Prominent finger pads	++	++
Simian crease	–	+
Camptodactyly	++	+
Broad thumbs	++	+
Thin, deep-set nails	++	++
Feet		
Clinodactyly, toes	+	+
Talipes equinovarus	++	–
Short fourth metatarsals	+	–
Limited early elbow and knee extension	+	+
Widened distal femurs and ulnae	++	++
Skin		
Excessive loose skin	++	++
Inverted nipples	+	+
Thin hair	+	+
Others		
Umbilical hernia	++	+
Inguinal hernias	++	–

*From Weaver, D. D., Graham, C. B., Thomas, I. T., et al.: A new overgrowth syndrome with accelerated skeletal maturation, unusual facies, and camptodactyly, J. Pediatr. **84**:547-552, 1974.
Key: + through ++++ = present, in varying degrees of severity; – = absent; ? = uncertain.

such as the trisomy 21 syndrome, is cytogenetically defined. In a *biochemical defect syndrome,* the specific enzymatic defect is known, for example, sulfoiduronate sulfatase in Hunter syndrome A. The term also refers to specific defects in structural proteins when these become known in some of the dominant disorders. An *environmentally induced syndrome,* such as the fetal alcohol syndrome or aminopterin syndrome, is defined in terms of the causative teratogen or environmental factor.

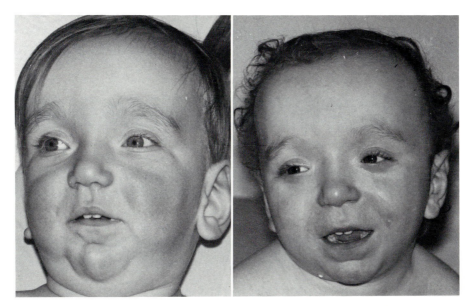

Fig. 17-4. Example of *repeated-pattern syndrome* in two patients. Note large bifrontal diameter, ocular hypertelorism, large ears, long philtrum, and relative micrognathia. (See Fig. 17-5 and Table 17-1.)

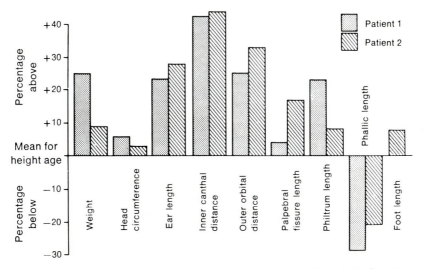

Fig. 17-5. Example of *repeated-pattern syndrome* in two patients. Note similarity of measurement patterns. (See Fig. 17-4 and Table 17-1.) (From Weaver, D., et al.: J. Pediatr. **84**:547, 1974.)

Several points should be clarified about syndrome delineation. In some instances, a syndrome may be delineated in one step, thus bypassing some of the stages discussed earlier. For example, if a new chromosomal abnormality is discovered during the laboratory investigation of a patient clinically defined as having a provisionally unique-pattern syndrome, the patient represents a known-genesis syndrome of the chromosomal type in a one-step delineation. However, the variability of the clinical features must await the discovery of more patients. In other instances, such as a large dominant pedigree with many affected individuals, a known-genesis syndrome of the pedigree type and much of its phenotypic variability can be determined in one step.

Finally, it should be carefully noted that some provisionally unique- and repeated-pattern syndromes are remarkably well described in the older literature. Many workers today (1) do not have access to much of the older literature before the turn of the century, (2) do not have the linguistic prowess to read different languages, or (3) do not have time to carry out such a literature search. Thus it frequently happens that after a "new" syndrome becomes well-delineated, a complete description of an affected patient is discovered in some eighteenth- or nineteenth-century reference. We owe a great deal to early investigators who were limited only as prisoners of history in not being able to understand pedigree analysis, chromosomal aberrations, or defects in enzymes and structural proteins.

TYPES OF SYNDROMES
Nosology of syndromes

Most syndrome classifications are arbitrary and reflect the interests of the authors proposing them.[5, 8] Syndromes have been grouped on the basis of general features, such as mental deficiency or short stature. Indeed, such features have served as the basis for whole monographs.[6, 7] Syndromes can also be grouped on the basis of striking anomalies, such as ocular hypertelorism, phocomelia, or tetralogy of Fallot. Each

clinician tends to view various syndromes according to his particular specialty. For example, a classification of cleft palate syndromes provides a useful differential diagnosis for the stomatologist.

Because classifications based on anatomical features are clinically useful, any one is as justifiable as any other. However, it should be recognized that both duplication and inadequate coverage occur when such classifications are employed. Is the Carpenter syndrome a craniosynostosis syndrome, a limb defect syndrome, or a cardiac anomaly syndrome? Obviously it is all three. Why does the Holt-Oram syndrome not exist in stomatology? Because there are no oral manifestations. Other limitations of anatomical classification include different types of syndromes described in similar terms and similar types of syndromes described in different terms.

To reiterate, the arbitrary nature of anatomical classifications should always be kept in mind. In the broader study of dysmorphic syndromes, there are no cleft palate syndromes. There are syndromes with cleft palate, but that is another matter.

Biological types of syndromes

In the broadest possible context, there are perhaps four general classes of syndromes. The syndrome models discussed here are based on the work of Opitz and Herrmann[11, 12] and Cohen.[9] Although some syndromes clearly can be assigned to one class or another, many have overlapping features. Thus the categories are not always mutually exclusive.

The term *syndrome model* is used to convey the notion that not necessarily every finding in a given syndrome can be accounted for. In fact, the power of any model is that it is an abstract conception, and, as such, it can ignore some of the realities in the same manner as the law of gravity ignores friction. "Science," says the noted philosopher Morris Cohen, "must abstract some phenomena and neglect others because not all things that exist together are relevant together."[10] Thus the models provide us with a framework

Table 17-2. Biological types of syndromes

Type	Level of disturbance	Features
Dysmetabolic syndrome	Metabolism	Frequently normal at birth with generalized progressive disturbances after birth
		Clinical features relatively uniform compared with other types of syndromes
		Not associated with congenital malformations
		Biochemically defined or potentially so
		Commonly recessive mode of inheritance
Dysplasia syndrome	Tissues	Simple dysplasia syndrome
		Characterized by involvement of only one germ layer
		Inheritance may be dominant or recessive
		Hamartoneoplasia syndrome
		Characterized by hamartomas, hyperplasias, and a propensity for neoplasia
		May involve one, two, or all three germ layers
		Inheritance is commonly dominant
Malformation syndrome	Organs	Two or more anomalies or anomalads in same patient
		Characterized by mosaic pleiotropy in which patterns of anomalies or anomalads are developmentally unrelated at the embryologic level
		Lack of biochemical definition; highest state of definition is a known-genesis syndrome of chromosomal or pedigree type
Deformation syndrome	Regions	Characterized by alterations in shape or structure of previously normal parts
		Most important cause is lack of fetal movement regardless of whether cause be a mechanical, functional, or malformational disturbance

for analyzing various types of syndromes by giving us convenient points from which to depart in our thinking.

The models set forth here include the dysmetabolic syndrome, the dysplasia syndrome, the malformation syndrome, and the deformation syndrome (Table 17-2). These models deal with disturbances in metabolism, tissues, organs, and regions, respectively.

It needs to be emphasized that different levels of organization exist and that problems can be analyzed at the molecular level, the tissue structure level, the organ structure level, or the regional level. Problems at different levels of organization demand different investigative techniques, different analyses, and different solutions because of the phenomenon of emergence that takes place in shifting to a higher level of organization. Analyses of genetic syndromes at different

levels of organization are urgently needed. To my knowledge, not a single textbook of medical genetics in any language to date attempts to deal with this problem or even acknowledges its existence. Instead, the approach consistently put forth is the archreductionistic model for inborn errors of metabolism. Any monogenic disorder that cannot be explained at this level, such as an autosomal recessive multiple anomaly syndrome, is either confined to the genetic wastebasket or ignored altogether.

Syndrome model 1: the dysmetabolic syndrome

In a *dysmetabolic syndrome,* an inborn error of metabolism is present that is either biochemically defined or potentially so. Such syndromes have enzymatic defects and are primarily recessively inherited. The Hurler syndrome and the Lesch-Nyhan syndrome are good examples. Some dominantly inherited dysmetabolic syndromes may be caused by a basic defect in a structural protein in some instances and by a regulator mutation, which results in excessive or reduced enzyme production rates in other instances.

The clinical manifestations of dysmetabolic syndromes depend on the metabolic pathways involved, the availability of alternate pathways, the solubility of metabolites, the particular organ systems involved, and a variety of other factors. Dysmetabolic syndromes are not associated with congenital malformations except coincidently.*

In "small molecular weight" dysmetabolic syndromes, the patient is usually normal at birth, since intrauterine compensation has taken place by placental or maternal metabolism. In "large molecular weight" dysmetabolic syndromes, abnormalities may be present during fetal life or at birth. Generalized progressive disturbances may appear after birth in some instances or considerably later in other instances or only under special circumstances in still other instances.

Although there may be a vast difference between the early and late stages of the same dysmetabolic syndrome, the comparable stages in different patients tend to be similar. Thus, compared with other types of syndromes, the clinical features of dysmetabolic syndromes tend to be relatively uniform from patient to patient.

---

*In general, malformations do not occur in metabolic disorders except for the defect in decussation of the optic nerve fibers in albinism. It is also possible for a malformation to occur coincidentally in a metabolic disorder, but the frequency would not be expected to be any more common than the frequency of isolated malformations in the general population.

Syndrome model 2: the dysplasia syndrome

The term *dysplasia* is used here to mean a developmental disturbance of tissue structure. There are two classes of dysplasia syndromes: simple dysplasia syndromes and hamartoneoplasia syndromes.[13] Their features are compared in Table 17-3. In *simple dysplasia syndromes* only one germ layer is involved, and either dominant or recessive inheritance may be encountered. The Marfan syndrome and achondroplasia are good examples of connective tissue dysplasias. Although not biochemically defined at the present time, elucidation of the basic defects in some of the simple dysplasia syndromes is much closer to realization than in the hamartoneoplasia syndromes.

In *hamartoneoplasia syndromes,* one, two, or all three germ layers may be involved, and dominant inheritance is characteristically observed. The major distinguishing features consist of hamartomas, hyperplasias, and a marked propensity for neoplasia. The Peutz-Jeghers syndrome, Gardner syndrome, and Sipple syndrome are good examples of hamartoneoplasia syndromes.

Hamartoneoplasia syndromes can be divided into unilaminar, bilaminar, or trilaminar dysplasias depending on which germ layers are involved. A classification is presented in Table 17-4.

In a *monomorphic dysplasia,* only one derivative of a germ layer is involved. For example, only cartilage (derived from mesoderm) is disturbed in the Ollier syndrome. In a *polymorphic dysplasia,* two or more derivatives of a germ layer are involved. For example, disturbances of both cartilage and vascular tissue (both derived from mesoderm) occur in the Maffucci syndrome. The terms can also be applied to bilaminar

Table 17-3. Comparison of simple dysplasia syndromes and hamartoneoplasia syndromes

Feature	Simple dysplasia syndrome	Hamartoneoplasia syndrome
Hamartomas, hyperplasia	−	+
Propensity for neoplasia	−	+
Germ layers involved	One	One, two, or three
Inheritance	Dominant or recessive	Characteristically dominant

and trilaminar hamartoneoplasia syndromes. Thus, in the Gardner syndrome, both ectoderm (epidermoid cysts and odontomas) and mesoderm (osteomas, fibromas, lipomas, and leiomyomas) show polymorphic involvement, and the entoderm (colonic polyposis) shows only monomorphic involvement.[13]

Under the heading of hamartoneoplasia syndromes, descriptive aspects should be considered briefly. In various dysplasias, such as hemangiomas, melanotic nevi, café-au-lait spots, or gastrointestinal polyps, lesions can be described as, for example, large or small, single or multiple, scattered or concentrated, localized or generalized. Four special types of dysplasia will now be discussed.

Heteroplasia is primary anomalous differentiation of a developing tissue.[16] Examples include gastric differentiation in a portion of the esophageal mucosa or in Meckel's diverticulum. The keratinized stratified squamous epithelium that may be found in the collecting tubules of infants with hypoplastic kidneys is another example. Heteroplasia should be carefully distinguished from metaplasia, which is acquired anomalous differentiation in a regenerating adult tissue or neoplastic tissue. Although heteroplastic tissues have been described in man, their incidence is unknown in various dysplasia and malformation syndromes. Many studies must be carried out to determine the incidence with which heteroplasia occurs, its frequency in dysplasia and malformation syndromes, and its significance.

Hamartoplasia refers to the formation of hamartomas, which are tumor-like, nonneoplastic admixtures of tissues indigenous to the part with an excess of one or more of these.[16] Hamartomas are either present at birth or appear later during postnatal maturation of the tissue. Thus, the overt manifestations of multiple osteochondromas, multiple enchondromas, or tuberous sclerosis may not appear until childhood, adolescence, or even adulthood in some instances. Hamartomatous tissue varies in its predisposition to neoplasia. The lesions of neurofibromatosis are prone to neurofibrosarcomatous degeneration. On the other hand, malignant transformation of angiomyolipomas of the kidney in tuberous sclerosis is uncommon, and neoplasia in the angiomatous lesions of the Klippel-Trénaunay-Weber syndrome has never been reported.

Hyperplasia, or excess cell formation, is a frequent finding in hamartoneoplasia syndromes. For example, hyperplastic ganglion cells in the neurenteric plexus are a feature of the Wagenmann-Froboese syndrome, and hyperplasia of the adrenal medulla precedes the development of pheochromocytoma in the Sipple syndrome.[13]

As already indicated, hamartoneoplasia syndromes have a propensity for *neoplasia.* In this context, neoplasia is viewed as a special type of dysplasia. Syndromes associated with various neoplasms are considered further on p. 521.

Table 17-4. Hamartoneoplasia syndrome classification

Number of germ layers involved	Specific germ layers	Example
Unilaminar	Ectoderm	Multiple trichoepitheliomas
	Mesoderm	Multiple osteochondromas
	Entoderm	Juvenile colonic polyposis
Bilaminar	Ectoderm/mesoderm	Neurofibromatosis
	Ectoderm/entoderm	Acanthosis nigricans/adenocarcinoma syndrome
	Mesoderm/entoderm	Distinctly uncommon. An example does not come to mind
Trilaminar	Ectoderm/meseoderm/entoderm	Gardner syndrome

Syndrome model 3: the malformation syndrome

The terms *anomaly* and *malformation* are often used interchangeably. A *malformation* may be defined as a primary structural defect resulting from a localized error of morphogenesis.[22] Malformations are defects of organ structure that arise during the formation or developmental placement of an organ. There are three classes of malformations.

Incomplete morphogenesis is the most common class, and, depending on the particular type, morphogenesis may proceed normally until the time of developmental arrest. Incomplete morphogenesis includes a variety of different processes, such as failure of induction resulting in aplasia (for example, renal agenesis), hypoplasia (for example, mandibular micrognathia), failure of programmed cell death (for example, syndactyly), failure of proper mesodermal migration (for example, exstrophy of the bladder), persistence of an earlier form (for example, Meckel's diverticulum), or persistence of an earlier location (for example, omphalocele).

Redundant morphogenesis is much less common. In this class of malformations, the redundant organ passes through the same stage of morphogenesis at the same time as its normal counterpart. Examples include polydactyly or supernumerary lateral incisor teeth.

Aberrant morphogenesis, which is rare, has no counterpart in normal morphogenesis. Examples include the unusual "phylogenetically derepressed" muscles that may occur in the trisomy 18 syndrome.[17] Transference of an organ to a location remote from the site of origin may be caused by developmental movement of a neighboring structure.[23] The rarely encountered paratesticular spleen is a good example of this type of aberrant morphogenesis.

Malformations or anomalies may be relatively simple or complex. In general, the earlier a defect takes place during organogenesis, the more far reaching the subsequently derived changes. Conversely, the

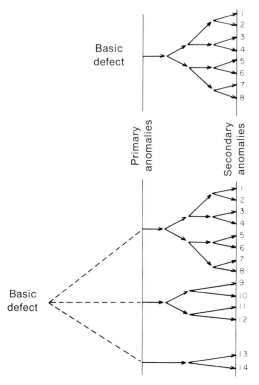

Fig. 17-6. Diagram comparing *anomalad, top,* with true *malformation syndrome, bottom.*

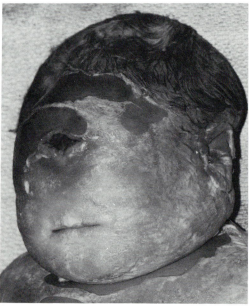

Fig. 17-7. Holoprosencephaly anomalad. Note single central eye and absent nose. (See Fig. 17-8.)

later the defect is initiated, the simpler the anomaly. An *anomalad* may be defined as a malformation together with its subsequently derived structural changes.[22] The primary defect sets off a morphological chain of secondary and tertiary events, resulting in what appear to be multiple anomalies. All such anomalies, however, are developmentally interrelated. The concept of an anomalad is diagrammed in the upper part of Fig. 17-6. An excellent example is the holoprosencephaly anomalad, which is illustrated in Fig. 17-7 and shows a single central eye and an absent nose; these occur together with absent nasal bones and a severe brain abnormality with failure of cleavage of the prosencephalon. All the anomalies encountered trace their origin developmentally to a single primary defect in morphogenesis as diagrammed in Fig. 17-8.

The holoprosencephaly anomalad is a *monotopic anomalad* because each anomaly is developmentally interrelated within a specific region of the body. In a *polytopic anomalad*, developmentally interrelated anomalies occur within different regions of the body and may appear to represent a true malformation syndrome.[19] However, close analysis reveals that all the seemingly disparate anomalies trace their origin to a single defect in morphogenesis. A good example is the Hanhart anomalad, which is diagrammed in Fig. 17-9.

A *malformation syndrome* may be defined as two or more anomalies or anomalads in the same individual and is diagramatically represented in the lower part of Fig. 17-6. The Carpenter syndrome and the Holt-Oram syndrome are good examples. A true malformation syndrome is characterized by *mosaic pleiotropy,* in which a pattern of developmentally unrelated anomalies or anomalads occurs.[18, 20, 21] This type of pleiotropy is well illustrated by the Meckel syndrome, in which there may be anomalies of the brain (encephalocele), limbs (polydactyly), and kidneys (polycystic kidneys). Mosaic pleiotropy characterizes not only monogenic malformation syndromes but chromosomal malformation syndromes as well. Perhaps the genetic imbalance at many loci produced by various aneuploidy states results in reduced genetic buffering, which produces generalized developmental instability with lack of develop-

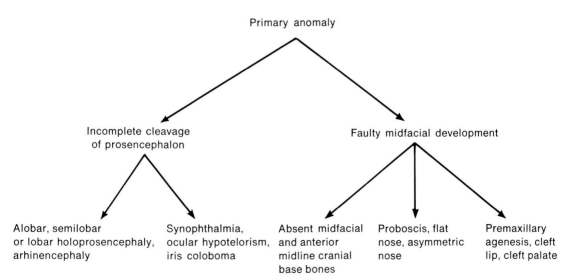

Fig. 17-8. Diagram of holoprosencephaly anomalad. Facial and central nervous system malformations can be variable in degree. (See Fig. 17-7.)

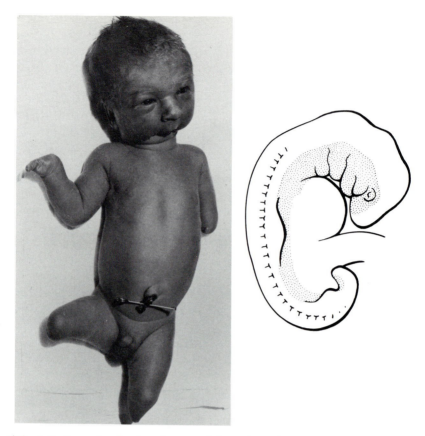

Fig. 17-9. *Left,* Example of polytopic anomalad: patient with Hanhart syndrome exhibiting severe micrognathia and peromelia of all four limbs. Anal atresia was also present. *Right,* Diagrammatic sketch of ectoderm ring (thickened band of ectoderm) (stippled) in 4.2 mm crown-rump embryo. Area of ectoderm ring includes mandible, limb buds, and area of future anus. Disturbance in interaction between ectoderm ring and underlying mesenchyme might result in mesenchymal deficiency in these areas, producing polytopic anomalad in which anomalies in different regions of body have common embryonic origin. (*Left* from Herrmann, J., et al.: Eur. J. Pediatr. **122**:19-55, 1976; *right* from Bersu, E. T., et al.: Eur. J. Pediatr. **122**:1-17, 1976.)

mental "canalization."* The existence of over a hundred anomalies in each of the three major autosomal trisomy syndromes illustrates this principle.

Malformation syndromes lack biochemical definition. The highest stage in malforma-

---

*Shapiro (Ann. N.Y. Acad. Sci. **171**:562, 1970) suggested the same concept for the Down syndrome and applied it to metric traits for the most part, noting greater variability in the Down syndrome than in the general population. However, the resultant instability can also be applied to the occurrence of malformations during organogenesis and can be extended to other autosomal aneuploidy states.

tion syndrome delineation is a known-genesis syndrome of the pedigree or chromosomal type. Pedigree syndromes may involve mutant embryonic proteins that are switched off before birth, thus masking the basic defect. Many other malformation syndromes remain unknown genesis syndromes of the provisionally unique- or repeated-pattern type.

Syndrome model 4: the deformation syndrome

A *deformation* is an alteration in the shape or structure of a previously normal part.[28] In contrast to most malformations, which arise during the period of organogenesis, most deformations arise during the fetal period. Thus malformations tend to be teratological embryopathies, whereas deformations are nonteratological fetopathies.[25] Also, in contrast, malformations tend to affect organs, and deformations tend to affect regions. Examples of deformations include clubfoot, postural scoliosis, and congenital sternomastoid torticollis.

Although the distinction between malformations and deformations based on the embryonic and fetal periods is useful, rigid adherence to these time periods can be misleading, since occasionally a deformation may occur during the embryonic period, many malformations are attributable to the fetal period, and many deformations occur after birth.

Since the process of deformation occurs much more readily during growth, it is not surprising that most deformations arise during the fetal period when the growth rate is five times faster than during childhood. The most important factor contributing to deformations is lack of fetal movement, whatever the cause.[28] Deformation may result from mechanical, functional, or malformational causes. Forces that produce deformation are usually slight but persistent over time; they may be extrinsic or intrinsic in origin.

One mechanical cause of deformation is oligohydramnios, which, in some instances, may be caused by a tear in the amnion. The resultant lack of amniotic fluid can lead to the multiple deformities of the Potter syndrome, which include compressed facies and abnormal positioning and bowing of the limbs.

Functional causes of deformation include the various forms of congenital hypotonia and the various neuromuscular types of arthrogryposis. Congenital hypotonia may be accompanied by micrognathia, microglossia, prominent secondary alveolar ridges, abnormal flexion creases, pes planovalgus, and other deformities. The arthrogryposes are characterized by congenital immobility of the limbs and fixation of the joints in certain positions.[26, 27]

Malformational causes of deformation include various central nervous system and urinary tract anomalies. For example, spina bifida may lead to hypoplastic lower limbs, hip dysplasia, hip dislocation, and clubfoot because the malformation produces partial paralysis of the legs. The resultant muscular imbalance is an intrinsic deforming force that limits the ability to kick and hence to change the position of the fetus to alter the direction along which extrinsic deforming forces may be acting. Hip dysplasia, hip dislocation, and clubfoot may be explained on this basis, as may the hypoplastic lower limbs (a growth disturbance caused by deficient innervation). Any malformation of the urinary tract that significantly reduces the output of fetal urine results in lack of amniotic fluid, thus producing the deformities of the Potter syndrome. Malformations such as bilateral renal agenesis, severe hypoplastic kidneys, or severe polycystic kidneys can cause oligohydramnios and its consequences.

A *deformity* may be defined as a single deformation, such as clubfoot. A *deformitad* consists of two or more deformities that have a common cause.[24] If the term is applied to a regional group of deformities, it may be called a *regional deformitad,* for example, the occurrence of plagiocephaly, mandibular asymmetry, and torticollis in a newborn infant. Several deformities secondary to a malformation constitute a *malformational deformitad,* for example, hip dysplasia, hip dislocation, and clubfoot secondary to spina bifida. Finally, if a deformitad is part of a broader pattern of abnormalities or occurs with another disorder, it may be referred to as a *component deformitad,* for example, a syndrome composed of several malformations and a deformitad secondary to one of them.[24] A second example is the postnatally acquired component deformitad of craniofacial deformity, scoliosis, and contractures that accompanies severe cerebral palsy.[26]

The term *deformation syndrome* should be reserved for conditions in which all the abnormalities are deformities. Although all the features of a regional deformitad are also deformities, a deformation syndrome and a regional deformitad differ in that the former is generalized and latter is regionalized. A good example of a deformation syndrome is the Rosenmann-Arad neurogenic type of arthrogryposis, which follows an autosomal recessive mode of transmission.[29] The disorder consists of immobility of the limbs, fixation of multiple joints in certain postures, and muscle wasting.

Comments on syndrome models

As was indicated earlier, some syndromes closely fit the models proposed, and many have overlapping features between one model and another. The Zellweger syndrome has features suggestive of a dysmetabolic syndrome and frank malformations. Are the recessively inherited hydroxylysine and procollagen peptidase deficiency forms of the Ehlers-Danlos syndrome connective tissue dysplasias or dysmetabolic syndromes?

In many syndromes with overlapping features, it is possible to use compound models. For example, the trisomy 13 syndrome is, technically speaking, a malformation/dysplasia syndrome because the nevus flammeus type of hemangioma found in the syndrome represents a dysplasia, although malformations predominate. In other conditions, such as the basal cell nevus syndrome, the dysplasia component is more extensive than the malformation component. Thus it is a dysplasia/malformation syndrome in which dysplasias such as basal cell carcinomas, aggressive keratocysts, medulloblastoma, and ovarian fibroma, occur together with malformations such as ocular hypertelorism, bifid ribs, and cervical spina bifida occulta.[30] The Pena-Punnett syndrome[31, 32] is an example of a compound malformation/deformation syndrome. Malformations include dysplastic low-set ears, ocular hypertelorism, epicanthal folds, and cryptorchidism; deformations include arthrogryposis, clubfoot, and camptodactyly.

To reiterate, models provide us with a framework for analyzing various syndromes by giving us convenient points from which to depart in our thinking.

SPECIAL CONSIDERATIONS
Syndrome nomenclature

The ideal way to designate a syndrome is to use the name of the basic defect, such as an enzymatic defect or chromosomal abnormality, when this is known. The basic defect in the Sanfilippo syndrome A is heparan sulfate sulfatase deficiency, which is also a suitable name for the disorder. Occasionally, the name of the basic defect can be unwieldy, as in hypoxanthine-guanine-phosphoribosyl-transferase deficiency or Lesch-Nyhan syndrome. All microscopically detectable chromosomal defects associated with malformation syndromes can be properly designated, such as trisomy 18 syndrome, 4p-syndrome, XXY syndrome, and so forth.

In the future, we can anticipate the elucidation of some dysmetabolic syndromes—and perhaps some dysplasia syndromes and deformation syndromes—and hence proper designations for them. However, the basic defect in most malformation syndromes (other than chromosomal syndromes) will remain unknown for a long time. Thus there is a bewildering variety of syndromes that must be designated by some method other than naming the condition after the basic defect.

In general, a new syndrome may be denoted by (1) an eponym, (2) one or more striking features, (3) an acronym, (4) a numeral, (5) a geographic term, or (6) some combination of the above. None of these systems of nomenclature is without fault. The advantages and disadvantages of each have been discussed elsewhere.[33] Standardized names for the many known malformation syndromes is a problem to resolve at some future international conference. Meanwhile, it is worth remembering that academicians are more likely to share each other's toothbrush than each other's nomenclature (Fig. 17-10).

Definitions of various types of abnormalities in dysmorphic syndromes

Gross abnormalities, whether malformations, deformations, or dysplasias are easily defined by their obvious discontinuity with

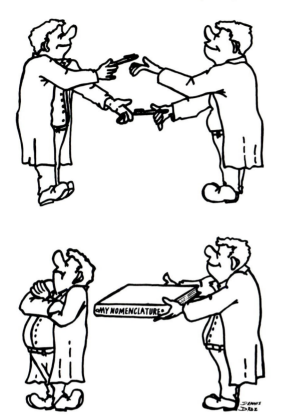

Fig. 17-10. Two academicians are more likely to share each other's toothbrush than each other's nomenclature.

the normal. Cleft lip, severe hypospadias, elbow contractures, talipes calcaneovalgus, and large hemangiomas are examples. Some abnormalities, such as patent ductus arteriosus and cryptorchidism, are defined in terms of timing, being normal at one point but abnormal at another. Other abnormalities are defined by the population in which they occur. Because a mongoloid spot in the sacral region is common in an Oriental population, it is considered normal. The same finding in a newborn from a North American Caucasian population is considered a minor abnormality, since it occurs rarely. Still other abnormalities, such as ocular hypertelorism, are assessed quantitatively, since the range, mean, standard deviation or percentiles by age, sex, and population are known.[34] Finally, some minor abnormalities that occur in the general population and in various syndrome populations, such as epicanthal folds or Brushfield spots, are determined subjectively by observation.[35] In some instances a grading system may be used, but such determinations are still subjective.

Major and minor abnormalities

Abnormalities may be considered major or minor, depending on their impact on the patient. There are three classes of abnormalities: anomalies (malformations), dysplasias, and deformities. Let us consider each class in turn.

Major anomalies are of surgical, medical, or cosmetic importance and may lead to secondary functional disturbances. Examples include congenital heart defect, cleft lip, and omphalocele. *Minor anomalies* are generally not of surgical or medical significance, although in some instances they may be of cosmetic concern, such as webbed neck, ptosis of the eyelids, or prominent epicanthal folds. Rarely, they may cause complications, as in an infected branchial arch fistula. A representative but by no means exhaustive list of minor anomalies is presented in Table 17-5. Photographic documentation of several minor anomalies is presented in Fig. 17-11. Of all minor anomalies, 71% occur in the head and neck region and the hand (Fig. 17-12).

The occurrence of single minor anomalies is common in the general population, being found in 15% of all newborns. However, the presence of two or especially three or more minor anomalies is distinctly unusual, occurring in less than 1% of all newborns. Of great interest is the occurrence of a major anomaly in association with 90% of all newborns with three or more minor anomalies.[37] The implication is clear. Any newborn with three or more minor anomalies should be carefully evaluated for possible hidden major anomalies, such as a cardiac, renal, or vertebral defect.

Minor anomalies often occur with high frequency in many malformation syndromes. For example, in the Down syndrome, 79% of all anomalies detectable by physical examination are minor anomalies; in trisomy 18 syndrome, 38%; in trisomy 13 syndrome, 50%;

Table 17-5. Minor abnormalities*

Area	Abnormality	Area	Abnormality
Head	Aberrant hair patterning	Neck	Mild webbing
	Scalp defect		Excess skin folds of posterior neck
	Third fontanel		Branchial sinus
	Frontal bossing	Chest	Accessory nipples
	Unusual occiput		Unusual placement of nipples
Eyes	Epicanthic folds		Absent or bifid xiphoid
	Upward-slanting palpebral fissures		Prominent sternum
	Downward-slanting palpebral fissures		Depressed sternum
	Short palpebral fissures	Abdomen	Single umbilical artery
	Minor hypertelorism		Diastasis recti
	Minor ptosis		Small umbilical hernia
	Medial hyperplasia of eyebrows		
Ears	Auricular tag	Genito-anal	Minor hypospadias
	Auricular pit		Chordee
	Overfolded helix		Shawl scrotum
	Lack of helical fold		Pilonidal sinus
	Posteriorly notched ear		Deep sacral dimple
	Absent tragus	Arms	Cubitus valgus
	Cup-shaped ears		Hypoplastic nails
	Protuberant ear		Hyperconvex nails
	Small ear		Clinodactyly
	Low-set ear		Unusual dermatoglyphics
	Posteriorly rotated ear		Dimple over bone (shoulder, elbow)
	Notched ear lobe		Rudimentary polydactyly
	Narrow external auditory meatus	Legs	Prominent calcaneus
Nose	Small nose		Genua valga
	Notched alas		Mild syndactyly (digits 2, 3)
	Flat nasal bridge		Recessed toes (digits 4, 5)
	Anteverted nostrils		Gap between toes (digits 1, 2)
	Long nasal septum		Hypoplastic nails
Oral	Asymmetric crying facies		Hyperconvex nails
	Cleft uvula	Skin	Hemangioma (other than face or neck)
	Absent uvula		Pigmented nevi (various types)
	Microform of cleft lip		Mongoloid spots (white population)
	Aberrant frenula		Depigmented spots
	Malformed teeth		
	Borderline small mandible		

*Most represent minor anomalies. However, a few minor dysplasias and minor deformities are also listed. The table, although fairly representative of external minor anomalies, is somewhat arbitrary in that other minor anomalies known to occur, especially internal anomalies, have not been included.

and in the Turner syndrome, 73%.[39] Certain minor anomalies have been found to be of more value as indicators of chromosomal syndromes than as indicators of nonchromosomal malformation syndromes. In decreasing order of value as an indicator are upslanting palpebral fissures, loose folds on the back of the neck in the newborn period, low-set ears, distal palmar triradius, and simian crease.[38] Thus minor anomalies serve as diagnostic aids for many malformation syndromes.

Finally, 42% of patients with idiopathic mental retardation have three or more

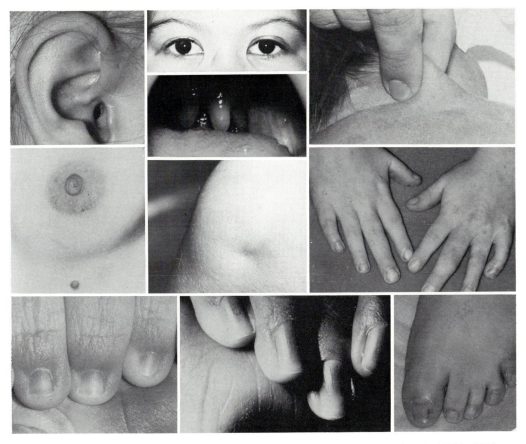

Fig. 17-11. Some examples of minor anomalies including auricular pit, epicanthal folds, bifid uvula, loose skin on posterior part of neck in infancy, supernumerary nipple, subacromial dimple, clinodactyly, deep-set nails, hyperconvex nails, and soft tissue syndactyly.

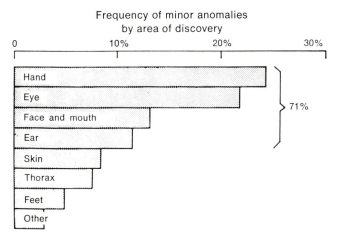

Fig. 17-12. Frequency of minor anomalies by region. Of all minor anomalies, 71% occur in head and neck region and hand. (From Smith, D. W., and Bostian, K. E.: J. Pediatr. **65:**189, 1964.)

anomalies, of which 80% are minor.[39] Thus minor anomalies may be considered an aid in the prognosis of mental deficiency. The significance of minor anomalies is summarized in Table 17-6.

Anomalies occur in fixed locations, but dysplasias occur in variable locations. The impact of a given dysplasia on the patient depends on (1) the type, (2) the location, (3) the size, and (4) the number. On this basis, dysplasias may be classified as major or minor.[36] A small hemangioma and an intradermal nevus are examples of minor dysplasias, and several others are listed under the heading "Skin" in Table 17-5. Minor dysplasias differ in frequency from minor anomalies, being extremely common in the general population. For example, the average Caucasian person has 20 melanotic nevi.[40] Hemangiomas are common and frequently occur internally (for example, hemangioma of the liver) as well as on the skin.

Deformities may also be classified as major or minor.[36] Talipes calcaneovalgus and severe contractures of the knees are examples of major deformities. Two minor deformities,

Table 17-6. Significance of minor anomalies

Fact	*Implication*
In newborns with three or more minor anomalies, 90% have major anomaly	Search for major anomaly
Minor anomalies are present in many multiple congenital anomaly syndromes	Aid in diagnosis
Of idiopathic mental retardation cases, 42% have three or more anomalies, of which 80% are minor anomalies	Aid in prognosis

Table 17-7. Nonspecificity of abnormalities

Examples of abnormalities	*Some conditions in which abnormalities appear*
Malformations	
Cleft palate	Isolated (polygenic)
	Stickler syndrome (autosomal dominant)
	Smith-Lemli-Opitz syndrome (autosomal recessive)
Holoprosencephaly anomalad	Isolated (sporadic, ?polygenic, ??teratogen-induced)
	Isolated (autosomal recessive)
	Isolated (autosomal dominant)
	Trisomy 13 syndrome
	13q– syndrome
	18p– karyotype
	Meckel syndrome (autosomal recessive)
Dysplasias	
Nevus flammeus	Isolated (sporadic)
	Klippel-Trénaunay-Weber syndrome (sporadic)
	Maffucci syndrome (sporadic)
	Trisomy 13 syndrome
Wilms' tumor	Isolated (most sporadic, few familial)
	Hemihypertrophy (sporadic)
	Beckwith-Wiedemann syndrome (most sporadic, few familial)
	Trisomy 18 syndrome
	Aniridia-Wilms' tumor syndrome (sporadic)
Deformations	
Clubfoot	Isolated (polygenic)
	Secondary to spina bifida (polygenic)
	With arthrogryposis (etiologically heterogeneous)

mild cubitus valgus and mild genua valga, are listed in Table 17-5.

Nonspecificity of abnormalities and patterns of abnormalities

All malformations, dysplasias, and deformities, whether major or minor, are nonspecific. Each may occur as an isolated abnormality; each may also occur as a component part of various syndromes. For example, ocular hypertelorism, ventricular septal defect, hemangiomas, and talipes equinovarus occur in many different disorders. The nonspecificity of abnormalities is further illustrated in Table 17-7.

Because abnormalities occur with various frequencies in different syndromes, they are facultative rather than obligatory,[42] that is, they may or may not be present. No abnormality should ever be thought of as obligatory for a given syndrome. For example, two common features of the Beckwith-Wiedemann syndrome are macroglossia and omphalocele, yet cases are known in which both anomalies were absent. Pathognomonic abnormalities for various syndromes are either nonexistent or extremely rare. One possible example is the bony pelvic spur of the nail-patella syndrome.

Since abnormalities are both nonspecific and facultative for various disorders, syndrome diagnosis is made from the overall pattern of abnormalities. It cannot be stressed strongly enough that diagnosis is never made on the basis of specific abnormalities but on the basis of the overall pattern.

The more abnormalities there are in a given syndrome, the easier the condition is to diagnose because, even if some of the features are not expressed, the overall pattern is still discernible. Conversely, the fewer abnormalities there are in a given syndrome, the more difficult the condition is to diagnose if some of the features are not expressed. In general, diagnosis of any syndrome with some of its features not expressed is more of a problem in a sporadic case than in a familial instance. For example, if an 8-year-old child has ocular hypertelorism and bifid ribs but no other abnormalities, the diagnosis of the

basal cell nevus syndrome is extremely probable if the child comes from a family in which one or more members are known to have the syndrome. It is highly likely that such a child will go on to develop other features of the syndrome, such as jaw cysts, bridging of the sella turcica, and basal cell carcinomas. On the other hand, the diagnosis is far from certain if a child with the same anomalies comes from a perfectly normal family.[41]

Three heterogeneous groups of nonspecific abnormalities—mental deficiency, abnormalities of growth and development, and neoplasia—are so important and so common in various syndromes that they will be considered separately.

Mental deficiency. Mental deficiency has a multiplicity of causes and is a feature of many syndromes. Depending on the particular syndrome, retardation may be mild, moderate, severe, or variable. In general, a specific diagnosis can be made more frequently in cases of severe mental deficiency (IQ < 50) than in cases of mild deficiency (IQ = 50 to 70). The latter group is primarily composed of individuals from mentally dull or socioeconomically deprived families. Polygenic and environmental factors play the major role in most of these cases. However, this group also contains a few individuals with X-aneuploidy states (especially the Klinefelter syndrome), malformation syndromes, milder defects of central nervous system development, metabolic disorders, or residual central nervous system insults.[44]

A subcategorization of severe mental deficiency, based on a large study,[43] is presented in Table 17-8. Of all such patients, 45% had either a single central nervous system malformation or a malformation syndrome in which a defect in brain morphogenesis also occurred or was thought to occur by inference. The total malformation group (45%) stood in marked contrast to metabolic disorders (5.8%). These two groups were mutually exclusive with respect to (1) major and minor anomalies, which occurred in the former but not in the latter, and (2) biochemical abnormalities which occurred in

Table 17-8. Study of a severely retarded population (1224 patients)*

Type of disorder	Frequency	
Malformation syndromes	45%	29 %
Primary central nervous system malformation		15.7%
Metabolic disorders	5.8%	
Hypothyroidism	0.7%	
Cerebral palsy, seizures, or hypotonia	31.4%	
Environmental damage	12.4%	
Pure mental deficiency	4.1%	
Psychosis and mental deficiency	1.2%	
	100%	

*Modified from Kaveggia, E. G., Durkin, M. V., Pendleton, E., and Opitz, J. M.: Diagnostic/genetic studies on 1,224 patients with severe mental retardation, Proceedings of the Third Congress of the International Association for the Scientific Study of Mental Deficiency, The Hague, 1973, pp. 82-93.

the latter but not in the former.* These findings are consistent with syndrome models 1 and 3 discussed earlier.

Patients with mental deficiency can be divided into four categories based on the age of onset of CNS dysfunction.[44] In the first and largest category are patients with a defect in prenatal morphogenesis of the brain. Included are patients discussed above who either have a single central nervous system malformation or a malformation syndrome.

In the second category are patients who have sustained an insult to the brain perinatally. Included in this group are patients with severe hypoglycemia, kernicterus, cerebral hemorrhage, perinatal hypoxia, and meningitis. Although problems in perinatal adaptation also occur in patients belonging to the first category, such problems are secondary and not the cause of the mental deficiency.

*Biochemical screening did not reveal a single biochemical abnormality in over 600 patients with either a major central nervous system malformation or a malformation syndrome.

The third category is made up of patients with a problem in brain function of postnatal onset. Included in this group are patients with central nervous system insults such as trauma, meningitis, encephalitis, hypernatremia, lead encephalopathy, in addition to patients with enzymatic defects in amino acid, carbohydrate, uric acid, mucopolysaccharide, and lipid metabolism. Although some of the metabolic disorders are of prenatal onset, clinical manifestations are usually of postnatal onset.

Patients for whom the time of onset of brain dysfunction cannot be established belong to the fourth category, which is the second largest category. In this group, developmental progress is slow, and spasticity, hypotonia, seizures, or aberrant behavior may accompany the developmental delay.

Finally, some disorders, such as rubella, toxoplasmosis, and hypothyroidism may present clinically in several of the four categories.

Abnormalities of growth and development. Many syndromes are characterized by abnormalities of growth and development. One of the most common abnormalities is *growth deficiency of prenatal onset,* in which the infant is born small for gestational age.[48, 49] Both major and minor anomalies are frequently associated. If this type of growth deficiency is regarded as a malformation, that is, as hypoplasia of the whole individual, it is not surprising that other malformations, especially those of incomplete morphogenesis, frequently accompany the growth deficiency. Organ formation and developmental placement are susceptible to malformation if hypoplasia occurs during the periods of rapid differentiation and growth. For example, the trisomy 18 syndrome, which is characterized by growth deficiency of prenatal onset, also has many anomalies of organ formation, developmental placement, and insufficient growth, such as microcephaly, short palpebral fissures, low-set hypoplastic ears, micrognathia, microstomia, short sternum, and ventricular septal defect.

Growth deficiency of prenatal onset is a *primary cellular type* of deficiency. It is in marked contrast to *secondary growth defi-*

Table 17-9. Classification of growth deficiency*

	Primary cellular growth deficiency	Secondary growth deficiency (humoral factors)
Onset of growth deficiency	Usually prenatal	Usually postnatal
Rate of maturation	Variable	Usually retarded
Associated anomalies	Frequent	Infrequent, except for a causative anomaly
Cause	Chromosomal disorders Mutant gene disorders Fetal infection Idiopathic	Environmental Anomaly (malformation) Mutant gene disorders Chronic infection Idiopathic
Therapy to increase eventual stature	None	Replacement Correction of cause

*Modified from Smith, D. W.: Growth deficiency: a new classification into primary cellular growth deficiency and secondary humoral growth deficiency, South. Med. J. (Suppl.) **64:**5-15, 1971.

ciency, which is mediated by humoral factors, such as the supply of nutrients, minerals, hormones, and oxygen and the removal of waste products.[48] Secondary growth deficiency such as that found in malnutrition, respiratory insufficiency, renal dysfunction, hypothyroidism, or hypopituitarism, is usually *growth deficiency of postnatal onset*. The features of primary cellular growth deficiency and secondary humorally mediated growth deficiency are compared in Table 17-9.

The opposite of growth deficiency, growth excess, characterizes a number of syndromes. In *overgrowth syndromes,* such as cerebral gigantism and the Beckwith-Wiedemann syndrome, the newborn is large for gestation age or has excessively rapid somatic growth during infancy or both.

Many syndromes, especially the skeletal dysplasias, exhibit various types of disproportionate size or growth of the limbs or both. The *Marfanoid habitus* is characterized by a disproportionately long lower segment (pubis to sole) in comparison to the upper segment (vertex to pubis). A Marfanoid habitus may be observed in the Marfan syndrome, homocystinuria, congenital contractural arachnodactyly, Klinefelter syndrome, and Wagenmann-Froboese syndrome.

In *disproportionate short stature,* there is a discrepancy between limb length and trunk length. In some conditions, such as achondroplasia, limb length is shortened, but trunk length is relatively normal. Depending on which segment is shortened, a limb may be rhizomelic (shortened proximal portions, that is, humerus and femur), as in achondroplasia, or mesomelic (shortened distal portion, that is, radius and ulna, tibia and fibula), as in the Ellis–van Creveld syndrome. In other conditions, for example, Morquio syndrome, trunk length is shortened and limb length is relatively normal.[45]

Asymmetry, hemihypertrophy, and hemiatrophy are features of some syndromes. *Asymmetry* may occur by itself but is also, by definition, found in both hemihypertrophy and hemiatrophy. Asymmetric limbs may be seen in some cases of multiple osteochondromas or the Langer-Giedion syndrome. Severe asymmetry with pronounced overgrowth of limbs may occur with the Ollier syndrome or the Maffucci syndrome. *Hemihypertrophy* involving the limbs usually implies a discrepancy in both length and circumference of one limb compared with the other. Hemihypertrophy can be observed in the Klippel-Trénaunay-Weber syndrome and in some cases of the Russell-Silver and Beckwith-Wiedemann syndromes. In *hemiatrophy* one limb is smaller than the other. A good example is the Sturge-Weber dysplasia, in which a limb may be atrophic on the side contralateral to brain involvement.[45]

Many syndromes are characterized by *dysharmonic maturation,* which is characterized by (1) unusual ossification sequences, (2) delay or advancement of specific ossifica-

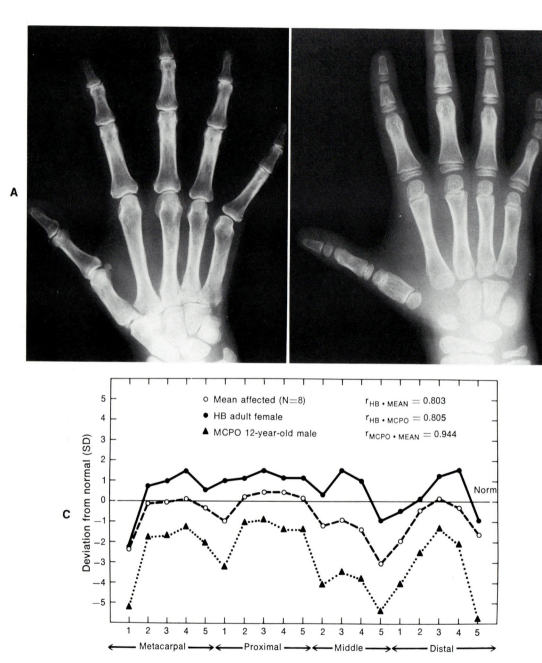

Fig. 17-13. Hand-wrist radiographs of **A**, woman, and **B**, 12-year-old boy, with hand-foot-uterus syndrome (HFUS). Note short first metacarpal in both hands. **C**, Metacarpophalangeal profile patterns of patients **A** and **B**. Note overall similarity of patterns. Also note relative shortening of first metacarpal, first proximal phalanx, second middle phalanx, fifth middle phalanx, and fifth distal phalanx. Profile pattern provides information beyond that visually observed in radiographs. Profiles are plotted against appropriate standards for age and sex. (From Poznanaski, A. K.: Radiology **104:**1, 1972.)

tion centers, (3) side-to-side asymmetry of ossification centers, or (4) abnormal bone configurations.[46] Several examples follow. An unusual ossification sequence occurs in patients with trisomy 18 syndrome who survive for several years; phalangeal epiphyses appear but carpal bones are absent. This sequence is never observed in the general population. Advanced skeletal age with disproportion in phalangeal and carpal ossification occurs in cerebral gigantism. Asymmetric skeletal maturation may occur in the Russell-Silver syndrome when hemihypertrophy is present. Finally, abnormal configurations of the epiphyses, short tubular bones, and cuboid bones may be seen in the hands and feet in the otopalatodigital syndrome.

The concept of dysharmonic maturation also includes the relative lengthening and shortening of various tubular bones with

Table 17-10. Syndromes with neoplasia*

Syndrome	Neoplasia
Acanthosis nigricans/adenocarcinoma syndrome	Adenocarcinoma (stomach abdominal cavity)
Aniridia–Wilms' tumor syndrome	Wilms' tumor
Ataxia-telangiectasia syndrome	Malignant lymphoma, leukemia
Basal cell nevus syndrome (Gorlin syndrome)	Basal cell carcinoma, medulloblastoma, other tumors
Beckwith-Wiedemann syndrome	Wilms' tumor, adrenal cortical carcinoma, other tumors
Bloom syndrome	Leukemia, malignant lymphoma
Cowden syndrome	Fibroadenoma and carcinoma (breast), adenocarcinoma (thyroid), other tumors
de Sanctis-Cacchione syndrome	Squamous cell carcinoma, basal cell carcinoma, malignant melanoma, other tumors
Down syndrome	Leukemia, retinoblastoma
Dyskeratosis congenita	Squamous cell carcinoma, leukemia
Fanconi syndrome	Leukemia
Gardner syndrome	Osteoma, odontoma, leiomyoma, lipoma, fibroma, adenocarcinoma (intestine), fibrosarcoma, leiomyosarcoma, papillary adenocarcinoma (thyroid)
Klinefelter syndrome	Carcinoma (breast)
Neurofibromatosis	Neurofibrosarcoma, pheochromocytoma, other tumors
Peutz-Jeghers syndrome	Adenomatous polyps (intestine) that rarely become malignant, granulosa cell tumor (ovary), other tumors
Rothmund-Thomson syndrome	Squamous cell carcinoma
Sebaceous nevus syndrome	Adnexal adenoma, basal cell carcinoma
Sipple syndrome	Medullary carcinoma (thyroid), pheochromocytoma
13q– syndrome	Retinoblastoma
Trisomy 13 syndrome	Leukemia
Trisomy 18 syndrome	Wilms' tumor
Tuberous sclerosis	Angiofibroma, glioma, angiomyolipoma, rarely angiomyoliposarcoma
Turner syndrome	Various low-frequency neoplasms, especially neurogenic tumors
von Hippel–Lindau syndrome	Pheochromocytoma
Wagenmann-Froboese syndrome	Medullary carcinoma (thyroid), pheochromocytoma, mucosal neuroma
Werner-Zollinger-Ellison syndrome	Islet cell tumor (pancreas), parathyroid adenoma, pituitary adenoma, bronchial carcinoid tumor
Werner syndrome	Hepatoma, carcinoma (breast), adenocarcinoma (thyroid), osteosarcoma

*This table, although representative, is not complete.

respect to each other. Analysis of this phenomenon in some syndromes has produced characteristic profile patterns. For example, hand-wrist radiographs of two patients with the hand-foot-uterus syndrome are illustrated in Fig. 17-13, *A* and *B,* and the metacarpophalangeal profile pattern analysis[47] of bone lengths is shown in Fig. 17-13, *C.* The similarity of the profile pattern is unmistakable despite the difference in age of the two patients.

Neoplasia. Teratogenesis and oncogenesis have some factors in common. The association of congenital malformations with neuroblastoma has been well documented,[51, 57] and soft tissue sarcoma, especially rhabdomyosarcoma, has been observed with single and multiple defects[56] in addition to well-delineated syndromes such as the basal cell nevus syndrome and Beckwith-Wiedemann syndrome.[53] Families have also been reported in which one member had a chromosomal syndrome and other members had a specific type of cancer. For example, sex chromosomal abnormalities and leukemia have shown familial aggregation.[50, 55] Cancer/chromosomal syndrome families have been reviewed elsewhere.[52]

Various syndromes known to be associated with neoplasia are listed in Table 17-10. The overwhelming majority are dysplasia syndromes of the hamartoneoplasia type and malformation syndromes of the chromosomal type. Some, such as the Peutz-Jeghers syndrome and the Gardner syndrome, are pure hamartoneoplasia syndromes. Others, such as the basal cell nevus syndrome, are compound hamartoneoplasia/malformation syndromes. In some, such as the Sipple syndrome and the Wagenmann-Froboese syndrome, every component of the disorder consists of hyperplasia or neoplasia or both. Chromosomal syndromes, such as the Down syndrome, trisomy 13 syndrome, trisomy 18 syndrome, 13q– syndrome, the Turner syndrome, and the Klinefelter syndrome, are known to be associated with a variety of neoplasms.

Monogenic disorders, such as ataxia-telangiectasia, the Bloom syndrome, and the Fanconi syndrome, are associated with chromosomal instability and breakage. The same genes in the homozygous state that cause these syndromes probably also produce the chromosomal instability that predisposes to leukemia and malignant lymphoma. With respect to the Fanconi syndrome, heterozygous carriers have been known to develop leukemia. In the de Sanctis-Cacchione syndrome, in which various skin cancers develop, the basic defect has been shown to be a failure of DNA excision repair of ultraviolet-induced thymine dimers.[54]

SYNDROMES

A great many syndromes are known, and with the discovery of new ones almost daily, the task of presenting them in one chapter or even in a whole textbook becomes extremely problematical. Generally speaking, only some of the more common syndromes with craniofacial or orofacial components are presented here. For extensive syndrome coverage, the reader is referred to other sources.[58-60] The disorders covered in this chapter are as follows:

> Achondroplasia
> Beckwith-Wiedemann syndrome
> *Branchial arch syndromes
> Cerebral gigantism
> *Cleft lip and palate syndromes
> Cleidocranial dysplasia
> Craniocarpotarsal dystrophy
> *Craniosynostosis syndromes
> Diastrophic dwarfism
> Ectodermal dysplasia
> Ellis–van Creveld syndrome
> Frontonasal dysplasia
> Gardner syndrome
> *Gingival fibromatosis syndromes
> Gorlin syndrome
> Hallermann-Streiff syndrome
> de Lange syndrome
> Marfan syndrome
> *Mucopolysaccharidoses
> Neurofibromatosis
> Oculodentoosseous dysplasia
> Osteogenesis imperfecta
> Prader-Willi syndrome
> Pyknodysostosis
> Rubinstein-Taybi syndrome
> Russell-Silver syndrome
> Sturge-Weber/Klippel-Trénaunay-Weber syndrome
> Tuberous sclerosis
> Williams syndrome

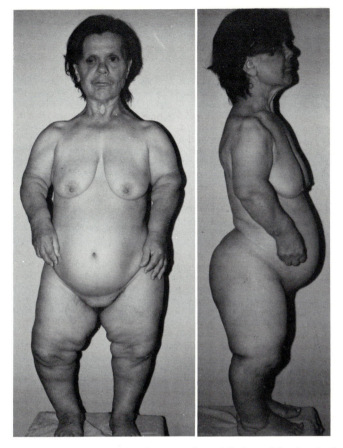

Fig. 17-14. Achondroplasia. Note rhizomelic shortening of limbs and lumbar lordosis with protuberant abdomen and buttocks.

The conditions with asterisks represent groups of disorders; the remaining conditions are single syndromes. Many conditions not presented in this chapter in detail appear elsewhere in the book. See Chapter 15 for chromosomal syndromes, Chapter 12 for mucocutaneous syndromes, Chapter 13 for metabolic syndromes, and Chapter 16 for a detailed discussion of cleft lip and palate.

Achondroplasia

The term *achondroplasia* was first used by Parrot in 1878 to describe a rhizomelic form of short-limbed dwarfism associated with enlarged head, depressed nasal bridge, short, stubby, trident hands, lordotic lumbar spine, prominent buttocks, and protuberant abdomen (Figs. 17-14 and 17-15). Achondroplasia is a misleading term because cartilage is, in fact, formed in the disorder. However,

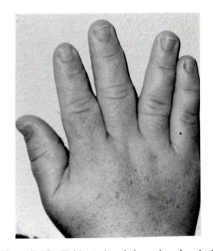

Fig. 17-15. Trident hand in achondroplasia.

the term is well established in the medical literature. Until relatively recently, a variety of chondrodystrophies were frequently confused with achondroplasia. Achondroplasia and hypochondroplasia may be allelic.

More than 80% of recorded cases of achondroplasia are sporadic, representing point mutations. Less than 20% of reported cases are familial, showing an autosomal dominant mode of transmission. Increased paternal age at time of conception is associated with sporadic cases.

The gene frequency of achondroplasia has been estimated to range between 0.00004 and 0.00014 in various populations. These are probably gross overestimates because various chondrodystrophies are undoubtedly included in these surveys.

Affected individuals are heterozygous for the achondroplasia gene. Presumed homozygosity has been reported in a few instances in which both parents were achondroplastic. Homozygous achondroplastic infants are more severely affected, both clinically and radiologically. The homozygous state resembles thanatophoric dwarfism in many respects, and the condition is lethal during infancy.

The possible existence of an autosomal recessive mode of transmission in achondroplasia has been the subject of numerous discussions. Most examples cited in support of this thesis either represent various recessively inherited chondrodystrophies or are insufficiently documented to establish diagnosis with certainty. The one known instance of affected sibs with normal parents can probably be explained by gonadal mosaicism, since one sib has subsequently produced an affected child.

Cases of achondroplasia within the same kindred that seemingly do not show complete penetrance have been reported on rare occasion. Such pedigrees may be explained by the inheritance of an unstable permutation, which could also explain instances of mosaic achondroplasia.

The basic defect is unknown. Early histological studies, which suggested gross disorganization of endochondral ossification, were misleading because they described patients with thanatophoric dwarfism, metatropic dwarfism, or achondrogenesis (Parenti-Fraccaro type), rather than true achondroplasia. Actually, well-organized endochondral ossification with longitudinal columns of cartilage has been found in the chondroosseous rib junctions in achondroplasia. These findings suggests that the abnormality might be quantitative, affecting the rate of cartilage growth. Defective oxidative energy formation with decreased phosphorylation at the NADH dehydrogenase region of the terminal respiratory system has been demonstrated in achondroplastic muscle.

Mean birth lengths are 47.7 cm for males and 47.2 cm for females. Mean birth weights are 3500 gm for males and 3150 gm for females. Both lengths and weights are somewhat less for achondroplastic offspring of dwarfed mothers.

Motor milestones are slow. Head control may not occur until 3 to 4 months, and affected children may not walk until 24 to 36 months. Ultimately, however, development is normal.

Final height attainment is 130 cm for males and 123 cm for females. Mean adult weights are 55 kg for males and 46 kg for females. There is a predilection for obesity.

Reproductive fitness is considerably reduced among achondroplastics because of social difficulties in finding mates and because of the obstetrical problems of achondroplastic women (prematurity and cesarean deliveries).

Craniofacial complex. The head is enlarged, with frontal bossing and depression of the nasal bridge (Fig. 17-16). These features occasionally may not be present at birth, but disproportionate growth of the head occurs during the first year of life and then parallels the normal curve. Midface hypoplasia with relative mandibular prognathism is commonly observed together with anterior crowding of teeth and class III malocclusion. Otitis media is common during the first 6 years of life and, if untreated, may lead to hearing loss.

Central nervous system. Intelligence is almost always normal, although the acquisition

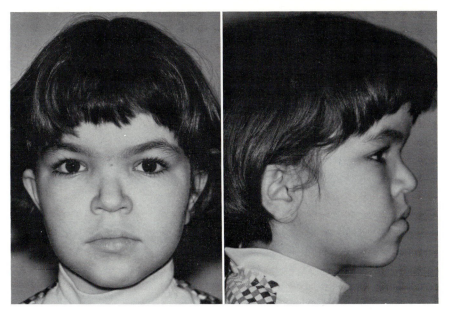

Fig. 17-16. Enlarged calvarium and depressed nasal bridge in achondroplasia.

of motor skills may be somewhat delayed because of the large head and short extremities. Enlargement of the head in achondroplasia may be due to true megalencephaly. Mild ventricular dilatation has been demonstrated by pneumoencephalographic studies. However, gross mechanical block caused by obliteration of the basal cisterns, by obliteration at the level of the foramen magnum, or by kinking of the cerebral aqueduct has not been demonstrated in most cases. Significant hydrocephaly (stepwise increase in the head-growth slope) with neurological signs and symptoms has occurred in a few instances and is probably caused by cerebrospinal fluid obstruction at the level of the foramen magnum.

The narrow spinal canal predisposes to neurological complications with age. Compression of the spinal cord and nerve rootlets results from osteophytes, prolapsed intervertebral discs, or deformed vertebral bodies.

Skeletal system. Enlarged calvarium with shortening of the cranial base and basilar kyphosis are constant features. The foramen magnum is small. Partial occipitalization of the first cervical vertebra occurs in most cases. The interpedicular distances in the upper to the lower lumbar spine are progressively narrowed, the pedicles are shortened in anteroposterior diameter, the posterior aspect of the vertebral bodies is concave, and the bony spinal canal diameters are decreased, especially in the lumbar region. Anterior wedging of the vertebral bodies (particularly in the region of the thoracolumbar junction) with resultant kyphosis may be prominent.

The lumbar spine appears to articulate low in relationship to the crests of the iliac bone. The sacrum is narrow and horizontally oriented. The pelvis is broad and short (Fig. 17-17). The superior acetabular margins are oriented horizontally, and the sacrosciatic notch is acute. The thoracic cage is relatively small in anteroposterior diameter. The legs are frequently bowed because of lax knee ligaments.

Limb bones are shortened (Fig. 17-18) in a rhizomelic pattern, which is more prominent in the upper extremities. There is incomplete extension at the elbows. The metacarpals and phalanges, although shortened, are disproportionately large in relation to the humerus, radius, and ulna. The fibula is long

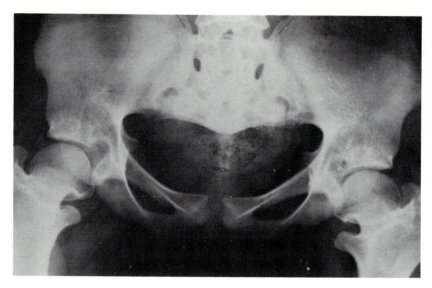

Fig. 17-17. Short squat pelvis of achondroplasia.

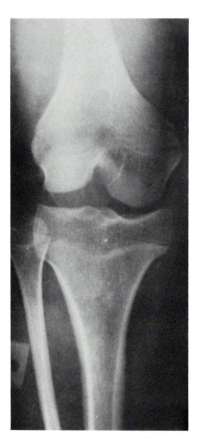

Fig. 17-18. Clubbing of long bones in achondroplasia.

at the ankle compared to the tibia, leading in some cases to varus foot deformity.[61-72]

Beckwith-Wiedemann syndrome

In 1963, Beckwith reported three cases of a newly recognized syndrome consisting of macroglossia, omphalocele, cytomegaly of the adrenal cortex, hyperplasia of the gonadal interstitial cells, renal medullary dysplasia, and hyperplastic visceromegaly. Subsequently, Beckwith enlarged his series of patients, noting postnatal somatic gigantism, mild microcephaly, and severe hypoglycemia. In 1964, Wiedemann independently reported the syndrome in three sibs and observed a further component, a dome-shaped defect of the diaphragm.

Most cases of the Beckwith-Wiedemann syndrome are sporadic. Affected sibs have been reported occasionally, and consanguinity has been established in one case. Several cases have occurred in more than one sibship in the same family. Based on familial cases, autosomal recessive, autosomal dominant, polygenic, and autosomal dominant sex-dependent inheritance have been proposed. Etiological heterogeneity is also possible.

The frequency of the syndrome has been estimated to be 1 per 13,700 births. The syn-

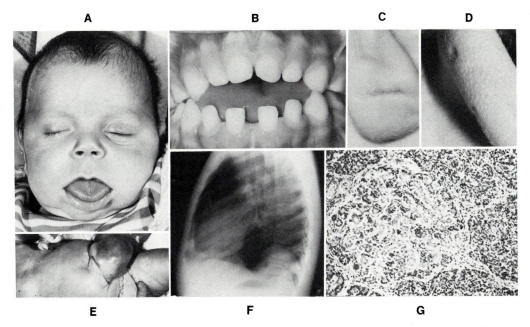

Fig. 17-19. Beckwith-Wiedemann syndrome. **A**, Macroglossia. **B**, Anterior open bite. **C**, Ear lobe groove. **D**, Circular depression on posterior rim of helix. **E**, Omphalocele. **F**, Diaphragmatic eventration. **G**, Hyperplasia of ducts and acini in pancreas.

drome may occur in more than 15% of all infants with omphalocele.

Because of the endocrine cytomegaly present in the syndrome, it has been suggested that the fetal adrenal cortex is either overactive or underactive, with excessive stimulation caused by a feedback mechanism similar to that found in the adrenogenital syndrome. Abnormalities of the hypophysis, gonads, islets of Langerhans, and paraganglia should be considered in evaluating the abnormal growth in this syndrome. Altered placental endocrine physiology could conceivably play a role in producing many of the features found during the neonatal period.

Hydramnios has been noted in about 60% of cases, and some infants have been premature. Placentas have also been large.

Symptomatic neonatal hypoglycemia may be present in a third to half of the patients. Some later become prediabetic.

Facies (Fig. 17-19, *A* to *D*). Macroglossia is evident at birth and later produces an open bite. Maxillary hypoplasia and relative mandibular prognathism are common.

Cleft palate and the Robin anomalad have been noted rarely. The occiput may be prominent. Mild microcephaly has been noted in about half the cases. Asymmetrical earlobe grooves and pits have been observed in about 60% of patients. Circular depressions on the posterior rim of the helices have been noted in about 50%. Facial nevus flammeus, a finding seen in over 90% of patients, tends to become less prominent during the first year of life. It occurs principally in the glabellar area and over the upper eyelids.

Gastrointestinal system. Omphalocele, or umbilical hernia, is a common feature (Fig. 17-19, *E*). Malrotation anomalies are present in most cases. Several patients have had diastasis recti. Hepatomegaly is common.

Skeletal system. Gigantism is not necessarily present at birth, but mean birth weight is about 3900 gm (range 2775 to 6235 gm). Growth may even be subnormal for a few months, but somatic gigantism eventually results. Height and weight are often above the ninetieth percentile. Advanced bone age is present in the majority of cases, and widening of the metaphyses and cortical thickening of long bones have been reported. Hemihypertrophy has been noted in about 15% of the cases.

Central nervous system. Mental deficiency, which occurs in some cases, is probably due, in part, to undetected hypoglycemia during infancy. Intelligence has been normal in many cases, although mild to moderate retardation was a regular feature in Beckwith's series. Hydrocephalus has been observed in two instances.

Other findings. Diaphragmatic eventration (Fig. 17-19, *F*) and clitoromegaly have been reported. Various other abnormalities, such as genitourinary tract anomalies, have been described.

Pathology. Nephromegaly is common, and pancreatomegaly may also occur. Hyperplasia of the bladder, uterus, liver, and thymus has also been reported. In Beckwith's autopsy series, increased renal lobulation was noted. Each lobule was capped by a wide, persistent nephrogenic activity zone. Medullary dysplasia was evident, with most pyramids showing an increased amount of stroma. The collecting tubules were immature. Hyperplasia of acini, islets, and ducts was evident in the pancreas (Fig. 17-19, *G*). Cytomegaly of the fetal adrenal cortex was a constant feature, the cells containing sudanophilic droplets. The adrenal cortex was cystic, and the medulla was hyperplastic. An increased number of amphophils was present in the pituitary gland. The gonadal interstitial cells were hyperplastic. The paraganglia were also hyperplastic.

Neoplasia. Wilms' tumor and adrenal cortical carcinoma occur with a frequency of about 5%. Hepatoblastoma, glioma, embryonal rhabdomyosarcoma, carcinoid tumor, myxoma, and fibroma have also been noted. The presence of hemihypertrophy does not increase the risk for malignancy.[73-91]

Branchial arch syndromes

The so-called branchial arch syndromes comprise an etiologically heterogeneous group of malformation syndromes. The literature is replete with oversimplifications about complexity and nosology. Many problems remain unresolved.

Terms such as branchial arch dysplasia, branchial arch syndrome, first arch syndrome, first and second branchial arch syndrome, and hemifacial microsomia impart the erroneous impression that involvement is limited to the face. In some cases, cardiac, renal and skeletal anomalies occur, and, when they do, they are just as much part of the syndrome as any brachial arch component; they do not occur coincidentally or by chance. The branchial arch syndromes will be considered in two major groups: syndromes with mandibulofacial dysostosis and syndromes with hemifacial microsomia.

Syndromes with mandibulofacial dysostosis. As used here, the term *mandibulofacial dysostosis* will refer to an anomalad (1) that may occur as an isolated finding or together with other anomalies resulting in various malformation syndromes (Table 17-11) and (2) that has bilateral, symmetrical facial involvement.

Poswillo has elucidated the pathogenesis of the branchial arch syndromes. The pathogenesis of mandibulofacial dysostosis may be based on focal death of preotic neural crest cells, creating a spatial rearrangement of the developing ears and a paucity of ectomesenchyme in the first and second branchial arches.

Treacher Collins syndrome. The most common syndrome with the mandibulofacial dysostosis anomalad is the Treacher Collins syndrome. The syndrome has autosomal dominant transmission with variable expressivity. The gene seems to have a lethal effect, since miscarriage or early postnatal death is common. A number of families have expressed the syndrome in several generations. Possibly 300 or more cases have been published.

CRANIOFACIAL COMPLEX. The facial appearance (Fig. 17-20) is striking, with downward-sloping palpebral fissures, depressed cheek bones, dysplastic ears, receding chin, and downturned mouth. Another feature seen in about 25% of affected individuals is a tongue-shaped process of hair that extends toward the cheek. The calvarium is essentially

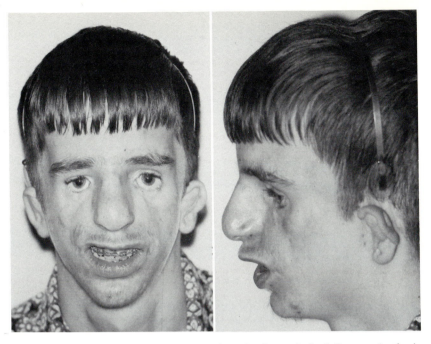

Fig. 17-20. Treacher Collins syndrome. Note downslanting palpebral fissures, dysplastic ears, and micrognathia.

normal, but radiographic studies reveal poorly developed supraorbital ridges and frequently increased digital markings in the presence of a normal suture relationship. The body of the malar bones may be totally absent but more often is grossly and symmetrically underdeveloped, with nonfusion of the zygomatic arches. The mastoids are not pneumatized and are frequently sclerotic. The paranasal sinuses are often small and may be completely absent.

Although vision is usually normal, the palpebral fissures slope laterally downward, and often there is a coloboma (in about 75%) in the outer third of the lower lid. About half of the patients have a deficiency of cilia medial to the coloboma. Iridial coloboma may also occur. The lower lacrimal points may be absent as well as the Meibomian glands and intermarginal strip. Radiographic studies have shown the lower orbital margins to be defective and the orbital cavity to be oval, with the roof inclining downward and outward.

The ear is often deformed, crumpled forward, or misplaced. Over a third of all patients have absence of the external auditory canal or ossicle defect accompanied by conductive deafness. Radiographic studies have shown sclerosis of the middle and, rarely, the inner ear, with poor delineation of their structures. The auditory ossicles and cochlear and vestibular apparatus have been observed to be absent or severely malformed. Surgical investigation has corroborated the radiographic findings, revealing such abnormalities as fixed malleus, fusion of malformed malleus and incus, monopodal stapes, absence of stapes and oval window, complete absence of the middle ear, and epitympanic space. The space may be filled with connective tissue.

Extra ear tags and blind-ended fistulas may occur anywhere between the tragus and the angle of the mouth. In one case, blind fistulas were found behind the ear lobes. The nasofrontal angle is usually obliterated and the bridge of the nose raised. The nose appears large because of the lack of malar development. The nares are often narrow and the alar cartilages hypoplastic. Choanal atresia has been reported.

Table 17-11. Syndromes with mandibulofacial dysostosis

Name	Features	Etiology
Treacher Collins syndrome	Mandibulofacial dysostosis, rarely other anomalies (especially of heart)	Autosomal dominant
Nager acrofacial dysostosis	Mandibulofacial dysostosis, preaxial upper limb deficiency, other anomalies	Autosomal recessive
Wildervanck-Smith syndrome	Mandibulofacial dysostosis, preaxial and postaxial upper and lower limb deficiency, other anomalies	Unknown; sporadic to date

The mandible is almost always hypoplastic. Radiographic studies have shown that the angle is more obtuse than normal and that the ramus may be deficient. The coronoid and condyloid processes are flat or even aplastic. The undersurface of the body of the mandible is often concave. The palate is cleft in about 30%. Macrostomia is observed in about 15% and may be unilateral or bilateral. Because of the poor development of the maxilla and the frequency of highly arched or cleft palate, dental malocclusion is frequent. The teeth may be widely separated, hypoplastic, displaced, or associated with open bite.

OTHER FINDINGS. Mental deficiency has been reported and may be secondary to hearing loss in some instances. Various low-frequency anomalies, such as ventricular septal defect and other cardiac malformations, may be associated. Other syndromes with the mandibulofacial dysostosis anomalad are presented in Table 17-11.

Nager acrofacial dysostosis. A distinct entity, *Nager acrofacial dysostosis,* has autosomal recessive inheritance. Mandibulofacial dysostosis occur in association with reduction defects of the preaxial side of the upper limbs (Figs. 17-21 and 17-22). The thumbs are hypoplastic or absent, the radius and ulna may be fused, or there may be absence or hypoplasia of the radius and/or one or more metacarpals. Lower lid colobomas are rarer, cleft palate more frequent, and the mandible more severely retarded in growth than in Treacher Collins syndrome. Other anomalies may also occur.

Wildervanck-Smith syndrome. The Wildervanck-Smith syndrome combines mandibulofacial dysostosis with reduction defects of both upper and lower limbs (Figs. 17-23 and 17-24). All known cases to date are sporadic.

Syndromes with hemifacial microsomia. The second general group of branchial arch syndromes is composed of patients with hemifacial microsomia. As used here, the term refers to (1) an anomalad that may occur as an isolated finding or together with other anomalies resulting in various malformation syndromes and (2) asymmetrical (but sometimes bilateral to some degree) facial involvement.

Goldenhar syndrome. The term *hemifacial microsomia* was used by Gorlin and associates to refer to patients with unilateral microtia, macrostomia, and failure of formation of the mandibular ramus and condyle. They suggested that the Goldenhar syndrome (oculoauriculovertebral dysplasia) was a variant of this complex, characterized in addition by vertebral anomalies and epibulbar dermoids.

Grabb suggested an incidence of at least 1 in 5600 births and Poswillo 1 in 3500 births. There may be a slight predilection for males (3:2 male/female ratio).

The cause is unresolved and probably complicated. On the one hand, there are many transitional forms between hemifacial microsomia and the Goldenhar syndrome. Invalid nosological splitting has been discussed by several authors in this connection. On the other hand, the great variability observed in

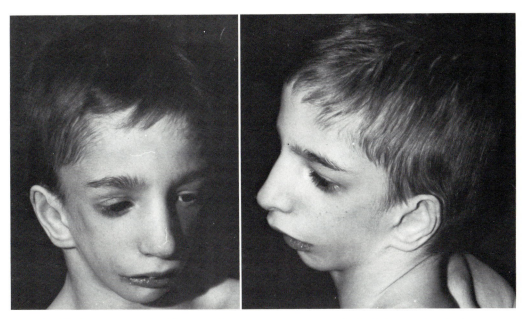

Fig. 17-21. Nager acrofacial dysostosis. Note downslanting palpebral fissures, dysplastic ears, and micrognathia. (Courtesy J. Herrmann, Madison, Wis.)

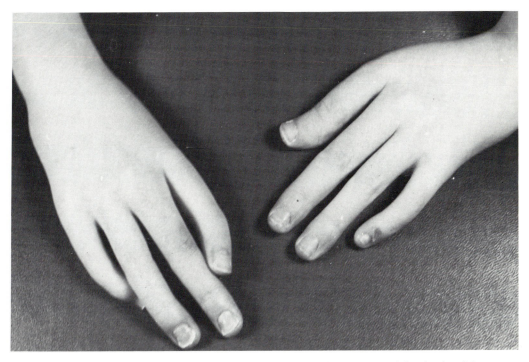

Fig. 17-22. Hands of patient with Nager acrofacial dysostosis. Note preaxial reduction defects. (Courtesy J. Herrmann, Madison, Wis.)

sporadic cases and the fact that familial instances that *seem* to have different modes of inheritance do occur, suggest etiological heterogeneity.

The overwhelming majority of cases are sporadic. However, several instances have been observed in successive generations. Affected sibs of normal parentage have been reported. Autosomal dominant, autosomal recessive, and multifactorial modes of inheritance are all possibilities to consider.

Concordance and discordance for the

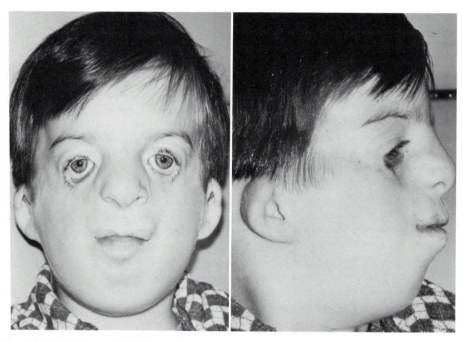

Fig. 17-23. Wildervanck-Smith syndrome. Note severe downslanting of palpebral fissures and dysplastic ears.

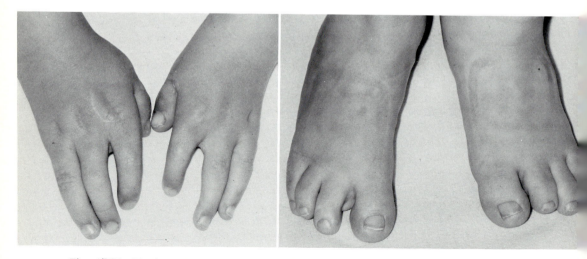

Fig. 17-24. Hands and feet of patient with Wildervanck-Smith syndrome. Note postaxial reduction defects.

Goldenhar variant have been recorded in identical twins. The zygosity of several other twin pairs discordant for the variant is less certain. The Goldenhar variant has also been seen with 5p– karyotype.

Poswillo, using an animal model of hemifacial microsomia, was able to show that destruction of differentiating tissues, in the region of the ear and jaw by an expanding hematoma, produced a branchial arch abnormality. The severity was related to the degree of local destruction. Thus a simple branchial arch defect sui generis should probably be regarded as an anomalad, whose pathogenesis probably has several different causes.

With further knowledge, several etiological and nosological entities may be delineated from this heterogeneous group of disorders. At least two entities within this group are distinctive even at the present time. First, the Summitt branchial arch syndrome seems to be a dominantly inherited disorder in which dysplastic ears occur with triangular facies, downslanting palpebral fissures, epibulbar dermoids, epicanthal folds, and congenital heart defects in some instances. Vertebral anomalies do not occur. Second, Herrmann and Opitz reported a dominantly inherited branchial arch syndrome. However, nosology for most of the asymmetrical branchial arch defects is far from clear.

In the present state of knowledge, it is best to evaluate each patient and his or her family on an individual basis. It is important to note that extreme variability of expression is characteristic. Some patients have an extensive range of anomalies and others have only a single minor anomaly such as a preauricular tag or slightly dysplastic ear. For the purposes of recurrent risk counseling, thorough evaluation for cardiac, skeletal, and renal anomalies should be carried out, first-degree relatives of the proband also being carefully scrutinized. A skeletal, cardiac, or renal anomaly in a relative probably has genetic significance regardless of whether facial abnormalities are present.

CRANIOFACIAL COMPLEX. The facies may be striking (Fig. 17-25) because of asymmetry; this is partly due to hypoplasia and/or displacement of the pinna, but the degree of involvement is markedly variable. The maxil-

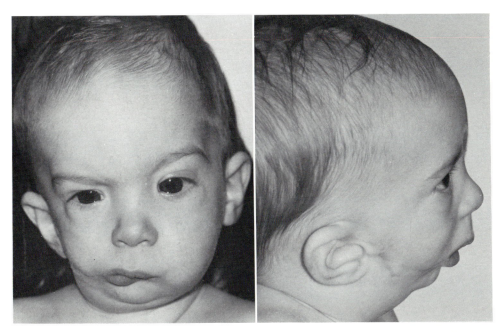

Fig. 17-25. Hemifacial microsomia. Note asymmetrical hypoplasia of ear and mandible. Ear tags have been surgically removed.

lary, temporal, and malar bones on the involved side are somewhat reduced in size and flattened, and the ipsilateral eye may be at a lower level than that on the opposite side. Further flattening may result from aplasia or hypoplasia of the mandibular ramus and condyle. Some patients manifest mild flattening of the mastoid region. Frequently there is frontal bossing. About 10% of patients have bilateral involvement, but the disorder is nearly always more severe on one side. Among 2000 cases, the right side was predominantly involved in 62%.

Malformation of the external ear may vary from complete aplasia to a crumpled, distorted pinna that is displaced anteriorly and inferiorly. Occasionally bilateral anomalous pinnae are noted. About 40% of patients with microtia have varying degrees of the syndrome. Conduction deafness due to middle ear abnormalities and/or absence or deficiency of the external auditory meatus has been noted in 30% to 50% of cases. Supernumerary ear tags may occur anywhere from the tragus to the angle of the mouth (Fig. 17-26). They are more commonly seen in patients with macrostomia and/or aplasia of the parotid gland. In the presence of epibulbar dermoids, the ear tags tend to be bilateral. Blind-ended fistulas are often found in the same area but not always bilaterally.

Often the palpebral fissure is somewhat lowered on the affected side, but marked downslanting of the palpebral fissures does not occur in this syndrome. Epibulbar dermoid and/or lipodermoid is a variable feature (Fig. 17-27). It is milky white to yellow, flattened or somewhat ellipsoidal, and usually solid rather than cystic. The surface is usually smooth but may be granular or covered by fine hairs. The dermoid is usually located at the limbus or corneal margin in the lower outer quadrant. The lipodermoid usually is found in the upper outer quadrant. Some patients have a dermoid and lipodermoid in the same eye. Generally these defects are bilateral, but about a third of patients who have epibulbar dermoids have unilateral lesions.

Unilateral coloboma of the superior lid is a common finding, occurring in about 50% to 60% of those with epibulbar dermoids. The defect usually occurs between the middle and inner third of the lid. Rarely there are colobomas of both upper and lower lids or bilateral involvement of upper lids. Choroidal or iridial coloboma and congenital cystic eye may occasionally be associated with the syndrome.

When unilateral microphthalmia or anophthalmia (Fig. 17-28) is present, mental deficiency occurs concomitantly.

Patients may have minimal underdevelopment of the condyle to unilateral aplasia of the mandibular ramus and/or condyle with absence of the glenoid fossa. Microtia oc-

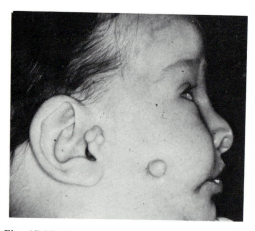

Fig. 17-26. Ear tags may appear anywhere from tragus to corner of mouth. (Courtesy M. D. Berkman, New York, N.Y.)

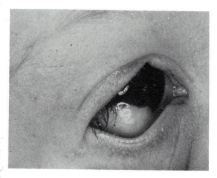

Fig. 17-27. Epibulbar dermoid in Goldenhar variant.

curs in over 70% of patients with agenesis of the ramus. Conversely, about 50% with microtia have ramus agenesis. The gonial angle is commonly flattened, and the maxilla is narrowed on the involved side. Intraorally, decreased palatal width is noted from the midline palatal raphe to the lingual surface of the teeth on the affected side. The muscles of the palate and tongue may be hypoplastic and/or paralyzed on one side. About 7% have associated cleft lip and/or palate.

At least a third of the patients with agenesis of the mandibular ramus have associated macrostomia, that is, lateral facial cleft, usually of mild degree. Occasionally a triangle of skin extends onto the inner surface of the cheek at the angle of the mouth. In the presence of epibulbar dermoids, the incidence of macrostomia may be somewhat higher. It is nearly always unilateral and on the side of the more affected ear. Occasionally there may be agenesis of the ipsilateral parotid gland, displaced salivary gland tissue, or salivary fistulas.

Failure of development or hypoplasia of muscles, such as the masseter, temporalis, pterygoideus, and those of facial expression on the involved side has been observed. In about 10% of cases, lower facial weakness

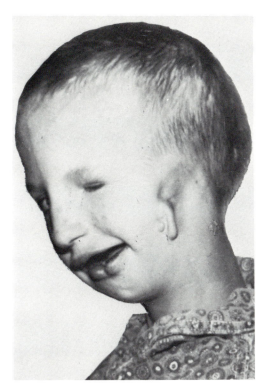

Fig. 17-28. Hemifacial microsomia with unilateral anophthalmia. Note cleft of lower lip.

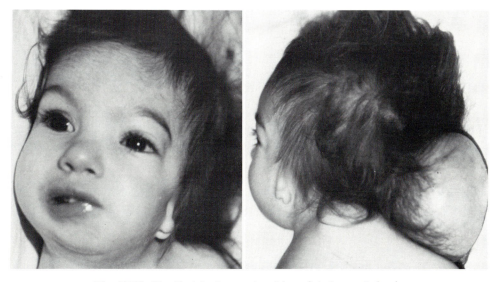

Fig. 17-29. Hemifacial microsomia with occipital encephalocele.

has been noted, possibly being related to bony involvement in the region of the facial canal.

NERVOUS SYSTEM. About 10% of patients have been mentally retarded. Occipital encephalocele has been noted in several cases (Fig. 17-29).

SKELETAL SYSTEM. Growth deficiency of prenatal onset may be observed in some instances. Bony anomalies, especially of the vertebral column, are seen in 40% to 60% of patients. The most common findings include occipitalization of the atlas, cuneiform vertebra, complete or partial cervical synostosis (Fig. 17-30) or block of two or more vertebras, supernumerary vertebras, hemivertebras, spina bifida, and anomalous ribs. Talipes equinovarus is noted in about 20% of cases. Limb reduction defects have been reported occasionally.

CARDIOVASCULAR SYSTEM. About 45% to 55% of patients have various forms of heart disease: ventricular septal defect and patent ductus arteriosus or a variant of this finding —right-sided aortic arch, connection of the ductus arteriosus with the left subclavian artery, which arises from a short but distinct common trunk, coarctation of the descending aorta, which occurs immediately distal to the obliterated ductus arteriosus, persistent left superior vena cava, and ventricular septal defect. The left subclavian artery may run behind the esophagus. Tetralogy of Fallot or Eisenmenger complex may also be found.

OTHER ANOMALIES. Pulmonary agenesis or hypoplasia has been noted in several cases, the missing lung occurring on the homolateral side. Various renal and genitourinary and other anomalies have been described as associated findings.[92-132]

Cerebral gigantism

In 1964, Sotos and associates defined cerebral gigantism, a syndrome of advanced height and bone maturation dating from infancy, mental deficiency, and unusual craniofacial appearance. The cause is not known. The syndrome has been concordant in monozygotic twins. Over seventy-five cases have been reported, about two thirds in males.

Growth hormone levels have been normal. Branched-chain essential amino acids in plasma have been found at higher levels than normal, the glycine:valine ratio being altered. Levels of 17-ketosteroids and gonadotropins have been elevated in several patients.

Craniofacial complex. The facies is characterized by macrocranium with dolichocephaly and ocular hypertelorism, with downslanting palpebral fissures. The frontal hairline is often receded. Highly arched palate (in over 90% of patients) and early dental eruption (in over 50%) have been observed. Mandibular prognathism has been noted in over 80% (Fig. 17-31).

Nervous system. Most patients have nonprogressive neurological dysfunction, manifested by unusual clumsiness, dull intelligence (mean IQ = 60), and, at times, aggressive behavior. Over 80% have dilated cerebral ventricles. About 40% have abnormal electroencephalographic studies. Convulsions and respiratory and feeding problems have been noted frequently. Delay in walking until after 15 months of age and delay in speech development until after 2½ years are usual.

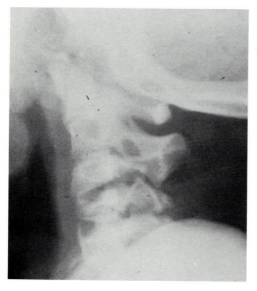

Fig. 17-30. Note fusion of cervical spinous processes.

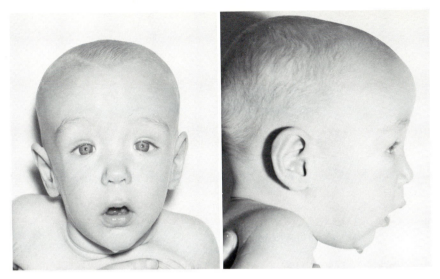

Fig. 17-31. Cerebral gigantism. Note macrocephaly, dolichocephaly, downslanting palpebral fissures, and pointed chin. (Courtesy D. W. Smith, Seattle, Wash.)

Skeletal system. Many patients are large at birth, the mean being about 4250 gm and 55 cm. Bone age is usually 2 to 3 years in advance of chronological age in the absence of obvious endocrine dysfunction in about 75%. Hands and feet are disproportionately large in over 80%. Head circumference and height are well above the ninety-seventh percentile for age, and frontal bossing is marked. The span is greater than the height in about 90% of cases. Kyphoscoliosis has been present in about 30%.[133-143]

Cleft lip–cleft palate syndromes

Both cleft lip and cleft palate are discussed in detail in Chapter 16. In this section, only syndromes with clefting are considered. All disorders associated with cleft lip–cleft palate are presented in Tables 17-12 to 17-15, including syndromes with cleft lip–cleft palate (Table 17-12), syndromes with isolated cleft palate (Table 17-13), syndromes associated with the nonspecific Robin anomalad (Table 17-14), and syndromes with median or pseudomedian cleft lip (Table 17-15). In each table, the striking features of each condition and the etiology are given. Table 17-16 lists the chromosomal syndromes known to be associated with clefting. They are considered in more detail in Chapter 15. Table 17-17 lists the nonrandom association of clefts with various other abnormalities.

In this section, only the Stickler syndrome, the van der Woude syndrome, orofaciodigital syndrome I, orofaciodigital syndrome II, otopalatodigital syndrome, and ectrodactyly-ectodermal dysplasia-clefting syndrome are considered in detail. Some syndromes with clefting are presented more fully in other sections of this chapter (Beckwith-Wiedemann syndrome, branchial arch syndromes, cleidocranial dysplasia, craniosynostosis syndromes, diastrophic dwarfism, frontonasal dysplasia, the Gorlin syndrome, the de Lange syndrome, and the Marfan syndrome). Detailed discussions of all syndromes with clefting are presented elsewhere.[150, 159, 160]

Stickler syndrome. The Stickler syndrome is a relatively common, autosomal dominant, connective tissue dysplasia composed of a *generalized skeletal complex,* including slender body habitus, joint hyperextensibility, prominence of large joints, arthropathy, and mild epiphyseal dysplasia, an *orofacial complex* including midfacial flattening (Fig. 17-32), cleft palate, and sometimes the Robin anomalad, and an *ocular complex* of myopia, retinal detachment, and cataracts.

Text continued on p. 551.

Table 17-12. Syndromes with cleft lip–cleft palate

Syndrome	Striking features	Relative frequency of cleft lip–cleft palate in syndrome	Etiology
Monogenic syndromes			
Appelt syndrome[1]	Ocular hypertelorism, tetra-phocomelia, enlarged penis or clitoris	Common	Autosomal recessive; some authorities consider this syndrome and the pseudo-thalidomide syndrome to be identical
Bixler syndrome[3]	Hypertelorism, microtia, ectopic kidneys, congenital heart defect, growth deficiency	Common	Autosomal recessive
Bowen-Armstrong syndrome[5]	Growth retardation, mental deficiency, abnormal electro-encephalogram, syndactyly of toes (2 and 3, 4 and 5), hyper-pigmented areas, oligodontia, ankyloblepharon filiforme adnatum	Apparently common	Autosomal recessive
Clefting/ankylo-blepharon syn-drome[9]	Ankyloblepharon filiforme adnatum	Common	Autosomal dominant
Clefting/enlarged parietal foram-ina syndrome[9]	Enlarged parietal foramina	Uncommon	Autosomal dominant

1. Appelt, J., et al.: Pädiat. Pädol. **2**:119, 1966.
2. Bergsma, D.: Snydrome Identification 3(1):7, 1975.
3. Bixler, D., et al.: Birth Defects 5(2):77, 1969.
4. Bixler, D., et al.: Clin. Genet. **3**:43, 1971.
5. Bowen, P., and Armstrong, H. B.: Clin. Genet. **9**:35, 1976.
6. Cervenka, J., et al.: Am. J. Hum. Genet. **19**:416, 1967.
7. Cohen, M. M., Jr.: Unpublished data, 1973.
8. Freire-Maia, N.: Am. J. Hum. Genet. 22:370, 1970.
9. Gorlin, R. J., Cervenka, J., and Pruzansky, S.: Birth Defects 7(7):3-49, 1971.
10. Gorlin, R. J., Pindborg, J. J., and Cohen, M. M., Jr.: Syndromes of the head and neck, ed. 2, New York, 1976, McGraw-Hill Book Co.
11. Gorlin, R. J., and Sedano, H. O.: Multiple nevoid basal cell carcinoma syndrome. In Vinken, P. J., and Bruyn, G. W., editors: Handbook of clinical neurology: the phakomatoses, vol. 14, New York, 1973, American Elsevier Publishing Co., pp. 455-473.
12. Gorlin, R. J., Sedano, H. O., and Cervenka, J.: Pediatrics 41:503-509, 1968.
13. Hanson, J. W., and Smith, D. W.: J. Pediatr. **87**:285, 1975.
14. Herrmann, J., et al.: Birth Defects 5(3):81, 1969.
15. Herrmann, J., et al.: Rocky Mt. Med. J. **66**:45, 1969.
16. Hsia, Y. E., et al.: Pediatrics 48:237, 1971.
17. Ide, C. H., and Wollschlaeger, P. B.: Arch. Ophthalmol. 81:640, 1969.
18. Jones, K. L., et al.: J. Pediatr. **84**:90, 1974.
19. Juberg, R. C., and Hayward, J. R.: J. Pediatr. **74**:755, 1969.
20. Opitz, J. M., et al.: Birth Defects 5(2):86, 1969.
21. Pallister, P. D., et al.: Birth Defects 10(7):51, 1974.
22. Pantke, O. A., and Cohen, M. M., Jr.: Birth Defects 7(7):147, 1971.
23. Pilotto, R. F., et al.: Birth Defects 11(2):51, 1975.
24. Rapp, R. S., and Hodgkin, W. E.: J. Med. Genet. 5:269, 1968.
25. Zackai, E. H., et al.: J. Pediatr. **87**:280, 1975.

Table 17-12. Syndromes with cleft lip–cleft palate—cont'd

Syndrome	Striking features	Relative frequency of cleft lip–cleft palate in syndrome	Etiology
Cryptophthalmos syndrome[17]	Cryptophthalmos, abnormal frontal hairline, variable syndactyly of hands and feet, coloboma of alae nasi, genitourinary anomalies	Uncommon	Autosomal recessive
Ectrodactyly-ectodermal dysplasia-clefting syndrome[4]	Ectrodactyly (hands and feet), sparse blond hair, oligodontia, nasolacrimal duct obstruction	Common	Autosomal dominant with reduced penetrance; may be etiologically heterogeneous with an autosomal recessive type
Freire-Maia syndrome[8]	Tetraperomelia, large deformed ears, sparse hair, hypoplastic nipples, oligodontia, conical crown form, hypogonadism, mental deficiency	Uncommon	Autosomal recessive
Fetal face syndrome[7]	Macrocephaly, ocular hypertelorism, flat nose, overfolding of helix, mesomelia, clinodactyly, vertebral anomalies, genital anomalies	Rare	Etiologically heterogeneous with common autosomal dominant type and rare autosomal recessive type
Gorlin syndrome[11]	Multiple basal cell carcinomas, jaw cysts, skeletal anomalies	Uncommon	Autosomal dominant
Hemifacial microsomia (Goldenhar syndrome)[10]	Unilateral dysplastic ear, ear tags and/or pit, unilateral hypoplasia of mandibular ramus, and variably epibulbar dermoids, vertebral anomalies, cardiac defects, renal anomalies, other abnormalities	Uncommon	Most cases sporadic; few familial instances; pedigrees compatible with autosomal dominant and autosomal recessive transmission
Hypertelorism-hypospadias syndrome[20]	Hypertelorism, hypospadias, other abnormalities	Uncommon	Autosomal dominant with predominantly male sex limitation
Juberg-Hayward syndrome[19]	Microcephaly, hypoplastic distally placed thumbs, short radii	Common	Autosomal recessive
Meckel syndrome[16]	Polydactyly, polycystic kidneys, encephalocele, cardiac anomalies, other abnormalities	Common	Autosomal recessive
Oculodentoosseous dysplasia[10]	Narrow nose, hypoplastic alae, microcornea, iris anomalies, syndactyly and camptodactyly of fourth and fifth fingers, enamel hypoplasia	Rare	Autosomal dominant
Popliteal pterygium syndrome[14]	Popliteal pterygia, musculoskeletal anomalies, especially hypoplastic digits, genitourinary anomalies, other abnormalities	Common	Probably autosomal dominant

Continued.

Table 17-12. Syndromes with cleft lip–cleft palate—cont'd

Syndrome	Striking features	Relative frequency of cleft lip–cleft palate in syndrome	Etiology
Pseudothalido-mide syndrome[12]	Tetraphocomelia, hypoplastic cartilages of alae and pinnae, facial hemangiomas, mental deficiency	Uncommon	Autosomal recessive
Rapp-Hodgkin syndrome[24]	Hypohidrosis, thin, wiry hair, dystrophic nails	Common	Autosomal dominant
W syndrome[21]	Mental deficiency, seizures, frontal prominence, anterior cowlick, ocular hypertelorism, downslanting palpebral fissures, strabismus, broad nasal tip, congenitally absent central incisors, prominent lower facial height, cubitus valgus, subluxation at radioulnar joints, camptodactyly, clinodactyly	Incomplete cleft lip, submucous cleft palate	Autosomal dominant?
van der Woude syndrome[6]	Lip pits	Common	Autosomal dominant
Waardenberg syndrome[22]	Dystopia canthorum, synophrys, heterochromia irides, deafness, poliosis, vitiligo	Uncommon	Autosomal dominant
Environmentally induced syndromes			
Amniotic band syndrome[18]	Ring constrictions and amputations of digits or limbs, distal syndactyly, cleft lip-palate, microcephaly, encephaloceles, microphthalmia, bizarre facial clefts, facial deformities, bands, other abnormalities	Uncommon	Amniotic bands
Fetal hydantoin syndrome[13]	Digit and nail hypoplasia, unusual facies, growth and psychomotor retardation, other anomalies	Uncommon	Phenytoin during pregnancy
Fetal trimethadi-one syndrome[25]	Mental deficiency, speech disorder, V-shaped eyebrows, epicanthal folds, low-set ears with overfolded helix, other anomalies	Uncommon	Trimethadione or para-methadione during pregnancy
Unknown genesis syndromes			
Clefting/ectropion syndrome[9]	Ocular hypertelorism, ectropion of lower eyelids, digital and/or limb reduction defects	Common	Almost all cases sporadic to date; one known familial instance
Herrmann syndrome II[15]	Microbrachycephaly, craniosynostosis, symmetrically malformed limbs, mental deficiency	?	? Sporadic to date

Table 17-12. Syndromes with cleft lip–cleft palate—cont'd

Syndrome	Striking features	Relative frequency of cleft lip–cleft palate in syndrome	Etiology
Pilotto syndrome[23]	Growth retardation, mental deficiency, microbrachycephaly, ocular hypertelorism, malformed ears, high nasal bridge, facial asymmetry, short neck, low posterior hairline, patent ductus arteriosus, hypoplastic external genitalia, scoliosis, rib defects, other skeletal anomalies	?	? Sporadic to date
Wildervanck-Smith syndrome[2]	Mandibulofacial dysostosis, preaxial and post-axial upper and lower limb deficiencies	?	? Sporadic to date

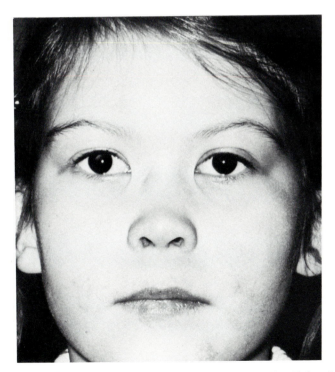

Fig. 17-32. Stickler syndrome. Note flat midface and epicanthal folds. Cleft palate and Robin anomalad are common. (From Cohen, M. M., Jr., et al.: Birth Defects 7[7]:143, 1971.)

Table 17-13. Syndromes with cleft palate

Syndrome	Striking features	Relative frequency of cleft palate in syndrome	Etiology
Monogenic syndromes			
Aase-Smith syndrome[1]	Hydrocephaly, Dandy-Walker malformation, hip dislocation, malformed ears, other malformations	?	? Autosomal dominant
Apert syndrome[7]	Craniosynostosis, ocular hypertelorism, downslanting palpebral fissures, proptosis, midface deficiency, symmetrical syndactyly	Common	Autosomal dominant

1. Aase, J. M., and Smith, D. W.: J. Pediatr. **73:**606, 1968.
2. Beare, J. M., et al.: Br. J. Dermatol. **81:**241, 1969.
3. Berg, J. M., et al.: The de Lange syndrome, New York, 1970, Pergamon Press.
4. Braun, F. C., Jr., and Bayer, J. F.: J. Pediatr. **60:**33, 1962.
5. Burgio, G. R., et al.: Arch. Fr. Pédiat. **31:**681, 1974.
6. Christian, J. C., et al.: Clin. Genet. **2:**95, 1971.
7. Cohen, M. M., Jr.: Birth Defects **11**(2):137, 1971.
8. Cohen, M. M., Jr., and Hanson, J. W.: Personal observation, 1975.
9. Daentl, D. L., et al.: J. Pediatr. **86:**106, 1975.
10. de la Chapelle, A., et al.: Arch. Fr. Pédiat. **29:**759, 1972.
11. Erikson, A.: Acta Paediatr. Scand. **63:**885, 1974.
12. Fontaine, G., et al.: J. Génét. Hum. **22:**289, 1974.
13. Fuhrmann, W., et al.: Humangenetik **14:**196, 1972.
14. Gareis, F. J., and Smith, D. W.: J. Pediatr. **79:**470, 1971.
15. Gordon, H., et al.: J. Med. Genet. **6:**266, 1969.
16. Gorlin, R. J., Alper, R., and Langer, L.: J. Pediatr. **83:**633, 1973.
17. Gorlin, R. J., Cervenka, J., Anderson, R. C., et al.: Am. J. Dis. Child. **119:**176, 1970.
18. Gorlin, R. J., Pindborg, J. J., and Cohen, M. M., Jr.: Syndromes of the head and neck, ed. 2, New York, 1976, McGraw-Hill Book Co.
19. Gorlin, R. J., et al.: Birth Defects **7:**87, 1971.
20. Gunderson, C. H., et al.: Medicine **46:**491, 1967.
21. Herrmann, J.: Eur. J. Pediatr. (In press.)
22. Herrmann, J., and Opitz, J. M.: Birth Defects **11**(2):76, 1975.
23. Ho, C.-K., et al.: Am. J. Dis. Child. **129:**714, 1975.
24. Jones, K. L., et al.: Lancet **1:** 1267, 1973.
25. Katcher, M., and Hall, J. G.: Am. J. Dis. Child. (In press.)
26. Langer, L. O., Jr., and Herrmann, J.: Birth Defects **10**(7):167, 1974.
27. Lowry, R. B., and Miller, J. R.: Lancet **1:** 1302, 1971.
28. Marden, P. M., and Walker, W. A.: Am. J. Dis. Child. **112:**225, 1966.
29. Maroteaux, P., et al.: Presse Méd. **78:**2371, 1970.
30. Nance, W. E., and Sweeney, A.: Birth Defects **6**(4):25, 1970.
31. Opitz, J. M., et al.: Birth Defects **10:**97, 1974.
32. Opitz, J. M.: Personal communication, 1976.
33. Palant, D. I., et al.: J. Pediatr. **78:**686, 1971.
34. Pantke, O. A., et al.: Birth Defects **11**(2):76, 1975.
35. Phillips, C. I., and Griffiths, D. L.: Br. J. Ophthalmol. **53:**346, 1969.
36. Rudiger, R. A., et al.: J. Pediatr. **79:**977, 1971.
37. Say, B., et al.: Humangenetik **26:**1, 1975.
38. Shaw, E. B., and Steinbach, H. L.: Am. J. Dis. Child. **115:**477, 1968.
39. Shepard, T. H.: Catalog of teratogenic agents, Baltimore, 1973, John Hopkins University Press.
40. Siggers, D. C., et al.: Birth Defects **10:**193, 432, 1974.
41. Spranger, J. W., and Langer, L. O., Jr.: Radiology **94:**313, 1970.
42. Walden, R. H., et al.: Plast. Reconstr. Surg. **48:**80, 1971.
43. Walker, B. A., et al.: Medicine **51:**41, 1972.
44. Wildervanck, L. S.: Ned. T. Geneesk. **104:** 2600, 1960.

Table 17-13. Syndromes with cleft palate—cont'd

Syndrome	Striking features	Relative frequency of cleft palate in syndrome	Etiology
	of hands and feet, minimally involving second, third, and fourth digits, mental deficiency		
Braun-Bayer syndrome[4]	Urinary tract anomalies, rudimentary distal phalanges with bifid ends, conduction deafness	Cleft uvula only (2/5)	? X-linked or autosomal recessive
Campomelic syndrome[29]	Flat face, hypertelorism, hypoplastic scapulae, thoracic vertebral defects, bowing of femora and tibiae, pretibial dimpling, valgus deformity of feet, other abnormalities, commonly lethal before 6 months of age	Common	Autosomal recessive; may be etiologically heterogeneous
Cerebrocostomandibular syndrome[25]	Microcephaly, posterior rib gap defects, other abnormalities, commonly lethal during neonatal period	Common	Autosomal recessive
de la Chapelle syndrome[10]	Micromelic dwarfism, low-set ears, ocular hypertelorism, flat natal root, short curved bones (especially radius and ulna), triangular fibula and ulna, double phalanges, vertebral anomalies, patent foramen ovale, patent ductus arteriosus, commonly lethal	2/2	Autosomal recessive
Chondrodysplasia punctata (rhizomelic type)[18]	Short femora and humeri, prominent forehead, flat face, cataracts, stippled epiphyses, other abnormalities, commonly lethal	Uncommon	Autosomal recessive
Christian sydrome I[6]	Craniosynostosis, microcephaly, arthrogryposis, adducted thumbs	Common	Autosomal recessive
Cleft palate/brachial plexus neuritis syndrome[11]	Recurrent brachial plexus neuritis, limited extension at elbows, winging of scapulae, facial asymmetry, downslanting palpebral fissures, deep-set hypoteloric eyes	Common	Autosomal dominant
Cleft palate/connective tissue dysplasia syndrome[8]	Cervical fusions, downslanting palpebral fissures, micrognathia, dislocated radial heads, clinodactyly, positional foot deformities	Only submucous clefts to date	? X-linked or autosomal recessive
Cleft palate/lateral synechiae syndrome[13]	Lateral synechiae	Common	Autosomal dominant

Continued.

Table 17-13. Syndromes with cleft palate—cont'd

Syndrome	Striking features	Relative frequency of cleft palate in syndrome	Etiology
Cleft palate/stapes fixation syndrome	Stapes fixation, hypodontia, skeletal anomalies	2/2	Autosomal recessive
Cleidocranial dysplasia[18]	Large calvaria, relatively small face, Wormian bones, persistent fontanels, supernumerary teeth, delayed eruption or failure of eruption, absent or hypoplastic clavicles, other skeletal anomalies	Highly arched palate, submucous cleft palate or complete cleft common	Autosomal dominant
Diastrophic dwarfism[43]	Short stature, contractures, clubfoot, hitchhiker's thumb, cystic ear, other defects	Common	Autosomal recessive
Dubowitz syndrome[18]	Growth deficiency, mild mental deficiency, microcephaly, blepharophimosis, micrognathia, eczema	Submucous cleft, bifid uvula, highly arched palate common	Autosomal recessive
Ectrodactyly-cleft palate syndrome[32]	Ectrodactyly and syndactyly (hands and feet)	Common	Autosomal dominant
Fontaine syndrome[12]	Micrognathia, dysplastic ears, ectrodactyly and syndactyly (feet), mental deficiency in some cases	Submucous cleft palate, common; sometimes cleft palate	Autosomal dominant
Gareis-Smith syndrome[14]	Short stature	Common	Dominant (X-linked ?)
Gordon syndrome[15]	Camptodactyly, clubfoot	Common	Autosomal recessive
Katcher-Hall syndrome[25]	Short stature, mental deficiency	Common	? Autosomal recessive
Larsen syndrome[18]	Multiple dislocations, skeletal defects, flat face	Uncommon	Autosomal recessive and autosomal dominant types
Lowry-Miller syndrome[27]	Persistent trucus arteriosus, abnormal right pulmonary artery, intrauterine death	2/2	Autosomal recessive
Marden-Walker syndrome[28]	Blepharophimosis, joint contractures, muscular hypotonia, other abnormalities	Uncommon	Autosomal recessive
Marfan syndrome[18]	Dolichostenomelia, arachnodactyly, ectopia lentis, aortic aneurysm	Uncommon; highly arched palate common	Autosomal dominant
Megepiphyseal dwarfism[16]	Enlarged joints, abbreviated long bones, large epiphyses, flared metaphyses	?	? Autosomal recessive
Micrognathic dwarfism[29]	Micromelic dwarfism, small mandible, cleft vertebrae	Common	Autosomal recessive

Table 17-13. Syndromes with cleft palate—cont'd

Syndrome	Striking features	Relative frequency of cleft palate in syndrome	Etiology
Multiple pterygia syndrome[18]	Multiple pterygia	Common	Autosomal recessive
Nance-Sweeney chondrodysplasia[30]	Rhizomelic dwarfism, dysplastic ears, thick leathery skin, soft tissue calcifications	?	Autosomal recessive
Nager acrofacial dysostosis[21]	Hypoplastic ears, downslanting palpebral fissures, micrognathia, preaxial upper limb deficiency	Uncommon	Autosomal recessive
Orofaciodigital syndrome I[18]	Dystopia canthorum, hypoplastic alar cartilages, milia, multiple frenula, laterally cleft palate, bifid tongue, malposed teeth, tooth anomalies, brachydactyly, syndactyly, clinodactyly	Common	X-linked dominant; lethal in male
Orofaciodigital syndrome II[18]	Lobed tongue, manual polydactyly, bilateral polysyndactyly of halluces	Uncommon	Autosomal recessive
Otopalatodigital syndrome[18]	Frontal prominence, ocular hypertelorism, broad nasal root, occipital prominence, conduction deafness, short terminal phalanges and short nails on fingers and toes, fifth finger clinodactyly, widely spaced curved toes, dislocation of radial heads, pectus excavatum	Common	X-linked
Palant syndrome[33]	Microcephaly, short stature, mental deficiency, almond-shaped deep-set eyes, bulbous nasal tip, clinodactyly of toes, prominence of anteromedial aspects of wrists	2/2	Autosomal recessive
Persistent left superior vena cava syndrome[17]	Persistent left superior vena cava, clubfeet	Common	X-linked recessive
Phillips-Griffiths syndrome[35]	Growth deficiency, macular colobomas, hallux valgus, flexion deformities of distal interphalangeal joint of fifth fingers, other abnormalities	Apparently common	? Autosomal recessive
Pseudodiastrophic dwarfism[5]	Flat nose, ocular hypertelorism, micrognathia, full cheeks, malformed ears, micromelia, talipes equinovarus, externally rotated hands, toe anomalies, other abnormalities	2/2	? Autosomal recessive

Continued.

Table 17-13. Syndromes with cleft palate—cont'd

Syndrome	Striking features	Relative frequency of cleft palate in syndrome	Etiology
Rudiger syndrome[36]	Growth retardation, flexion contractures of hands, simian creases, small fingers and fingernails, ureteral stenosis, coarse facies, lethal during first year of life	2/2	Autosomal recessive
Saethre-Chotzen syndrome[34]	Craniosynostosis, facial asymmetry, low-set frontal hairline, ptosis of eyelids, deviated nasal septum, variable brachydactyly, variable cutaneous syndactyly, especially of second and third fingers	Rare	Autosomal dominant
Say syndrome[37]	Small head size, large ears, short stature, tapering fingers, hypoplastic distal phalanges, proximally placed thumbs	Apparently common	Autosomal dominant
Smith-Lemli-Opitz syndrome[18]	Growth deficiency, mental deficiency, broad nasal tip, anteverted nostrils, ptosis of eyelids, broad alveolar ridges, micrognathia, hypospadias, cryptorchidism, syndactyly of second and third toes	Common if submucous cleft and cleft uvula included	Autosomal recessive
Spondyloepiphyseal dysplasia congenita[41]	Disproportionate short stature involving neck and trunk, myopia, retinal detachment	Common	Autosomal dominant
Stickler syndrome[22]	Myopia, retinal detachment, flat midface, prominent joints with degenerative joint disease, mild epiphyseal dysplasia, overtubulation of long bones, other abnormalities	Common	Autosomal dominant
Treacher Collins syndrome[18]	Dysplastic low-set ears, downslanting palpebral fissures, micrognathia	Common	Autosomal dominant
Wildervanck syndrome[44]	Cervical fusion, deafness, abducens paralysis	Apparently common	Autosomal dominant
Environmentally induced syndromes			
Aminopterin syndrome[38]	Cranial dysplasia, craniosynostosis, micrognathia, clubfoot, hypodactyly	Uncommon	Aminopterin as abortifacient during first trimester of pregnancy
Fetal alcohol syndrome[24]	Growth deficiency, mental deficiency, microcephaly, narrow palpebral fissures, congenital heart defects, joint anomalies, other abnormalities	Uncommon	Chronic alcoholism during pregnancy

Table 17-13. Syndromes with cleft palate—cont'd

Syndrome	Striking features	Relative frequency of cleft palate in syndrome	Etiology
Thalidomide syndrome[39]	Phocomelia, dysplastic ears, facial hemangioma, atresia of esophagus or duodenum, tetralogy of Fallot, renal agenesis	Rare	Thalidomide during pregnancy
Unknown genesis syndromes			
Beckwith-Wiedemann syndrome[18]	Macroglossia, omphalocele, neonatal hypoglycemia, postsomatic gigantism, other abnormalities	Rare	Most cases sporadic; few familial instances
Charlie M. syndrome[18]	Ocular hypertelorism, seventh nerve paralysis in some cases, absent or conical incisors, variable limb anomalies from oligodactyly to peromelia	?	Sporadic to date
Cleft palate/acanthosis nigricans syndrome[2]	Cutis gyratum, acanthosis nigricans, ocular hypertelorism, neonatal teeth, hypodontia, bifid nipples, hypogonadism	?	Sporadic to date
Coffin-Siris syndrome[18]	Coarse facies, absent fifth fingernails and toenails, growth deficiency, mental deficiency, other abnormalities	Uncommon	Most cases sporadic to date; one known instance of affected sibs
Femoral hypoplasia-unusual facies syndrome[9]	Upslanting palpebral fissures, short nose with hypoplastic alar cartilages, long philtrum, short or absent femurs and fibulae, other defects	Common	Sporadic to date
Glossopalatine ankylosis syndrome[18]	Glossopalatine ankylosis, micrognathia, hypodontia, variable limb anomalies from oligodactyly to peromelia	Uncommon	All cases sporadic to date
Ho syndrome[23]	Micrognathia, Wormian bones, congenital heart defect, dislocated hips, absent tibiae, bowed fibulae, preaxial polydactyly (feet), simian creases, ulnar deviation of fingers	?	Sporadic to date
Klippel-Feil syndrome[18, 20]	Block fusion of cervical vertebrae	Fairly common	Almost all cases sporadic; few familial instances (autosomal recessive)
Kniest syndrome[40]	Disproportionate dwarfism, round face, flat midface, short neck, lordosis, kyphoscoliosis, tibial bowing, progressively enlarged, stiff and painful joints, clubfeet, severe myopia, retinal detachment, cataracts, deafness, recurrent respiratory infections	Common	Almost all cases sporadic to date; one known familial instance (autosomal dominant ?)

Continued.

Table 17-13. Syndromes with cleft palate—cont'd

Syndrome	Striking features	Relative frequency of cleft palate in syndrome	Etiology
de Lange syndrome[3]	Microbrachycephaly, confluent eyebrows, anteverted nostrils, long philtrum, thin lips, growth deficiency, mental deficiency, limb anomalies, other abnormalities	Fairly common	Most cases sporadic; few familial instances
Walden syndrome[42]	Short humeri and femora, long radii and tibiae	?	Sporadic to date

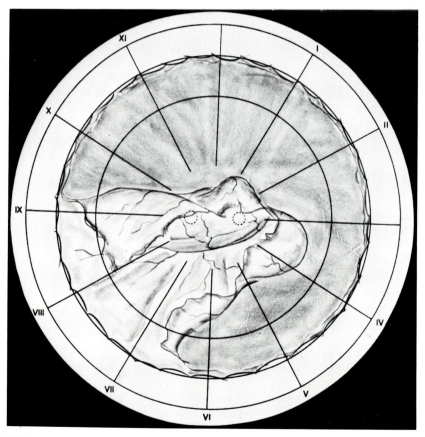

Fig. 17-33. Stickler syndrome. Retinal sketch of 12-year-old patient showing rolled-over retina with 270° disinsertion. (From Cohen, M. M., Jr., et al.: Birth Defects 7[7]:143, 1971.)

Table 17-14. Conditions associated with the Robin anomalad

Condition	Striking features	Frequency of Robin anomalad in given condition	Mode of inheritance or cause
Monogenic syndromes			
Beckwith-Wiedemann syndrome[2]	Macroglossia, omphalocele, visceromegaly, neonatal hypoglycemia, postsomatic gigantism, other defects	Uncommon; isolated cleft palate uncommon	Most cases sporadic, few familial instances
Campomelic syndrome[15]	Flat face, hypertelorism, hypoplastic scapulas, thoracic vertebral defects, bowing of femurs and tibias, pretibial dimpling, valgus deformity of foot, other abnormalities	Common	Autosomal recessive; may be etiologically heterogeneous
Cerebrocostomandibular syndrome[11]	Microcephaly, posterior rib gap defects, other abnormalities	Common	Autosomal recessive
Diastrophic dwarfism[6, 16]	Short stature, contractures, clubfoot, hitchhiker's thumb, cystic ear, and other defects	Uncommon; isolated cleft palate common	Autosomal recessive
Femoral hypoplasia–unusual facies syndrome[3, 6]	Upslanting palpebral fissures, short nose with hypoplastic alar cartilages, long philtrum, short or absent femurs and fibulas, other defects	Micrognathia and cleft palate common; glossoptosis uncommon	Sporadic, cause unknown
Myotonic dystrophy (severe congenital)[12]	Myotonia, progressive muscle wasting, cataracts, various other abnormalities	Uncommon	Autosomal dominant
Persistent left superior vena cava syndrome[4]	Persistent left superior vena cava, atrial septal defect, talipes equinovarus	Common	X-linked recessive
Radiohumeral synostosis syndrome[5, 6]	Radiohumeral synostosis, anosmia	? Too few cases known	? Autosomal dominant
Spondyloepiphyseal dysplasia congenita[9, 14]	Disproportionately short stature involving neck and trunk, myopia, retinal detachment	Uncommon; isolated cleft palate common	Autosomal dominant

1. Aurias, A., and Laurent, C.: Ann. Génét. **18:** 189, 1975.
2. Cohen, M. M., Jr., et al.: Am. J. Dis. Child. **122:**515, 1971.
3. Daentl, D. L., et al.: J. Pediatr. **86:**106, 1975.
4. Gorlin, R. J., et al.: Am. J. Dis. Child. **119:** 176, 1970.
5. Hanson, J. W.: Personal communication, 1975.
6. Hanson, J. W., and Smith, D. W.: J. Pediatr. **87:**30, 1975.
7. Hanson, J. W., and Smith, D. W.: J. Pediatr. **87:**285, 1975.
8. Herrmann, J., and Opitz, J. M.: Birth Defects **11**(2):76, 1975.
9. Holthusen, W.: Ann. Radiol. (Paris) **15:**253, 1972.
10. Jones, K. L., et al.: Lancet **1:**1267, 1973.
11. Langer, L. O., Jr., and Herrmann, J.: Birth Defects **10**(7):167, 1974.
12. Opitz, J. M.: Personal communication, 1975.
13. Shah, C. V., et al.: Am. J. Dis. Child. **119:** 238, 1970.
14. Spranger, J. W., and Langer, L. O., Jr.: Radiology **94:**313, 1970.
15. Storer, J., and Grossman, H.: Radiology **111:** 673, 1974.
16. Walker, B. A., et al.: Medicine **51:**41, 1972.
17. Zackai, E. H., et al.: J. Pediatr. **87:**280, 1975.

Continued.

Table 17-14. Conditions associated with the Robin anomalad—cont'd

Condition	Striking features	Frequency of Robin anomalad in given condition	Etiology
Stickler syndrome[8]	Myopia, retinal detachment, flat midface, prominent joints with degenerative joint disease, mild epiphyseal dysplasia, overtubulation of long bones, other abnormalities	Common; isolated cleft palate common	Autosomal dominant
Chromosomal syndromes			
Trisomy 11q[1]	Axial hypotonia, limb hypertonia, wrinkled face, beaked nose, low-set malformed ears, short neck, narrow chest, widely spaced nipples, congenital heart defect, renal agenesis, malformations of urinary tract, micropenis, acetabular dysplasia, clubfoot	Micrognathia most common; cleft palate second most common; glossoptosis least common	Trisomy for distal segment of long arm of chromosome 11
Teratogenically induced syndromes			
Fetal alcohol syndrome[10]	Growth deficiency, mental deficiency, microcephaly, narrow palpebral fissures, congenital heart defects, joint anomalies, other abnormalities	Uncommon	Chronic alcoholism during pregnancy
Fetal hydantoin syndrome[7]	Digit and nail hypoplasia, unusual facies, growth and psychomotor retardation, other anomalies	Uncommon; cleft lip and palate also observed	Phenytoin during pregnancy
Fetal trimethadione syndrome[17]	Mental deficiency, speech disorders, V-shaped eyebrows, epicanthus, low-set posteriorly rotated ears with overfolded helix, cardiac anomalies, irregular teeth, other defects	Uncommon; cleft lip and palate also observed	Trimethadione or paramethadione during pregnancy
Associations			
Cleft palate–accessory metacarpal of index finger association[9]	Bilateral accessory metacarpal of index finger with clinodactyly, pectus carinatum	? Too few cases known	Sporadic; cause unknown
Cleft palate–amelia association[9]	Amelia	? Too few cases known	Sporadic; cause unknown
Cleft lip–cleft palate and associated congenital heart disease[13]	Patent ductus arteriosus, atrial septal defect, ventricular septal defect, ventricular hypertrophy, cor triloculare, coarctation of aorta, biventricular aorta, dextrocardia	Uncommon; cleft lip–cleft palate or isolated cleft palate more commonly associated than Robin anomalad	Sporadic; cause unknown

Table 17-15. Conditions with median cleft lip

Conditions	Striking features	Relative frequency of median cleft lip in condition	Etiology
Frontonasal dysplasia[2]	Ocular hypertelorism, widow's peak, anterior cranium bifidum occultum, wide-set nostrils, lack of elevation of nasal tip, notching or colobomas of nostrils, other abnormalities	Uncommon	Most cases sporadic; few familial instances; probably etiologically heterogeneous
Majewski syndrome[3]	Short narrow thorax, preaxial and postaxial polydactyly of hands and feet, short tibias, protuberant abdomen, cardiac anomalies, genital anomalies, cleft lip and/or palate, other abnormalities, death from respiratory distress	Common	All cases sporadic to date
Orofaciodigital syndrome I[2]	Dystopia canthorum, hypoplastic alar cartilages, milia, multiple frenula, laterally cleft palate, bifid tongue, malposed teeth, tooth anomalies, brachydactyly, syndactyly, clinodactyly	Common	X-linked dominant; lethal in male
Orofaciodigital syndrome II[2]	Lobed tongue, manual polydactyly, bilateral polysyndactyly of halluces	Common	Autosomal recessive
Premaxillary agenesis[1]	Median cleft lip, flat nose, ocular hypotelorism, holoprosencephaly, other abnormalities, amentia, seizures, apnea, neonatal demise	Common	Etiologically heterogeneous (trisomy 13 syndrome, 18p– karyotype, other chromosomal aberrations, Meckel syndrome, autosomal recessive, autosomal dominant with markedly variable expressivity)

1. Cohen, M. M., Jr., and Hohl, T. H.: Etiologic heterogeneity in the holoprosencephalic disorders. In Bosma, J. F., editor: The cranial base, Washington, D.C., U.S. Government Printing Office. (In press.)

2. Gorlin, R. J., Pindborg, J. J., and Cohen, M. M., Jr.: Snydromes of the head and neck, ed. 2, New York, 1976, McGraw-Hill Book Co.

3. Spranger, J., et al.: Z. Kinderheilkd. **116:**73, 1974.

Features of the syndrome are variably expressed. First recognized by Stickler, the condition has been described under a variety of different names. The most extensive discussion of the disorder was presented by Herrmann and associates.

The joints are enlarged, often hyperextensible, and sometimes painful to use, becoming stiff with rest. Rarely they may be reddened and warm. Radiographically, multiple epiphyseal ossification disturbances, moderate flattening of the vertebral bodies, and thinning of the diaphyses of the tubular bones are noted. The pelvic bones are hypoplastic. The femoral necks are poorly modeled and plump.

Congenital myopia, as great as 18 diopters, is characteristic. Before the tenth year of life, broad zones of retinal detachment may occur (Fig. 17-33), which, if untreated, may lead to blindness, cataracts, keratopathy, and glaucoma.

Text continued on p. 556.

Table 17-16. Chromosomal syndromes with clefts and palatal anomalies

Karyotype	Striking features	Cleft lip	Cleft palate	Bifid uvula	Narrow and/or highly arched palate
1q+	Beaked nose, prominent ears, micrognathia, long, tapered fingers, congenital heart defect, involuted or absent thymus[20]	+?	+?	–	–
3p+	Microbrachycephaly, frontal bossing, high forehead, ocular hypertelorism, epicanthic folds, large mouth, short neck, congenital heart defect[4]	–	++	–	–
3p–, q+	Distorted forehead, low-set ears, upslanting palpebral fissures, short nose, anteverted nostrils, low nasal bridge, micrognathia, omphalocele or umbilical hernia, talipes equinovarus, congenital heart defects, renal anomalies, cryptorchidism, failure to thrive, frequent early demise[1]	+	++	±	–
4p+	Microcephaly, prominent forehead, ocular hypertelorism, thin upper lip, cylindrical thorax, hypoplastic pelvis, limb anomalies, growth deficiency, mental deficiency[10]	–	–	–	+?

Key for karyotype: p, short arm; q, long arm; + or – after karyotype number or letter, trisomy or deletion of chromosome or chromosome segment; 13q+p, partial trisomy for proximal part of long arm of chromosome 13; 13q+d, partial trisomy for distal part of long arm of chromosome 13; *karyotype in italics,* more well-known chromosomal syndromes or most common chromosomal syndromes or both. *Key for right four columns:* –, absent or not reported to date; ±, rare; +?, reported but relative frequency unknown since syndrome is incompletely delineated; +, uncommon; ++, common (>15%).

1. Allderdice, P. W., et al.: Am. J. Hum. Genet. 27:699, 1975.
2. Aurias, A., and Laurent, C.: Ann. Génét. 18:189, 1975.
3. Baccichetti, C., et al.: J. Med. Genet. 12:425, 1975.
4. Ballesta, F., and Behi, L.: Ann. Génét. 17:287, 1974.
5. Bijlsma, J. B., et al.: Helv. Paediatr. Acta 27:281, 1972.
6. Bowen, P., et al.: J. Pediatr. 85:95, 1974.
7. Bühler, E. M., et al.: Humangenetik 15:150, 1972.
8. Centerwall, W. R., and Beatty-DeSana, J. W.: Pediatrics 56:748, 1975.
9. Cohen, M. M., Sr., and Cohen, M. M., Jr.: Birth Defects 7(7):241, 1971.
10. Crisalli, M., et al.: J. Génét. Hum. 23:187, 1975.
11. deCicco, F., et al.: J. Pediatr. 83:836, 1973.
12. deGrouchy, J.: Birth Defects 5:74, 1969.
13. Escobar, J. I., and Yunis, J. J.: Am. J. Dis. Child. 128:221, 1974.
14. Gorlin, R. J., Pindborg, J. J., and Cohen, M. M., Jr.: Syndromes of the head and neck, ed. 2, New York, 1976, McGraw-Hill Book Co.
15. Lejeune, J., et al.: Ann. Génét. 11:171, 1968.
16. Lurie, I. W., and Lazjuk, G. I.: Humangenetik 15:203, 1972.
17. McPherson, E., et al.: Humangenetik. (In press.)
18. Muldal, S., et al.: Clin. Genet. 4:480, 1973.
19. Nakagome, Y., and Kobayashi, H.: J. Med. Genet. 12:412, 1975.
20. Norwood, T. H., and Hoehn, H.: Humangenetik 25:79, 1974.
21. Opitz, J. M., and Patau, K.: Birth Defects 11(5):191, 1975.
22. Orbeli, D. J., et al.: Humangenetik 12:296, 1971.
23. Penchaszadeh, V. B., and Coco, R.: J. Med. Genet. 12:193, 1975.
24. Sanchez, O., et al.: Humangenetik 22:59, 1974.
25. Schinzel, A., et al.: Humangenetik 22:287, 1974.
26. Sedano, H. O., et al.: Birth Defects 7(7):89, 1971.
27. Short, E. M., et al.: J. Med. Genet. 9:367, 1972.
28. Smith, D. W.: Birth Defects 5(5):67, 1969.
29. Vogel, W., et al.: Ann. Génét. 16:227, 1973.
30. Yunis, J. J., and Sanchez, O.: J. Pediatr. 84:567, 1974.

Table 17-16. Chromosomal syndromes with clefts and palatal anomalies—cont'd

Karyotype	Striking features	Cleft lip	Cleft palate	Bifid uvula	Narrow and/or highly arched palate
4p–	Severe growth and psychomotor retardation, seizures, hypotonia, small head, ocular hypertelorism, prominent glabella, downslanting palpebral fissures, preauricular dimple, short philtrum, downturned mouth, micrognathia, congenital heart defects, cryptorchidism, hypospadias, dimpling at sacrum[26]	++	++	–	–
4q+	Growth retardation, mental deficiency, small head circumference, frontal bossing, small eyes, low nasal bridge, wide, flat nose, long philtrum, micrognathia, large, prominent posteriorly angulated ears, clinodactyly of toes, simian creases, incompletely delineated phenotype[3]	–	–	–	+?
5p+	Variable central nervous system anomalies, dolichocephaly, mental deficiency, respiratory difficulties, renal/ureteral malformations, short first toes[21]	–	–	–	+?
5p–	Catlike cry during infancy, microcephaly, round face, ocular hypertelorism, downslanting palpebral fissures, strabismus, low-set ears, mild micrognathia, mental deficiency, growth deficiency[26]	±	±	±	±
7p–	Craniosynostosis, other variable anomalies, incompletely delineated phenotype[17]	–	–	+?	+?
7q+	Low birth weight, mental deficiency, fuzzy hair, wide anterior fontanel, small palpebral fissures, ocular hypertelorism, small nose, large tongue, malformed, low-set ears, skeletal anomalies[29]	–	++	–	–
8+	Mild to moderate mental deficiency, asymmetrical skull or scaphocephaly, strabismus, malformed ears, long, slender trunk with sloping shoulders, slender pelvis, vertebral and rib anomalies, reduced joint mobility, absent patellas, deep linear grooves on palms and soles[5]	–	–	–	++
9+	Microcephaly, small palpebral fissures, prominent nose, low-set ears, micropenis, cryptorchidism, long contracted fingers, dislocated hips, congenital heart defects, early demise[6]	–	–	–	++
9p+	Microcephaly and brachycephaly, mental deficiency, downslanting palpebral fissures, ocular hypertelorism, enophthalmos, globular prominent nose, downturned mouth, micrognathia, single palmar crease, low total ridge count, hypoplastic nails with short phalanges, short stature, delayed puberty[8]	–	–	–	++
10p+	Ocular hypertelorism, low-set, malformed ears, micrognathia, pes varus, anal atresia, rectovaginal fistula, absent lung lobe, incompletely delineated phenotype[19]	+?	+?	–	–
10q+	Growth deficiency, psychomotor retardation, microcephaly, flat, rounded face, arched eyebrows, narrow palpebral fissures, microphthalmia, malformed ears,	–	++	–	++

Continued.

Table 17-16. Chromosomal syndromes with clefts and palatal anomalies—cont'd

Karyotype	Striking features	Cleft lip	Cleft palate	Bifid uvula	Narrow and/or highly arched palate
	small nose, micrognathia, short neck, proximally placed thumbs and great toes, overlapping fingers, soft tissue syndactyly, camptodactyly, deep plantar furrows, reduced renal function[30]				
11p+	Mental deficiency, hypotonia, frontal bossing, downslanting palpebral fissures, strabismus, nystagmus, broad fingers and toes[24]	−	++	−	++
11q+	Axial hypotonia, limb hypertonia, wrinkled face, large, beaked nose, micrognathia, malformed, low-set ears, short neck, narrow chest, widely spaced nipples, micropenis, renal agenesis, urinary tract malformations, acetabular dysplasia, clubfoot, congenital heart defects, genital anomalies[2]	−	++	−	++
13+	Holoprosencephaly, seizures, apneic episodes, severe mental deficiency, early demise, severe facial dysmorphia (including ocular hypotelorism, flat nose, microphthalmia), iris coloboma, malformed ears, glabellar hemangioma. scalp defects, polydactyly, congenital heart defects, genital anomalies[28]	++	++	−	−
13q+[p]	Psychomotor retardation, low-set ears, clinodactyly, simian creases, microphthalmia, iris coloboma[13]	−	+	−	−
13q+[d]	Psychomotor retardation, microcephaly, narrow temples, prominent forehead, long, incurving eyelashes, delayed or abnormal dentition, low-set or malformed ears, polydactyly, hernias, hemangiomas, increased fetal hemoglobin level, may live beyond first year of life[25]	−	−	−	++
13q−	Microcephaly, lobar holoprosencephaly, trigonocephaly, mental deficiency, microphthalmia, iris coloboma, retinoblastoma, malformed ears, micrognathia, hypoplastic thumbs, imperforate anus, hypospadias, cryptorchidism, congenital heart defects[22]	−	+	±	−
14q+	Mental deficiency, failure to thrive, seizures, microcephaly, microphthalmia, flat nasal bridge, low-set or malformed ears, micrognathia, cryptorchidism[18, 27]	−	++	−	++
18+	Prominent occiput, narrow bifrontal diameter, low-set malformed ears, micrognathia, growth deficiency, mental deficiency, hypertonicity, overlapping fingers, congenital heart defects, early demise[28]	+	+	−	−
18p−	Mental deficiency, failure to thrive, epicanthic folds, ptosis, ocular hypertelorism, micrognathia, short neck, variable phenotype from Turner-like features to holoprosencephaly with facial dysmorphia[12, 16]	+	+	−	+
18q−	Short stature, microcephaly, mental deficiency, midface hypoplasia, deep-set eyes, prominent antihelix, carp-shaped mouth, tapering fingers, increased digital whorls, congenital heart defects[15, 16]	+	+	−	−

Table 17-16. Chromosomal syndromes with clefts and palatal anomalies—cont'd

Karyotype	Striking features	Cleft lip	Cleft palate	Bifid uvula	Narrow and/or highly arched palate
21+	Brachycephaly, flat midface, upslanting palpebral fissures, Brushfield spots, epicanthic folds, small, malformed ears, protruding tongue, loose skin on posterior neck, delayed dentition, minor tooth anomalies, malocclusion, periodontal disease, brachydactyly, clinodactyly, simian creases, increased ulnar loops, congenital heart defects, hypotonia, hyperflexibility, short stature, mental deficiency[9]	±	±	−	++
21q−	Psychomotor and mental deficiency, hypertonia, growth deficiency, microcephaly, downslanting palpebral fissures, broad nasal root, prominent low-set ears, large external auditory canals, micrognathia, hypospadias, cryptorchidism, inguinal hernia, pyloric stenosis, skeletal anomalies[14]	+?	++	−	++
22+	Growth deficiency, mental deficiency, hypotonia, underdeveloped musculature, microcephaly, craniofacial asymmetry, long, beaked nose, long philtrum, micrognathia, large, low-set, malformed ears, preauricular tags and pits, strabismus, long, slender fingers, fingerlike thumbs, congenital heart defects, hip dislocation, cryptorchidism[23]	−	++	−	−
22q+	Psychomotor retardation, coloboma of iris and choroid, downslanting palpebral fissures, ocular hypertelorism, preauricular tags or pits, and atresia, rectovaginal fistula, cardiac, genitourinary, and skeletal anomalies[7]	−	+?	−	−
22q−	Mental deficiency, hypotonia, epicanthic folds, flat nasal bridge, soft tissue syndactyly of second and third toes, clinodactyly of fifth finger[11]	−	−	++	++
XO	Short stature, ovarian agenesis, infantile vagina and breasts, widely spaced nipples, webbed neck, low posterior hairline, prominent ears, micrognathia, cubitus valgus, short fourth metacarpals, peripheral lymphedema during infancy, coarctation of aorta, renal anomalies, hypoplastic nails, multiple pigmented nevi[14]	−	±	−	++
XXXXY	Mild microcephaly, severe mental deficiency, hypotonia, upslanting palpebral fissures, ocular hypertelorism, epicanthic folds, short neck, redundant posterior neck skin, taurodontism, mandibular prognathism, micropenis, small testes, cryptorchidism, radioulnar synostosis, cubitus valgus, genua valga[14]	−	+	−	−
Triploidy	Growth deficiency, mental deficiency, hypotonia, asymmetry, microphthalmia, iris and choroid colobomas, mild ocular hypertelorism, anomalous low-set ears, micrognathia, syndactyly of third and fourth fingers, simian creases, clubfoot, congenital heart defects, genital anomalies[14]	++	++	−	−

Table 17-17. Association of clefts with other abnormalities

Type of cleft	Association	Comment
Cleft lip or palate or both	Thoracopagus twins[1]	
Cleft palate	Oral duplication[1]	
Cleft lip or palate or both	Anencephaly[1]	
Cleft palate	Congenital oral teratoma[1]	Cleft probably secondary to teratoma
Cleft lip or palate or both	Nasal glioma or meningo-encephalocele[1]	Cleft probably secondary to glioma or meningoencephalocele
Cleft lip or palate or both	Congenital neuroblastoma[1]	Other associated anomalies frequent
Cleft lip or palate or both	Congenital heart defects (ASD, VSD, pulmonary valvular atresia, tetralogy of Fallot, tricuspid stenosis, coarctation of aorta)[2]	
Cleft lip or palate or both	Forearm bone aplasia[1]	Other associated anomalies frequent
Cleft palate	Amelia[1]	
Cleft lip and palate	Sacral agenesis[1]	
Cleft palate	Accessory metacarpal of index finger[1]	
Cleft lip and palate	Cleft larynx[1]	
Cleft lip and palate	Laryngeal web[1]	
Cleft lip and palate	Lateral proboscis[1]	Usually occurs with absent nostril on ipsilateral side
Cleft palate	Persistent buccopharyngeal membrane[1]	
Cleft palate	Aniridia[1]	
Cleft palate	Aplasia of trochlea[1]	

1. Gorlin, R. J., et al.: Birth defects 7(7):3, 1971. 2. Shah, C. V., et al.: Am. J. Dis. Child. **119**:238, 1970.

The craniofacial spectrum has varied from a reasonably normal face to midfacial flattening and the Robin anomalad. Herrmann and associates indicated that a sizable proportion of newborns with the Robin anomalad may have the Stickler syndrome. Isolated cleft palate, submucous cleft palate, and abnormal palatal mobility have also been observed. Epicanthal folds, sensorineural deafness, and dental abnormalities have been noted in some cases.[163, 177, 178]

Van der Woude syndrome. The van der Woude syndrome is an autosomal dominant disorder characterized by cleft lip or cleft palate or both, together with fistulas of the lower lip. Penetrance is approximately 80%, and expression is variable. Cervenka

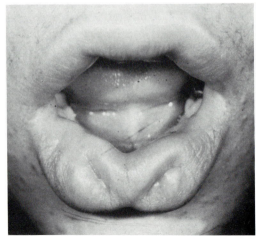

Fig. 17-34. Symmetrical lip pits in van der Woude syndrome.

and co-workers estimated the frequency of the syndrome to be 1:75,000 to 1:100,000 in the white population.

Usually, bilateral, symmetrically placed depressions are observed on the vermilion portion of the lower lip, one on each side of the midline (Fig. 17-34). They are circular, or they may be located at the apex of nipple-like elevations. Rarely, the elevations may fuse in the midline, producing a snoutlike structure. The depressions represent blind sinuses that descend through the orbicularis oris muscle to a depth of 0.5 to 2.5 cm and communicate with the underlying minor salivary glands through their excretory ducts. They often transport a viscid saliva to the surface, either spontaneously or on pressure. Nipple-like processes occasionally occur without demonstrable fistulas. Although usually bilateral and symmetrically placed, variations may be seen, such as an asymmetrical single pit, central single pit, or pits of the upper lip and frenum. It has been suggested that the congenital fistulas arise from arrested development, that is, persistence of a median and/or lateral sulcus or sulci, which normally are evanescent structures. These median and lateral grooves appear in the 5 to 6 mm embryo and disappear at the 10 to 16 mm stage. The grooves disappear at about the same time that fusion occurs between several facial processes.

Syngnathia, absence of second premolars, talipes equinovarus, syndactyly, and accessory nipples have been noted occasionally.[149, 181]

Orofaciodigital syndrome I. The orofaciodigital syndrome I consists of abnormally developed frenula, cleft tongue, hypoplasia of the nasal alar cartilages, median pseudocleft of the upper lip, asymmetrical cleft palate, various malformations of digits, and mental deficiency. To date, approximately 125 cases have appeared in the literature. It has been suggested that the incidence of the syndrome is probably about 0.0225 per 1000 live births. OFD I syndrome follows an X-linked dominant mode of transmission trait limited to females and lethal in males.

Craniofacial complex. The facies is remarkably distinctive with euryopia, dystopia canthorum, some aquiline thinning of the nose, due at least in part to hypoplasia of the alar cartilages, a pseudocleft in the midline of the upper lip, which is usually short, and a broad nasal root. One nostril may be smaller than the other, and there may be flattening of the nasal tip (Fig. 17-35). Be-

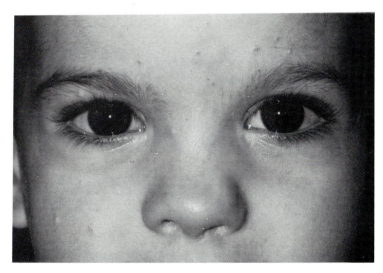

Fig. 17-35. Asymmetrical hypoplasia of alar cartilages and dystopia canthorum in child with orofaciodigital syndrome I.

cause of zygomatic hypoplasia the midfacial region is flattened in most cases.

The most striking oral manifestations are the "clefts" associated with hyperplastic frenula (Fig. 17-36). There is often a small midline "cleft" in the upper lip extending through the vermilion border. On retraction of the short upper lip, a wide, thickened or hyperplastic reduplicated frenum is seen to be associated with the pseudocleft. This, in part, eradicates the mucobuccal fold in the area. Because of these bands, complete retraction is often not possible.

The palate is cleft laterally, deep bilateral grooves extending medially from the maxillary buccal frenula, dividing the palate into an anterior segment containing the incisors and the canines and two lateral palatal processes. The soft palate is completely and asymmetrically cleft in most patients. A large bony ridge extends from the alveolar crest medially to the midline in the canine-premolar area in some cases.

Numerous thick fibrous bands are evident in the lower mucobuccal fold, eliminating the sulcus, clefting the hypoplastic mandibular alveolar processes, and, by extension, bifurcating, trifurcating, or tetrafurcating the tongue. Bifurcation occurs in about 30% of cases. Three or more lobes are present in the rest. On the ventral surface of the tongue, between the tongue halves or lobules, a small whitish hamartomatous mass is seen in most affected individuals. This consists of fibrous connective tissue, salivary gland tissue, a few striated muscle fibers, and, rarely, cartilage. Ankyloglossia or tonguetie of a diffuse nature is present in at least a third of the cases.

Malposition of the maxillary canine teeth, supernumerary maxillary canines and premolars, and infraocclusion are common. The supernumerary canines are often separated by the clefts. The canine crown form is often T-shaped. Aplasia of mandibular lateral incisors occurs in about half the affected persons and appears to be predicated on the

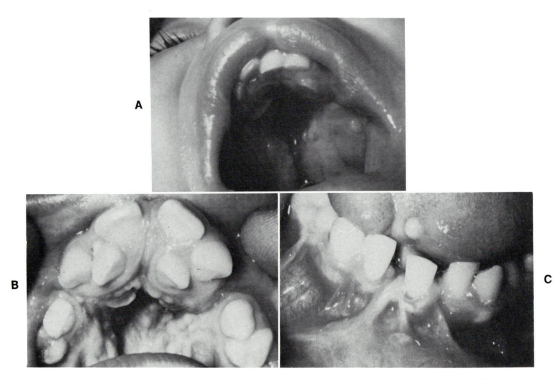

Fig. 17-36. Orofaciodigital syndrome I. **A,** Hypoplastic frenula and palatal clefting. **B,** Palatal clefts and malposed teeth in another patient. **C,** Note bifurcated tongue, white hamartoma, and hyperplastic frenula.

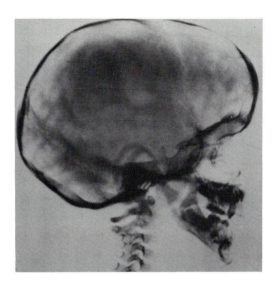

Fig. 17-37. Skull in orofaciodigital syndrome I. Note increased nasion-sella-basion angle, retrusion of maxilla and mandible with respect to cranial base, normal relationship between maxilla and mandible, and increased gonial angle.

effect of the fibrous bands on the developing tooth germs. The mandible is small or hypoplastic with a short ramus.

Central nervous system. Mental deficiency is seen in over half the patients. The intelligence quotient usually ranges from 70 to 90. Various central nervous system alterations have been described, including hydrocephaly, porencephaly, hydranencephaly, and partial agenesis of the corpus callosum. Decreased hearing has been noted in some patients.

Skeletal manifestations. The nasion-sella-basion angle is increased, being about 144° and exceeding the normal value of 131° (S.D. = 4.5°) by almost three standard deviations (Fig. 17-37).

On radiographic examination, the short tubular bones of the hands and feet appear irregularly short and thick. Irregular reticulated areas of radiolucency or osteoporosis are observed in the metacarpals and, especially, in the phalanges.

Malformations of the fingers, in decreasing frequency of appearance, are clinodactyly, syndactyly, and brachydactyly (Fig. 17-38). Toe malformations, which are considerably

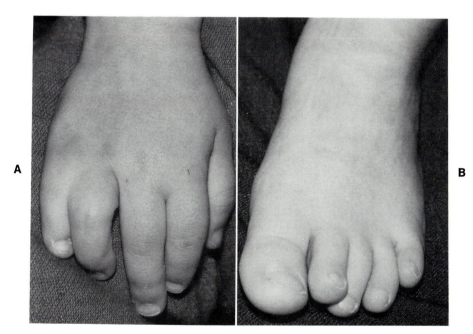

Fig. 17-38. Hands and feet in orofaciodigital syndrome I. **A,** Note syndactyly and clinodactyly. **B,** Note irregularity of toes.

less common, include unilateral hallucal polysyndactyly, syndactyly, and brachydactyly. The hallux is often bent in a fibular direction, with brachydactyly and hypoplasia of the second to fifth toes. Occasionally there is a postminimus toe. Some patients have cone-shaped epiphyses in the digits.

Skin and skin appendages. Commonly there are evanescent milia of the face and ears, which usually disappear before the third year of life (Fig. 17-39). Dryness and alopecia of the scalp are common.

Dermatoglyphic studies have revealed a preponderance of whorls. Increased arches have also been noted.*

Orofaciodigital syndrome II. The orofaciodigital syndrome II is characterized by lobed tongue, manual polydactyly, and bilateral polysyndactyly of the halluces. The syndrome clearly follows an autosomal recessive mode

*See references 144, 151-153, 156, 158, 161, 165, 166, 172, 176, 180, 182.

of transmission. Parental consanquinity has been observed, and there have been several examples of the syndrome occurring in sibs.

Orofacial complex (Figs. 17-40 and 17-41). Frequently there is a midline cleft of the upper lip. Cleft tongue is commonly observed, and ankyloglossia has been described. In a few cases, cleft palate or bifid uvula has been noted. However, in most patients the palate has been intact. Multiple frenula are occasionally present and far less frequent than in OFD I syndrome. Fatty hamartomas on the dorsum of the tongue have been present in several cases.

Central nervous system. Mental deficiency has been reported in several cases. Various other abnormalities have been described, including microcephaly, porencephaly, internal hydrocephaly, conduction deafness, choroid coloboma, and muscular hypotonia with poor coordination.

Skeletal alterations. Bony changes appear to be limited to the hands and feet. Bilateral manual ulnar hexadactyly and bilateral polysyndactyly of the halluces are characteristic. Patients have also had one or more postminimus digits. Bimanual hexadactyly may be present, although in some cases there have been five fingers with ulnar deviation of the fifth finger, syndactyly of third and fourth

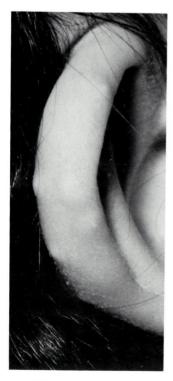

Fig. 17-39. Milia of ears in orofaciodigital syndrome I.

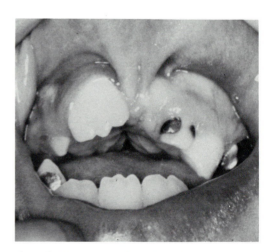

Fig. 17-40. Orofaciodigital syndrome II. Note hyperplastic frenula. (Courtesy R. E. Stewart, Los Angeles, Calif.)

fingers with extra bones in the web, or hexadactyly of only one hand.

Other findings. There would appear to be increased susceptibility to respiratory infection, which in several patients has resulted in death during infancy. Tachypnea has also been reported.

Cryptorchidism and inguinal hernia have also been noted.[173]

Otopalatodigital syndrome. The otopalato-

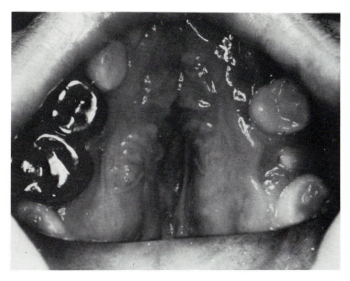

Fig. 17-41. Orofaciodigital syndrome II. Note palatal defect. (Courtesy R. E. Stewart, Los Angeles, Calif.)

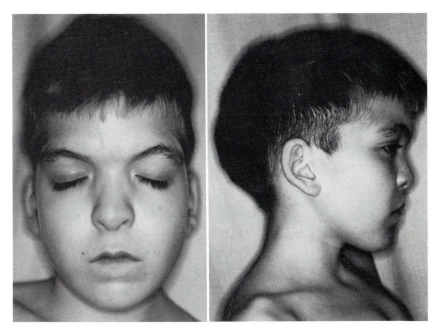

Fig. 17-42. Otopalatodigital syndrome. Prominent supraorbital ridges, downslanting palpebral fissures, broad nasal root, flat midface, and prominent occiput.

digital syndrome has characteristic facies, conduction deafness, short stature, cleft palate, and generalized bone dysplasia. The inheritance pattern is X-linked recessive. Although most patients have been male, affected females have been described, who exhibit milder stigmata of the syndrome, in accord with the Lyon hypothesis.

Craniofacial complex. The facies in the male is rather distinctive (Fig. 17-42). Overhanging brow with prominent supraorbital ridges and downslanting palpebral fissures are noted. The corners of the mouth are often downturned. Ocular hypertelorism with associated broad nasal root gives the patient

a pugilistic appearance. A slight notching may be noted at the medial third of the upper eyelid margin. All male patients have had cleft palate. The mandible is small, with obtuse angulation. Facial features in the female carrier are variable. Most constant is overhanging brow with prominent supraorbital ridges, depressed nasal bridge, and flat midface.

Central nervous system. All male patients have been mildly retarded, their intelligence quotient ranging from 75 to 90 and perhaps reflecting hearing loss. Speech development has been slow, but this may also be related to bilateral conductive hearing loss.

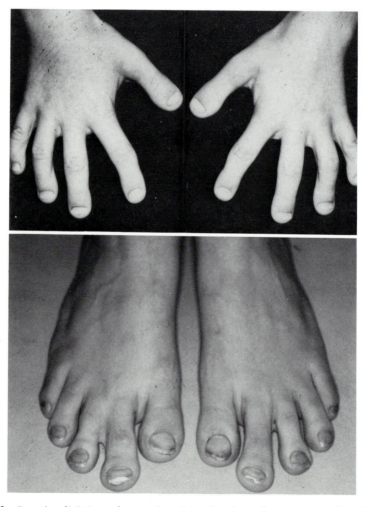

Fig. 17-43. Otopalatodigital syndrome. Spatulate thumbs and great toes, short fingernails, syndactyly between second and third toes, and irregular curvature of fingers and toes.

Skeletal anomalies. Skeletal growth is retarded, all patients being below the tenth percentile and often below the third percentile. The trunk is small, with pectus excavatum. Limited elbow extension and wrist supination have been noted in several patients, and some have exhibited subluxation of the radial head.

The appearance of the hands and feet is striking (Fig. 17-43). The thumb and hallux are spatulate and especially abbreviated. The clefting between the hallux and the rest of the toes is exaggerated. The toes and fingers are irregular in form and in direction of curvature, resembling those of a tree frog. The second and third fingers may deviate to the ulnar side, and the fifth finger often bends to the radial side.

Radiographic alterations are marked. Frontal and occipital bossing and thickening give the skull a mushroom-like appearance. The skull base is thick, the facial bones are hypoplastic, and the paranasal sinuses and mastoids are poorly pneumatized. The nasion-sella-basion angle is about 116° (normal mean = 132°), and the mandibular plane angle is increased. The clivus, or basisphenoid, lies further posterior than normal in relation to the cervical spine. These changes are essentially limited to affected males.

The iliac bones are small, with decreased flare. Coxa valga is a common finding. The lower tibia is laterally bowed. Failure of fusion of several vertebral arches is common.

Distinctive changes in the hands of males (Fig. 17-44) include shortening of the radial

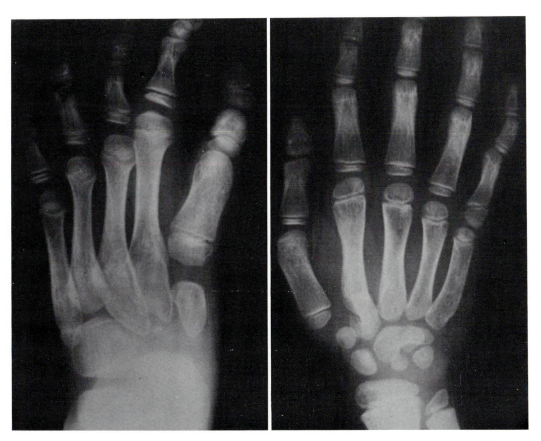

Fig. 17-44. Otopalatodigital syndrome. Clinodactyly of fifth finger with short curved middle phalanx, short distal thumb phalanx, accessory ossification center of second metacarpal, short phalanges and metatarsal of great toe, and abnormally shaped second and third metatarsals. (Courtesy L. O. Langer, Jr., Minneapolis, Minn.)

side of the middle phalanx of the fifth finger, clinodactyly, short distal thumb phalanx (which, during development, has a cone-shaped epiphysis), accessory ossification center of the second metacarpal, teardrop-shaped lesser multangular, and transverse capitate. Females may have greater multangular-navicular fusion.

In the male, alterations in the feet (Fig. 17-44) include short phalanges and metatarsals of the great toes and, because of their fusion with the cuneiform bones, long, abnormally shaped second and third metatarsals. The fifth metatarsal may be prominent, with an extra ossification center. Tarsal fusions are common, and males usually have two ossification centers for the navicular bone.[154, 157, 162, 164, 179]

Ectrodactyly–ectodermal dysplasia clefting syndrome. Most cases of the ectrodactyly–ectodermal dysplasia clefting syndrome have been isolated examples, although there have been affected sibs with normal parents, and several cases in which the disorder has been transmitted from a parent to one or more children. The syndrome appears to have autosomal dominant inheritance with reduced penetrance and variable expressivity, although a recessive form may also exist.

Craniofacial complex. The facies is characterized by cleft lip, dacryocystitis, keratoconjunctivitis, tearing, and photophobia. The scalp hair, lashes, and eyebrows may be sparse (Fig. 17-45). Cleft lip and palate, more often bilateral, has been described in many cases but has been absent in others. Lack of permanent incisors has been observed, as well as anodontia, severe oligodontia or enamel hypoplasia (Fig. 17-46). Xerostomia and deeply furrowed tongue have also been noted. The mucous membranes are predisposed to candidiasis.

Absent lacrimal punctas have been noted in most cases. This is associated with tearing, blepharitis, dacryocystitis, keratoconjunctivitis, and photophobia. Primary telecanthus has been observed, and a reduction in the number of meibomian orifices has been noted.

Central nervous system. Microcephaly and mental deficiency have been described in several cases. Conduction deafness has also been noted.

Limbs. The lobster-claw deformity (ectrodactyly) usually involves all four limbs (Fig. 17-47), but there have been exceptions. Occasionally there has been some degree of soft-tissue syndactyly, especially of the toes.

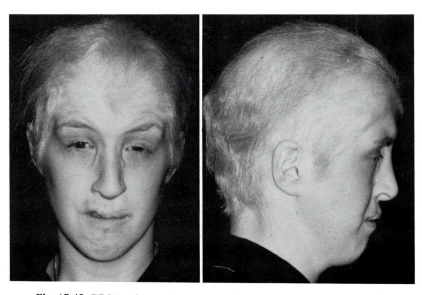

Fig. 17-45. EEC syndrome. Sparse hair, blepharitis, and repaired cleft lip.

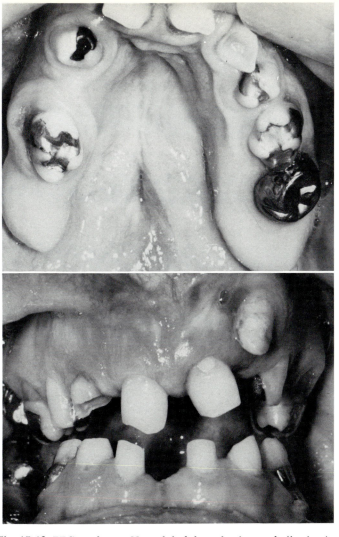

Fig. 17-46. EEC syndrome. Note cleft defect of palate and oligodontia.

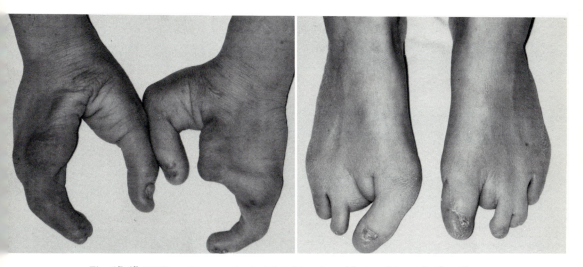

Fig. 17-47. EEC syndrome: ectrodactyly of hands and feet and hypoplastic nails.

Skin. An albinoid alteration in the skin and hair has been noted in a few cases. The scalp hair, eyebrows, and lashes have been sparse and the nails may be hypoplastic and brittle. Skin biopsy has shown an absence of sebaceous glands. Several patients have had numerous pigmented nevi.

Other findings. Inguinal hernia, absent kidney, hydronephrosis, hydroureter, and cryptorchidism have been noted.*

Cleidocranial dysplasia

Over 700 cases of cleidocranial dysplasia have been documented in the medical literature. The disorder consists of aplasia or hypoplasia of one or both clavicles, exaggerated development of the transverse diameter of the cranium, delayed ossification of fontanels, delayed dental eruption, and supernumerary teeth. Over 100 associated abnormalities have been recorded. The disorder follows an autosomal dominant mode of transmission.

Craniofacial complex (Fig. 17-48). The appearance is usually striking. The neck appears long, and the shoulders are narrow and droop markedly. The skull is brachy-

---

*See references 145-148, 155, 169-171, 174, 175, 183, 184.

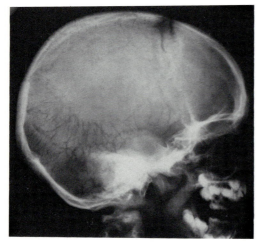

Fig. 17-48. Cleidocranial dysplasia. Note relatively large skull, small face, Wormian bones, and open anterior fontanel.

cephalic, with pronounced frontal and parietal bossing, causing the face to appear small. The nose is broad at the base and the bridge depressed. The skull is large and short, the cephalic index being usually in excess of 80. Usually a groove, overlying the metopic suture, extends from the nasion to the sagittal suture. Because of the failure of various bones to unite, closure of the fontanels and sutures is delayed, often for life. Secondary centers of ossification appear in the suture lines, and many Wormian bones are formed. The sagittal diameter of the cranial base is short. The accessory sinuses are often undeveloped or absent. The mastoids are usually not pneumatized because of altered function of the sternocleidomastoid muscles. The orbital height may be great compared with the width, and the orbital ridges may overhang the orbits. Mild exophthalmos associated with a depressed orbital roof may be observed.

The palate is highly arched and may have submucous cleft or even complete palatal cleft involving both the hard and soft tissues. Nonunion at the mandibular symphysis has also been noted. Development of the premaxilla is poor, and since growth of the mandible is usually normal, relative prognathism results.

The failure of eruption of the deciduous and permanent teeth, which in some cases is total, results in pseudoanodontia. The jaw bones may possibly have increased density, which may inhibit tooth eruption. Cyst formation around impacted, inverted, or displaced teeth is common. There is also a tendency for nonexfoliation of deciduous teeth. Teeth without deciduous predecessors seem to have a greater chance to erupt. Extraction of deciduous teeth does not seem to promote eruption of the permanent teeth. Gemination and dilaceration of roots are also common.

Supernumerary teeth are common. The crown form of many such teeth is similar to a flattened premolar. Extracted teeth have been found to be severely deformed with hypoplastic enamel. Roots lack a layer of cellular cementum.

Skeletal alterations. Short stature is generally present, males measuring 156.6 cm and females, 144.6 cm. The clavicle may be unilaterally or bilaterally absent (Figs. 17-49 and 17-50), but more frequently it is dysplastic at the acromial end. Some patients have manifested a central gap (pseudoarthrosis) with bone replacement by fibrous connective tissue. The deficiency of the clavicle is responsible for the long appearance of the neck and the narrow shoulders. The range of shoulder movements is often remarkable, frequently allowing the individual to approximate his shoulders in front of his chest. There are variations in size, origin, and insertion of muscles related to the clavicles, especially the sternocleidomastoid, trapezius, deltoid, and pectoralis major, yet function is remarkably good.

Although cleidocranial dysplasia was originally believed to involve only bones of membranous origin, involvement of bones of both intramembranous and endochondral origin has been recognized. The most frequent deformities include delayed closure of the pubic symphysis, coxa vara or, less often, coxa valga, spina bifida occulta of the cervical, thoracic, or lumbar spine, pseudoepiphyses at the base of one or more metacarpals, abnormally pointed terminal digits of the hands and feet, and cone-shape epiphyses of the distal phalanges.

Conduction deafness has been described in several patients.[185-198]

Craniocarpotarsal dysplasia

In 1938, Freeman and Sheldon described a syndrome characterized by microstomia and flat midface, talipes equinovarus, and ulnar deviation of the fingers. Although most cases are sporadic, there are several examples of the syndrome in two generations, and, in view of established male-to-male transmission, it would appear to have autosomal dominant inheritance.

Facies (Fig. 17-51). The stiff, immobile, flattened midface and long philtrum are extremely characteristic. The eyes appear deeply sunken. Convergent strabismus, epicanthus, and ocular hypertelorism have been noted in several cases. Several patients have exhibited downslanting palpebral fissures and ptosis of the upper lids. The nose is small and

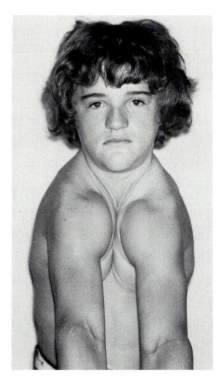

Fig. 17-49. Cleidocranial dysplasia. Shoulders can be approximated in severe cases.

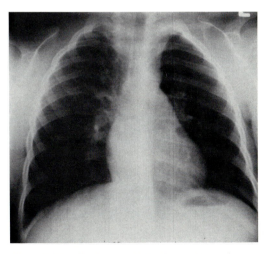

Fig. 17-50. Cleidocranial dysplasia. Note absence of clavicles.

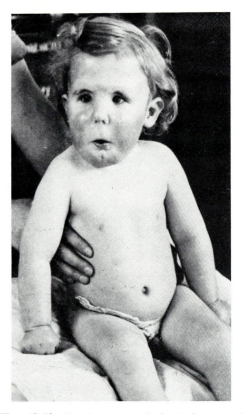

Fig. 17-51. Craniocarpotarsal dysplasia: pursed lips, narrow nostrils, and grooved chin. (Courtesy R. J. Gorlin, Minneapolis, Minn.)

the philtrum long. The nostrils are narrow, the alae often being bent, thus stimulating nostril colobomas. Near the tip, the alae are of normal thickness, but they thin dorsally to be inserted close to the columnella. The nasolabial folds are evident only near the sides of the nose.

There is marked microstomia (Fig. 17-52), the interangular or intercommissural distance being about two thirds of that for a child of the same age. The lips are pursed or held as in whistling, which accounts for this disorder being frequently referred to as the "whistling face syndrome." The palate is highly arched, the mandible tends to be small, and the tongue is small. Extending from the middle of the lower lip to the chin is a fibrous band or elevation demarcated by two paramedian grooves, forming an H- or V-shaped scarlike structure. Biopsy of buccinator muscles has shown fibrous connective tissue replacement of muscle bundles.

Skeletal system. Growth has been below the third percentile in about half the cases. Flexion contractures of the fingers are a constant feature, the thumbs being especially involved at the metacarpophalangeal joints.

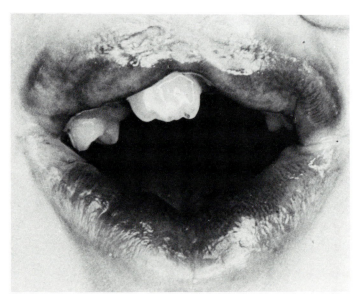

Fig. 17-52. Craniocarpotarsal dysplasia. Note narrow intercommissural distance. (From Burzynski, N. J.: Oral Surg. **39:**893, 1975.)

There is ulnar deviation of the fingers without bony abnormalities.

Talipes equinovarus is common. Occasionally this is unilateral. Other less frequently found anomalies include moderate to severe scoliosis, spina bifida occulta, and inguinal hernia.

The facial skeleton is small. The anteroposterior length of both face and cranium is short, whereas the height is relatively great. Most patients have shown a steep cranial base.

Other findings. Atrophy of one kidney and hydronephrosis of the other have been noted.[199-205]

Craniosynostosis syndromes

Craniosynostosis is a nonspecific abnormality that may occur as a primary anomalad but may also occur in association with other abnormalities, producing various craniosynostosis syndromes. In the past, a great deal of confusion in the nosology of craniosynostosis syndromes has been apparent. History shows that the English and American literature was characterized by a tendency to lump various disorders together until the appearance of the classic paper by Blank in 1960.[208] An early notable exception was the magnificent monograph of Park and Powers.[222] In contrast, the European literature, particularly the German literature, tended to split various disorders. Recent classifications of craniosynostosis syndromes have been proposed by McKusick,[221] Herrmann and associates,[216] and Cohen.[211]

The craniosynostosis syndromes discussed in this section are classified on the basis of clinical similarity and genetic considerations. They should never be classified on the basis of which sutures are synostosed nor on the presence or absence of mental deficiency. Various sutures may be involved in different patients with the same syndrome. Thus, in some instances, the cranial malformation may be different in patients with the same disorder.

It cannot be stated categorically that mental retardation occurs in one craniosynostosis syndrome but not in another. The risk of retardation is probably present to some extent in all craniosynostosis syndromes. Some have a higher frequency of retardation and, in some, the degree of retardation tends to be more severe. For example, retardation accompanies the Apert syndrome much more frequently than it accompanies the Crouzon syndrome. On the other hand, some patients with the Apert syndrome have normal intelligence, and patients with the Crouzon syndrome may be retarded.

The craniosynostosis syndromes are listed in Table 17-18. Some, such as the Crouzon syndrome and the Apert syndrome, are well known. Others are less well known. Within this latter group, some syndromes need further study to delineate the phenotypic spectrum, natural history, and etiology. Only the Crouzon syndrome, the Apert syndrome, the Pfeiffer syndrome, the Saethre-Chotzen syndrome, and the Carpenter syndrome are discussed here. Detailed presentation of other craniosynostosis syndromes can be found elsewhere.[211, 215] The cloverleaf skull malformation (Fig. 17-53), once thought to be a syndrome sui generis, is now known to be nonspecific, and can be found as an isolated anomalad or as a component part of various syndromes.[209] Presenting features of the cloverleaf skull malformation are as follows[212]:

Isolated anomalad
With bony ankylosis of limbs
With Crouzon syndrome
With Apert syndrome
With Pfeiffer syndrome
With Carpenter sydrome
Iatrogenic anomalad

Crouzon syndrome. The Crouzon syndrome is characterized by craniosynostosis, maxillary hypoplasia, and shallow orbits with ocular proptosis. First described by Crouzon in 1912, the syndrome clearly follows an autosomal dominant mode of transmission. Impressive pedigrees have been reported by various authors. In most affected families reported to date, penetrance has been complete. Sporadic cases, representing fresh mutations, have also been observed.

The possibility of an autosomal recessive form of the Crouzon syndrome has been

Text continued on p. 574.

Table 17-18. Syndromes with craniosynostosis

Syndrome	Striking features	Relative frequency of craniosynostosis in syndrome	Etiology
Chromosomal syndromes			
5p+ syndrome[21]	Variable central nervous system anomalies, dolichocephaly, craniosynostosis, mental deficiency, respiratory difficulties, renal/ureteral malformations, short first toes; phenotype not completely delineated at present	?	Trisomy for most of short arm of chromosome 5
7p– syndrome[18]	Craniosynostosis and variable anomalies; phenotype not completely delineated at present	Apparently common	Deletion of short arm of chromosome 7
13q– syndrome[22]	Microcephaly, lobar holoprosencephaly, trigonocephaly, craniosynostosis, mental deficiency, microphthalmia, iris coloboma, retinoblastoma, malformed ears, micrognathia, hypoplastic thumbs, imperforate anus, hypospadias, cryptorchidism, congenital heart defects	8/44	Deletion of long arm of chromosome 13

1. Andersen, T. H., and Pindborg, J. J.: Odontol. T. **55**:472, 1947.
2. Antley, R., and Bixler, D.: Birth Defects **11** (2):397, 1975.
3. Armendares, S., et al.: J. Pediatr. **85**:872, 1974.
4. Berant, M., and Berant, N.: J. Pediatr. **83**:88, 1973.
5. Christian, J. C.: Personal communication, 1975.
6. Christian, J. C., et al.: Clin. Genet. **2**:95, 1971.
7. Cohen, M. M., Jr.: Personal observations, 1972-1975.
8. Cohen, M. M., Jr.: Birth Defects **11**(2):137, 1975.
9. Cohen, M. M., Jr.: J. Maxillofacial Surg. (In press.)
10. Elejalde, B. R., et al.: Eur. J. Pediatr. (In press.)
11. Fairbanks, T.: An atlas of general affections of the skeleton, Edinburgh, 1951, E. & S. Livingstone, Ltd.
12. Gorlin, R. J., et al.: J. Pediatr. **56**:778, 1960.
13. Hall, J. G.: Personal communication, 1974.
14. Herrmann, J., and Opitz, J. M.: Birth Defects **5**(3):39, 1969.
15. Herrmann, J., et al.: Rocky Mt. Med. J. **66**: 45, 1969.
16. Hootnick, D., and Holmes, L. B.: Clin. Genet. **3**:128, 1972.
17. Lowry, R. B.: J. Med. Genet. **9**:227, 1972.
18. McPherson, E., et al.: Humangenetik. (In press.)
19. Opitz, J. M.: Personal communication, 1975.
20. Opitz, J. M., and Kaveggia, E. G.: Z. Kinderheilkd. **117**:1, 1974.
21. Opitz, J. M., and Patau, K.: Birth Defect **11** (5):191, 1975.
22. Orbeli, D. J., et al.: Humangenetik **13**:296, 1971.
23. Pantke, O. A., et al.: Birth Defects **11**(2):190, 1975.
24. Pederson, G.: Personal communication, 1975.
25. Sakati, N., et al.: J. Pediatr. **79**:104, 1971.
26. Shaw, E. B., and Steinbach, H. L.: Am. J. Dis. Child. **115**:477, 1968.
27. Smith, D. W.: Birth Defects: Proceedings of the Fourth International Conference, Amsterdam, 1974, Excerpta Medica Foundation, p. 309.
28. Summitt, R. L.: Birth Defects **5**(2):35, 1969.
29. Waardenburg, P. J.: Klin. Monatsbl. Augenheilkd. **92**:29, 1934.

Table 17-18. Syndromes with craniosynostosis—cont'd

Syndrome	Striking features	Relative frequency of cranio-synostosis in syndrome	Etiology
Monogenic syndromes			
Apert syndrome[5]	Craniosynostosis, proptosis, downslanting palpebral fissures, strabismus, ocular hypertelorism, midface deficiency, highly arched palate, complete symmetrical syndactyly of hands and feet minimally involving second, third, and fourth digits	Almost all cases	Autosomal dominant
Armendare syndrome[3]	Craniosynostosis, microcephaly, retinitis pigmentosa, ptosis of eyelids, malformed ears, micrognathia, highly arched palate, clinodactyly, simian creases, short stature	Apparently common	Probably autosomal or X-linked recessive
Baller-Gerold syndrome[8]	Craniosynostosis, radial aplasia, absent or hypoplastic carpal bones and preaxial digits	Apparently common	Probably autosomal recessive
Berant syndrome[4]	Craniosynostosis involving sagittal suture, radioulnar synostosis	Apparently common	Probably autosomal dominant
Carpenter syndrome[8]	Craniosynostosis, mental deficiency, preaxial polysyndactyly of feet, variable soft tissue syndactyly with brachymesophalangy of hands, displacement of patellae, genua valga, congenital heart defects, short stature, obesity	All reported cases	Autosomal recessive
Christian syndrome I[6]	Craniosynostosis, microcephaly, ocular hypertelorism, downslanting palpebral fissures, cleft palate, arthrogryposis	Apparently common	Autosomal recessive
Christian syndrome II[5]	Craniosynostosis, involving metopic suture, ocular hypertelorism, epicanthal folds, downslanting palpebral fissures, C 2-3 fusion, hemivertebrae, anomalous ears, clinodactyly, simian creases, foot abduction, imperforate anus, short stature	Apparently common	X-linked semidominant
Craniofacial dyssynostosis[19]	Craniosynostosis involving lambdoidal and posterior sagittal sutures and variably coronal suture, prominent forehead, ocular hypertelorism, frequent Spanish ancestry	All known cases	?Autosomal recessive
Crouzon syndrome[8]	Craniosynostosis, shallow orbits with proptosis, strabismus, midface deficiency	Almost all cases	Autosomal dominant
Elejalde syndrome[10]	Craniosynostosis, swollen face, epicanthic folds, ocular hypertelorism, hypoplastic nose, malformed ears, redundant neck tissue, gigantism at birth, short limbs, polydactyly, omphalocele, lung hypoplasia, cystic renal dysplasia, sponge kidney, redundant connective tissue in skin and many viscera, proliferation of perivascular nerve fibers	Apparently common	Autosomal recessive

Continued.

Table 17-18. Syndromes with craniosynostosis—cont'd

Syndrome	Striking features	Relative frequency of craniosynostosis in syndrome	Etiology
FG syndrome[9]	Variable growth problems, disproportionately large head circumference, mental deficiency, congenital hypotonia, high narrow palate, imperforate anus, sacral dimple, partial syndactyly of second and third toes, various other findings, including craniosynostosis and frontal bossing	Apparently uncommon	X-linked
Frontonasal dysplasia[9]	Ocular hypertelorism, cranium bifidum occultum, widow's peak, broad nasal root, flat nasal tip or bifid nose, notching or colobomas, of nostrils, and median cleft lip in variable combinations; occurrence of many low-frequency anomalies, including craniosynostosis	Uncommon	Etiologically heterogeneous, probably representing many poorly delineated entities; some cases are consistent with autosomal dominant inheritance
Gorlin-Chaudhry-Moss syndrome[12]	Craniosynostosis, midface deficiency, hypertrichosis, downslanting palpebral fissures, upper eyelid colobomas, patent ductus arteriosus, hypoplastic labia majora	Apparently common	Probably autosomal recessive
Hootnick-Holmes syndrome[16]	Frontal bossing, dolichocephaly, craniosynostosis involving sagittal suture, ocular hypertelorism, strabismus, preaxial and postaxial polysyndactyly of hands, preaxial polysyndactyly of feet	?	Probably autosomal dominant
Lowry syndrome[17]	Craniosynostosis, prominent eyes, strabismus, highly arched or cleft palate, fibular aplasia, talipes equinovarus, simian creases	Apparently common	Probably autosomal recessive
Pfeiffer syndrome[8]	Craniosynostosis, proptosis, strabismus, ocular hypertelorism, downslanting palpebral fissures, midface deficiency, broad thumbs and great toes, mild cutaneous syndactyly of fingers and toes (variable)	All known cases	Autosomal dominant
Saethre-Chotzen syndrome[23]	Craniosynostosis, facial asymmetry, low-set frontal hairline, ptosis of eyelids, deviated nasal septum, variable brachydactyly and cutaneous syndactyly especially of second and third fingers, normal thumbs and great toes	All known cases	Autosomal dominant
Summitt syndrome[28]	Craniosynostosis, strabismus, variable symmetrical syndactyly of hands and feet from partial to complete with clinodactyly, normal-sized thumbs and great toes, genua valga, obesity	Apparently common	Probably autosomal recessive

Table 17-18. Syndromes with craniosynostosis—cont'd

Syndrome	Striking features	Relative frequency of cranio-synostosis in syndrome	Etiology
Washington syndrome I[7]	Craniosynostosis involving sagittal suture, short fourth and fifth metacarpals	Apparently common	Probably autosomal recessive
Washington syndrome II[7]	Craniosynostosis, midface hypoplasia, lack of extension of distal interphalangeal joints	Apparently common	Probably autosomal recessive
Weiss syndrome[27]	Craniosynostosis, medially deviated great toes, altered tarsal morphogenesis, mild syndactyly, wide variability of craniofacial involvement	Common	Autosomal dominant
Teratogenically induced syndromes			
Aminopterin syndrome[26]	Craniosynostosis, hypoplasia of cranial and facial bones, low-set ears, cleft palate, micrognathia, hypodactyly of feet, mild syndactyly of hands	Apparently common	Aminopterin or methotrexate during pregnancy
Sporadic, incompletely delineated syndromes			
Andersen-Pindborg syndrome[1]	Craniofacial dysostosis, ectodermal dysplasia, short stature	?	?
Antley-Bixler syndrome[2]	Trapezoidocephaly, deformed ears and nose, elongated hands and feet, radiohumeral synostosis, digit contractures	?	?
Fairbank syndrome[11]	Craniosynostosis, proptosis, short stature, brachydactyly, failure of tooth eruption	?	? (two sporadic cases known)
Hall syndrome[13]	Craniosynostosis and Turner-like phenotype	?	?
Herrmann syndrome I[14]	Craniosynostosis, mental deficiency, hypoplastic supraorbital ridges, bitemporal flattening, ocular hypertelorism, ear anomalies, micrognathia, partial soft tissue syndactyly of second to fourth fingers, absent toes		
Herrmann syndrome II[15]	Craniosynostosis, microbrachycephaly, mental deficiency, anomalous ears, cleft lip and palate, symmetrical limb reduction defects with absent four and fifth fingers, short forearms, valgus positioning of hands, ankylosis at knees, and varus positioning of feet	?	?
Idaho syndrome I[7]	Craniosynostosis, scaphocephaly, strabismus, mental deficiency, congenital heart defect, umbilical hernia, complete anterior dislocation of tibia and fibula, talipes equinovarus, camptodactyly of second to fifth fingers, deviation of fingers to ulnar side, proximally placed thumbs	?	?

Continued.

Table 17-18. Syndromes with craniosynostosis—cont'd

Syndrome	Striking features	Relative frequency of cranio- synostosis in syndrome	Etiology
Idaho syndrome II[7]	Craniosynostosis, scaphocephaly, mental deficiency, downslanting palpebral fissures, beaked nose, micrognathia, small low-set posteriorly angulated ears, preauricular tags, long neck, sloping shoulders, narrow thorax, pectus carinatum, winging of scapulae, cubitus valgus	?	?
Pederson syndrome[24]	Craniosynostosis, exostoses of skull, premature exfoliation of deciduous teeth, linear verrucous nevi of neck, scaly patches on hands	?	?
Sakati syndrome[25]	Craniosynostosis, disproportionately small face, anomalous ears, patches of alopecia with atrophic skin, short limbs, polysyndactyly of feet, polydactyly of hands, congenital heart defect	?	?
Waardenburg craniosynostosis syndrome[29]	Craniosynostosis, hydrophthalmos, downslanting palpebral fissures, cleft palate, micrognathia, low-set ears, malposed clavicles, contractures at elbows and knees, soft-tissue syndactyly of second to fourth fingers, absent distal phalanx of thumb with absent nail, double nail with bifid terminal phalanx on second fingers, clinodactyly of fourth and fifth fingers, four toes, soft tissue syndactyly of fourth and fifth toes, hammertoes, ambiguous external genitalia, patent ductus arteriosus	?	?
Wisconsin syndrome[19]	Craniosynostosis, mental deficiency, upslanting palpebral fissures, microtia, short fourth metatarsals	?	? (two sporadic cases known)

raised by several authors. Genetic heterogeneity should always be kept in mind. However, that an autosomal recessive form of the Crouzon syndrome exists still remains equivocal.

In the Crouzon syndrome, craniosynostosis commonly begins during the first year of life and is usually complete by 2 to 3 years of age (Fig. 17-54). In some cases, craniosynostosis may be evident at birth. Occasionally, no sutural involvement may be noted.

Cranial deformity depends on the order and rate of progression of sutural synostosis. There is no characteristically shaped calvarium in the Crouzon syndrome. Brachycephaly, scaphocephaly, trigonocephaly and, rarely, the cloverleaf skull malformation may be observed. Palpable ridging is usually evident. A prominent bulge may be present at the bregma.

Radiographically, the coronal, sagittal, lambdoidal, and metopic sutures may be involved. Other findings may include digital impressions (Fig. 17-55), basilar kyphosis, widening of the hypophyseal fossa, and small paranasal sinuses.

Increased intracranial pressure and mental deficiency may be observed in some cases.

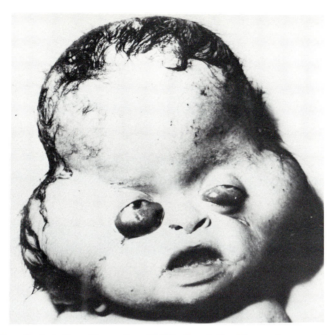

Fig. 17-53. Cloverleaf skull malformation. Trilobular skull with craniosynostosis is nonspecific and can be found in several different syndromes. (From Cohen, M. M., Jr., Birth Defects 11 [2]:137, 1975.)

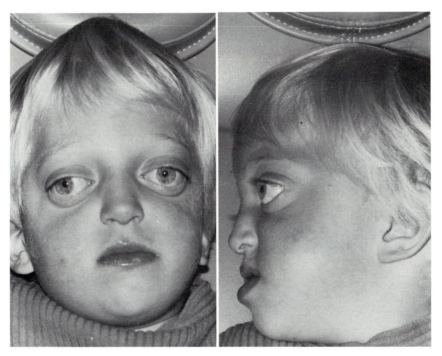

Fig. 17-54. Crouzon syndrome. Craniosynostosis, shallow orbits, proptosis, and midface hypoplasia.

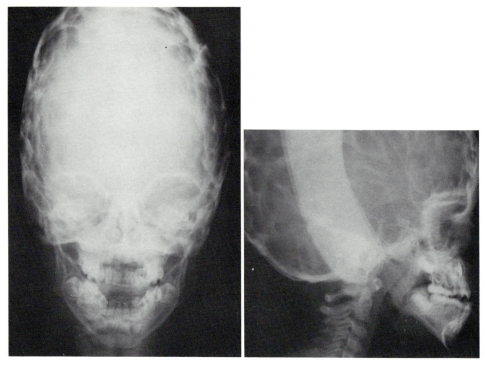

Fig. 17-55. Crouzon syndrome. Radiographs showing digital impressions. (From Cohen, M. M., Jr.: Birth Defects **11**[2]:137, 1975.)

Epilepsy has been noted in a few instances.

In the Crouzon syndrome, ocular proptosis is secondary to shallow orbits. Divergent strabismus and hypertelorism are commonly found. Optic nerve involvement and even luxation of globes have been noted. Low-frequency anomalies may include nystagmus, iris coloboma, aniridia, anisocoria, corectopia, microcornea, megalocornea, cataract, ectopia lentis, blue sclera, and glaucoma.

Maxillary hypoplasia is observed. This is usually, but not always, accompanied by relative mandibular prognathism with drooping lower lip, short upper lip, and parrot-beaked nose.

Deviation of the nasal septum and bilateral atresia of the auditory meatus have been reported occasionally. Ankylosis at the elbows and subluxation of the radial head have been described.

Oral manifestations include narrow highly arched palate, crowding of the upper teeth, V-shaped maxillary dental arch, and class III malocclusion. Oligodontia, macrodontia, peg-shaped, teeth and widely spaced teeth have been reported occasionally.[207, 211, 214, 219, 229]

Apert syndrome. The Apert syndrome is characterized by craniosynostosis and symmetrical syndactyly of the hands and feet, minimally involving the second, third, and fourth digits. Over 200 cases have been reported to date. Advanced paternal age as a factor in producing fresh mutations for the Apert syndrome has been confirmed. Although most cases of the Apert syndrome are sporadic, affected females have given birth to affected children in four instances. No instance of male-to-male transmission has been observed. However, the four familial cases, the equal number of affected males and females, and the increased paternal age effect in sporadic instances strongly suggest autosomal dominant transmission. The rarity of familial cases is explained by the reduced fitness of affected individuals.

The mutation rate in the Apert syndrome was estimated to be 3×10^{-6} per gene per generation by Blank and 4×10^{-6} per gene

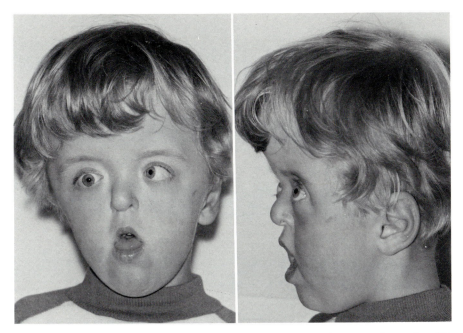

Fig. 17-56. Apert syndrome. Note turribrachycephaly, proptosis, esotropia, and midface deficiency.

per generation by Tünte and Lenz. Blank noted that the disorder occurs once in 160,000 births and, because of the high mortality rate in the neonatal period, occurs once in 2 million times in the general population. The incidence of the Apert syndrome was estimated as one in 100,000 births by Tünte and Lenz.

In the Apert syndrome, there is irregular early obliteration of cranial sutures, especially the coronal suture. The anterior fontanel may remain open longer than normal. Accentuation of digital markings may be observed with age. Because sutural involvement is variable, craniofacial appearance and degree of asymmetry is also variable. Turribrachycephaly is commonly observed, and the occiput is flattened. The forehead is steep, and, during infancy, a horizontal groove that disappears with age may be present above the supraorbital ridges. Bulging at the bregma or slightly anterior to the bregma may be noted in some cases. The middle third of the face is hypoplastic, resulting in relative man-

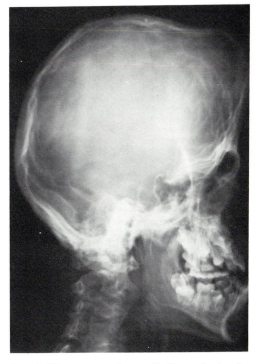

Fig. 17-57. Apert syndrome. Radiograph showing turribrachycephaly and midface hypoplasia.

dibular prognathism. When the nasal bridge is depressed, the nose may have a parrot-beaked appearance, but nasal morphology may be variable (Figs. 17-56 and 17-57).

Hypertelorism, proptosis, antimongoloid obliquity and, frequently, strabismus may be observed. Optic atrophy has been noted and, rarely, keratoconus, ectopia lentis, congenital glaucoma, lack of pigment in the fundi, and luxation of the eyeglobes have been reported.

The ears may appear to be low-set in some instances, and other minor anomalies of the pinnae have been noted. Conductive hearing loss, congenitally fixed stapes, and abnormally patent cochlear aqueduct have been documented in several patients.

In the relaxed state, the lips frequently assume a trapezoidal configuration. The palate is highly arched (Fig. 17-58), constricted, and may have a median furrow. Cleft soft

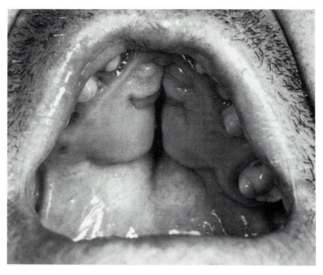

Fig. 17-58. Apert syndrome. Byzantine arch palate.

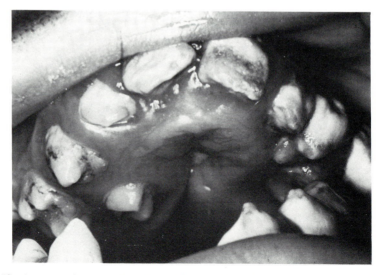

Fig. 17-59. Apert syndrome. V-shaped maxillary arch, malposed teeth, and bulging alveolar ridges.

palate or bifid uvula may be observed in over 30% of the cases. The maxillary dental arch may be V-shaped with severely crowded teeth and bulging alveolar ridges (Fig. 17-59). Class III malocclusion is usually present with anterior openbite or crossbite and unilateral or bilateral posterior crossbite. Retarded dental eruption is a common finding. Supernumerary teeth have been observed.

Mental deficiency has been found in many patients, although normal intelligence has also been observed. Ventricular dilatation has been reported, but the frequency of this finding is uncertain because of ascertainment bias. In both reported series, hydrocephalus was variable and the underlying mechanism unknown, both aqueductal stenosis and communicating hydrocephalus being noted. In some instances, hydrocephalus was nonprogressive and became compensated. In other patients, significant hydrocephalus was correlated with elevated cerebrospinal fluid pressure and increased digital markings. However, it is important to note that in still other patients with significant hydrocephalus, cerebrospinal fluid pressure was normal, head circumference remained unchanged, and no alterations in the optic fundi were observed.

Thus patients with the Apert syndrome warrant careful observation for other signs of hydrocephalus such as behavioral regression and increased tone in the lower limbs.

Malformations of the hands and feet are symmetrical (Fig. 17-60). A middigital hand mass minimally involving the second, third, and fourth fingers is always observed. Associated synonychia is variable in degree. The first and fifth fingers may be joined to the middigital hand mass or may be separate. When the thumb is free, it is broad and deviates radially. Some degree of brachydactyly involving all five fingers is usually present. The interphalangeal joints become stiff by 4 years of age.

Radiographically, the first metacarpal is normal. The proximal phalanx of the thumb is short, frequently narrow, and sometimes delta shaped. The distal phalanx of the thumb is enlarged and trapezoidal. In approximately half the cases, only the distal phalanx is present in the thumb. The second to fifth metacarpals are shorter than normal and tend to be uniform in length. The proximal ends of the fourth and fifth metacarpals are frequently fused. Symphalangism of the proximal interphalangeal joints occurs by 4

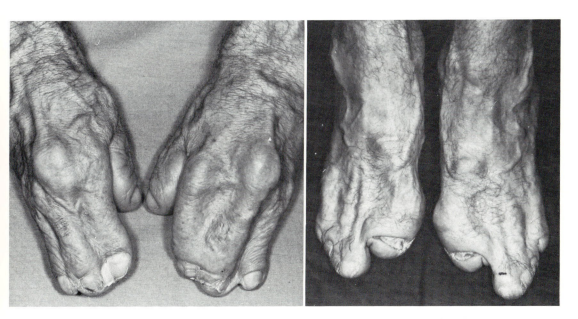

Fig. 17-60. Hands and feet in Apert syndrome showing extensive syndactyly.

to 6 years of age. The distal interphalangeal joints are less frequently fused. Synostosis of adjacent distal phalanges occurs with age, most frequently between the third and fourth distal phalanges, but also between the second to fourth or between the second to fifth distal phalanges. Fusion of carpal bones, especially the hamate and capitate bones, may be observed. Other bony abnormalities of the hands have also been noted.

In the feet, syndactyly involves the second, third, and fourth toes. The first and fifth toes are sometimes free and sometimes joined by soft tissue union to the second and fourth toes, respectively. Toenails may be separate or partially continuous. The great toes are broad, and hallux varus is commonly observed.

The distal phalanx of the great toe is enlarged and trapezoidal. The proximal phalanx of the great toes is malformed. The second phalanges of the second to fifth toes are often absent. The first metatarsal is broad, shortened in some instances, and may exhibit partial or complete duplication. Symphalangism, fusion of tarsal bones, and other bony abnormalities may be observed in the feet.

Aplasia or ankylosis of joints, including the elbow, shoulder, and hip, is common. Rhizomelia may be observed, especially involving the humerus. Progressive synostosis of the bones of the hands, feet, and cervical spine has been documented. Abnormalities of the pelvis and other skeletal defects have also been noted.

A large number of low-frequency visceral anomalies have been reported, including cardiovascular and renal abnormalities. Other abnormalities have included an increased frequency of acne vulgaris with unusual extension to the forearms.*

Pfeiffer syndrome. The Pfeiffer syndrome consists of craniosynostosis, broad thumbs and great toes, and partial soft tissue syndactyly of the hands and feet, which is a variable feature. Autosomal dominant in-

heritance with complete penetrance and variable expressivity characterize the disorder.

The Pfeiffer syndrome and Apert-type acrocephalosyndactyly are noteworthy for their close similarity, the former being less severe in degree. It has been suggested that the Pfeiffer syndrome may in fact represent a mild form of Apert-type acrocephalosyndactyly. Clinical differences have been explained by later onset of the gene's action. However, on the basis of pedigree studies reported to date, no transition from one type to the other has been observed within families despite the presence of variability in expression. Thus the two disorders appear to be nosologically and genetically distinct. An allelic mutant gene to account for the differences between the two disorders was postulated by Pfeiffer.

The skull is usually turribrachycephalic. Craniofacial asymmetry may be present in some instances. Maxillary hypoplasia and relative mandibular prognathism are observed. The nasal bridge is depressed. Ocular hypertelorism, downslanting palpebral fissures, proptosis, and strabismus are common (Fig. 17-61). The nose may be beaked. The palate is highly arched, and the alveolar ridges are broad. Class III malocclusion and crowded teeth have been noted. The syndrome has been reported in association with the cloverleaf skull malformation. All such cases to date have been sporadic, and none have occurred within an affected family. Therefore etiological heterogeneity cannot be ruled out.

Intelligence is usually normal, but mental deficiency has been observed in some instances. Hydrocephalus, Arnold-Chiari malformation, and seizures have been noted.

The thumbs and great toes are broad, usually with varus deformity (Figs. 17-62 and 17-63). Mild soft-tissue syndactyly may involve especially the second and third digits and sometimes the third and fourth digits of both hands and feet. Brachydactyly may be observed, and in some cases syndactyly is absent. Clinodactyly has also been noted.

Low-frequency abnormalities have included pyloric stenosis, umbilical hernia,

---

*See references 206, 210, 213, 214, 217, 218, 224, 226-228, 230.

malpositioned anus at the scrotal base, bifid scrotum, widely spaced nipples, choanal atresia, preauricular tag, absent external auditory canals, hearing loss, bifid uvula, supernumerary teeth, and gingival hypertrophy.

Radiographic aspects of the Pfeiffer syndrome include craniosynostosis, especially involving the coronal suture, turribrachycephaly, and increased digital markings with age. Maxillary hypoplasia, shallow orbits, and depressed nasal bridge are also observed.

Brachymesophalangy of both hands and

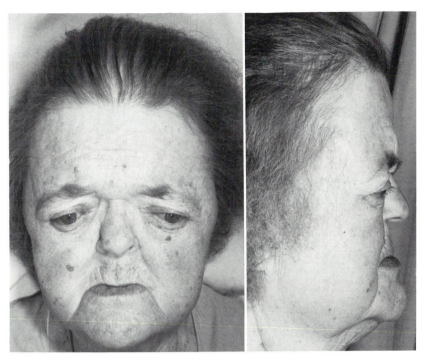

Fig. 17-61. Pfeiffer syndrome. Note brachycephaly, proptosis, downslanting palpebral fissures, and midface deficiency.

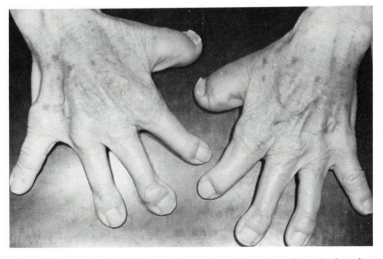

Fig. 17-62. Hands in Pfeiffer syndrome: broad thumbs and brachydactyly.

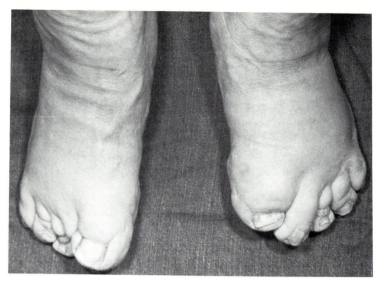

Fig. 17-63. Feet in Pfeiffer syndrome: broad great toes and crooked digits.

feet are frequently present. Middle phalanges may be absent in some cases. The distal phalanx of the thumb is broad, and the proximal phalanx is triangular in some instances or absent. The distal phalanx of the great toe is broad and the proximal phalanx malformed. The first metarsal is broad, may be shortened, and may be duplicated in some cases.

Accessory epiphyses in the first and second metatarsals and double ossification centers in the proximal phalanx of the great toe have been reported. Partial duplication of the great toe may be observed occasionally. Symphalangism of both hands and feet has been reported. Fusion of carpals and tarsals, in some instances involving the proximal ends of the metacarpals and metatarsals respectively, has also been noted.

Fused cervical vertebrae and lumbar vertebrae have been described. Shortened humerus, cubitus valgus, radiohumeral and radioulnar synostosis, abnormalities of the pelvis, coxa valga, and talipes calcaneovarus have been reported occasionally.[220, 223, 225, 231]

Saethre-Chotzen syndrome. The Saethre-Chotzen syndrome is characterized by craniosynostosis, low-set frontal hairline, facial asymmetry, ptosis of the eyelids, deviated nasal septum, and, variably, some degree of brachydactyly and partial cutaneous syndactyly, especially of the second and third fingers. Autosomal dominant inheritance is evident with a high degree of penetrance and variable expressivity.

First recognized as an entity in 1931 by Saethre and in 1932 by Chotzen, the syndrome has been reported by several authors since that time under a variety of different terms. The most extensive discussion has been published by Pantke and associates.[225] The Saethre-Chotzen syndrome is relatively common among craniosynostosis syndromes per se. Relatively few cases have been recognized and reported for two reasons. First, some cases with relatively mild involvement never come to medical attention. The physical appearance may not be especially bothersome to affected individuals in many cases. Furthermore, complications of craniosynostosis do not seem to ensue in most instances. Second, those cases that do come to medical attention are often erroneously diagnosed as examples of simple craniosynostosis, Crouzon syndrome, "pseudo-Crouzon syndrome," or the Pfeiffer syndrome.

In the Saethre-Chotzen syndrome the degree of craniosynostosis is variable. Involvement is often asymmetrical, producing plagiocephaly and facial asymmetry. Acro-

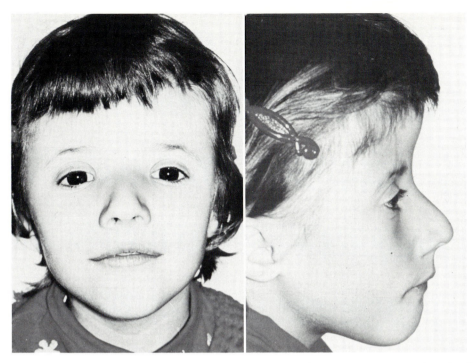

Fig. 17-64. Saethre-Chotzen syndrome. Note brachycephaly, broad flat forehead, and ptosis of eyelids. (From Cohen, M. M., Jr.: Birth Defects 11[2]:137, 1975.)

cephaly is frequently observed, but scapho-cephaly has been noted in some instances. Frontal bossing, parietal bossing, and flattened occiput have been reported in various cases. The head circumference is reduced, and a low-set frontal hairline is frequently observed (Figs. 17-64 and 17-65).

Ptosis of the eyelids and hypertelorism are common. Esotropia are exotropia have been reported. In some instances lacrimal duct abnormalities have been noted. Optic atrophy has also been reported. The ears may be low-set, small, and posteriorly angulated, or they may have folded helices or prominent antihelical crura. A minor degree of hearing loss is common. The nasofrontal angle may be flattened in some instances. Narrow or highly arched palate is frequently observed.

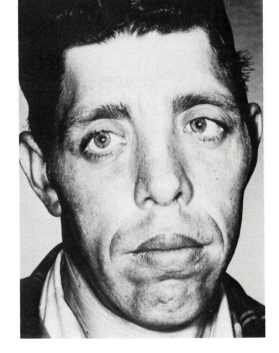

Fig. 17-65. Saethre-Chotzen syndrome. Craniofacial asymmetry, low-set frontal hairline, ptosis of eyelids, and esotropia. (From Cohen, M. M., Jr.: Birth Defects 11[2]:137, 1975.)

Cleft palate has been noted in several instances. Relative mandibular prognathism, class III malocclusion, enamel hypoplasia, and other dental defects have been noted.

Intelligence is frequently normal. However, mild-to-moderate mental deficiency has been observed in a number of cases. Moderate dilatation of the lateral ventricles was demonstrated in one case. Epilepsy and schizophrenia have also been noted.

Some degree of brachydactyly may be observed. Partial cutaneous syndactyly is present in some instances, most frequently between the second and third fingers (Fig. 17-66), but sometimes extending from the second to fourth fingers. Clinodactyly, especially of the fifth finger, has been noted in some cases. Dermatoglyphic findings have included simian creases, distally placed axial triradii, an increased frequency of thenar and hypothenar patterns, and low total ridge count.

Partial cutaneous syndactyly between the second and third toes but occasionally involving other toes has been reported. Hallux valgus has been noted in some instances, and dorsiflexion of the fourth toe has been observed.

Short stature has been documented in some instances. Defects of the cervical and lumbar spine have been reported by several authors. Radioulnar synostosis has been noted, and shortened fourth metacarpals have also been recorded. Other findings have included cryptochidism, renal anomalies, and congenital cardiac defects.[206, 222, 225, 228]

Carpenter syndrome. The Carpenter syndrome is characterized by craniosynostosis, polysyndactyly of the feet, short hands with variable soft tissue syndactyly, and other abnormalities. First described by Carpenter in 1901 and 1909, the syndrome was not recognized as a distinct nosological and genetic entity until Temtamy's report in 1966. The disorder is frequently confused with the Apert syndrome and the Laurence-Moon syndrome. It clearly follows an autosomal recessive mode of transmission.

Craniosynostosis usually involves the sagittal and lambdoidal sutures first, the coronal suture being last to close. The calvarium is grossly malformed (**Fig. 17-67**) but variable in shape. In many cases, unilateral involvement of the coronal or lambdoidal suture produces marked cranial asymmetry. The cloverleaf skull malformation has been observed in association with the Carpenter syndrome. Wormian bones in the anterior fontanel have been noted. To date, mental de-

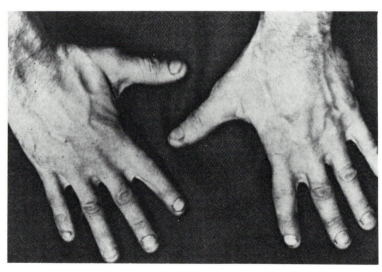

Fig. 17-66. Hands in Saethre-Chotzen syndrome. Note soft tissue syndactyly. (From Bartsocas, C. S., et al.: J. Pediatr. **77**:267, 1970.)

ficiency has been apparent in all cases except one.

The nasal bridge is flattened, and dystopia canthorum is usually observed. Epicanthal folds, microcornea, corneal opacity, slight optic atrophy, and blurring of the disk margins have been reported in some instances. The ears appear to be low-set, and the neck is short. The mandible may be somewhat small, and the palate may be narrow or highly arched.

The hands are short and the fingers stubby. Marked soft tissue syndactyly may be present, especially between the third and fourth fingers, with less marked involvement between other fingers. In some cases, minimal or no syndactyly may be evident. Clinodactyly, single flexion crease, and occasionally postminimus digits may be observed. Radiographically, brachymesophalangy or agenesis of middle phalanges is evident. A tongue-shaped projection may extend from the radial side of the epiphysis of the proximal phalanx of the second finger. Two ossification centers in the proximal phalanx of the thumb have been reported.

Abnormalities of the feet include bilateral varus deformities and preaxial polydactyly with duplication of the second toes or, less commonly, duplication of the halluces. Soft tissue syndactyly may be observed between the toes, and only two phalanges are present in each toe.

Genua valga and lateral displacement of the patellae are common. Other skeletal findings have included decreased hip joint mobility, flaring of the ilia with poor development of the acetabula, coxa valga, absent coccyx, spina bifida occulta, and scoliosis.

Height is usually below the twenty-fifth percentile, but weight is often above average.

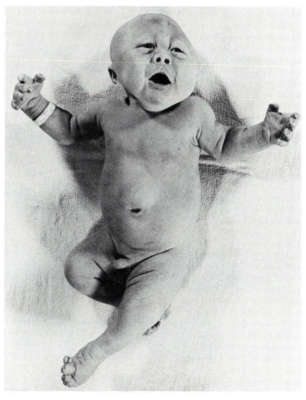

Fig. 17-67. Carpenter syndrome. Note bizarre skull shape and polysyndactyly of feet. (From Cohen, M. M., Jr.: Birth Defects **11**[2]:137, 1975.)

Obesity involves the trunk, proximal limbs, face, and neck.

Congenital heart defects have been reported in several cases. Ventricular septal defect, atrial septal defect, patent ductus arteriosus, pulmonic stenosis, and tetralogy of Fallot have been described. Other findings have included cryptorchidism, omphalocele, accessory spleen, hydronephrosis, hydroureter, and inguinal hernia.[237, 238]

Diastrophic dwarfism

Diastrophic dwarfism consists of micromelic dwarfism, contractures, progressive scoliosis, bilateral talipes equinovarus, hip dysplasia, characteristic external ear deformities and, frequently, cleft palate (Figs. 17-68 to 17-70). Over 120 cases have been described. The most complete survey is that of Walker and associates.[246] The syndrome follows an autosomal recessive mode of transmission.

About 25% die in infancy of aspiration pneumonia or respiratory distress. The somewhat hoarse cry and respiratory distress may be related to abnormal laryngeal cartilages. Intelligence is normal.

Craniofacial complex. The face tends to be square with a narrow nasal bridge, broad midnose, flared nostrils, and circumoral fullness. The lower lip is slightly larger than the upper lip. The mandible tends to be small. Cleft palate is common.

The external auditory canals may be narrowed. Bilateral but at times asymmetrical deformity of the ear is frequently observed. It may be evident within the first few days or weeks of life as a cystic swelling from which serosanguinous fluid may be extracted. This resolves within a month, but the ear

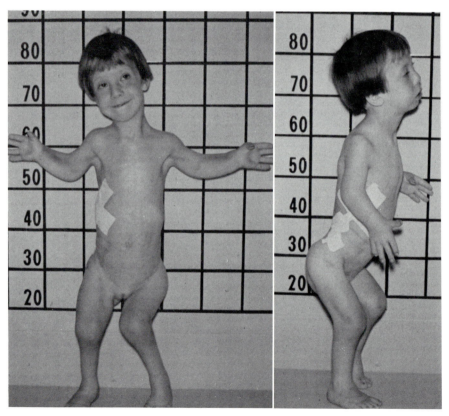

Fig. 17-68. Diastrophic dwarfism: short stature and contractures. (Courtesy R. E. Stewart, Los Angeles, Calif.)

becomes distorted with calcification of the cartilage.

Musculoskeletal alterations. Mean adult height is about 44 inches (112 cm) with men ranging from 34 to 50 inches and women ranging from 41 to 48 inches. The diastrophic variant is taller, general skeletal deformity is less marked, and clubfoot is not so resistant to treatment.

Mesomelic dwarfism is a constant feature.

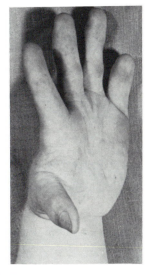

Fig. 17-69. Proximally placed thumb in diastrophic dwarfism.

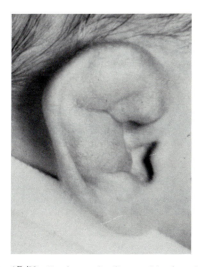

Fig. 17-70. Cystic ear in diastrophic dwarfism.

Mean birth length is about 13 inches. There is shortening of all limbs; bilateral talipes equinovarus is severe, becomes worse with age, is resistant to treatment, and tends to recur after therapy. The patients bear their weight on their toes, so walking is limited.

The thumbs are proximally inserted, hypermobile, and laterally displaced. The broad hands and shortened fingers often exhibit ulnar deviation, and frequently webbing, contractures, and fixation of the interphalangeal finger joints occur.

Scoliosis is not present at birth but is progressive and often is present by the first few years of life. Kyphosis is occasionally associated, and lordosis is frequent. Flexion contracture and/or subluxation or dislocation, especially of the hips, and to a lesser extent of the knees and shoulders are common and progressive, further reducing height. Inguinal hernia has also been described.

Radiographic changes include shortening and thickening of nearly all tubular bones. The epiphyses have delayed appearance and are flattened and distorted. With time the metaphyses become widened, irregular, and deformed. The humerus is less shortened than the radius and ulna. The thumb is proximally placed, and the first metacarpal is small and rounded. Synostosis of the proximal interphalangeal joints is a constant feature. Carpal development is accelerated, but secondary centers for the metacarpals, metatarsals, and phalanges are retarded in appearance. The metacarpals are broader at the distal end than at the proximal end. The first metatarsal is broader and wider than other metatarsals.

Dislocation or subluxation of the hips and coxa vara is associated with flattening of the acetabular roof and delayed appearance and poor development of the capital femoral epiphysis. The patella is often subluxated. Progressive kyphosis of the cervical spine with subluxation of C_2 on C_3 is frequent and may result in spinal cord compression.

Precocious ossification of costal cartilages and calcification of pinnal cartilage occur. Intracranial calcification has also been described.[239-247]

Ectodermal dysplasia

In the past, the term *ectodermal dysplasia* was used to refer to a specific entity, hypohidrotic ectodermal dysplasia. More recently, the term has been applied to many genetic syndromes that have various ectodermal abnormalities. Although both uses of the term are justified, only the common hypohidrotic type is discussed in this section. The disorder consists of hypohidrosis, hypotrichosis, and hypodontia.

Analysis of over 300 cases reveals an X-linked mode of transmission, the gene being carried by the female and manifest in the male. However, at least thirty-five females have manifested the complete disorder, and it is probable that most of these cases are examples of the autosomal recessive form of the condition. In the X-linked form, the carrier mothers exhibit minimal expression of the gene in the form of hypodontia and/or conical teeth and spottily reduced sweating. This is consistent with the Lyon hypothesis for variability of expression.

Craniofacial complex (Fig. 17-71). The condition may not be apparent until the sec-

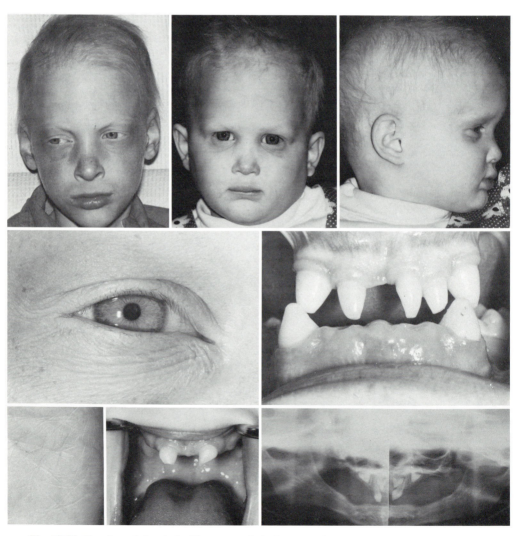

Fig. 17-71. Ectodermal dysplasia. Note sparse hair, low nasal bridge, linear wrinkling under eye, wrinkling of palm, oligodontia, and conically shaped teeth.

ond year of life. The combination of frontal bossing, low nasal bridge, protuberant lips, and in some cases obliquely inserted ears is striking. Lacrimal gland function has been diminished in a few cases. Congenital glaucoma has been occasionally noted.

The most characteristic oral alteration is hypodontia or, in many cases, anodontia, reflecting complete suppression of dental ectoderm. The few teeth that may be present are often retarded in eruption. Because of the hypodontia and the resultant loss of vertical dimension, the lips are protuberant. The vermilion border is indistinct, and pseudorhagades may be present. The alveolar process does not develop in the absence of teeth and, hence, is missing. The incisors, canines, and premolars, when present, often have conical crowns. The oral mucosa appears dry. Histopathological studies have shown aplasia of the labial, buccal, and lower respiratory glands. Pharyngeal and laryngeal mucosa may be atrophic, resulting in dysphonia. Atrophy of the nasal mucosa associated with severe crusting and marked ozena have been described.

Skin and skin appendages. Because the physical features may not be apparent during the first year, the child may present a fever of unknown origin. The inability to sweat, predicated on marked aplasia of the eccrine sweat glands, results in intolerance to heat, with severe incapacitation and hyperpyrexia after only mild exertion or even after meals. The skin is soft and thin. Dryness is often severe, because of the absence of sebaceous glands, and atopic flexural eczema is common, especially during the early years of life. Fine, linear wrinkles and increased pigmentation are often noted about the eyes and mouth. The palms and soles are frequently the sites of small hyperkeratoses. The body is usually devoid of lanugo hair, and after puberty, although the beard is usually normal, the axillary and pubic hair is frequently scant. The scalp hair is often blond, fine, stiff, and short. The eyelashes and especially the eyebrows are often missing.

The nails are usually normal or somewhat spoon-shaped, but the mammary glands have been noted by several observers to be aplastic or hypoplastic. Dermatoglyphic alterations have been recorded.[240-246]

Ellis–van Creveld syndrome

The Ellis–van Creveld syndrome consists of bilateral manual postaxial polydactyly, mesomelic dwarfism, ectodermal dysplasia affecting principally the nails and teeth (Figs. 17-72 to 17-75), and congenital heart malformations. More than 100 cases have been reported to date. The syndrome follows an autosomal recessive mode of transmission with parental consanguinity in about 30% of cases. This condition is the most common type of dwarfism among the Amish.

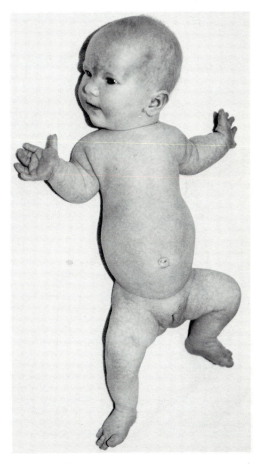

Fig. 17-72. Ellis–van Creveld syndrome: mesomelic shortening of limbs and postaxial polydactyly of hands. (Courtesy D. W. Smith, Seattle, Wash.)

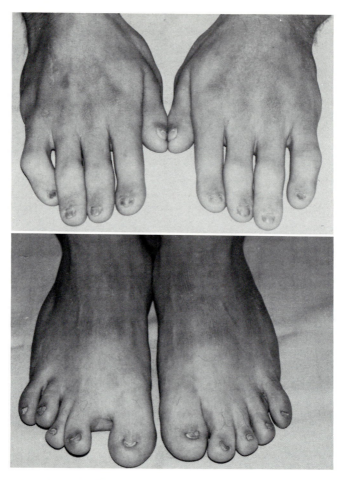

Fig. 17-73. Hands and feet in Ellis–van Creveld syndrome. Note short digits and hypoplastic nails.

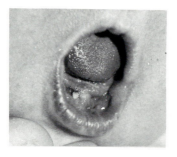

Fig. 17-74. Ellis–van Creveld syndrome. Note serrated lower anterior alveolar ridge and natal tooth. (Courtesy D. W. Smith, Seattle, Wash.)

Skeletal anomalies. The limbs exhibit mesomelia (Fig. 17-72). Bilateral manual hexadactyly is frequent, the extra digit being present on the ulnar side. Heptadactyly has also been noted. Frequently the patient cannot make a tight fist. Only rarely are there extra toes. A widened space frequently is present between the hallux and the second toe. Genua valga, curvature of the humerus, talipes equinovarus, talipes calcaneovalgus, and pectus carinatum with thoracic constriction have also been reported.

Radiographically, the tubular bones are short and thickened. The diaphyseal ends of the humerus and the femur are plump. Shortening of the radius and ulna is even more marked than that of the humerus. The

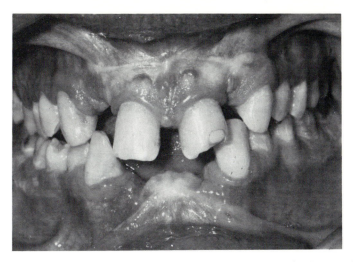

Fig. 17-75. Ellis–van Creveld syndrome. Note missing teeth and thick frenula.

proximal end of the ulna and the distal end of the radius are unusually large, and the proximal end of the radius and the distal end of the ulnar are unusually small. The widened end of the tibial shaft is irregular, and the ossification centers in the proximal epiphysis are hypoplastic. There is peaking of the proximal tibia, with a long lateral and a short medial slope, resulting in genua valga after the age of 6 years. The fibula is most severely shortened, being only about half the normal length. Phalangeal bones are often missing, and syncarpalism involving the hamate and capitate bones, synmetacarpalism, and polymetacarpalism are common. Cone-shaped epiphyses of the hands are also observed. In infancy the pelvis is dysplastic with low iliac wings and hooklike downward projection of the medial acetabulum. The capital femoral epiphysis may ossify prematurely. In childhood, the pelvic shape normalizes.

Hair and nails. The hair (especially the eyebrows and pubic hair) is thin and sparse. Nearly all patients have severe dystrophy of the fingernails (Fig. 17-73). They are markedly hypoplastic, thin, and often wrinkled or spoon-shaped.

Heart. Congenital heart defect has been noted in 40% to 50% of the cases reported to date. Most patients have demonstrated single atrium and endocardial cushion defect. Some patients have had cor triloculare or even cor biloculare.

Genitalia. About a third of male patients have had genital anomalies. Cryptorchidism, mild epispadias, and hypospadias have been reported.

Mental status. Some patients have been noted to be mentally retarded, but it has been suggested that mental retardation is not an integral part of the disorder. Hydrocephalus has been reported in several instances.

Oral manifestations. The most striking oral finding is fusion of the middle portion of the upper lip to the maxillary gingival margin so that no mucobuccal fold or sulcus exists anteriorly. Because of this fusion, the middle portion of the upper lip appears hypoplastic, resembling a lip that has undergone cheiloplasty.

Natal teeth (Fig. 17-74) have been observed in at least 25% of infants. Oligodontia is also common, especially in the mandibular anterior region (Fig. 17-75). In this area, the alveolar ridge is often serrated, which may represent persistence of the normally serrated ridge during the third to seventh months in utero. The teeth are usually small, conically crowned, and irregularly spaced. The crown form of many of the

teeth is distinctive. Those that are not conical are somewhat bicuspid in form with accentuated cuspal height and steep fissures.
The enamel has been noted to be hypoplastic
in about half the cases.[255-263]

Frontonasal dysplasia

Frontonasal dysplasia is an anomalad consisting of ocular hypertelorism, broad nasal
root, lack of formation of the nasal tip,
widow's peak scalp-hair anomaly, anterior
cranium bifidum occultum, median clefting
of the nose and/or lip, and unilateral or bilateral notching or clefting of the nasal alae
(Figs. 17-76 and 17-77). The most complete
reviews are those of Sedano and associates,[268]
who called the condition *frontonasal dysplasia,* and deMyer,[266] who used the term
median cleft face syndrome. Embryologically,
if the nasal capsule fails to develop properly,
the primitive brain vesicle fills the space normally occupied by the capsule, thus producing anterior cranium bifidum occultum, a
morphokinetic arrest in the positioning of
the eyes, lack of formation of the nasal tip,
and sometimes median clefting of the nose
and lip. The widow's peak scalp-hair anomaly results from ocular hypertelorism, since
the two periocular fields of hair-growth suppression are also further apart than usual.
Thus the fields fail to overlap sufficiently
high up on the forehead, resulting in a
widow's peak.

Almost all cases are sporadic. However,
the condition has been observed in half-sibs
and through two generations. Although
dominant inheritance (with most cases representing fresh mutations together with reduced genetic fitness) and polygenic inheritance are both possible, the condition is most
likely etiologically heterogeneous with a multiplicity of causes. For example, the same set
of facial features may be observed with large
anterior encephalocele, frontal lipoma, or
frontal teratoma. Furthermore, the varied
low-frequency anomalies found with frontonasal dysplasia suggest that a variety of multiple congenital anomaly syndromes may be

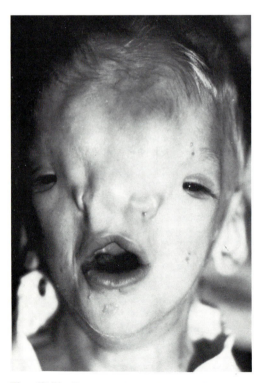

Fig. 17-76. Frontonasal dysplasia: ocular hypertelorism, secondary telecanthus, wide-set nostrils,
and lack of elevation of nasal tip. (From Cohen,
M. M., Jr.: Birth Defects **7**[7]:117, 1971.)

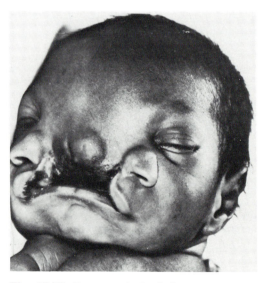

Fig. 17-77. Frontonasal dysplasia: ocular hypertelorism, widow's peak scalp hair anomaly, and
median clefting of nose and mouth. (From deMyer,
W.: Neurology **17**:961, 1967.)

present within the frontonasal dysplasia category. To date, however, no true multiple congenital anomaly syndromes have been isolated or identified.

The number of instances of twinning is greater in families with frontonasal dysplasia than in the general population. No explanation for this phenomenon is known. Although some clinicians have maintained that frontonasal dysplasia represents an incomplete form of twinning, this view cannot be accepted. Twinning of the head results from anterior duplication of the notochord. Doubling of the hypophysis constitutes the mildest form of anterior duplication. In diprosopia, a more extensive duplication, there may be doubling of the hypophysis, mouth, and nose. Doubling may lead to formation of two lateral eyes and a median eye. There is no evidence of duplication of any structure in frontonasal dysplasia.

Craniofacial complex. The clinical appearance of the face has been classified on a somewhat different basis by deMyer[266] and by Sedano and co-workers.[268] Facial malformation can be graded from mild to severe. Ocular hypertelorism is a constant finding. Secondary telecanthus or narrowing of the palpebral fissures may be observed in severe cases. Epibulbar dermoids and upper eyelid colobomas have been observed in several instances. Rarely observed are congenital cataracts, microphthalmia, and anophthalmia. In severe cases, the nose may be flattened with widely spaced nostrils and broad nasal root. In other cases, clefting of the nose may be observed. Notching or clefting of the nasal alae is present in some cases. When notching occurs bilaterally, the nose appears square. Nose tags have also been noted. Median cleft of the upper lip is present in some cases. Rarely, cleft palate is observed. Preauricular tags have been recorded. Also reported have been low-set ears, absent tragus, and conductive deafness.

Central nervous system. Mental deficiency is present in some cases. Of clinical importance, especially at birth, is deMyer's observation that when extracephalic anomalies occur or when hypertelorism is severe, the probability of mental deficiency is increased. Conversely, when extracephalic anomalies are absent and hypertelorism is mild, the probability of mental deficiency is lower.

Anterior cranium bifidum is present radiographically. The frontal sinuses have been noted to be hypoplastic in a number of instances. Large anterior encephalocele and, rarely, lipoma or teratoma may be associated with the condition.

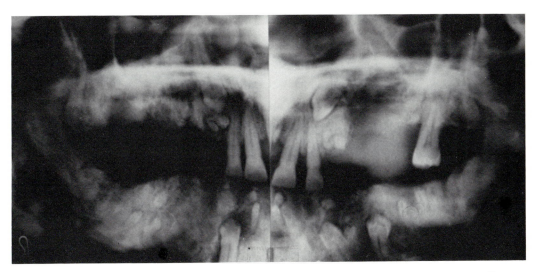

Fig. 17-78. Gardner syndrome: supernumerary teeth. (Courtesy C. J. Witkop, Jr., Minneapolis, Minn.)

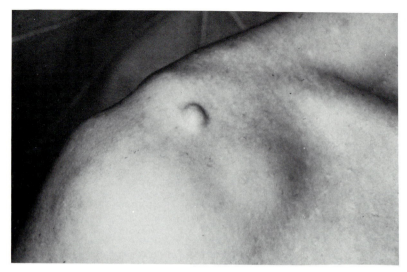

Fig. 17-79. Gardner syndrome: epidermoid cyst. (Courtesy A. F. Morgan, Seattle, Wash.)

Coronal craniosynostosis and brachycephaly have been noted in several patients. Also reported have been absence of the corpus callosum, hydrocephalus, and early occlusive anterior and middle cerebral artery disease.

Other findings. Occasionally polydactyly, syndactyly, clinodactyly, brachydactyly, umbilical hernia, cryptorchidism, and other anomalies have been reported.[264-270]

Gardner syndrome

Gardner and co-workers, in 1953, recognized a syndrome of multiple osteomas, epidermoid cysts of the skin, multiple polyposis of the large bowel, desmoids, fibromas, lipomas, leiomyomas, and odontomas (Figs. 17-78 to 17-81). The syndrome follows an autosomal dominant mode of transmission with at least 80% penetrance and markedly variable expressivity. The incidence has been estimated at 1 per 14,000 people.

Skin and skin appendages. Epidermoid inclusion cysts of the skin occur in about 50% of the cases but may be present in nearly all affected in some families. These may appear anywhere on the scalp, face, trunk, or extremities. The age at which the cysts first appear is variable, although on the average they become manifest about the age of 18

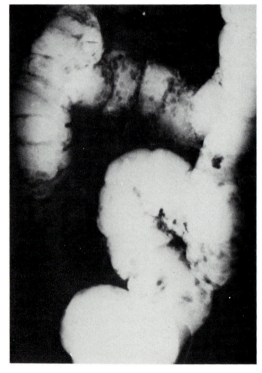

Fig. 17-80. Gardner syndrome: barium study demonstrating polyposis. (Courtesy A. F. Morgan, Seattle, Wash.)

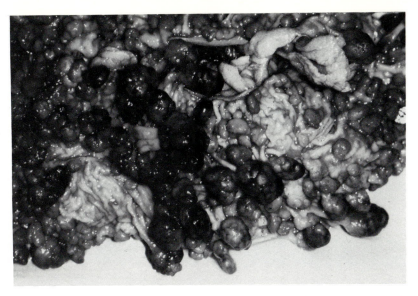

Fig. 17-81. Gardner syndrome: polyposis of colon. (Courtesy A. F. Morgan, Seattle, Wash.)

years, before the appearance of the intestinal polyposis. New cysts appear periodically.

Fibrous tumors of the skin (fibromas and desmoids) commonly occur in association with polyposis of the colon. The desmoid tumors frequently arise in the abdominal scar after resection for colonic surgery. They may, however, arise on the skin in the absence of any prior surgery. Lipoma or lipofibroma of the skin may also be found.

Gastrointestinal system and allied structures. Multiple intestinal polyposis of the colon and rectum, with a marked tendency to rapid malignant degeneration, is characteristic. Small bowel involvement has been reported by only a few investigators, but there is marked malignant propensity at this site. The polyps may occur before puberty. By 20 years, about 50% have demonstrated polyps and at the time of surgery about half of the patients exhibit malignant degeneration of one or more polyps. Lymphoid hyperplasia of the terminal ileum has been reported.

Desmoid tumors may be found scattered throughout the mesentery. They may be single or multiple and may be found in 10% to 30%. Postoperative adhesions are especially severe, frequently resulting in obstruction. Leiomyomas, both retroperitoneal and within the stomach and ileum, have also been observed.

Oral manifestations. Multiple osteomas may be scattered throughout the calvaria and facial skeleton. In most cases, the osteomas appear around puberty and precede the intestinal polyposis. The frontal bone, maxilla, mandibular angle, and the lower border of the mandible are most frequently involved. The osteomas may project into the paranasal sinuses. Microscopically, the bone is mature, consisting of well-developed Haversian systems.

Long bones, most often the radius, ulna, and metacarpals, may be the site of small osteomas, but involvement, in contrast to that of the facial skeleton, is minimal, and bony thickening is usually subperiosteal and rather diffuse. In a few cases, however, the osteomas have been small and well defined. Early involvement may stimulate osteomyelitis.

Compound odontomas, supernumerary teeth, and/or hypercementoses have been described in about 50% of affected individuals.

Other findings. Papillary adenocarcinoma of the thyroid has been documented occasionally.[271-282]

Gingival fibromatosis syndromes

Gingival fibromatosis is a nonspecific disorder that is most frequently caused by the use of phenytoin. In addition, it may occur as an isolated autosomal dominant trait. The binary combination of gingival fibromatosis and hypertrichosis also follows an autosomal dominant mode of transmission. The combination of gingival fibromatosis, hypertrichosis, mental deficiency, and/or epilepsy is genetically heterogeneous with autosomal dominant and autosomal recessive types. Known gingival fibromatosis syndromes include the Murray syndrome, the Rutherfurd syndrome, the Laband syndrome, the Cross syndrome, the Jones syndrome, and the Byars-Jurkiewicz syndrome. The last-named disorder is incompletely delineated at the present time but is probably distinct from the Cowden syndrome. Conditions with gingival fibromatosis together with their striking features and inheritance patterns are listed in Table 17-19. Figs. 17-82 to 17-85 demonstrate a provisionally unique-pattern syndrome with gingival fibromatosis that also needs to be further delineated. Findings include gingival fibromatosis, hirsutism, prominent frontal bone, axillary pterygium, swollen ribs, and other abnormalities.[283-293]

Gorlin syndrome

The Gorlin syndrome has been designated by a variety of different terms, including the basal cell nevus syndrome, nevoid basal cell carcinoma syndrome, epitheliomatose multiple generalisée (type Ferrari), syndrome of jaw cysts, basal cell tumors, and skeletal anomalies, polycystoma, fünfte Phakomatose, hereditary cutaneomandibular polyoncosis, the Gorlin syndrome, the Gorlin-Goltz syn-

Table 17-19. Conditions with gingival fibromatosis

Name	Features	Etiology
Isolated gingival fibromatosis	Gingival fibromatosis only	Autosomal dominant
Gingival fibromatosis dyad	Gingival fibromatosis and hypertrichosis	Autosomal dominant
Gingival fibromatosis tetrad	Gingival fibromatosis, hypertrichosis, mental deficiency and/or epilepsy	Genetically heterogeneous with autosomal dominant and autosomal recessive types
Murray syndrome	Gingival fibromatosis; hyaline fibrous tumors of scalp, back and limbs; contractures at knees, hips, elbows and shoulders; thoracolumbar scoliosis; osteolysis of terminal phalanges; small cystic lesions of long bones; generalized osteoporosis	Autosomal recessive
Rutherfurd syndrome	Mild gingival enlargement, mental deficiency, aggressive behavior, corneal opacities, failure of tooth eruption, root resorption, dentigerous cysts	Autosomal dominant
Laband syndrome	Gingival fibromatosis, hypoplastic or absent nails and terminal phalanges, joint hypermobility, hepatosplenomegaly, mild hirsutism, soft cartilage of nose and ears	Autosomal dominant
Cross syndrome	Gingival fibromatosis, microphthalmia, cloudy corneae, hypopigmented skin, mental deficiency, athetosis	?Autosomal recessive
Jones syndrome	Gingival fibromatosis, sensorineural deafness	
Byars-Jurkiewicz syndrome	Gingival fibromatosis, hypertrichosis, giant fibroadenomas of breast	?

drome, and the Ward syndrome. The *basal cell nevus syndrome* and *nevoid basal cell carcinoma syndrome* are the most commonly used names in the United States. However, only half of all affected adults reported actually have basal cell carcinomas. Furthermore, there is probably a strong ascertainment bias favoring syndrome patients who do manifest skin tumors. Thus these designations are singularly inappropriate. On the other hand, the condition is known throughout Europe as the Gorlin syndrome because of his many contributions to our understanding of the condition. In keeping with a recent international

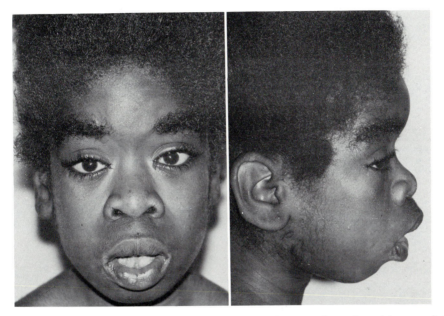

Fig. 17-82. Provisionally unique-pattern syndrome: hirsutism, prominent frontal bone, and deformed lips caused by gingival fibromatosis. (From Cohen, M. M., Jr., et al.: Syndrome Identification 2:12, 1974.)

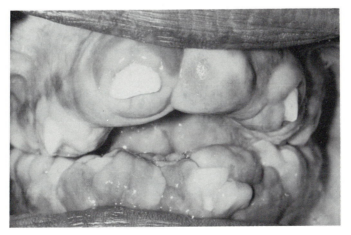

Fig. 17-83. Provisionally unique-pattern syndrome: severe gingival fibromatosis. (From Cohen, M. M., Jr., et al.: Syndrome Identification 2:12, 1974.)

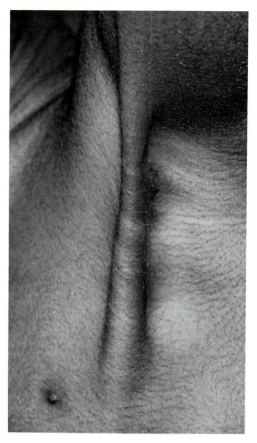

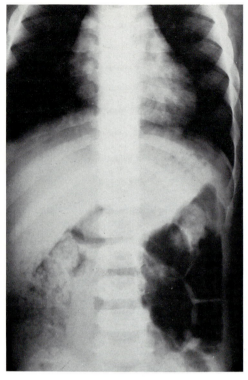

Fig. 17-85. Provisionally unique-pattern syndrome: note swollen ribs. (From Cohen, M. M., Jr., et al.: Syndrome Identification 2:12, 1974.)

Fig. 17-84. Provisionally unique-pattern syndrome: axillary pterygium. (From Cohen, M. M., Jr., et al.: Syndrome Identification 2:12, 1974.)

nomenclature meeting, I should like to propose that henceforth the condition be known universally as the Gorlin syndrome.

The disorder is a complex dysplasia/malformation syndrome with over a hundred different signs and symptoms primarily involving the skin, central nervous system, and skeletal system. An excellent historical review of the syndrome is provided by Gorlin and Sedano.[240] Gorlin has also provided several systematic surveys.[238, 239, 241, 242] Autosomal dominant inheritance with high penetrance and variable expressivity is characteristic. Many sporadic instances have been reported. These represent fresh mutations for the Gorlin syndrome. Preliminary evidence seems to indicate an increased paternal age effect in these cases.

Skin. In the Gorlin syndrome, basal cell carcinomas differ in several respects from the classic basal cell carcinoma. First, the lesions tend to be multiple rather than single. Second, they may occur on nonexposed as well as sun-exposed areas of the skin. Third, they tend to occur at an earlier age than the classic basal cell carcinoma. Fourth, the lesions are more commonly associated with an inflammatory infiltrate and have minute areas of calcification and/or metaplastic bone formation. Fifth, the biological behavior may differ slightly, since some lesions are quiescent for long periods of time before aggressive behavior ensues.

Histological study has revealed a wide spectrum of adnexal tumors, ranging from those with a benign trichoepitheliomatous appearance to frank, aggressive, ulcerating basal cell carcinomas. Solid basal cell carcinomas occur most frequently (Fig. 17-86),

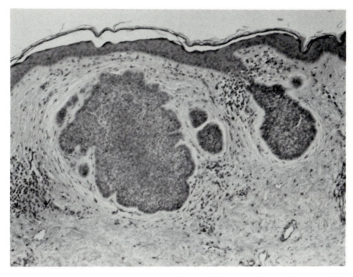

Fig. 17-86. Gorlin syndrome: histological section of basal cell carcinoma. Note peripheral palisading and "cracking-away" artifact.

but adenoid, cystic, morphea-like, and superficial basal cell carcinomas also occur.

As mentioned earlier, only half of reported adults with the Gorlin syndrome exhibit basal cell carcinomas. Approximately a third of the patients who have skin tumors exhibit two or more histological types. Lesions usually appear around puberty but may appear earlier or later and may persist for the entire lifetime of the patient. Only one, several, hundreds, or even thousands may appear. Metastases are rare but have been recorded.

Lesions are flesh-colored papules, nodules, or plaques. They may also be pigmented, and ulceration is frequently observed. The midface and especially the periorbital areas are commonly involved, but lesions also appear on the neck, chest, abdomen, back, and upper arms. Rarely, a basal cell carcinoma arises at the base of a palmar pit.

It has been shown that malignant transformation of cells in vitro with acetylaminofluorene occurs at a faster rate in cells from patients with the Gorlin syndrome than in cells from normal individuals. This test, known as the Elejalde test, needs confirmation. It may possibly be useful as a diagnostic aid in suspected sporadic instances of the dis-

order, in which basal cell carcinomas and/or jaw cysts have not yet developed.

Skin cysts are observed in some patients. They may be minute milia involving the face but are more commonly found on the limbs. Comedones have been noted in some. Occasional skin findings include café-au-lait pigmentation and hirsutism.

Parakeratosis on the palmar and plantar surfaces of the hands and feet (Fig. 17-87) may be observed in some instances after adolescence. The tiny pits represent focal failure in maturation of the basal cell layer.

Craniofacial complex. The facial appearance may be striking in some cases with enlarged head circumference (Fig. 17-88), frontal and biparietal bossing, ocular hypertelorism or dystopia canthorum, prominent supraorbital ridges with sunken eyes, and mild mandibular prognathism. These features have become stereotyped through the years. However, it is important to note that many patients lack mandibular prognathism. The most common features seem to be enlarged head circumference and ocular hypertelorism or dystopia canthorum.

Several patients have been noted to have mildly slanted auricles, although this feature has frequently been overlooked. Cleft lip

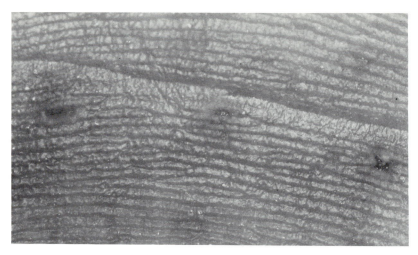

Fig. 17-87. Gorlin syndrome: palmar pits.

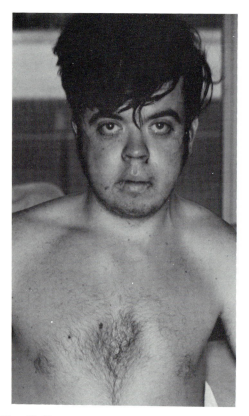

Fig. 17-88. Gorlin syndrome. Note macrocephaly, ocular hypertelorism, and pectus excavatum.

and/or palate has been a feature in at least nine reported cases. Other occasionally noted abnormalities include strabismus, congenital blindness due to corneal opacity, colobomas of the choroid and optic nerve, and chalazion.

Keratocysts are a common feature; 80% occur in the mandible, especially the third molar region, and 20% occur in the maxilla (Fig. 17-89). They may develop during the first decade of life but are more frequent during adolescence and thereafter. Symptoms may include swelling of the jaws, dull pain, or drainage of the cyst intraorally. If a cyst develops during the formation of a tooth root, dilaceration occurs. As cysts enlarge, adjacent teeth may be displaced. Keratocysts are aggressive, and recurrences after curettage are common, being seen in 40% of the cases. Cysts are frequently associated with unerupted teeth, the stated incidence being approximately 40%.

Histological evaluation of cysts (Fig. 17-90) shows a regular, continuous lining of stratified squamous epithelium, usually six to eight cells thick. The basal cells are somewhat columnar, often showing features suggestive of reversed polarity. Parakeratosis is commonly observed. Keratin is sometimes found sloughed into the cyst cavity (Fig. 17-90), but orthokeratinization is usually not found in the cyst lining itself. The connec-

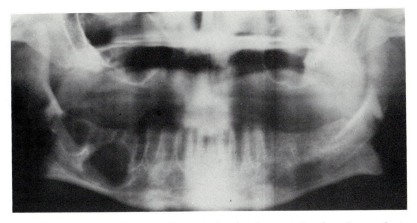

Fig. 17-89. Gorlin syndrome: radiograph showing jaw cysts in edentulous patient.

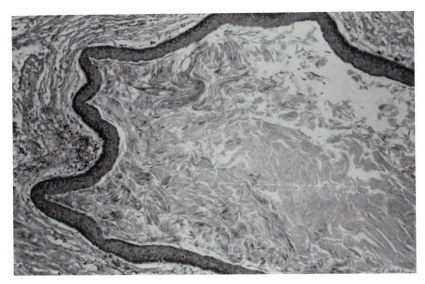

Fig. 17-90. Gorlin syndrome: histological section of keratocyst. Note sloughed keratin in cyst cavity.

tive tissue capsule tends to be freer of inflammatory cell infiltrates and cholesterol clefts than other types of jaw cysts. The presence of ciliated and mucous secreting cells, which arise by metaplasia, is also uncommon in keratocysts.

About 70% of cysts associated with an unerupted tooth are not true dentigerous cysts when examined histologically. Usually a layer of fibrous tissue separates the crown from the adjacent cyst cavity. Some of the larger keratocysts expand in size to include tooth follicles.

The continuous parakeratinized epithelial lining acts as a more efficient semipermeable membrance than the epithelium of other odontogenic cysts. Hence the osmolality, rate of growth, and aggressiveness are greater in keratocysts than in other odontogenic cysts.

The Stoelinga hypothesis is a particularly attractive explanation for the histogenesis of keratocysts in the Gorlin syndrome. When keratocysts and overlying epithelium are removed together, the cysts are adherent to the overlying soft tissue through a perforation in the bone. In most cysts removed in association with the overlying soft tissue, epithelial islands, cords, and microcysts are observed. Although sporadic islands and microcysts are found surrounding keratocysts, they are observed in large numbers consistently in the pathway between the overlying epithelium and the cyst itself. Occasionally a connection can be established between a microkeratocyst and the basal cell layer of the oral epithelium (Fig. 17-91).

The Stoelinga hypothesis states that jaw cysts in the Gorlin syndrome arise directly from the basal cell layer of the oral epithelium. The consistent observation of islands and microcysts between the bony keratocysts and the overlying surface epithelium supports this notion.

Corroborating evidence that suggests the soft tissue origin of keratocysts is provided by two reports of cyst formation within bone grafted from the iliac crest to the mandible.

If keratocysts arise from the oral epithe-

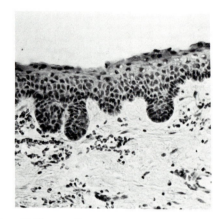

Fig. 17-92. Gorlin syndrome: keratocyst lining showing budding into connective tissue.

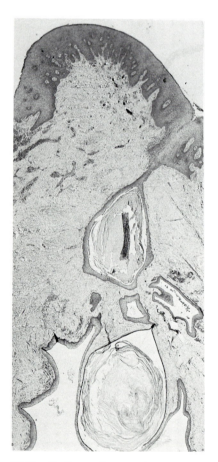

Fig. 17-91. Gorlin syndrome: histological section showing microkeratocyst arising from surface epithelium. Note other microkeratocysts below surface.

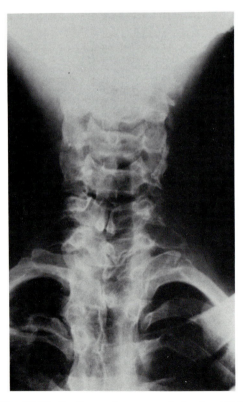

Fig. 17-93. Gorlin syndrome: cervical spina bifida occulta.

lium, how do they come to lie within bone? Resorption of bone caused by mechanical pressure is most likely a contributing factor only. Inductive bone resorption is probably the major factor.

Some keratocysts may arise directly from budding of the keratocyst lining itself (Fig. 17-92) or from odontogenic rests. Both are, of course, derivatives of the oral epithelium.

Skeletal system. The true incidence of skeletal anomalies (Figs. 17-93 to 17-95) is not known, since most of them are commonly asymptomatic, and radiographic surveys have not always been carried out in all reported families. Bifid ribs are a common feature, although splaying, synostosis, partial agenesis rudimentary cervical ribs, and pseudoarthroses have been described. Spina bifida occulta in the cervical or upper thoracic region, scoliosis, and cervical or upper thoracic vertebral fusions have been observed. The fourth and fifth metacarpals are commonly shortened. Also noted in some cases have been Wormian bones, platybasia, pectus excavatum, pectus carinatum, Sprengel deformity, medial hooking of the scapula, defective medial aspect of the clavicle, pes planus, hallux valgus, syndactyly, oligodactyly, polydactyly of the thumbs and halluces, extra hallucal fused terminal phalanges, short distal thumb phalanx, and supernumerary metatarsal. A Marfanoid habitus has been observed in several patients. Jaw cysts have been discussed above under craniofacial complex.

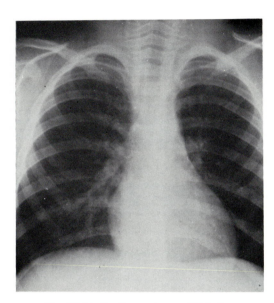

Fig. 17-94. Gorlin syndrome: bifid ribs.

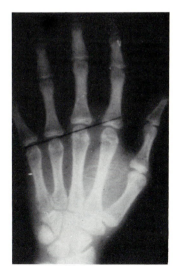

Fig. 17-95. Gorlin syndrome: short fourth metacarpal.

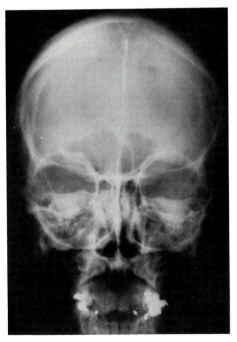

Fig. 17-96. Gorlin syndrome: calcification of falx cerebri.

Calcifications; calcium and phosphorus metabolism. Various calcifications have been described. Common are bridging of the sella turcica and calcifications of the falx cerebri, especially the lamellar type (Figs. 17-96 and 17-97). Involvement of the parietal dura and petroclinoid ligament has also been reported. Other calcifications have been noted in ovarian fibromas and cysts, lymphomesenteric cysts, and the uterus.

It has been suggested that shortened fourth metacarpals and calcifications in various parts of the body might indicate abnormal calcium and phosphorus metabolism. Using the Ellsworth-Howard test, an almost complete lack of end-organ responsiveness to parathormone has been noted. However, interpretation of the Ellsworth-Howard test is fraught with danger, since phosphaturia after the administration of parathormone can be minimal even in some normal individuals. Since calcemic and phosphaturic responses to parathormone are mediated by cyclic AMP, and since cyclic AMP is a more sensitive measure of responsiveness than phosphaturia, it follows that testing with cyclic AMP is preferable to the use of the Ellsworth-Howard test. On this basis, normal responsiveness to parathormone has been reported in patients with the Gorlin syndrome (Fig. 17-98).

Central nervous system. Mental deficiency is a variable feature. When present, it is usually mild in degree. Psychosis has also been reported. Congenital communicating hydrocephalus has been noted by several authors. Other low-frequency findings include sensorineural deafness, hyposmia, cysts of the choroid plexus, glial nodules, and partial agenesis of the corpus callosum.

Neoplasms. The commonly observed basal cell carcinomas have already been discussed. Various low-frequency neoplasms are also part of the Gorlin syndrome. Especially noteworthy is medulloblastoma, which has a dismal prognosis. The tumor spreads through the cerebrospinal fluid to the subarachnoid space and seeds intracranially or along the spinal cord. Since medulloblastoma occurs during the first few years of life in the Gorlin syndrome, the patient usually dies before the onset of many other manifestations of the syndrome.

Other tumors found with low frequency include meningioma, neurofibroma, fibroma, fibrosarcoma, leiomyoma, leiomyosarcoma,

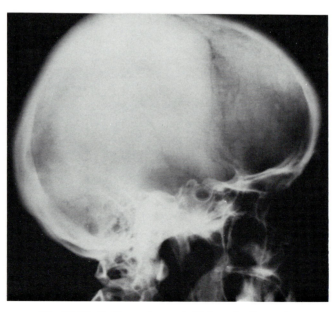

Fig. 17-97. Gorlin syndrome: bridging of sella turcica.

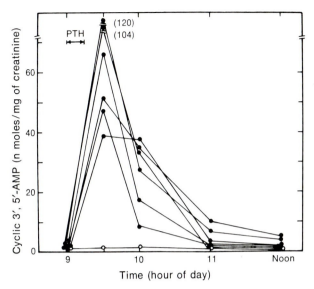

Fig. 17-98. Gorlin syndrome: effect of parathyroid hormone (PTH) on urinary excretion of $3^1,5^1$-AMP. PTH (200 to 300 units) was infused from 9 to 9:15 A.M. Results are plotted to coincide with end of each test period. Each set of closed circles represents patient with basal cell nevus syndrome. All are responsive to PTH. Open circles represent patient with pseudo-hypoparathyroidism, who is not responsive to PTH. (From Kaufman, R. L., and Chase, L. R.: Birth Defects 7[8]:149, 1971.)

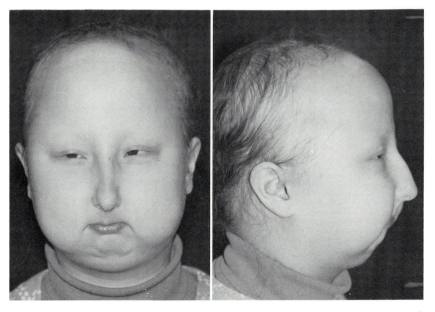

Fig. 17-99. Hallermann-Streiff syndrome: hypotrichosis, small palpebral fissures, beaked nose, and micrognathia.

embryonal rhabdomyosarcoma, "carcinoma," thecal cell tumor, adrenal cortical adenoma, ameloblastoma, craniopharyngioma, and odontogenic myxoma.

Other findings. A variety of other findings have been reported, including renal malformations, bicornuate uterus, female escutcheon with scanty facial hair and gynecomastia in males, cryptorchidism, absent testis, inguinal hernia, and amenorrhea.[294-431]

Hallermann-Streiff syndrome

The Hallermann-Streiff syndrome consists of dyscephaly, beaked nose, mandibular hypoplasia, hypotrichosis, and blue scleras (Fig. 17-99). Virtually all cases have been sporadic. There is no sex predilection. The syndrome has been described as concordant and discordant in identical twins, and an affected female has had two normal children. Although the disorder has been described in a father and daughter, these cases are probably not examples of the syndrome.

Narrow upper air passages may cause feeding problems during infancy. Pneumonia and/or severe feeding difficulties have led to the death of the infant in several instances.

Body growth is diminished proportionately, being at least 2 to 5 S.D. below the mean. Adult height for women is about 152.4 cm (5 feet), with men about 2.5 to 5 cm taller.

Craniofacial complex. The face is small, with a long, thin, tapering, beaklike nose, receding chin, and an odd-shaped, often bulging skull. Brachycephaly is often accompanied by bossing, especially of the frontal or parietal areas. Mild microcephaly and malar bone hypoplasia also occur but are not constant features. Gaping or dehiscence of the sagittal and lambdoidal sutures, as well as delayed closure of fontanels, has been described by nearly all authors.

Microphthalmia of variable severity and bilateral congenital cataract are virtually constant features. The cataracts are rather unusual, since they often spontaneously resorb. Secondary glaucoma may occur. Blue scleras have been described in about 15% to 25% of cases, as well as posterior synechiae

and prepupillary membrane. Because of diminished vision, most patients have nystagmus and/or strabismus.

The nose is thin, pointed, and often curved. Several authors have remarked on the tendency to septal deviation.

Micrognathia is often accompanied by a double chin with a central cleft or dimple. The ascending ramus is usually short, and the condyle may be missing or the glenoid fossa hypoplastic. The temporomandibular joint is displaced approximately 2 cm forward. The palate is high and narrow, and the paranasal sinuses are small.

Absence of teeth, persistence of deciduous teeth, malocclusion, malformation of teeth, and severe dental caries have been reported. Supernumerary teeth have been seen as well as natal teeth.

Skin and skin appendages. Hypotrichosis, especially of the scalp, brows, and cilia, has been a frequent feature. Axillary and pubic hair may also be scant. Alopecia is most prominent about the frontal and occipital areas but is especially marked along suture lines.

Cutaneous atrophy is largely limited to the scalp and nose. The skin is thin and taut, and the scalp veins are prominent.

Mental status. Mental deficiency has been noted in about 15% of the cases.

Other findings. Skeletal anomalies are infrequent and have included osteoporosis, syndactyly, lordosis and/or scoliosis, and spina bifida. The scapulas are commonly winglike. Hypogenitalism has also been reported.[432-444]

de Lange syndrome

The syndrome of primordial growth deficiency, severe mental retardation, anomalies of the extremities, and characteristic facies was independently described by Brachmann[448] in 1916 and by de Lange[450] in 1933. Excellent reviews are those of Ptacek and associates[458] and Berg and co-workers.[447] At least 250 examples have been reported.

Most cases have been sporadic. The frequency of affected sibs among reported cases is between 2% and 5%. There has been no increased rate of parental consanguinity. In a few cases, various inconsistent chromosomal abnormalities have been noted. The disorder has been observed in identical twins.

Birth weight is usually less than 2500 gm, and both height and weight remain below the third percentile for age. There are often recurrent respiratory tract infections and gastrointestinal upsets. Sucking and swallowing ability are diminished. In most cases, the intelligence quotient has been below 50. Seizures have been observed in about 20% of the cases. Speech maturation is especially retarded. Most patients die before the age of 6 years.

Craniofacial complex. The skull is micro-brachycephalic. The eyebrows are confluent (synophrys), the eyelashes are long and curly, and the hairline is low. The nose is small with a flat bridge. The nostrils are anteverted, and there is a long philtrum. A bluish hue is often noted about the eyes, nose, and mouth. The temporal and scalp veins may be prominent. The typical facies may not be evident during the first year of life (Fig. 17-100).

Micrognathia and a prominent mental spur are characteristically present. The lips are thin, with the corners of the mouth downturned. Delayed tooth eruption has been reported, and several authors have remarked on the smallness of the teeth, although no measurements have been published to date.

Central nervous system. Mental deficiency has been a feature of all cases. The cry is usually low-pitched and growling. Oral self-mutilation has been described.

Musculoskeletal alterations. In about 35% of cases there is initial hypertonia. Generally, the hands and feet are small. The fingers are often short and tapering, with clinodactylous fifth digits, which have only a single flexion crease. The thumbs are proximally placed. About 15% to 20% of the patients exhibit oligodactyly or more severe reducing defects of the upper limbs (Fig. 17-101). Flexion contractures of the elbow are present in at least 80% of cases. Soft-tissue syndactyly of the second and third toes is an almost constant feature.

Radiographic examination shows the skull to be small, with the dorsum sella enlarged. Bone age is delayed, and there is often discrepancy in the sequence of development of

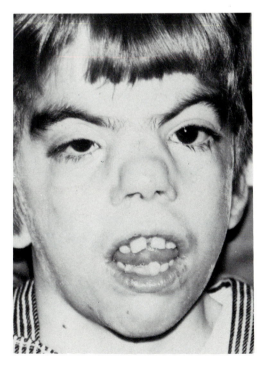

Fig. 17-100. de Lange syndrome: characteristic facial features.

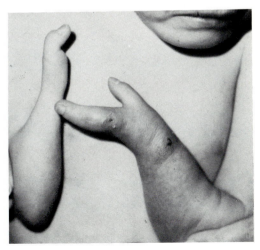

Fig. 17-101. de Lange syndrome: reduction defects of upper limbs.

various centers of ossification. The humerus, radius, and ulna are shortened. Hypoplasia and dorsal dislocation of the radial head are noted. Often the neck of the humerus is elongated. In some cases, the forearm bones are absent. The first metacarpal and middle phalanx of the fifth finger are frequently hypoplastic. The acetabular angle is low, especially when the child is less than a year of age. The sternum is short with a reduced number of ossification centers, and the ribs are rather thin.

Skin. Hirsutism is often generalized, but is especially marked by low hairline, synophrys, long and curly eyelashes, and hair whorls over the shoulders, lower back, and extremities (Fig. 17-102). The nipples and umbilicus are frequently hypoplastic. Cutis marmorata is present in at least 50% of patients.

Dermatoglyphic findings include hypoplastic ridge patterns, simian creases, and increased "atd" palmar angle. There is also an increase in radial loops on the third and fourth fingertips and a palmar interdigital triradius.

Genitourinary system. The kidneys are often hypoplastic, dysplastic, or cystic. The testes are undescended in over 70% of males, and in some, there is hypospadias. Female

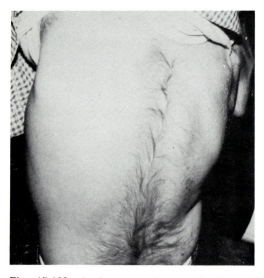

Fig. 17-102. de Lange syndrome: hirsutism of back.

patients commonly have bicornuate or septate uterus and long, narrow ovaries.

Other findings. Malrotation of the intestine and various congenital heart defects have been described. A variety of miscellaneous findings have been reported.[445-465]

Marfan syndrome

The main features of the Marfan syndrome include disproportionate skeletal growth with dolichostenomelia and arachnodactyly (Fig. 17-103), ectopia lentis, and fusiform and dissecting aneurysms of the aorta. Although it has been suggested that Marfan's original patient had cystathionine synthase deficiency (homocystinuria), a more convincing argument has been made for congenital contractural arachnodactyly.

The disorder has autosomal dominant inheritance with a high degree of penetrance and variable expressivity. Roughly 85% of the cases are familial, the rest arising as fresh mutations. Advanced paternal age at time of conception is associated with isolated cases. The prevalence of the Marfan syndrome is at least 1.5 per 100,000 in the general population, with both sexes being equally affected.

The syndrome is thought to result from a structural defect in protein, particularly the elastic fiber. Collagen production is disturbed at the cellular level, and an increase in the ratio of soluble to insoluble collagen has been reported.

Craniofacial complex. Dolichocephaly usually occurs with prominent supraorbital ridges. Frontal bossing is common, and the eyes often appear sunken, giving the patient a wizened appearance.

Eyes. Eye changes seem to be more common in males. Iridodonesis may occur as an early sign of lens dislocation. Ectopia lentis, resulting from weakened or broken suspensory ligaments, is present bilaterally in at least 70% of patients. The dislocated lenses are displaced superiorly, superonasally, or superotemporally in about 70% of the cases. There are alterations in the chamber angle, ciliary body, and pupil. Increased transillumination of the iris diaphragm has been noted. Megalocornea, blue scleras, microphakia, sphero-

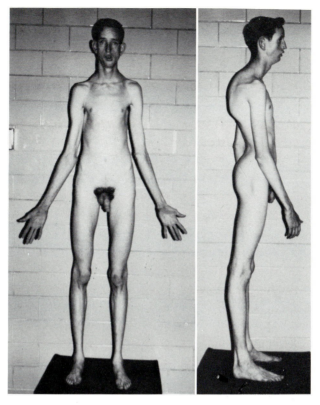

Fig. 17-103. Marfan syndrome: disproportionate skeletal pattern with dolichostenomelia and arachnodactyly.

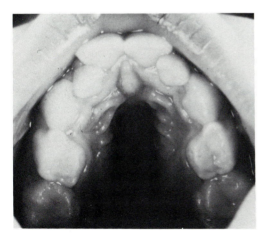

Fig. 17-104. Marfan syndrome: highly arched, narrow palate.

phakia, and retinal detachment may be observed. Myopia is common.

Although earlier authors estimated the prevalence of high palatal vault to be between 15% and 40%, some have observed this condition in all their patients (Fig. 17-104). Cleft palate or bifid uvula has been noted in several instances.

The teeth have been noted to be long and narrow and frequently maloccluded. Mandibular prognathism is common. Radiographically, the maxillary sinuses may be enlarged.

Musculoskeletal system. Dolichostenomelia and arachnodactyly are common features, with the halluces disproportionately elongated. Hallux valgus and hammer toe are frequent.

The lower segment (pubis to sole) is greater than the upper segment (vertex to pubis). The US/LS ratio in the Marfan syndrome averages 0.85, in comparison with the average normal Caucasian value of 0.93. Pectus excavatum and carinatum, late-developing kyphoscoliosis, elongated patellar ligament, spina bifida, and weakness of joint capsules manifested by pes planus and hyperextensibility of joints with habitual dislocation (hips, patella, clavicle) are commonly observed. Enlarged vertebrae and widened spinal cord have also been noted. Inguinal or femoral hernia is frequent.

Cardiovascular system. Diffuse, generally progressive dilatation of the ascending aorta with or without dissecting aneurysm may occur and may be a common cause of sudden death in affected individuals even in early adulthood. These changes are preceded by aortic regurgitation and floppy mitral valve with mitral regurgitation in at least 65% of patients. Aneurysms of the thoracic or abdominal aorta or pulmonary artery are less common. An angina-like chest pain is common. Aortic coarctation has also been noted with increased frequency. Alterations of the renal artery leading to severe hypertension have been reported. Microscopically, medial necrosis and intimal thickening of blood vessels have been observed. Occasionally, pulmonary malformations may increase susceptibility to infection in the lower part of the respiratory tract and lead to emphysema.

Abnormal bleeding tendency with easy bruising has been observed. Defective giant platelets and an increased number of immature granulocytes have been reported in the peripheral blood.

Skin. Deficiency of subcutaneous fat and striae distensae have been noted. Miescher's elastoma, especially on the neck, has been noted with increased frequency.[466-488]

Mucopolysaccharidoses

The mucopolysaccharidoses are inherited disorders of mucopolysaccharide metabolism. Defective activity of various genetically controlled pathways of lysosomal degradation leads to intracellular storage of undegraded acid mucopolysaccharides and to a relatively uniform clinical and skeletal phenotype. This phenotype is most pronounced in the Hurler and the Maroteaux-Lamy syndromes and is less severe in other mucopolysaccharidoses.

A classification of the various mucopolysaccharidoses (types I-VII) is presented in Table 17-20. With the exception of the Hunter syndrome, which has X-linked recessive inheritance, the other mucopolysaccharidoses have autosomal recessive inheritance. In this section, only the Hurler and the Morquio syndromes are considered in detail. All are presented in synoptic form in Table 17-20, however. In addition, the oral manifestations of the various mucopolysaccharidoses are summarized in Table 17-21.

Hurler syndrome (MPS I H). The Hurler syndrome is characterized by growth failure after infancy, marked mental deficiency, characteristic craniofacial appearance and body habitus (Fig. 17-105), dysostosis multiplex, corneal clouding, intracellular storage of acid mucopolysaccharides, and excessive urinary excretion of acid mucopolysaccharides.

In the first months of life there are a few relatively nonspecific findings, such as hernias, macrocephaly, limited hip abduction, and recurrent respiratory infections. The full clinical picture usually develops in the second year of life. Death usually occurs before 10 years of age from pneumonia and cardiac failure.

The frequency of mucopolysaccharidosis I H is approximately 1 in 100,000 births. The basic biochemical defect is absence of α-L-iduronidase activity, which inhibits intralysosomal degradation of α-L-iduronide–containing mucopolysaccharides. Intracellular accumulation of undegraded or partially degraded AMPS interferes with normal function of the affected cells and leads to the characteristic clinical symptoms.

Craniofacial complex. Slight coarsening of facial features at 3 to 6 months of age is usually the first abnormality noted. The head is large, and the frontal bones bulge. Premature closure of the sagittal and metopic sutures and hyperostosis frequently lead to scaphocephaly. Synophrys is commonly present. The nasal bridge is depressed, the tip of the nose is broad, and the nostrils are wide

Table 17-20. The mucopolysaccharidoses

Syndrome designation		Clinical deformity	Skeletal dysplasia	Corneal opacity	Mental deficiency	Excessive urinary acid mucopolysaccharide excretion	Enzymatic defect	Mode of inheritance
Numeral	Eponym							
I H	Hurler syndrome	Severe	Severe	Yes	Yes	Dermatan sulfate, heparan sulfate	α-L-iduronidase	Autosomal recessive
I S	Scheie syndrome	Mild	Mild	Yes	No	Dermatan sulfate, heparan sulfate	α-L-iduronidase	Autosomal recessive
II A	Hunter syndrome A	Late, moderate	Moderate	No	No	Heparan sulfate, dermatan sulfate	Sulfoiduronate sulfatase	X-linked recessive
II B	Hunter syndrome B	Early, moderate	Moderate	No	Yes	Dermatan sulfate, heparan sulfate	Sulfoiduronate sulfatase	X-linked recessive
III A	Sanfilippo syndrome A	Mild	Minimal	No	Yes	Heparan sulfate	Herparan sulfate-N-sulfatase	Autosomal recessive
III B	Sanfilippo syndrome B	Mild	Minimal	No	Yes	Heparan sulfate	N-acetyl-α-gluco-saminidase	Autosomal recessive
IV	Morquio syndrome	Severe	Severe	Yes	No	Keratan sulfate	Chondroitin-6-sulfate-n-acetyl-hexosamine sulfate sulfatase	Autosomal recessive
VI A	Maroteaux-Lamy syndrome A	Mild to moderate	Moderate	Yes	No	Dermatan sulfate	Aryl sulfatase B	Autosomal recessive
VI B	Maroteaux-Lamy syndrome B	Severe	Severe	Yes	Mild	Dermatan sulfate	Aryl sulfatase B	Autosomal recessive
VII	None	None	None	None	Late	?Chondroitin-4-sulfate	β-glucuronidase	Autosomal recessive

Table 17-21. Oral manifestations of the mucopolysaccharidoses

	Mucopolysaccharidosis	*Oral manifestations*
I H	Hurler syndrome	Macroglossia, widely spaced teeth, hyperplastic alveolar ridges, retarded dental eruption, frequent distoangular positioning of molar teeth, especially in mandibles, bony radiolucent defects thought to represent pooling of dermatan sulfate in hyperplastic dental follicles
I S	Scheie syndrome	None
II A	Hunter syndrome A	Macroglossia, widely spaced teeth
II B	Hunter syndrome B	Macroglossia, widely spaced teeth, bony radiolucent defects thought to represent pooling of dermatan sulfate in hyperplastic dental follicles
III A	Sanfilippo syndrome A	None
III B	Sanfilippo syndrome B	None
IV	Morquio syndrome	Dull, gray teeth with thin, pitted enamel that flakes off, leaving diastemas, frequent dental caries
VI A	Maroteaux-Lamy syndrome A	Macroglossia, widely spaced teeth, retarded eruption of permanent molars (some may be deeply buried and angulated in mandible), bony radiolucent defects thought to represent pooling of dermatan sulfate in hyperpalstic dental follicles
VI B	Maroteaux-Lamy syndrome B	
VII	β-Glucuronidase deficiency	Widened alveolar ridges

and anteverted. The interpupillary distance is greater than normal. Corneal clouding appears during the third year of life, rarely earlier. The lower eyelids and nasolabial folds are prominent, and the cheeks are full. The earlobes are thick. The lips are enlarged and patulous, and the mouth is usually held open with protruding tongue, especially after the age of 3 years. Chronic nasal discharge is usually marked even between the frequent bouts of upper respiratory infection. Nasal congestion with labored breathing through the mouth is severe, being related to hyperplastic adenoid tissue and a deep cranial fossa that narrows the airway between the sphenoid bone and the hard palate. Gag and swallowing reflexes become progressively diminished.

The teeth are widely spaced, often exhibiting severe attrition. The incisors may exhibit conical crown form to some extent. Because of macroglossia, there may be anterior open bite. Eruption is probably delayed in at least half the patients, especially in areas of bone destruction. The second primary molars or

first and second permanent molars are often distoangularly positioned, with the distal surface of the crown being situated more deeply than the mesial. In some cases, there is dilaceration of the distal roots. These changes occur more frequently in the mandible.

Extremely common are localized areas of bone destruction, which have been designated as *dentigerous cysts*. These are often present by 3 years of age and more often involve the second primary molar and first and second permanent mandibular molars. The margins of the radiolucencies are usually smooth and clearly defined. These seem to represent pooling of dermatan sulfate in hyperplastic dental follicles, since they also occur in MPS VI but not in MPS III.

The alveolar ridges are nearly always hyperplastic. Some patients exhibit hyperplastic gingivitis because of poor oral hygiene and mouth breathing.

The mandible is short and broad, with wide bigonial distance. The rami are short and narrow, and the condyle is replaced by a

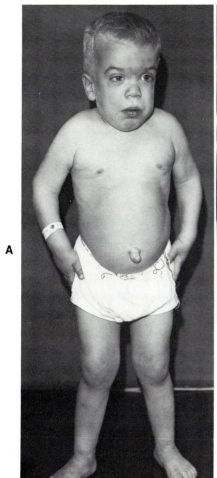

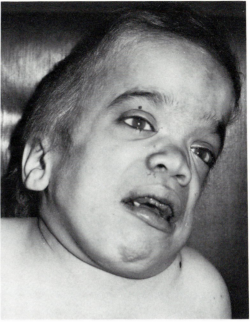

Fig. 17-105. A, Hurler syndrome in 10-year-old patient. Note coarse facial features and umbilical hernia. **B,** Same patient at 18 years of age. Note progressive coarsening of facial features, corneal clouding, and open mouth with hyperplastic maxillary gingiva. (Courtesy J. M. Opitz, Madison, Wis.)

flat, inclined surface or cup-shaped excavation. The mandibular notch is irregular or cleft. The temporomandibular joint may exhibit limited motion.

Musculoskeletal system. Length at birth is not decreased below the norm. Most patients are at or above the eighty-seventh percentile for length. Growth ceases before 3 years of age. By 3 years of age, all patients are below the third percentile for height. The neck is short. Both pectus carinatum and pectus excavatum occur, and usually there is lumbodorsal kyphosis or gibbus. Range of motion is limited in the joints, resulting in a clawhand deformity.

Radiographically, in infancy, bone trabeculation is seen to be coarse. In late infancy and early childhood, a pattern of skeletal changes called *dysostosis multiplex* emerges: the skull becomes large and deformed; the sphenoidal plane is depressed; and the sella is J-shaped, possibly from arachnoid cysts. The sagittal and lamboidal sutures close prematurely. The cranial base and orbital roofs are especially thick and dense. The orbits are shallow. Communicating hydrocephalus is often present. The ribs are wide in their lateral and ventral portions, with overconstriction at their paravertebral ends. The vertebral bodies are dysplastic, with biconvex end plates and hook-shaped, configuration of the lower thoracic and upper lumbar bodies after 12 to 18 months of age. The basilar portions of the ilia are underdeveloped, with flaring of the iliac wings. The long tubular bones show marked diaphyseal widening and distortion, with small and deformed epiphyses. The shafts of the short tubular bones are underconstricted, with bullet-shaped phalanges and proximal pointing of the second to fifth metacarpals.

The abdomen protrudes because of hepatic and splenic enlargement, deformity of the chest, shortness of the spine, and laxity of the abdominal wall. These changes are noted during the second year of life. Hepatomegaly may be detected as early as 6 to 12 months of age.

Inguinal hernia, present at birth or developing within the first 3 months of life, is a constant feature in boys. Umbilical hernias, usually small at birth in both sexes, gradually reach major proportions. Rarely, intraabdominal complications occur.

Other findings. The skin is pale, coarse, and dry. It is covered by fine, lanugo-like hair, particularly on the back and extremities. Mental deficiency is progressive. Moderate cardiomegaly, due to deposition of acid mucopolysaccharides in the myocardium and valves, is usually present.

Morquio syndrome. Marked growth failure, progressive spinal deformity, short neck, pectus carinatum, and other skeletal anomalies such as genua valga and pes planus (Fig. 17-106) characterize the Morquio syndrome. The disorder has autosomal recessive inheritance. Its frequency has been estimated to be about 1 per 40,000 births. The basic defect is a deficiency of chondroitin-6-sulfate N-acetyl-glucosamine-4-sulfate sulfatase.

Craniofacial complex. The facies is not specific, but the lower half of the face is often striking because of shortness and hyperextension of the neck.

The corneas become slowly but diffusely opacified as a filmy haze. This is rarely obvious to the unaided eye before the tenth year of life.

Intelligence is nearly always normal. Progressive deafness usually begins during adolescence.

Both the deciduous and permanent teeth have dull, gray crowns with thin, pitted

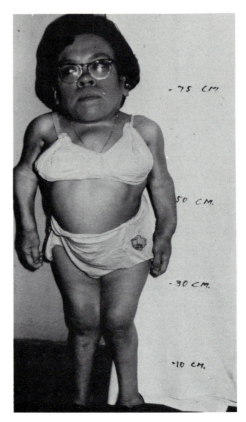

Fig. 17-106. Morquio syndrome: disproportionate short stature, short neck, and genua valga. (Courtesy L. O. Langer, Jr., Minneapolis, Minn.)

enamel (Fig. 17-107), which has a tendency to flake off, causing small diastemas between the teeth. The cusps are small, flattened, and poorly formed, and caries is frequent. The mandibular condyles may be flat or concave.

Musculoskeletal system. Birth length is normal, but by 2 years of age, growth is stunted. There is reduced height because of shortening of the neck and trunk and, to a lesser extent, the extremities. Adult height rarely exceeds 100 cm (range 80 to 120 cm). The head is essentially normal, but mild scaphocephaly may be present because of premature closure of sutures. The head seems to rest directly on the shoulders. The neck is greatly shortened, with exaggerated cervical curvature and restricted movement. The thorax, after the second year of life, exhibits marked kyphosis or kyphoscoliosis, with gen-

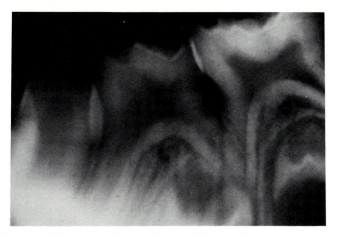

Fig. 17-107. Morquio syndrome: dental radiograph showing thin enamel.

eral flattening of vertebras and a character-istic pectus carinatum, the sternum extend-ing almost horizontally from its clavicular junction, then angling downward in mid-section. The lumbar region of the spine fre-quently exhibits a gibbus-like kyphosis or, less often, lordosis in the region of the first lum-bar vertebra. Spinal cord compression may result in death. It may occur in the upper cervical segment as a complication from either atlantoaxial dislocation or subluxation at the thoracolumbar gibbus.

Extremities appear disproportionately long. There may be excessive joint mobility, and the wrists are usually enlarged. Genua valga, thickened knee joints, and pes planus are nearly constant findings. The stance is semi-crouched. Usually there is a prominent abdomen.

Radiographically, generalized platyspondyly occurs with hypolasia of the last thoracic and first lumbar vertebrae, coxa valga, flared ilia, and progressive flattening and fragmentation of the femoral head. In the young child, the vertebral bodies are ovoid, and the superior acetabula are poorly ossified. The odontoid process is hypoplastic or absent. The bases of the second to fifth metacarpals are conical, but their shafts are normally constricted. The distal ends of the radius and ulna are in-clined toward each other. All the bones be-come markedly osteoporotic.

Other findings. Aortic regurgitation has been reported.[489, 490]

Neurofibromatosis

The syndrome of multiple neurofibromas, cutaneous pigmentation, skeletal anomalies, central nervous system involvement, and pre-dilection to malignancy was classically pre-sented by von Recklinghausen[534] in 1882, al-though it was described earlier by several other authors.

The syndrome follows an autosomal domi-nant mode of transmission, with approxi-mately 50% of the cases representing fresh mutations. The mutation rate has been cal-culated to be 10^{-4} per gamete per generation, the highest rate known in man. Neurofi-bromatosis appears with a frequency of one case per 2500 to 3300 births in the general population and occurs approximately once in 200 mental defectives.

It is incorrect to categorize the disorder as a neurocutaneous syndrome because not all defects are attributable to neural crest de-rivatives. For example, certain bony altera-tions occur in the absence of tumors from the region, thus implicating mesenchymal deriva-tives.

The syndrome has protean manifestations. The complexity of the clinical spectrum is compounded by the fact that the disorder may evolve slowly and may present in a variety of ways. Over 40% of patients have manifestations at birth and over 60% by the second year of life. Incomplete forms are common and may go unrecognized. A sporadic case without neurofibromas and without the requisite number of café-au-lait spots can present great difficulty in diagnosis during childhood.

Tumors. The most distinctive and common skin tumor is the neurofibroma (Fig. 17-108), especially the plexiform variety. Tumors may be present at birth or appear during childhood or even later. They vary greatly in size, with localized enlargement of many nerve trunks in larger neurofibromas. They are most striking on the skin, with some patients manifesting hundreds or even thousands of individual neurofibromas and others having unilateral pendulous masses. Many organs may be involved, including stomach,

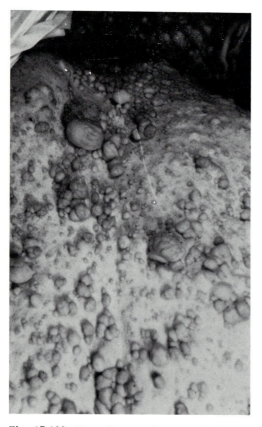

Fig. 17-108. Neurofibromatosis: multiple skin tumors of back.

intestine, kidney, bladder, larynx, and heart. Neurofibrosarcomatous transformation has been reported in 3% to 12% of cases.

Schwannomas and fibromas are also known to occur. Meningiomas, neuromas of the cranial nerves (especially optic and acoustic) and spinal nerves, and gliomas (astrocytomas and ependymomas) have been reported. The incidence of pheochromocytoma is increased. Various other low-frequency tumors, both malignant and benign, may occur.

Skin. In addition to nodular tumors of the skin, café-au-lait spots (Fig. 17-109) are common, appearing in 90% of patients. The smooth-edged pigmented spots usually appear during the first decade, most often preceding the tumors. The color varies from yellowish to chocolate-brown. Lesions are observed especially on the unexposed areas of the body. The presence of six or more café-au-lait spots greater than 1.5 cm in diameter should arouse a strong suspicion of neurofibromatosis. Axillary freckling (Fig. 17-110) is present in approximately a third of the cases. Pigmented hairy nevi may also be observed.

Central nervous system. Mental deficiency is usually absent, but retardation may occur, the stated incidence varying from 8% to 50%. Seizures frequently accompany the syndrome. Hydrocephalus has been noted in some cases.

In addition to neuromas, gliomas, and meningiomas, distortion of cortical architecture from glial proliferation and neuronal heterotopias deep in the cerebral white matter have been reported.

Craniofacial complex. Any part of the eye may be involved. Neurofibromas of the eyelids have been observed in some cases. Intraorbital lesions may produce proptosis and muscle palsies. Phakoma, congenital glaucoma, fibroma of the iris, corneal opacity, detached retina, and optic atrophy have been noted.

Oral involvement is not common, the incidence probably lying between 4% and 7%. Tumors may involve any oral soft tissue, although there is some predilection for the tongue (Fig. 17-111).

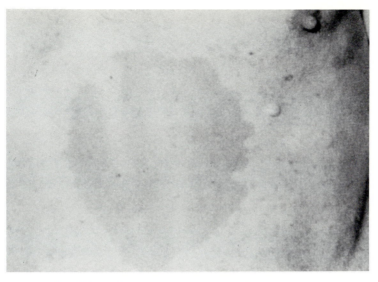

Fig. 17-109. Neurofibromatosis: café-au-lait spot on chest.

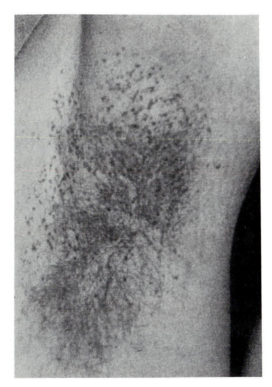

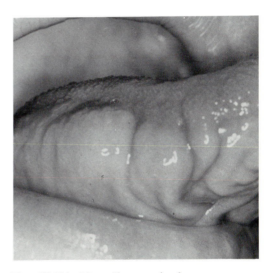

Fig. 17-111. Neurofibromatosis: large tumor on lateral border of tongue.

Fig. 17-110. Neurofibromatosis: axillary freckling.

Skeletal system. Commonly observed are subperiosteal erosive changes caused by pressure from proliferating neurofibromatous tissue in the periosteum and overlying soft parts. Central so-called cystic lesions of bone result from expansive growth of neurofibromas within the medullary cavity in some cases. In other cases, no cause for central lesions can be found.

Kyphoscoliosis and pseudoarthroses (especially with bowing of the tibia and fibula) are also common. Bony defects of the skull, especially of the posterosuperior orbital wall, have been reported. Overgrowth of cranial bones, craniofacial asymmetry, and macrocephaly have been noted. A variety of other anomalies may be observed, including hemihypertrophy of a limb or digit, spina bifida, absent patella, elevated scapulae, congenital dislocations (especially of the hip, radius, and ulna) clubfoot, syndactyly, and complete or partial absence of limb bones.

Endocrine system. Pheochromocytoma is the most common endocrine lesion in adult patients. Of patients with pheochromocytoma, 5% have neurofibromatosis. In childhood, the most common endocrine abnormality is sexual precocity. Other findings have included hypopituitarism, hypogonadism, gigantism, acromegaly, delayed sexual development, obesity, hypoglycemia, diabetes insipidus, goiter, myxedema, and hyperparathyroidism.

Cardiovascular system. Although this fact is not often appreciated, cardiovascular anomalies may occur in low frequency, including pulmonic valvular stenosis, supravalvular aortic stenosis, coarctation of the aorta, atrial septal defect, congenital heart block, stenotic renal arteries, and other defects.[491-538]

Oculodentoosseous dysplasia

Oculodentoosseous dysplasia consists of narrow nose with hypoplastic alae and thin nostrils, microcornea with iris anomalies, syndactyly and camptodactyly of the fourth and fifth fingers, certain bony anomalies of the middle phalanx of the fifth finger and toes, and enamel hypoplasia, resembling amelogenesis imperfecta (Fig. 17-112). The disorder follows an autosomal dominant mode of transmission.

Craniofacial complex. Ocular hypertelorism, epicanthal folds, and thin nose with absent alar flare produce a characteristic physiognomy. Head circumference may be somewhat reduced (Fig. 17-113).

Eye defects consist of microcornea (6 to 10 mm in diameter), iris anomalies, and, in some cases, secondary glaucoma and small

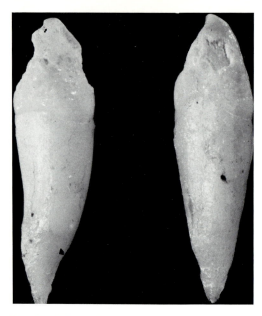

Fig. 17-112. Oculodentoosseous dysplasia: enamel hypoplasia. (From Gorlin, R. J., et al.: J. Pediatr. **63:**69, 1963.)

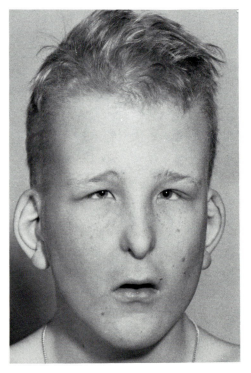

Fig. 17-113. Oculodentoosseous dysplasia: hypoplastic alae and small palpebral fissures. (From Gorlin, R. J., et al.: J. Pediatr. **63:**69, 1963.)

palpebral fissures. Microphthalmia with small orbits has been noted. The pupil may be eccentric. The iris consists of fine, porous, spongy tissue. Between the frill and the pupillary rim are crypts and lacunae, and the iris frill may overlie the pupillary rim. Remnants of the pupillary membrane are present along the iris margin rather than across the pupil. Narrowing of visual fields has also been observed.

Generalized enamel hypoplasia is common. In addition, the alveolar ridge of the mandible may be wider than normal. Cleft lip and palate have been noted.

Dry, lusterless hair that fails to grow to normal length has been described but is not a constant feature.

The ears may be somewhat abnormally modeled, and conduction deafness has been described.

Extremities. The most common finding appears to be camptodactyly of the fifth or, less often, of the fourth and fifth fingers (Fig. 17-114). Clinically, the fifth finger appears to be shortened. Bilateral syndactyly of the fourth and fifth fingers with ulnar clinodactyly and syndactyly of the third and fourth toes is usually present.

Radiographic examination of the middle phalanx shows a cube-shaped or deltoid appearance. The feet are clinically normal but on radiographic examination exhibit aplasia or hypoplasia of the middle phalanx of one or more toes. There is lack of modeling of the metaphyseal area of the long bones.[539-546]

Osteogenesis imperfecta

Osteogenesis imperfecta consists of fragile bones, blue scleras, deafness, loose ligaments, and frequently dentinogenesis imperfecta–like changes in the teeth (Figs. 17-115 to 17-118). Most reported cases (about 90%) represent the tarda form with blue scleras (90%), brittle bones (60%), impaired hearing (60%), dentin defect (50%), hyperelasticity of joints and ligaments, and capillary fragility. This type has autosomal dominant inheritance, with variable expressivity and incomplete penetrance. The incidence varies from about 2 to 5 per 100,000 births in different populations.

Since the congenital form has been observed in families also exhibiting the tarda

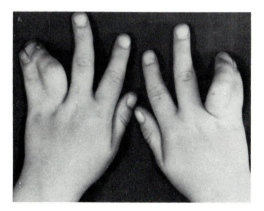

Fig. 17-114. Oculodentoosseous dysplasia: syndactyly and camptodactyly of fourth and fifth fingers. (From Gorlin, R. J., et al.: J. Pediatr. **63:**69, 1963.)

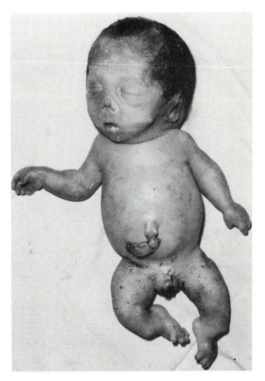

Fig. 17-115. Osteogenesis imperfecta. Note fractures of lower limbs. (Courtesy I. Emanuel, Seattle, Wash.)

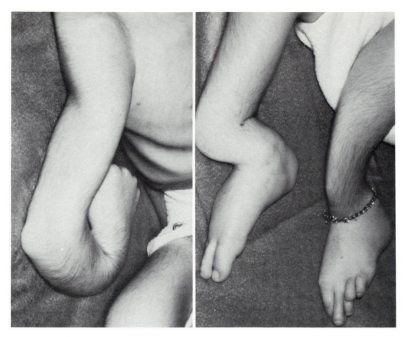

Fig. 17-116. Osteogenesis imperfecta: limb deformities in severe case.

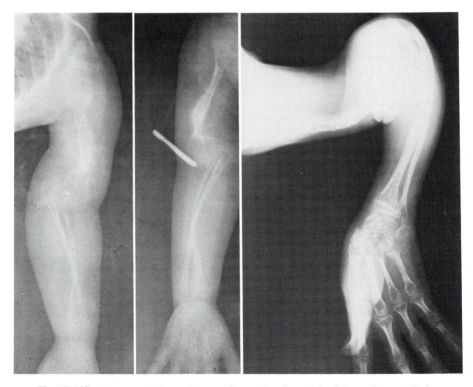

Fig. 17-117. Osteogenesis imperfecta: radiographs of severely deformed upper limbs.

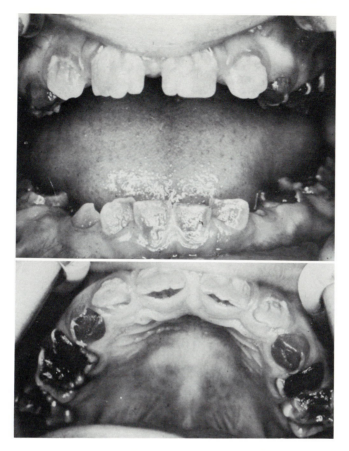

Fig. 17-118. Osteogenesis imperfecta: dentinogenesis imperfecta–like changes. (Courtesy W. K. Smith, Baltimore, Md.)

form, clinical distinction based on age of onset of fractures makes little genetic sense.

Brittle bones not associated with the other classic signs may be inherited as an isolated autosomal dominant trait, with a greater proportion of males being affected.

A congenital lethal type follows an autosomal recessive mode of transmission. A fourth distinct form, also exhibiting autosomal recessive inheritance, most likely represents a renal tubular defect. Anomalies in this type are limited to the skeletal system.

The basic defect in osteogenesis imperfecta has been stated to be a generalized mesenchymal change in maturation of collagen beyond the reticulum fiber stage. Fine structural study of the cornea suggests that the defect lies in tropocollagen synthesis or in extracellular collagen aggregation. It has

been suggested that in classic osteogenesis imperfecta, the production of normally cross-linked collagen is reduced, whereas in the type with only bone involvement, the collagen is unstable but is produced in normal amounts. Bone formation rates have been found to be at least three times the normal rate. It is still unkown whether altered levels of tissue mucopolysaccharide and abnormal amino acid ratios in the collagen are responsible for the defect or simply represent the expression of a metabolic disturbance. Bone collagen from patients with this disorder inhibits calcification in vitro. However, normal biosynthesis, maturation, and excretion of collagen have been found in cultured fibroblasts from patients with classic osteogenesis imperfecta.

Craniofacial complex. The skull appears

disproportionately large, with a temporal bulge that causes the ears to be thrown outward and forward. The forehead is broad and domed, and the occiput is protuberant.

Blue scleras are one of the most common features of the syndrome and may be the only expression. The intensity of the blueness varies from family to family and from case to case. The blue color may be due in part to thinning of the sclera, allowing the color of the choroid to be transmitted, but it also may be due to increased translucency related to a deficiency of collagen fibers or to an increase in mucopolysaccharide content. Some reports have, in fact, indicated that the blue sclera may be thicker than that of normal controls. The sclera adjacent to the limbus often appears to be whitish, resulting in a so-called Saturn's ring. Hypermetropia, arcus juvenilis, keratoconus, megalocornea, and dislocation of lenses have been observed.

Severely impaired hearing is found in 60% of patients with the tarda type. Fewer than half the patients exhibit the classic triad of deafness, blue scleras, and bone disease. Rarely is complete deafness observed, but hearing appears to be more severely impaired in patients with marked bone involvement. Deafness usually begins in the third decade and increases progressively with time, the footplate of the stapes being slightly fixed with a heavy growth of white chalky material, although there may be underlying malformation of the stapes as well. The deafness, usually conductive, may be mixed or purely sensorineural. In some patients the tympanic membrane has been found to be thinned and bluish.

The dentin is chiefly affected; although the enamel frequently cracks off, it is not considered to be involved. In the tarda type, the deciduous teeth are affected in only 35% of patients. The teeth formed early in life or during fetal development are the more severely affected. There seems to be no correlation between dentin impairment and the degree of bone involvement.

The tooth crowns may be smaller than normal, especially in the incisocervical dimension. On eruption, they are noted to be translucent or opalescent. The crowns darken with age, so that they assume a gray, pink, amber, or bluish color. The teeth are prone to abrasion down to the gingival margin. Hypertrophy of the alveolar bone takes place as a compensatory measure.

On radiographic examination, the changes in the teeth are found to be striking. The roots are thin, fine, and disproportionately shortened. The pulp chamber and canal are greatly diminished in size or totally obliterated by the formation of irregular dentin.

Microscopically, the dentinoenamel junction seems to be flattter, lacking the normal scalloping. The normal tubular dentin may be partially or totally replaced by a more laminated dentin that is traversed by tubules of abnormal size and shape. There are comet-shaped structures that appear to be remnants of blood vessels entrapped in the dentin matrix. In contrast, in hereditary opalescent dentin, all the dentin is abnormal except for the mantle dentin adjacent to the enamel or cementum. In osteogenesis imperfecta, the amount of normal-appearing dentin is variable. Microscopic evidence of poor calcification of the dentin (interglobular calcification) has been corroborated by chemical and physical studies.

Musculoskeletal system. In the congenital type, intrauterine fractures may be so numerous that the child may be born dead or may survive for only a short time. Micromelia with broad long bones is often striking. Bones massive at birth may become gracile with age. The diagnosis has been made in utero on radiographic examination of the abdomen.

The skull is large, the forehead being especially broad and bossed, with a temporal bulge, an overhanging occiput, decreased vertical dimension, and platybasia, giving the skull the appearance of a soldier's helmet.

Radiographic examination may reveal a remarkably thin calvaria (caput membranaceum), these patients succumbing from intracranial hemorrhage through birth injury. Numerous Wormian bones are evident in the occipital area.

The long bones, especially those of the lower extremities, are bowed or unevenly shortened, with thinned cortices. Subperiosteal fractures of the shaft and multiple microfractures at the epiphyses, due to minor trauma or sudden muscle pulls, are frequently observed. Hypercallosity at the site of healing fractures may be interpreted erroneously as osteogenic sarcoma or as a rachitic bone. Instead of compact cortical bone, there is a thin, loose, poorly formed and arranged spongy layer. The vertebrae are markedly osteoporotic, with a codfish appearance.

On histological section, the bony plates are seen to be small, irregular, and nonanastomosing. They are poorly endowed with osteoblasts and osteoid matrix. The mucoid component of the connective tissue seems to be increased, resembling that in ascorbic acid deficiency.

Spinal cord compression resulting from abnormally shaped vertebrae, kyphoscoliosis, pectus carinatum and excavatum, and pseudoarthroses are frequently encountered.

The tendency toward fractures decreases after puberty, although pregnancy, lactation, or senile involution may enhance their likelihood. Laxity of ligaments or rupture of tendons, resulting in habitual dislocation of joints, flatfoot, and distortions, is observed in at least 25% of the cases. Hernia occurs with high frequency, sometimes in combination with cryptorchidism.

Skin. Clinically, the skin may be thin and translucent, resembling that of the aged. Histologically, increased amounts of mucopolysaccharides have been found. Healing is often poor, with wide hypertrophic scarring being common. Elastosis perforans has been found with increased frequency. Subcutaneous hemorrhage tends to occur even after minor trauma.

Cardiovascular system. Premature atherosclerosis has been reported. The connective tissue of the myocardium, cardiac valves, and aorta shows increased amounts of mucoid material. Several patients have had aortic or mitral regurgitation.[547-588]

Prader-Willi syndrome

The Prader-Willi syndrome is characterized by mental deficiency, muscular hypotonia, obesity, short stature, and hypogonadism (Figs. 17-119 to 17-121). The syndrome is rather common, and over 100 cases have been reported. The preponderance of reported males probably reflects the easy recognition of the rudimentary scrotum.

The etiology is unknown. Almost all cases are sporadic. The disorder has been reported in sibs, cousins, and identical twins. Autosomal recessive inheritance, polygenic inheritance, and etiological heterogeneity have been suggested. Karyotypes have been normal in most cases, although various inconsistent chromosomal aberrations have been found.

Delivery usually occurs at term, with birth weight being almost always below 3000 gm. Prolonged gestation periods and complicated

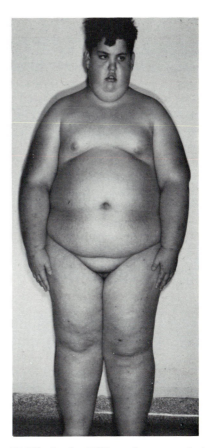

Fig. 17-119. Prader-Willi syndrome: marked obesity. (From Cohen, M. M., Jr., and Gorlin, R. J.: Am. J. Dis. Child. **117**:213, 1969.)

deliveries have been noted in several instances.

Many endocrine and metabolic studies have been carried out with normal or inconsistent results. A hypothalamic-hypophyseal disorder or primary dysfunction of the adrenal cortex or both have been suggested.

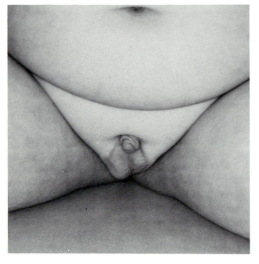

Fig. 17-120. Prader-Willi syndrome: micropenis and hypoplastic scrotum.

The hyperphagia often manifested in the Prader-Willi syndrome is reminiscent of the behavior of experimental animals with destructive lesions of the ventromedial hypothalamic nucleus.

Generalized obesity becomes apparent during the second and third years of life and in some patients may be less pronounced in later childhood. The distribution of fat is particularly marked on the lower part of the trunk and buttocks.

During childhood and adolescence, diabetes mellitus frequently develops; it differs from the usual type by the absence of weight loss and acidosis, the presence of insulin resistance, and good response to oral hypoglycemic drugs.

Craniofacial complex. Bifrontal diameter is reduced. Marked obesity is present around the cheeks and under the chin. The palpebral fissures are almond shaped with slightly overhanging lids. Strabismus and mild ear dysplasia may be observed. The nose is retroussé, and the mouth is fishlike with a triangular upper lip.

Marked dental caries, possibly due to xerostomia, has been noted. Hypoplastic

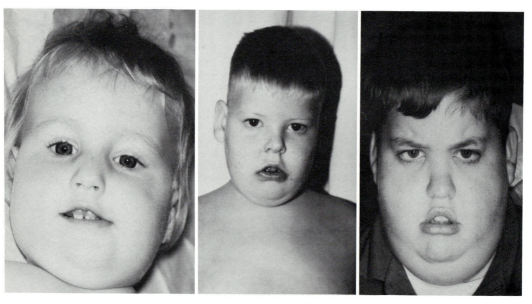

Fig. 17-121. Prader-Willi syndrome: characteristic facial appearance in three patients of different ages.

enamel (Fig. 17-122), supernumerary teeth, delayed eruption, micrognathia, extreme narrowing of the mandibular dental arch, and highly arched palate have been observed.

Nervous system. In the newborn there is marked hypotonia, almost certainly a continuation of the diminished intrauterine movements so frequently reported. Little spontaneous activity, poor sucking and swallowing reflexes, a weak cry, and sometimes episodes of asphyxia are characteristic. Cortical atrophy has been documented in a few cases by pneumoencephalography. Poor thermoregulation with a tendency to hyperpyrexia and convulsions have been reported.

Mental deficiency is almost always observed. The friendly nature of these patients is striking. Psychiatric problems, however, have been noted in the postadolescent period. Waddling gait is characteristic.

Skeletal system. Short stature, retarded bone age, and small hands and feet are almost always observed. There is an increased frequency of scoliosis. Less common findings include clinodactyly, partial syndactyly, genua valga, fusion of lumbar vertebrae, displaced thumbs, and poor mineralization.

Genitourinary system. In males, the genitalia are poorly developed. The penis is small, the testes are ectopic or infantile, and the scrotum is rudimentary. Pubertal changes are both delayed and diminished. In females, no genital abnormalities have been observed. The menarche is usually normal, although puberty may be delayed.[589-608]

Pycnodysostosis

The characteristic features of pycnodysostosis include short stature, osteopetrosis, partial agenesis of the terminal digits of the hands and feet, cranial anomalies, such as persistence of fontanels and failure of closure of cranial sutures, and hypoplasia of the angle of the mandible.

Affected sibs have been reported in several instances. Parental consanguinity has been noted in more than 30%, and autosomal recessive inheritance is clearly indicated.

Craniofacial complex. The head is dolichocephalic with frontal and occipital bossing (Fig. 17-123). Characteristic are parrot-like nose with mild exophthalmos and micrognathia. Blue scleras have been observed.

Agenesis of the angle of the mandible is a constant feature. Facial bones are usually underdeveloped with relative mandibular prognathism.

Oral and dental anomalies include premature or delayed eruption, enamel hypoplasia, malposed teeth, and grooved palate.

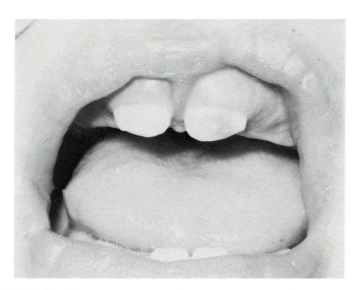

Fig. 17-122. Prader-Willi syndrome: enamel defect of maxillary deciduous central incisor.

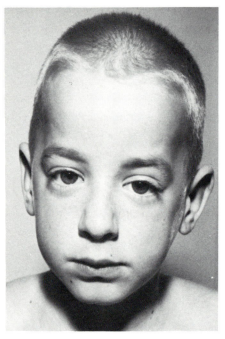

Fig. 17-123. Pycnodysostosis: dolichocephaly and frontal bossing. (Courtesy D. W. Smith, Seattle, Wash.)

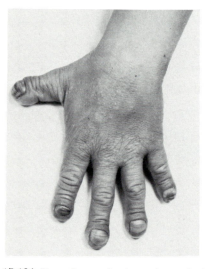

Fig. 17-124. Pycnodysostosis: shortening and widening of terminal digits. (Courtesy D. W. Smith, Seattle, Wash.)

Skeletal alterations. Adult height is reduced, being 134 to 152 cm (53 to 60 inches) because of shortness of the limbs. The trunk is not shortened but often exhibits marked pectus excavatum. The terminal digits of the fingers and toes are reduced and widened, often presenting a drumstick appearance. The acromial end of the clavicle has been noted to be somewhat hypoplastic. Bilateral genua valga is frequent.

On radiographic examination, there is increased radiopacity of all bones, especially of the long bones, spine, and skull base. The terminal phalanges of the fingers and toes are markedly hypoplastic, exhibiting fragmentation of the distal ends with preservation of the bases (Fig. 17-124).

Most cranial sutures and fontanels are open, especially the parietooccipital. The bones of the calvaria are thin, dense, and without diploic markings. Wormian bones are common. The frontal sinuses are absent, and other paranasal sinuses are hypoplastic or missing. The mastoid air cells are often not pneumatized (Fig. 17-125).

Microscopic studies of the involved bones show reduction in osteoclastic and osteoblastic activity.[609-618]

Rubinstein-Taybi syndrome

The constellation of features that make up the Rubinstein-Taybi syndrome consists of broad thumbs and great toes, characteristic facial features, growth retardation, and mental deficiency (Fig. 17-126). Over 120 cases have been recorded to date. The incidence in the general population is unknown. In various diagnostic clinics and mental retardation groups, the frequency varies from 1 in 300 to 1 in 700 individuals.

The etiology is unknown. No affected individual has reproduced. Almost all cases have been sporadic. Affected sibs and identical twins have rarely been reported. Consanguinity has been noted in two instances. Normal karyotypes have been observed in almost all cases, although inconsistent chromosomal variations have been observed occasionally.

Major medical difficulties include neonatal

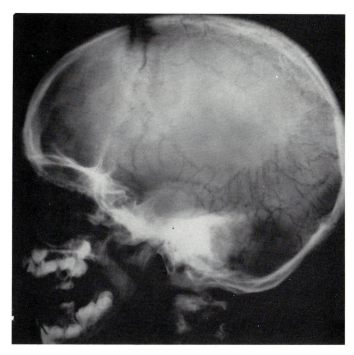

Fig. 17-125. Pycnodysostosis: open anterior fontanel, Wormian bones, increased radiopacity of cranial base, hypoplastic sinuses, nonpneumatized mastoid air cells, and flattened gonial angle. (Courtesy D. W. Smith, Seattle, Wash.)

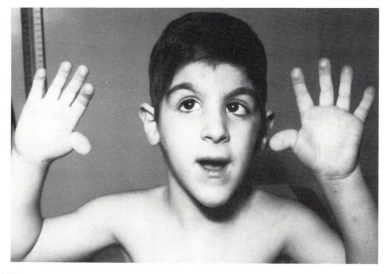

Fig. 17-126. Rubinstein-Taybi syndrome: microcephaly, downslanting palpebral fissures, strabismus, beaked nose with nasal septum extending below alae, and broad deviated thumbs. (Courtesy D. W. Smith, Seattle, Wash.)

distress, recurrent respiratory infections, feeding difficulties during infancy, and allergy-like manifestations, including hay fever, asthma, and eczema.

Craniofacial complex. The facial appearance is striking with microcephaly, prominent forehead, downslanting palpebral fissures, epicanthal folds, strabismus, broad nasal bridge, beaked nose with nasal septum extending below the alae, and mild micrognathia. Grimacing or unusual smile has been observed frequently. Other findings may include long eyelashes, nasolacrimal duct obstruction, ptosis of the eyelids, refractive error, and minor abnormalities in the shape, position, and degree of rotation of the auricles.

The mouth has been stated to be small in some cases. Highly arched palate has been observed in most instances. Irregular, crowded teeth have also been reported. Low-frequency abnormalities have included bifid uvula, bifid tongue, macroglossia, short lingual frenum, and thin upper lip.

Central nervous system. Mental deficiency has been present in all cases. In most evaluations, IQ was reported as less than 50. In several instances, language and speech have been retarded to a greater extent than expected on the basis of IQ. Electroencephalographic abnormalities, seizures, and absence of the corpus callosum have been reported. In a number of cases, hyperactive deep tendon reflexes have been noted.

Hands and feet. Broad thumbs and great toes have been present in all reported cases. In most instances, the terminal phalanges of the fingers are also broad. Clinodactyly of the fifth fingers and overlapping toes are present in over half of all cases. Angulation deformities of the thumbs and great toes together with abnormally shaped proximal phalanges occur in some instances. Abnormally shaped first metatarsals and duplication of the proximal or distal phalanx of the halluces have also been reported. Rarely, hexadactyly of the feet, partial cutaneous syndactyly involving the toes, and absence of the distal phalanx of the hallux have been noted.

Alterations in the frequency of various fingerprint patterns have been observed, but the findings have been inconsistent. Increased frequencies of loops, whorls, or arches have been reported. Significant dermatoglyphic findings have included as increased frequency of thenar, interdigital, and hypothenar patterns. Simian creases have been observed in many cases. Thumb tip triradius, thumb double pattern, distally placed axial triradius, deep plantar crease, and large hallucal loop with laterally displaced f triradius with or without associated e^1 triradius have also been noted.

Skeletal system. Growth retardation and delayed bone age have been observed. Large anterior frontanel or delay in its closure, large foramen magnum, and parietal foramina have been reported in some cases. Other skeletal anomalies have included pectus excavatum, rib defects, scoliosis, kyphosis, lordosis, spina bifida, flat acetabular angles, flaring of the ilia, and notched ischia.

The gait has been stated to be stiff. Hypotonia, lax ligaments, and hyperextensible joints have also been noted.

Genitourinary system. Incomplete or delayed descent of the testes has been reported in most males. Anomalies of the urinary tract, including duplication of the kidney and ureter, renal agenesis, and other abnormalities have been recorded in a number of cases. Rarely, angulated penis and hypospadias have been noted.

Other findings. A variety of congenital heart defects, abnormal lung lobulation, supernumerary nipples, nevus flammeus of the forehead, nape of neck, or back, hirsutism, and other abnormalities have been reported.[619-621]

Russell-Silver syndrome

The Russell-Silver syndrome of short stature of prenatal onset, triangular facies, asymmetry, variation in the pattern of sexual development, and other abnormalities including café-au-lait pigmentation and clinodactyly was independently described by Silver and associates[664] in 1953 and by Russell in 1954.[660] Most authors regard the Russell-Silver syndrome as a single entity, although a few separate the Russell syndrome from the Silver syndrome.

The etiology is unknown. Almost all cases are sporadic, although an occasional familial instance has been noted. In two instances, the mother was stated to be short. Autosomal dominant inheritance with most cases representing fresh mutations is possible. Monozygotic twins have been reported. The syndrome has also been observed with 45,X/46,XY mosaicism and with XXY karyotype.

Birth weight is usually less than 2200 gm at full term. Short stature is maintained throughout childhood, height usually being below the third percentile. There is some catch-up growth, with adult height not being grossly retarded.

Craniofacial complex. The facies is characterized by pseudohydrocephaly. This is due to relative smallness of the face, the normal-sized calvaria appearing large. The forehead

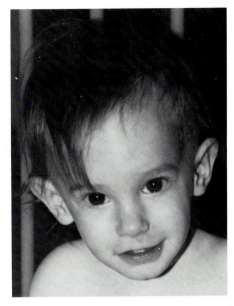

Fig. 17-127. Russell-Silver syndrome: triangular facies.

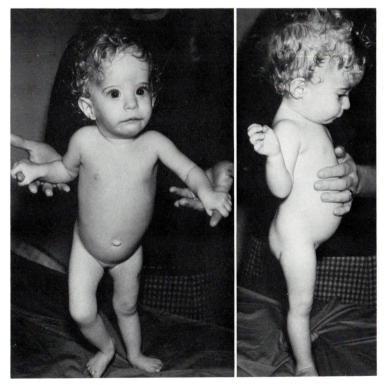

Fig. 17-128. Russell-Silver syndrome: asymmetry of lower limbs. (From Gareis, F., et al.: J. Pediatr. **79:**775, 1971.)

is prominent, sometimes bossed with the face triangular in form and the chin small and pointed. The corners of the mouth are often turned downward. Appearance becomes markedly less striking with age. The palate may be high and narrow and the teeth crowded and somewhat small (Fig. 17-127).

Musculoskeletal system. Asymmetry has been noted in about 80% of cases (Fig. 17-128). Although occasionally total, it may involve only the head, trunk, or limbs. In some cases, the asymmetry becomes evident only with growth. Poor muscular development is usually a feature.

Delayed closure of the anterior fontanel is common. Bone age is retarded in relation to sexual development and chronological age. Occasionally, there is hip or elbow dislocation. The humerus may be somewhat shortened. The fifth fingers are abbreviated and exhibit clinodactyly in over 75% of cases.

Radiographically, there is hypoplasia of the middle phalanx of the fifth finger. Pseudoepiphyses are found more often at the base of the second metacarpal than in the normal population. Soft tissue syndactyly between the second and third toes is observed in about a third of the cases.

Genital anomalies. Variation in sexual development has been found in over 30% of all patients. There may be premature puberty and rarely, cryptorchidism, enlarged clitoris, or hypospadias. Urinary gonadotropins have been elevated in about 10% of the cases. Elevation in both FSH and LH levels has been reported in some cases. In other cases, there has been premature estrogenation of the urethral or vaginal mucosa.

Other findings. Café-au-lait spots have been noted in about 45% of the cases. Rarely there is mild mental deficiency. Hyperhidrosis is a common finding. Hypoglycemia after short periods of fasting has been described in many cases.[653-672]

Sturge-Weber dysplasia/Klippel-Trénaunay-Weber syndrome

Sturge-Weber dysplasia is characterized by angiomatosis of the leptomeninges. Other findings most often include ipsilateral facial angiomatosis, ipsilateral gyriform calcifications of the cerebral cortex, seizures, mental deficiency, hemiplegia, and ocular defects (Figs. 17-129 and 17-130).

All cases to date have been sporadic. Although a few reports have suggested incomplete forms in first-degree relatives who presented single features such as seizures, mental deficiency, or vascular nevi, no instance of full-blown Sturge-Weber dysplasia has ever been recorded in more than one individual within the same family. Neither sex preponderance nor predilection for left- or right-sided involvement has been found.

The Sturge-Weber dysplasia can be explained on the basis of an embryological abnormality with secondary consequences. During the sixth week of intrauterine development, a vascular plexus develops around the cephalic portion of the neural tube and under the ectoderm destined to become facial skin. Normally, this vascular plexus regresses during the ninth week, but in the Sturge-Weber dysplasia, it persists, resulting in an-

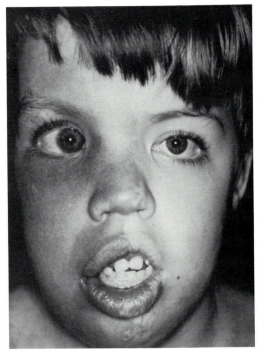

Fig. 17-129. Sturge-Weber dysplasia: unilateral facial involvement. Note buphthalmos.

giomatosis of the leptomeninges overlying the cerebral cortex together with facial angiomatosis on the ipsilateral side. Variation in the degree of persistence or regression of the vascular plexus account for cases of bilateral involvement and for unilateral cases in which an angioma of the leptomeninges occurs in the absence of facial involvement.

Other features of the Sturge-Weber dysplasia seem to be secondary to the leptomeningeal lesion. A poorly understood alteration in the vascular dynamics of the angioma results in the precipitation of calcium deposits in the cerebral cortex underlying the angioma. Seizures and mental deficiency are probably secondary to this process.

Since angiomas of the skin and, in some cases, the viscera may be observed in the Klippel-Trénaunay-Weber syndrome, it is not surprising that the Sturge-Weber dysplasia occurs in association with this syndrome. Over twenty such cases have been noted in the literature. Since angiomas may occur anywhere in the Klippel-Trénaunay-Weber syndrome, it is possible that this syndrome and the Sturge-Weber anomaly represent the same basic disorder, with the Sturge-Weber phenomenon occurring whenever an angioma happens to be present in the leptomeninges.

The characteristic lesion in the Sturge-Weber dysplasia consists of a unilateral thin-walled angioma in the leptomeninges overlying the posterior temporal, posterior parietal, and occipital areas. Occasionally, bilateral involvement may be present. An abnormal cerebral venous drainage pattern, caused by lack of functioning superficial cortical veins beneath the angioma, has been reported. Whether these veins become thrombosed or are truly absent remains to be determined.

Gyriform, double-contoured lines of calcification develop in the underlying cerebral cortex after the second year of life, although rarely calcification has been present at birth (Fig. 17-131). The radiographic appearance is pathognomonic. Calcific deposition becomes stationary usually by the end of the second decade. Asymmetry of the skull has been noted. Macrocephaly has been observed in a few cases associated with the Klippel-Trénaunay-Weber syndrome.

A nevus flammeus lesion occurs on the ipsilateral side of the face in approximately 90% of all cases. In some instances, the nevus may extend onto the neck, chest, and

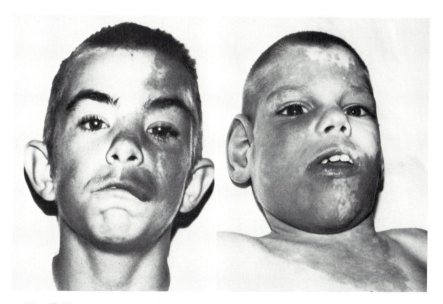

Fig. 17-130. Sturge-Weber dysplasia. Compare patients for extent of involvement.

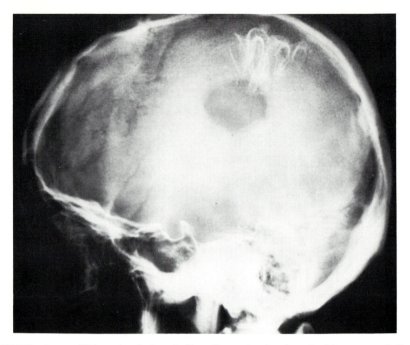

Fig. 17-131. Sturge-Weber dysplasia: skull radiograph showing double-contoured lines of calcification.

back. Occasionally, bilateral facial nevus or no facial nevus may occur. The color varies from pink to purplish red and may decrease in intensity with age in some cases. The lesion is sharply demarcated and usually flat.

Seizures were observed in 90% of the cases in one series. Symptoms appear during infancy, with seizures occurring contralateral to the angiomatosis. They are most often focal, but generalized convulsions may occur. Hemiparesis occurs less frequently, and the paretic limb is sometimes hypotrophic.

At least 30% exhibit mental deficiency. With extensive cerebral changes, deficiency may be pronounced.

Choroidal angioma is common, and buphthalmos, glaucoma, and hemianopia have been reported.

Intraoral angiomatosis occurs most frequently on the buccal mucosa and lips, with macrocheilia occurring when the lips are affected. The palate is less frequently affected. Tongue involvement may be accompanied by hemihypertrophy. Gingival lesions, when present, may range from slight vascular hyperplasia to monstrous overgrowth, mak-

ing closure of the mouth impossible. Vascular gingival hyperplasia, which blanches on pressure, should be distinguished from fibrous hyperplasia, which may accompany medication with diphenylhydantoin.

Both unilateral hypertrophy and hypotrophy of the alveolar process have been reported. Ipsilateral premature eruption of permanent teeth, ipsilateral delayed eruption, and ipsilateral normal eruption have been noted. Unilateral premature eruption causes irregular positioning of teeth, leading to malocclusion. The size of the teeth may vary in the affected area, macrodontia being most frequently observed.

The *Klippel-Trénaunay-Weber* syndrome is the most complex of all vascular syndromes. Features include unilateral leg hypertrophy with cutaneous and subcutaneous hemangiomas, varicosities, phlebectasia, arteriovenous fistula in some cases, lymphangiomatous anomalies, macrodactyly, syndactyly, polydactyly, oligodactyly, and internal hemangiomas.

Pathological evaluation of the vascular lesions has shown no consistent pattern. Ve-

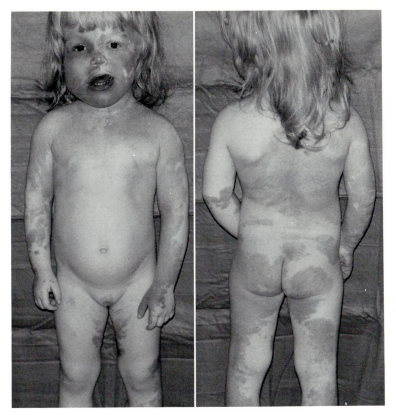

Fig. 17-132. Klippel-Trénaunay-Weber syndrome combined with Sturge-Weber dysplasia. Note macrocephaly and facial asymmetry. Intelligence was normal in this case.

nous abnormalities such as phlebectasia of the superficial and deep veins predominate, but arterial defects are not unusual. Because of the variability of the vascular defects, Klippel-Trénaunay-Weber syndrome is a clinical diagnosis and not a pathological one.

Most patients are of normal mentality, the exceptions occurring when the vascular abnormalities involve the craniofacial area. Most of these patients present features of the Sturge-Weber dysplasia as part of the Klippel-Trénaunay-Weber syndrome (Fig. 17-132).

Almost all cases of the Klippel-Trénaunay-Weber syndrome are sporadic. So-called familial instances usually include relatives of the proband who have findings common to the general population, such as birthmarks on the posterior neck or isolated varicosities. A number of inadequately documented familial instances may represent neurofibroma-tosis. Among so-called familial cases in the literature, only one instance of affected sibs is convincing. The great variety of findings observed in sporadic cases may mean etiological heterogeneity.

Unilateral leg hypertrophy is the most frequent finding. However, the hypertrophy can symmetrically or asymmetrically involve any or all limbs. The hypertrophy is usually noted at birth but may occur at any age and progressively increase in degree. Extremity circumference and/or length are usually increased, but rarely, only the proximal or distal limb segment may be disproportionately large. Infrequently, atrophy of a limb may occur, or a hypertrophied limb may become atrophic over many years. Ultimate height is rarely excessive or stunted except in severe cases.

In most instances, a visible vascular abnormality is present in the hypertrophied area.

However, this is not always the case. Hemangiomatous lesions of almost every variety have been noted, but varicosities, phlebectasia, nevus flammeus, and vascular masses predominate. These lesions may minimally involve the extremity, but they can cause severe distortion. The longer vascular masses can sometimes cause a generalized bleeding diathesis of the Kasabach-Merritt variety. The occurrence of an arteriovenous fistula has been reported in a number of cases. Lymphectasia in association with the vascular abnormalities can result in marked limb swelling with recurrent cellulitis.

Macrodactyly may involve one or more digits, some assuming gigantic proportions (Fig. 17-133). When the digits are not enlarged, they are often of unequal length. Clinodactyly and brachydactyly have been noted in some cases. Cutaneous syndactyly is common but rarely involves more than two digits on any one limb. Polydactyly and oligodactyly are relatively uncommon.

Radiographic studies of the hypertrophied limbs usually show enlargement of subcutaneous tissue, muscle, and bone. However, only one of these tissues may be hypertrophied. Phlebectasia, phleboliths, arteriovenous fistulas, hyperostosis, bony sclerosis, and bone atrophy can readily be demonstrated when present.

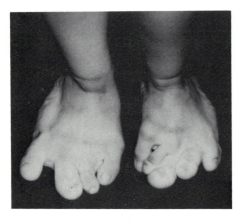

Fig. 17-133. Klippel-Trénaunay-Weber syndrome: macrodactyly involving both feet. One toe on right foot was so large that it had to be surgically removed.

Typical distribution of the various vascular lesions usually includes the lower limb with frequent extension to the buttocks and less often involvement of the lower back, flank, lateral chest, and axillary area. The upper limbs are sometimes involved, as are the abdomen, chest, neck, and craniofacial region (Sturge-Weber dysplasia). Melanotic streaks and spots have been noted in some cases.

Involvement of the viscera is not rare. The major manifestations are hemangiomatous lesions of the gastrointestinal tract, urinary system, visceral organs, mesentery, and pleura. Abdominal lymphectasia can occur, and protein-losing enteropathy secondary to lymphectasia has been described.

Lipodystrophy involving the upper limbs has occurred in a few cases. Scoliosis secondary to unequal leg length has been noted.[673-721]

Tuberous sclerosis

Tuberous sclerosis is characterized by epilepsy, mental deficiency, and cutaneous angiofibromas. The components of the triad may appear in any order. Some patients may manifest signs at birth, but in the majority of cases, seizures and skin changes first appear from 2 to 6 years of age. The syndrome is found in about 0.1% to 0.6% of persons institutionalized for epilepsy and mental deficiency and in about 1 in 100,000 to 200,000 in the general population. Autosomal dominant inheritance with variable expressivity has been demonstrated. About 70% are isolated cases, representing fresh mutations.

Most patients die before they are 20 years old, but some survive into middle age. The usual cause of death is pneumonia, cachexia, status epilepticus, or acute heart failure.

Skin and skin appendages. The skin lesions are of several types. Most common are the small, reddish, flat or rounded, seedlike masses composed of hyperplastic connective and vascular tissues that are located over the nose, cheeks, nasolabial furrows, and chin (Fig. 17-134). These angiofibromas have been misnamed "adenoma sebaceum" frequently in the past. They are present in 90% of patients over 4 years of age. The number seems to increase at puberty. Less commonly observed are soft polypoid fibromatous masses over the dorsal trunk or scalp. Subungual fibromas (Fig. 17-134) also occur less commonly. Round, flat plaques of fibrous connective tissue (shagreen patches) may be noted in the lumbar area in over 20% of patients.

Many other types of cutaneous lesions may be observed, including areas of vitiligo (about 70%) (Fig. 17-134) and café-au-lait spots (about 7%). The white leukodermic areas may be an extremely helpful diagnostic sign at birth or in early infancy. The fingernails may be discolored and misshapen because of the subungual fibromas.

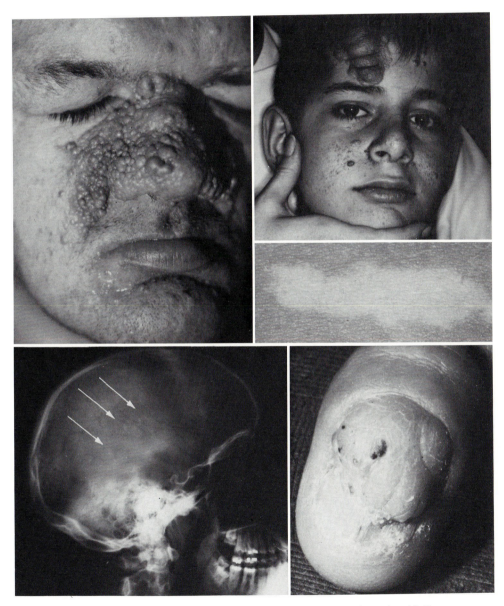

Fig. 17-134. Tuberous sclerosis. *Upper left,* angiofibromas; *upper right,* polypoid fibrous masses of forehead; *lower left,* skull radiograph showing intracranial calcifications; *lower right,* subungual fibroma; *right middle,* patch of vitiligo. (*Lower right* courtesy W. W. Lockwood, Spokane, Wash.)

Central nervous system. The name *tuberous sclerosis* is derived from the numerous, smooth, hard, potato-like masses of proliferated glial elements and ganglion cells located throughout the cerebral cortex, ependymal lining of the ventricles, and other areas of the brain. Rarely, malignancy may arise in the glial tissue. About 50% of those affected manifest intracranial calcification, and 60% manifest mental deficiency. Petit mal or grand mal seizures or Jacksonian-type epilepsy usually begin within the first 2 years of life and occur with variable frequency in over 90% of all patients. The degree of severity seems to increase with time.

Craniofacial complex. In addition to facial angiofibromas, the eyes and mouth may have unusual findings. Present in about 50% of all cases is unilateral or, less frequently, bilateral retinal tumor (phakoma), which may be large and nodular or, more commonly, flat and oval. Such tumors are gray or yellowish gray in color and are composed of glial cells, nerve cells, and vascular tissue. Epicanthus is also common.

The oral mucosa may be the site of fibrous growths in approximately 10% of affected individuals. Most frequently they are located on the anterior gingiva, but they may occur on the oral mucosa. They are usually the color of normal oral mucosa but may be bluish, red, or yellow, ranging in size from that of a pin point to that of a small pea.

Skeletal system. In about half the cases, the skull exhibits thickened calvaria with an irregular outer table, and exostoses are often seen on the inner table of the frontal bone. Areas of increased density appear throughout the skull, especially in the parietal region after puberty.

About 65% of all patients have cystlike areas in the phalanges and irregular periosteal new bone formation along the shafts of the metacarpals and metatarsals. Less frequently, long bones are involved.

Genitourinary system. About 40% have renal hamartomas, usually angiomyolipoma and less commonly angioleiomyolipoma. Rarely there is malignant change.

Other findings. Rhabdomyomas of the heart are common. Hamartomas may be noted in many organs, including the lungs, liver, thyroid, testes, and pancreas.[722-754]

Williams syndrome

The syndrome of characteristic facial appearance, mental retardation, growth deficiency, cardiovascular anomalies, and infantile hypercalcemia was described independently by Fanconi and Girardet[767] and by Schlesinger and associates[791] in 1952. A good historical review of the condition was presented by Myers and Willis.[784]

Naming the syndrome has been problematical. The disorder is probably best known as the idiopathic hypercalcemia–supravalvular aortic stenosis syndrome despite the fact that both features are frequently absent. Furthermore, the term is cumbersome. The name *elfin-face syndrome* presents a problem by naming the disorder after a mythical being. The currently accepted designation, the *Williams syndrome,* ignores the historical precedent mentioned earlier.

Delineating the phenotypic spectrum of abnormalities has also been problematical. Defining a syndrome on the basis of sporadic occurrence when the basic defect is unknown truncates the phenotype toward the severe end of the spectrum. Thus reported frequencies of various findings are not especially meaningful. The problem is further compounded by ascertainment on the basis of cardiovascular anomalies in some reports and on the basis of facial features in others. It has been suggested that the syndrome may represent a spectrum that overlaps with hypercalcemia with and without mental retardation, and supravalvular aortic stenosis with and without mental retardation. However, few families have been reported in which more than one of these phenotypes is present.

All so-called severe cases reported to date are seemingly sporadic, except for one pair of monozygotic twins. The etiology and pathogenesis are unknown. Similar craniofacial, dental, and cardiovascular anomalies have been produced in the offspring of rabbits treated with excessive vita-

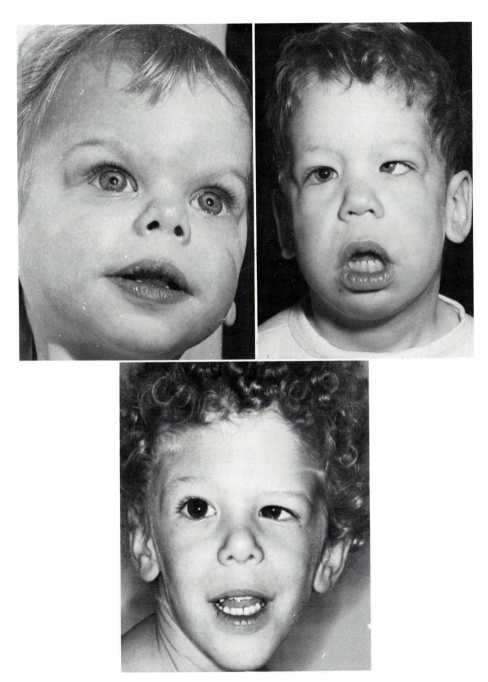

Fig. 17-135. Williams syndrome: ocular hypotelorism, strabismus, flat midface, low nasal bridge, anteverted nostrils, long philtrum, thick lips, and wide intercommissural distance. (Courtesy J. M. Opitz, Madison, Wis.)

min D during pregnancy. Hypotheses for the human syndrome have included vitamin D hypersensitivity or excess, an abnormality of cholesterol metabolism, and delayed turnover or degradation of vitamin D. It has been demonstrated that the ability of normocalcemic children with the Williams syndrome to handle large intravenous calcium loads efficiently is impaired, suggesting deficiency of calcitonin. All available human studies to date are limited by the inability to evaluate vitamin D or calcium metabolism during early fetal development.

Craniofacial complex (Fig. 17-135). Facial features are distinctive and become more striking with age. The combination of flat midface, depressed nasal bridge, anteverted nostrils, long philtrum, thick lips, wide intercommissural distance, and open mouth is characteristic. Ocular findings may include medial eyebrow flaring, short palpebral fissures, ocular hypotelorism, epicanthal folds, periorbital fullness, strabismus (especially esotropia), and a high percentage of blue-eyed individuals with a stellate iris pattern. Uncommonly, corneal and/or lenticular opacities and ptosis of the eyelids may be observed. In some cases, the ears may be prominent. The thyroid cartilage becomes more prominent with age.

The maxillary arch has been described as being too broad for the mandibular arch. Hypodontia, microdontia, small slender roots, and dens invaginatus have been reported. Hypoplastic bud-shaped maxillary deciduous second molars and mandibular permanent first molars have been noted by some authors. In a series of seventeen patients studied metrically, microdontia was not observed nor were hypoplastic bud-shaped teeth present in any patient. However, absence of teeth, especially the lower second premolars, was observed in some. Mild micrognathia, widened mandibular angle, osteosclerotic changes in the lamina dura (especially in the premolar-molar region), delayed mineralization of teeth, folding and thickening of the buccal mucous membranes, and prominent and accessory labial frenula have also been noted. The voice is often hoarse.

Central nervous system. Mild microcephaly (most striking in bifrontal diameter), mental retardation, mild neurological dysfunction, and unusual personality are characteristic features. Intelligence quotients have varied from 41 to 80 with an average of 56 among fourteen noninstitutionalized patients. In childhood, patients have been described as friendly, loquacious, or as having a "cocktail party manner."

Hypercalcemia. Hypercalcemia has not been documented in most cases. When present, it usually disappears during the second year of life. Retrospective interviewing may reveal a history of failure to thrive, hypotonia, anorexia, constipation, or renal impairment.

Skeletal and limb abnormalities. Mild to moderate growth deficiency of prenatal onset with more striking growth deficiency during the postnatal period is a feature in most cases.

The hypercalcemic phase may result in widespread osteosclerotic changes that regress in time. Craniosynostosis (secondary to microcephaly), retarded bone age, and increased density of the metaphyses, epiphyses, and skull base may be present in some instances.

Pectus excavatum, hallux valgus, fifth finger clinodactyly, and hypoplastic, deepset nails have been reported.

Cardiovascular system. Findings have included supravalvular aortic stenosis, valvular aortic stenosis, aortic hypoplasia, coarctation of the aorta, pulmonary artery stenosis, peripheral artery stenoses (cardiac, celiac, subclavian, mesenteric, and renal), atrial septal defect, ventricular septal defect, anomalous pulmonary venous return, arteriovenous fistula (lung), interruption of the aortic arch, and aplasia of the portal vein. Arterial hypertension and heart murmur have been noted frequently. There is no apparent correlation between the degree of mental retardation and the severity of the cardiovascular abnormalities.

Other findings. Small penis, inguinal hernia, and umbilical hernia have also been reported.[756-795]

REFERENCES
Syndrome delineation

1. Cohen, M. M., Jr.: Human dysmorphic syndromes. (To be published.)
2. Marden, P. M., Smith, D. W., and McDonald, M. J.: Congenital anomalies in the newborn infant, including minor variations, J. Pediatr. 64:358-371, 1964.
3. Cohen, M. M., Jr.: Human dysmorphic syndromes. (To be published.)
4. Opitz, J. M., Herrmann, J., and Dieker, H.: The study of malformation syndromes in man, Birth Defects 5(2):1-10, 1969.

Types of syndromes
Nosology of syndromes

5. Cohen, M. M., Jr.: Human dysmorphic syndromes. (To be published.)
6. Holmes, L. B., Moser, H. W., Hallorsson, S., et al.: Mental retardation: an atlas of diseases with associated physical abnormalities, New York, 1972, The Macmillan Co.
7. Smith, D. W.: Compendium on shortness of stature, J. Pediatr. 70:463, 1967.
8. Warkany, J.: Congenital malformations, Chicago, 1971, Year Book Medical Publishers, Inc.

Biological types of syndromes

9. Cohen, M. M., Jr.: Human dysmorphic syndromes. (To be published.)
10. Cohen, M. R.: Preface to logic, New York, 1958, Meridian Book Co.

Syndrome model 1: the dysmetabolic syndrome

11. Herrmann, J., and Opitz, J. M.: Naming and nomenclature of syndromes, Birth Defects 10(7):69-86, 1974.
12. Opitz, J. M., and Herrmann, J.: The study of genetic diseases and malformations, Birth Defects. (In press.)

Syndrome model 2: the dysplasia syndrome

13. Cohen, M. M., Jr.: Human dysmorphic syndromes. (To be published.)
14. Herrmann, J., Gilbert, E. F., and Opitz, J. M.: Dysplasia, malformations and cancer especially with respect to the Weidemann-Beckwith syndrome, Procedures of the Conference on Cell Aging, Institute for Medical Research, Camden, N.J., 1975.
15. Opitz, J. M., and Herrmannn, J.: The study of genetic diseases and malformations, Birth Defects. (In press.)
16. Willis, R. A.: The borderland of embryology and pathology, ed. 2, London, 1962, Butterworth & Co. (Publishers), Ltd.

Syndrome model 3: the malformation syndrome

17. Barash, B. A., Freedman, L., and Opitz, J. M.: Anatomic studies in the 18-trisomy syndrome, Birth Defects, 6(4):3-15, 1970.

18. Herrmann, J., and Opitz, J. M.: Naming and nomenclature of syndromes, Birth Defects 10(7):69-86, 1974.
19. Opitz, J. M.: Personal communication, 1975.
20. Opitz, J. M., and Herrmann, J.: The study of genetic diseases and malformations. Birth Defects. (In press.)
21. Opitz, J. M., Herrmann, J., and Dieker, H.: The study of malformation syndromes in man, Birth Defects 5(2):1-10, 1969.
22. Proposed guidelines for the classification, nomenclature, and naming of morphologic defects, Syndrome Identification 3:1-3, 1975.
23. Willis, R. A.: The borderland of embryology and pathology, ed. 2, London, 1962, Butterworth & Co. (Publishers), Ltd.

Syndrome model 4: the deformation syndrome

24. Cohen, M. M., Jr.: Human dysmorphic syndromes. (To be published.)
25. Dunn, P. M.: Congenital postural deformities: perinatal associations, Proc. R. Soc. Med. 65:735-738 (Section of Orthopedics 11-14), 1972.
26. Herrmann, J., and Opitz, J. M.: Naming and nomenclature of syndromes, Birth Defects 10(7):69-86, 1974.
27. Opitz, J. M., and Herrmann, J.: The study of genetic diseases and malformations, Birth Defects. (In press.)
28. Proposed guidelines for the classification, nomenclature, and naming of morphologic defects, Syndrome Identification 3:1-3, 1975.
29. Rosenmann, A., and Arad, I.: Arthrogryposis multiplex congenita: neurogenic type with autosomal recessive inheritance, J. Med. Genet. 11:91-93, 1974.

Comments on syndrome models

30. Cohen, M. M., Jr.: Human dysmorphic syndromes. (To be published.)
31. Pena, S. D. J., and Shokeir, M. H. K.: Syndrome of camptodactyly, multiple ankyloses, facial anomalies, and pulmonary hypoplasia: a lethal condition, J. Pediatr. 85:373-375, 1974.
32. Punnett, H. H., Kistenmacher, M. L., Valdes-Dapena, M., and Ellison, R. T.: Syndrome of ankylosis, facial anomalies, and pulmonary hypoplasia, J. Pediatr. 85:375-377, 1974.

Special considerations
Syndrome nomenclature

33. Cohen, M. M., Jr.: Syndrome designations, J. Med. Genet. (In press.)

Definitions of various types of abnormalities in dysmorphic syndromes

34. Cohen, M. M., Jr.: Human dysmorphic syndromes. (To be published.)

35. Opitz, J. M., Herrmann, J., and Dieker, H.: The study of malformation syndromes in man, Birth Defects 5:1-10, 1969.

Major and minor abnormalities

36. Cohen, M. M., Jr.: Human dysmorphic syndromes. (To be published.)
37. Marden, P. M., Smith, D. W., and McDonald, M. J.: Congenital anomalies in the newborn infant, including minor variations, J. Pediatr. 64:358-371, 1964.
38. Smith, D. W.: Minor anomalies. In Hook, E. B., Janerich, D. T., and Porter, I. H., editors: Monitoring birth defects and environment, New York, 1971, Academic Press, Inc.
39. Smith, D. W., and Bostian, K. E.: Congenital anomalies associated with idiopathic mental retardation, J. Pediatr. 65:189-196, 1964.
40. Willis, R. A.: The borderland of embryology and pathology, ed. 2, London, 1962, Butterworth & Co. (Publishers), Ltd.

Nonspecificity of abnormalities and patterns of abnormalities

41. Cohen, M. M., Jr.: Human dysmorphic syndromes. (To be published.)
42. Opitz, J. M., Herrmann, J., and Dieker, H.: The study of malformation syndromes in man, Birth Defects 5:1-10, 1969.

Mental deficiency

43. Kaveggia, E. G., Durkin, M. V., Pendleton, E., and Opitz, J. M.: Diagnostic/genetic studies on 1,224 patients with severe mental retardation, Proceedings of the Third Congress of the International Association for the Scientific Study of Mental Deficiency, The Hague, 1973.
44. Smith, D. W., and Simons, F. E. R.: Rational diagnostic evaluation of the child with mental deficiency, Am. J. Dis. Child. 129:1285-1290, 1975.

Abnormalities of growth and development

45. Cohen, M. M., Jr., and Lemire, R. J.: Malformations of the extremities, In Kelley, V. C., editor: Brennemann's practice of pediatrics, vol. 4, New York, 1976, Harper & Row, Publishers, Inc.
46. Poznanski, A. K., Garn, S. M., Kuhns, L. R., and Sandusky, S. T.: Dysharmonic maturation of the hand in the congenital malformation syndromes, Am. J. Phys. Anthropol. 35:417-432, 1971.
47. Poznanski, A. K., Garn, S. M., Nagy, J. M., and Gall, J. C., Jr.: Metacarpophalangeal pattern profiles in the evaluation of skeletal malformations, Radiology 104:1-11, 1972.
48. Smith, D. W.: Growth deficiency: a new classification into primary cellular growth deficiency and secondary humoral growth

deficiency, South. Med. J. (Suppl.) 64:5-15, 1971.
49. Warkany, J., Monroe, B. B., and Sutherland, B. S.: Intrauterine growth retardation, Am. J. Dis. Child. 102:249-261, 1961.

Neoplasia

50. Baikie, G. G., Court Brown, W. M., Buckton, K. E., and Harnden, D. G.: Two cases of leukemia and a case of sex chromosome abnormality in the same sibship, Lancet 2:1003, 1961.
51. Beckwith, J. B., and Perrin, E. V.: In situ neuroblastoma—a contribution to the natural history of neural crest tumors, Am. J. Pathol. 43:1089-1104, 1963.
52. Cervenka, J., and Koulischer, L.: Chromosomes and Cancer, Springfield, Ill., 1973, Charles C Thomas, Publisher.
53. Cohen, M. M., Jr.: Syndromes with hamartomas and neoplasms. (To be published.)
54. German, J., editor: Chromosomes and cancer, New York, 1974, John Wiley & Sons, Inc.
55. Mamumes, P., Lapidus, P. H., Abbott, F. A., and Roath, S.: Acute leukemia and Klinefelter's syndrome, Lancet 2:26-27, 1962.
56. Sloane, J. A., and Hubbell, M. M.: Soft tissue sarcomas in children associated with congenital anomalies, Cancer 23:175-182, 1969.
57. Sy, W. M., and Edmonson, J. H.: The developmental defects associated with neuroblastoma—etiologic implications, Cancer 22:234-238, 1968.

Syndromes

58. Gorlin, R. J., Pindborg, J. J., and Cohen, M. M., Jr.: Syndromes of the head and neck, ed. 2, New York, 1976, McGraw-Hill Book Co.
59. Holmes, L. B., Moser, H. W., Halldórsson, S., et al.: Mental retardation: an atlas of diseases with associated physical abnormalities, New York, 1972, The Macmillan Co.
60. Smith, D. W.: Recognizable patterns of human malformation, ed. 2, Philadelphia, 1976, W. B. Saunders Co.

Achondroplasia

61. Cohen, M. M., et al.: Neurological abnormalities in achondroplastic children, J. Pediatr. 71:367-376, 1967.
62. Dennis, J. P., et al.: Megencephaly, internal hydrocephalus and other neurological aspects of achondroplasia, Brain 84:427-445, 1961.
63. Hall, J. G., et al.: Two probable cases of homozygosity for the achondroplasia gene, Birth Defects 5(4):24-34, 1969.
64. Langer, L. O., et al.: Achondroplasia, Am. J. Roentgenol. 100:12-26, 1967.

65. Mackler, B., et al.: Oxidative energy deficiency. II. Human achondroplasia, Arch. Biochem. Biophys. **159**:885-888, 1973.

66. Maroteaux, P., and Lamy, M.: Achondroplasia in man and animals, Clin. Orthop. **33**:91-103, 1964.

67. McKusick, V. A., et al.: Observations suggesting allelism of the achondroplasia and hypochondroplasia genes, J. Med. Genet. **10**:11-16, 1973.

68. Murdoch, J. L., et al.: Achondroplasia—a genetic and statistical survey, Ann. Hum. Genet. **33**:227-244, 1970.

69. Opitz, J. M.: Delayed mutation in achondroplasia? Birth Defects **5**(5):20-23, 1969.

70. Rimoin, D. L.: Histopathology and ultrastructure of cartilage in the chondrodystrophies, Birth Defects **10**(9):1-18, 1974.

71. Rimoin, D. L., et al.: Somatic mosaicism in an achondroplastic dwarf, Birth Defects **5**(4):17-19, 1969.

72. Rimoin, D. L., et al.: Endochondral ossification in achondroplastic dwarfism, N. Engl. J. Med. **283**:728-735, 1970.

Beckwith-Wiedemann syndrome

73. Beckwith, J. B.: Extreme Cytomegaly of the adrenal fetal cortex, omphalocele, hyperplasia of kidneys and pancreas, and Leydig-cell hyperplasia: another syndrome? Presented at Annual Meeting of Western Society for Pediatric Research, Los Angeles, 1963.

74. Beckwith, J. B.: Macroglossia, omphalocele, adrenal cytomegaly, gigantism, and hyperplastic visceromegaly, Birth Defects **5**(2):188-196, 1969.

75. Cohen, M. M., Jr.: Comments on the macroglossia-omphalocele syndrome, Birth Defects **5**(2):197, 1969.

76. Cohen, M. M., Jr.: Macroglossia, omphalocele, visceromegaly, cytomegaly of the adrenal cortex and neonatal hypoglycemia, Birth Defects **7**:226-232, 1971.

77. Cohen, M. M., Jr., et al.: The Beckwith-Wiedemann syndrome: seven new cases, Am. J. Dis. Child. **122**:515-520, 1971.

78. Combs, J. T., et al.: New syndrome of neonatal hypoglycemia, N. Engl. J. Med. **275**:236-243, 1966.

79. Filippi, C., and McKusick, V. A.: Beckwith-Wiedemann syndrome (exomphalos-macroglossia-gigantism syndrome): report of two cases and review of the literature, Medicine **49**:279-298, 1970.

80. Irving, I.: Exomphalos with macroglossia: a study of 11 cases, J. Pediatr. Surg. **2**:499-507, 1967.

81. Irving, I.: The E.M.G. syndrome (exomphalos, macroglossia, gigantism). In Rickham, P. P., Hacker, W. C., and Prevolt, J., editors, Progress in pediatrics, vol. 1, Munich, Germany, 1970, Urban Schwarzenberg, pp. 1-61.

82. Kosseff, A. L., et al.: The Wiedemann-Beckwith syndrome: genetic considerations and a diagnostic sign, Lancet **1**:844, 1972.

83. Lubinsky, M., et al.: Autosomal dominant sex-dependent transmission of the Wiedemann-Beckwith syndrome, Lancet **1**:932, 1974.

84. Sotelo-Avila, C.: Personal communication, 1975.

85. Sotelo-Avila, C., and Singer, D. B.: Syndrome of hyperplastic fetal visceromegaly and neonatal hypoglycemia (Beckwith's syndrome): a report of seven cases, Pediatrics **46**:240-251, 1970.

86. Thorburn, M. J., et al.: Exomphalos-macroglossia-gigantism syndrome in Jamaican infants, Am. J. Dis. Child. **119**:316-321, 1970.

87. Wiedemann, H. R.: Complexe malformatif familial avec hernie ombilicale et macroglossie—un syndrome nouveau? J. Génét. Hum. **13**:223-232, 1964.

88. Wiedemann, H. R.: Das EMG Syndrom: Exomphalos, Makroglossie, Gigantismus und Kohlenhydratstoffwechselstörung, Z. Kinderheilkd. **102**:1-36, 1968.

89. Wiedemann, H. R.: Über das "Kerbenohr" beim Exomphalos-Makroglossie-Gigantismus Syndrom, über Ohrläppchen-Fisteln und über das Vorkommen entsprechender Erscheinungen bei anderweitigen Syndromen sowie bei Gesenden, Z. Kinderheilkd. **115**:95-110, 1973.

90. Wiedemann, H. R.: Exomphalos-Makroglossie-Gigantismus-Syndrom, Berardinelli-Seip-Syndrom und Sotos-Syndrom—ein vergleichende Betractung unter ausgewählten Aspekten, Z. Kinderheilkd. **115**:193-207, 1973.

91. Wiedemann, H. R., et al.: Über das Syndrom Exomphalos-Makroglossie-Gigantismus, über generalisierte Muskelhypertrophie, progressive Lipodystrophie und Miescher-Syndrom im Sinne diencephaler Syndrome, Z. Kinderheilkd. **102**:1-36, 1968.

Branchial arch syndromes

92. Bergsma, D.: Case report 28: syndrome identification **31**:7-13, 1975.

93. Berkman, M. D., and Feingold, M.: Oculoauriculovertebral dysplasia (Goldenhar's syndrome), Oral Surg. **25**:408-417, 1968.

94. Berry, G. A.: Note on a congenital defect (coloboma?) of the lower lid, R. Lond. Ophthalmol. Hosp. Rep. **12**:255-257, 1889.

95. Bock, R. H.: Ein Fall von epibulbarem Dermolipom mit Missbildungen einer Ge-

sichtshälfte. Diskordantes Vorkommen bei einem eineiigen Zweillingspaar, Ophthalmologica **122**:86-90, 1961.

96. Cohen, M. M., Jr.: Variability versus "incidental findings" in the first and second branchial arch syndrome: unilateral variants with anophthalmia, Birth Defects **7**(7):103-108, 1971.

97. Collins, E. T.: Cases with symmetrical congenital notches in the outer part of each lid and defective development of the malar bones, Trans. Ophthalmol. Soc. U.K. **20**: 190-192, 1900.

98. Franceschetti, A., and Klein, D.: Mandibulofacial dysostosis: new hereditary syndrome, Acta Ophthalmol. (Kbh.) **27**:143-224, 1949.

99. Franceschetti, A., et al.: Dysostose mandibulo-facial unilatérale avec déformations multiples du squelette (processus paramastöide, synostose des vertèbres, sacralisation, etc.) et torricolis clonique, Ophthalmologica **118**:796-814, 1949.

100. Franceschetti, A., et al.: La dysostose mandibulo-faciale dans le cadre des syndrome du premier arc branchial, Schweiz. Med. Wochenschr. **89**:478-483, 1959.

101. François, J., and Haustrate, L.: Anomalies colobomateuses du globe oculaire et syndrome du premier arc, Ann. Ocul. (Paris) **187**:340-368, 1954.

102. Goldenhar, M.: Association malformatives de l'oeil et de l'oreille, en particulier le syndrome dermoide epibulbaire–appendices auriculaires–fistula auris congenita et ses relations avec la dysostose mandibulofaciale, J. Génét. Hum. **1**:243-282, 1952.

103. Gorlin, R. J., et al.: Oculoauriculovertebral syndrome, J. Pediatr. **63**:991-999, 1963.

104. Grabb, W. C.: The first and second branchial arch syndrome, Plast. Reconstr. Surg. **36**:485-508, 1965.

105. Greenwood, R. D., et al.: Cardiovascular malformations in oculoauriculovertebral dysplasia (Goldenhar syndrome), J. Pediatr. **85**:816-821, 1974.

106. Gross, W.: Ein Fall von Agenesie der lunken Lunge, Beitr. Pathol. Anat. **37**:487-501, 1905.

107. Herrmann, J., and Opitz, J. M.: A dominantly inherited first arch syndrome, Birth Defects **5**(2):110-112, 1969.

108. Herrmann, J., et al.: Acrofacial dysostosis type Nager, Birth Defects. (In press.)

109. Kirke, D. K.: Goldenhar's syndrome: two cases of oculoauriculo-vertebral dysplasia occurring in full-blood Australian aboriginal sisters, Aust. Paediatr. J. **6**:213-214, 1970.

110. Klein, D., et al.: Sur un forme extensive de dysostose mandibulo-faciale (Franceschetti)

accompagnée de malformations des extremitiés), Rev. Otoneurophtalmol. **42**:422-440, 1970.

111. Krause, V. H.: The syndrome of Goldenhar affecting two siblings, Acta Ophthalmol. (Kbh.) **48**:494-499, 1970.

112. Ladekarl, S.: Combination of Goldenhar's syndrome with the cri-du-chat syndrome, Acta Ophthalmol. (Kbh.) **46**:605-610, 1968.

113. Mandelcorn, M. S., et al.: Goldenhar's syndrome and phocomelia, Am. J. Ophthalmol. **72**:618-621, 1971.

114. Manfredini, U.: Le considett sindrome del primo acro branchiale, Ann. Ottal. **91**:689-704, 1965.

115. Nager, F. R., and de Reynier, J. P.: Das Gehörorgan bei den angeborenen Kopfmissbildungen, Pract. Otorhinolaryngol. (Basel), Suppl. 2, **10**:1-128, 1948.

116. Opitz, J. M., and Faith, G. C.: Visceral anomalies in an infant with the Goldenhar syndrome, Birth Defects **5**(2):104-105, 1969.

117. Parish, J. G.: Treacher Collins syndrome with features of the Marfan syndrome, Proc. R. Soc. Med. **53**:515, 1960.

118. Pashayan, H., et al.: Hemifacial microsomia: oculoauriculo-vertebral syndrome: a patient with overlapping features, J. Med. Genet. **7**:185-188, 1970.

119. Poswillo, D.: The pathogenesis of the first and second branchial arch syndrome, Oral Surg. **35**:302-329, 1973.

120. Poswillo, D.: Otomandibular deformity: pathogenesis as a guide to reconstruction, J. Maxillofacial Surg. **2**:64-72, 1974.

121. Poswillo, D.: The pathogenesis of the Treacher Collins syndrome (mandibulo-facial dysostosis), Br. J. Oral Surg. **13**:1-26, 1975.

122. Proto, F., and Scullica, L.: Contributo allo studio della ereditarieta dei dermoidi epibulbari, Acta Genet. Med. (Roma) **15**:351-363, 1966.

123. Rovin, S., et al.: Mandibulofacial dysostosis: a familial study of five generations, J. Pediatr. **65**:215-221, 1964.

124. Saraux, H., et al.: À propos d'une observation familiale de syndrome de Franceschetti-Goldenhar, Bull. Soc. Ophtalmol. Fr. **63**: 705-707, 1963.

125. Sugar, H. S.: An unusual example of the oculoauriculo-vertebral dysplasia syndrome of Goldenhar, J. Pediatr. Ophthalmol. **4**: 9-12, 1967.

126. Sugiura, Y.: Congenital absence of the radius with hemifacial microsomia, ventricular septal defect and crossed renal ectopia, Birth Defects **7**(7):109-116, 1971.

127. Summitt, R.: Familial Goldenhar syndrome, Birth Defects **5**:(2):106-109, 1969.

128. ter Haar, B.: Oculo-auriculo-vertebral dysplasia (Goldenhar's syndrome) concordant in identical twins, Acta Med. Genet. (Roma) **21:**116-124, 1972.

129. Vatre, J.: Étude génétique et classification clinique de 154 cas de dysostose mandibulo-faciale (syndrome de Francechetti) avec description de leurs associations malformatives, J. Genet. Hum. **10:**17-1000, 1971.

130. Walker, F. A.: Apparent autosomal recessive inheritance of the Treacher Collins syndrome, Birth Defects **10**(8):135-139, 1974.

131. Weyers, H., and Thier, C. J.: Malformations mandibulo-faciales et délimitation d'un syndrome oculo-vertébral, J. Génét. Hum. **7:** 143-173, 1958.

132. Wildervanck, L. S.: Dysostosis mandibulofacialis (Francechetti-Zwahlen) in four generations, Acta Genet. Med. (Roma) **9:** 447-451, 1960.

Cerebral gigantism

133. Abraham, J. M., and Snodgrass, G.: Sotos' syndrome of cerebral gigantism, Arch. Dis. Child. **44:**203-210, 1969.

134. Bejar, R. L., et al.: Cerebral gigantism: concentrations of amino acids in plasma and muscle, J. Pediatr. **76:**105-111, 1970.

135. Cohen, M. I.: Cerebral gigantism in childhood, N. Engl. J. Med. **271:**635, 1964.

136. Cohen, M. M., Jr.: Diagnostic problems in cerebral gigantism, J. Med. Genet. **13:**80, 1976.

137. Hook, E. B., and Reynolds, J. W.: Cerebral gigantism, J. Pediatr. **70:**900-914, 1967.

138. Jaeken, J., et al.: Cerebral gigantism syndrome, Z. Kinderheilkd. **112:**332-346, 1972.

139. Kjellman, B.: Cerebral gigantism, Acta Paediatr. Scand. **54:**603-609, 1965.

140. Kowlessar, M.: Cerebral gigantism, abnormal urinary corticoid excretion, Minn. Med. **48:**1610-1614, 1965.

141. Ludwig, G. D., et al.: Cerebral gigantism with intermittent fractional hypopituitarism and normal sella turcica, Ann. Intern. Med. **67:**123-131, 1967.

142. Marie, J., et al.: Gigantisme avec encéphalopathie et dysmorphie craniofaciale, Ann. Pediatr. **12:**682-691, 1965.

143. Milunsky, A., et al.: Cerebral gigantism in childhood, Pediatrics **40:**395-402, 1967.

Cleft lip–cleft palate syndromes

144. Aduss, H., and Pruzansky, S.: Postnatal craniofacial development in children with the OFD syndrome, Arch. Oral Biol. **9:** 193-203, 1954.

145. Bixler, D., et al.: The ectrodactyly-ectodermal dysplasia-clefting (EEC) syndrome, Clin. Genet. **3:**43-51, 1971.

146. Brill, C. B., et al.: The syndrome of ectrodactyly, ectodermal dysplasia and cleft lip and palate, Clin. Genet. **3:**293-302, 1972.

147. Brunn, C.: Et tilfaelde af dysplasia acrodentalis, Tandlaegebladet **72:**162-167, 1968.

148. Bystrom, E. B., et al.: The syndrome of ectrodactyly ectodermal dysplasia and clefting (EEC), J. Oral Surg. **33:**192-198, 1975.

149. Cervenka, J., et al.: The syndrome of pits of the lower lip and cleft lip and/or palate: genetic considerations, Am. J. Hum. Genet. **19:**416-432, 1967.

150. Cohen, M. M., Jr.: The Robin anomalad—its nonspecificity and associated syndromes, J. Oral Surg. **34:**587-593, 1976.

151. Dodge, J. A., and Kernohan, D. C.: Oral-facial-digital syndrome, Arch. Dis. Child. **42:** 214-219, 1967.

152. Doege, T. C., et al.: Studies of a family with the oral-facial-digital syndrome, N. Engl. J. Med. **271:**1073-1080, 1964.

153. Doege, T. C., et al.: Mental retardation and dermatoglyphics in a family with the oral-facial-digital syndrome, Am. J. Dis. Child. **116:**615-622, 1968.

154. Dudding, B. A., et al.: The oto-palato-digital syndrome, Am. J. Dis. Child. **113:**214-221, 1967.

155. Fried, K.: Ectrodactyly-ectodermal dysplasia syndrome, Clin. Genet. **3:**396-400, 1972.

156. Fuhrmann, W., et al.: Das oro-facio-digitale Syndrom, Humangenetik **2:**133-164, 1966.

157. Gall, J. C., Jr., et al.: Oto-palato-digital syndrome: comparison of clinical and radiographic manifestations in males and females, Am. J. Hum. Genet. **24:**24-36, 1972.

158. Gorlin, R. J.: The oral-facial-digital (OFD) syndrome, Cutis **4:**1345-1349, 1968.

159. Gorlin, R. J., Cervenka, J., and Pruzansky, S.: Facial clefting and its syndromes, Birth Defects **7:**3-49, 1971.

160. Gorlin, R. J., Pindborg, J. J., and Cohen, M. M., Jr.: Syndromes of the hand and neck, ed. 2, New York, 1976, McGraw-Hill Book Co.

161. Gorlin, R. J., and Psaume, J.: Orodigitofacial dysostosis: a new syndrome: a study of 22 cases, J. Pediatr. **61:**520-530, 1962.

162. Gorlin, R. J., et al.: The oto-palato-digital (OPD) syndrome in females: heterozygotic expression of an X-linked trait, Oral Surg. **35:**218-224, 1973.

163. Herrmann, J., et al.: The Stickler syndrome (hereditary arthroophthalmopathy), Birth Defects **11:**76-103, 1975.

164. Langer, L. O.: The roentgenologic features of the oto-palato-digital (OPD) syndrome, Am. J. Roentgenol. **100:**63-70, 1967.

165. Mohr, O. L.: A hereditary sublethal syn-

drome in man, Nor. Vidensk. Akad. Oslo I. Mat.-Naturv. Klasse **14:**1-18, 1941.

166. Papillon-Leage (Mme.) and Psaume, J.: Une malformation héréditaire de la muqeuse buccale et freins anormaux, Rev. Stomatol. (Paris) **55:**209-227, 1954.

167. Pashayan, H. M., et al.: The EEC syndrome, Birth Defects **10:**105-127, 1974.

168. Pfeiffer, R. A., and Verbeck, C.: Spalthand und Spaltfuss, ektodermale Dysplasie und Lippen-Kiefer-Gaumen-Spalte: ein autosomal dominant vererbtes Syndrom, Z. Kinderheilkd. **115:**235-244, 1973.

169. Pries, C., et al.: The EEC syndrome, Am. J. Dis. Child. **127:**840-844, 1974.

170. Preus, M., and Fraser, F. C.: The lobster claw defect with ectodermal defects, cleft lip–palate, tear duct anomaly and renal anomalies, Clin. Genet. **4:**369-375, 1973.

171. Reed, W. B., et al.: The Reed syndrome, Birth Defects **10**(8):61-73, 1974.

172. Reinwein, H., et al.: Untersuchungen an einer Familie mit Oral-Facial-Digital Syndrom, Humangenetik **2:**165-177, 1966.

173. Rimoin, D. L., and Edgerton, M. T.: Genetic and clinical heterogeneity in the oral-facial-digital syndrome, J. Pediatr. **71:**94-102, 1967.

174. Robinson, G. C., et al.: Ectrodactyly, ectodermal dysplasia and cleft lip–palate syndrome, J. Pediatr. **82:**107-109, 1973.

175. Rudiger, R. A., et al.: Association of ectrodactyly, ectodermal dysplasia and cleft lip–palate: the EEC syndrome, Am. J. Dis. Child. **120:**160-163, 1970.

176. Stah, A., and Fuhrmann, W.: Oro-facio-digitales syndrome, Dtsch. Med. Wochenschr. **93:**1224-1228, 1968.

177. Stickler, G. B., et al.: Hereditary progressive arthroophthalmopathy, Mayo Clin. Proc. **40:**433-455, 1965.

178. Stickler, G. B., and Pugh, D. G.: Hereditary progressive vertebral anomalies, a hearing defect and a report of a similar case, Mayo Clin. Proc. **42:**495-500, 1967.

179. Taybi, H.: Generalized skeletal dysplasia with multiple anomalies, Am. J. Roentgenol. **88:**450-457, 1962.

180. Thuline, H. C.: Current status of a family previously reported with the oral-facial-digital syndrome, Birth Defects **5**(2):102-104, 1969.

181. van der Woude, A.: Fistula labii inferioris congenita and its association with cleft lip and palate, Am. J. Hum. Genet. **6:**244-256, 1954.

182. Wahrman, J., et al.: The oral-facial-digital syndrome: a male lethal condition in a boy with 47/XXY chromosomes, Pediatrics **37:**812-821, 1966.

183. Walker, J. C., and Clodius, L.: The syndromes of cleft lip, cleft palate and lobster-claw deformities of hands and feet, Plast. Reconstr. Surg. **32:**627-636, 1963.

184. Wiegmann, O. A., and Walker, F. A.: The syndrome of lobster claw deformity and nasolacrimal obstruction, J. Pediatr. Ophthalmol. **7:**79-85, 1970.

Cleidocranial dysplasia

185. Eldridge, W. W., et al.: Cleidocranial dysostosis, Am. J. Roentgenol. **34:**41-49, 1935.

186. Fitchet, S. M.: Cleidocranial dysostosis: hereditary and familial, J. Bone Joint Surg. **11:**838-866, 1929.

187. Fitzwilliams, D. C. L.: Hereditary cranio-cleido-dysostosis; with a review of all the published cases of this disease: theories of the development of the clavicle suggested by this condition, Lancet **2:**1466-1475, 1910.

188. Forland, M.: Cleidocranial dysostosis, Am. J. Med. **33:**792-799, 1962.

189. Job, J. C., et al.: La dysostose cleidocrânienne, son polymorphisme, Arch. Fr. Pediatr. **22:**669-686, 1965.

190. Marie, P., and Sainton, P.: Observation d'hydrocéphalie héréditaire (père et fils) par vice de developpement du crâne et du cerveau, Bull. Soc. Med. Hop. Paris **14:**706-712, 1897.

191. Miles, P. W.: Cleidocranial dysostosis: a survey of six new cases and 126 from the literature, J. Kansas Med. Soc. **41:**462-468, 1940.

192. Rushton, M. A.: The dental condition in cleidocranial dysostosis, Guy's Hosp. Rep. **87:**354-361, 1937.

193. Rushton, M. A.: The failure of eruption in cleidocranial dysostosis, Br. Dent. J. **63:**641-645, 1937.

194. Rushton, M. A.: An anomaly of cementum in cleidocranial dysostosis, Br. Dent. J. **100:**81-83, 1956.

195. Schuch, P., and Fleischer-Peters, A.: Zur Klinik der Dysostosis cleidocranialis, Z. Kinderheilkd. **98:**107-132, 1967.

196. Soule, A. B., Jr.: Mutational dysostosis, J. Bone Joint Surg. **28:**81-102, 1946.

197. Winkler, H.: Ein eigenartiger Fall von Dysostosis cleidocranialis bei einem siebenjahrigen Kinde, Jb. Kinderheilkd. **149:**238-260, 1937.

198. Winter, G. R.: Dental conditions in cleidocranial dysostosis, Am. J. Orthodont. **29:**61-89, 1943.

Craniocarpotarsal dysplasia

199. Burian, F.: The "whistling face" characteristic in a compound cranio-facio-carpal syndrome, Br. J. Plast. Surg. **16:**140-163, 1963.

200. Cervenka, J., et al.: Cranio-carpo-tarsal dysplasia or the whistling face syndrome. II. Oral intercommissural distance in children, Am. J. Dis. Child. **117**:434-435, 1969.

201. Cervenka, J., et al.: Craniocarpotarsal dysplasia or whistling face syndrome, Arch. Otolaryngol. **91**:183-187, 1970.

202. Fraser, F. C., et al.: Cranio-carpo-tarsal dysplasia, J.A.M.A. **211**:1374-1376, 1970.

203. Freeman, E. A., and Sheldon, J. H.: Cranio-carpo-tarsal dystrophy—an undescribed congenital malformation, Arch. Dis. Child. **13**:277-283, 1938.

204. Pfeiffer, R. A., et al.: Das Syndrom von Freeman und Sheldon, Z. Kinderheilkd. **112**:43-53, 1972.

205. Weinstein, S., and Gorlin, R. J.: Cranio-carpo-tarsal dysplasia or the whistling face syndrome. I. Clinical considerations, Am. J. Dis. Child. **117**:427-433, 1969.

Craniosynostosis syndromes

206. Bartsocas, C. S., et al.: Chotzen's syndrome, J. Pediatr. **77**:267-272, 1970.

207. Bergstrom, L., Neblett, L. M., and Hemenway, W. G.: Otologic manifestations of acrocephalosyndactyly, Arch. Otolaryngol. **96**:117-123, 1972.

208. Bertelsen, T. I.: The premature synostosis of the cranial sutures, Acta Ophthalmol. (Suppl.), vol. 51, 1958.

209. Blank, C. E.: Apert's syndrome (a type of acrocephalosyndactyly): observations on a British series of thirty-nine cases, Ann. Hum. Genet. **24**:151-164, 1960.

210. Cohen, M. M., Jr.: Cardiovascular anomalies in Apert type acrocephalosyndactyly, Birth Defects **8**:132-133, 1972.

211. Cohen, M. M., Jr.: The Kleeblattschädel phenomenon—sign or syndrome? Am. J. Dis. Child. **124**:944, 1972.

212. Cohen, M. M., Jr.: An etiologic and nosologic overview of craniosynostosis syndromes, Birth Defects **11**:137-189, 1975.

213. Crouzon, O.: Dysostose cranio-faciale héréditaire, Arch. Med. Enf. **18**:529-539, 1915.

214. Crouzon, O.: Une nouvelle famille atteinte de dysostose cranio-faciale héréditaire, Arch. Med. Enf. **18**:540-543, 1915.

215. Erickson, J. D., and Cohen, M. M., Jr.: A study of parental age effects on the occurrence of fresh mutations for the Apert syndrome, Ann. Hum. Genet. **38**:89-96, 1974.

216. Fishman, M. A., Hogan, G. R., and Dodge, P. R.: The concurrence of hydrocephalus and craniosynostosis, J. Neurosurg. **34**:621-629, 1971.

217. Gorlin, R. J., Pindborg, J. J., and Cohen, M. M., Jr.: Syndromes of the head and neck, ed. 2, New York, 1976, McGraw-Hill Book Co.

218. Herrmann, J., Pallister, P. D., and Opitz, J. M.: Craniosynostosis and craniosynostosis syndromes, Rocky Mt. Med. J. **66**:45-56, 1969.

219. Hogan, G. R., and Bauman, M. L.: Hydrocephalus in Apert's syndrome, J. Pediatr. **79**:782-787, 1971.

220. Hoover, G. H., Flatt, A. E., and Weiss, M. W.: The hand and Apert's syndrome, J. Bone Joint Surg. **52A**:878-895, 1970.

221. Jones, K. L., and Cohen, M. M., Jr.: The Crouzon syndrome, J. Med. Genet. **10**:398, 1973.

222. Kreigborg, S., et al.: The Saethre-Chotzen syndrome, Teratology **6**:287-294, 1972.

223. Martsolf, J. T., Cracco, J. B., Carpenter, G. G., and O'Hara, A. E.: Pfeiffer syndrome, Am. J. Dis. Child. **121**:257-262, 1971.

224. McKusick, V. A.: Mendelian inheritance in man, ed. 3, Baltimore, 1971, The Johns Hopkins University Press.

225. Pantke, O. A., et al.: The Saethre-Chotzen syndrome, Birth Defects **11**:190-225, 1975.

226. Park, E. A., and Power, G. F.: Acrocephaly and scaphocephaly with symmetrically distributed malformations of the extremities, Am. J. Dis. Child. **20**:235-315, 1920.

227. Pfeiffer, R. A.: Dominant erbliche Akrocephalosyndaktylie, Z. Kinderheilkd. **90**:301-320, 1964.

228. Pruzansky, S., et al.: Roentgencephalometric studies of the premature craniofacial synostoses: report of a family with the Saethre-Chotzen syndrome, Birth Defects **11**:226-237, 1975.

229. Roberts, K. B., and Hall, J. G.: Apert's acrocephalosyndactyly in mother and daughter: cleft palate in the mother, Birth Defects **7**:262-264, 1971.

230. Saldino, R. M., Steinbach, H. L., and Epstein, C. J.: Familial acrocephalosyndactyly (Pfeiffer syndrome), Am. J. Roentgenol. **116**:609-617, 1972.

231. Schauerte, E. W., and St.-Aubin, P. M.: Progressive synostosis in Apert's syndrome (acrocephalosyndactyly), Am. J. Roentgenol. **97**:67-73, 1966.

232. Solomon, L. M., Cohen, M. M., Jr., and Pruzansky, S.: Pilosebaceous abnormalities in Apert type acrocephalosyndactyly, Birth Defects **7**:193-195, 1971.

233. Tünte, W., and Lenz, W.: Zur Haufigkeit und Mutationsrate des Apert-Syndroms, Humangenetik **4**:104-111, 1967.

234. Vulliamy, D. G., and Normandale, P. A.: Craniofacial dysostosis in a Dorset family, Arch. Dis. Child. **41**:375-382, 1966.

235. Weech, A. A.: Combined acrocephaly and syndactylism occurring in mother and

daughter, Bull. Johns Hopkins Hosp. **40:** 73-76, 1927.

236. Zippel, H., and Schuler, K.-H.: Dominant vererbte Akrozephalosyndaktylie (ACS), Forschr. Roentgenstr. **110:**234-245, 1969.

Diastrophic dwarfism

237. Amuso, S. J.: Diastrophic dwarfism, J. Bone Joint Surg. **50A:**113-122, 1968.

238. Carpenter, G.: Case of acrocephaly with other congenital malformations, Proc. R. Soc. Med. (Part 1) **2:**45-53, 199-201, 1909.

239. Cohen, M. M., Jr.: An etiologic and nosologic overview of craniosynostosis syndromes, Birth Defects **11**(2):137-189, 1975.

240. Lamy, M., and Maroteaux, P.: Le nanisme diastrophique, Presse Med. **68:**1977-1980, 1960.

241. Langer, L. O.: Diastrophic dwarfism in early infancy, Am. J. Roentgenol. **93:**399-404, 1965.

242. Spranger, J., and Gerken, H.: Diastrophischer Zwergwuchs, Z. Kinderheilkd. **98:** 227-234, 1967.

243. Stover, C. N., et al.: Diastrophic dwarfism, Am. J. Roentgenol. **89:**914-922, 1963.

244. Taybi, H.: Diastrophic dwarfism, Radiology **80:**1-10, 1963.

245. Temtamy, S. A.: Carpenter's syndrome: acrocephalopolysyndactyly, an autosomal recessive syndrome, J. Pediatr. **69:**111-120, 1966.

246. Walker, B. A., et al.: Diastrophic dwarfism, Medicine **51:**41-59, 1972.

247. Wilson, D. W., et al.: Diastrophic dwarfism, Arch. Dis. Child. **44:**48-59, 1969.

Ectodermal dysplasia

248. Everett, F. G., et al.: Anhidrotic ectodermal dysplasia with anodontia: a study of two families, J. Am. Dent. Assoc. **44:**173-186, 1952.

249. Gorlin, R. J., et al.: Hypohidrotic ectodermal dysplasia in females: a critical analysis and argument for genetic heterogeneity, Z. Kinderheilkd. **108:**1-11, 1970.

250. Kerr, C. B., et al.: Genetic effect in carriers of anhidrotic ectodermal dysplasia, J. Med. Genet. **3:**169-176, 1966.

251. Lowry, R. B., et al.: Hereditary ectodermal dysplasia, Clin. Pediatr. **5:**395-402, 1966.

252. Passarge, E. C., et al.: Anhidrotic ectodermal dysplasia as autosomal recessive trait in an inbred kindred, Humangenetik **3:**181-185, 1966.

253. Reed, W. B., et al.: Clinical spectrum of anhidrotic ectodermal dysplasia, Arch. Derm. **102:**134-143, 1970.

254. Weech, A. A.: Hereditary ectodermal dysplasia, Am. J. Dis. Child. **37:**766-790, 1929.

Ellis–van Creveld syndrome

255. Biggerstaff, R. H., and Mazaheri, M.: Oral manifestations of the Ellis–van Creveld syndrome, J. Am. Dent. Assoc. **77:**1090-1095, 1968.

256. Blackburn, M. G., and Belliveau, R. E.: Ellis–van Creveld syndrome: a report of previously undescribed anomalies in two siblings, Am. J. Dis. Child. **122:**267-270, 1971.

257. Douglas, W. F., et al.: Chondroectodermal dysplasia (Ellis–van Creveld syndrome): report of two cases in sibship and review of literature, Am. J. Dis. Child. **97:**472-478, 1959.

258. Ellis, R. W. B., and Andrew, J. D.: Chondroectodermal dysplasia, J. Bone Joint Surg. **44B:**626-636, 1962.

259. Ellis, R. W. B., and van Creveld, S.: A syndrome characterized by ectodermal dysplasia, polydactyly, chondrodysplasia and congenital morbus cordis, Arch. Dis. Child. **15:**65-84, 1940.

260. Lynch, J. I., et al.: Congenital heart disease and chondroectodermal dysplasia, Am. J. Dis. Child. **115:**80-87, 1968.

261. McKusick, V. A., et al.: Dwarfism in the Amish. I. The Ellis–van Creveld syndrome, Bull. Johns Hopkins Hosp. **115:**306-336, 1964.

262. Metrakos, J. D., and Fraser, F. C.: Evidence for a hereditary factor in chondroectodermal dysplasia (Ellis–van Creveld syndrome), Am. J. Hum. Genet. **6:**260-269, 1954.

263. Mitchell, F. N., and Waddell, W. W., Jr.: Ellis–van Creveld syndrome: report of 2 cases in siblings, Acta Paediatr. **47:**142-151, 1958.

Frontonasal dysplasia

264. Burian, F.: Median clefts of the nose, Acta Chir. Plast. (Praha) **2:**180-189, 1960.

265. Cohen, M. M., Jr., et al.: Frontonasal dysplasia (median cleft face syndrome): comments on etiology and pathogenesis, Birth Defects **7**(7):117-119, 1971.

266. deMyer, W.: The median cleft face syndrome: differential diagnosis of cranium bifidum occultum, hypertelorism, and median cleft nose, lip, and palate, Neurology **17:** 961-971, 1967.

267. Peterson, M. Q., et al.: Comments on frontonasal dysplasia, ocular hypertelorism, and dystopia canthorum, Birth Defects **7**(7): 120-124, 1971.

268. Sedano, H. O., et al.: Frontonasal dysplasia, J. Pediatr. **76:**906-913, 1970.

269. Smith, D. W., and Cohen, M. M., Jr.: Widow's peak scalp–hair anomaly and its

relation to ocular hypertelorism, Lancet **2:** 1127-1128, 1973.

270. Warkany, J., et al.: Median cleft face syndrome in half-sisters, Teratology **8:**273-286, 1973.

Gardner syndrome

271. Camiel, M. R., et al.: Thyroid carcinoma with Gardner's syndrome in siblings, N. Engl. J. Med. **278:**1056-1058, 1968.

272. Chang, C. H., et al.: Bone abnormalities in Gardner's syndrome, Am. J. Roentgenol. **102:**645-652, 1968.

273. Coli, R. D., et al.: Gardner's syndrome, Am. J. Dig. Dis. **15:**551-568, 1970.

274. Fader, M., et al.: Gardner's syndrome (intestinal polyposis, osteomas, sebaceous cysts) and a new dental discovery, Oral Surg. **15:** 153-172, 1962.

275. Fitzgerald, G. M.: Multiple composite odontomas coincidental with other tumorous conditions, J. Am. Dent. Assoc. **30:**1408-1417, 1943.

276. Gardner, E. J.: Follow-up study of a family group exhibiting dominant inheritance for a syndrome including intestinal polyposis, osteomas, fibromas and epidermal cysts, Am. J. Hum. Genet. **14:**376-390, 1962.

277. Gardner, E. J., and Richard, R. C.: Multiple cutaneous and subcutaneous lesions occurring simultaneously with hereditary polyposis and osteomatosis, Am. J. Hum. Genet. **5:**139-147, 1953.

278. Gorlin, R. J., and Chaudhry, A. P.: Multiple osteomatosis, fibromas, lipomas, and fibrosarcomas of the skin and mesentery, epidermoid inclusion cysts of the skin, leiomyomas and multiple intestinal polyposis, N. Engl. J. Med. **263:**1151-1158, 1960.

279. McKusick, V. A.: Genetic factors in intestinal polyposis, J.A.M.A. **182:**271-277, 1962.

280. Smith, E. G.: Multiple polyposis, Gardner's syndrome and desmoid tumors, Dis. Colon Rectum **1:**323-332, 1958.

281. Thomas, K. E., et al.: Natural history of Gardner's syndrome, Am. J. Surg. **115:**218-226, 1968.

282. Trygstad, C. W., et al.: Resistance to parathyroid extract of Gardner's syndrome, J. Clin. Endocrinol. **28:**1153-1159, 1968.

Gingival fibromatosis syndromes

283. Cohen, M. M., Jr., Scott, C. R., and Smith, D. W.: A new syndrome with gingival fibromatosis, Syndrome Identification **2:**12-13, 1974.

284. Cross, H. E., et al.: A new oculocerebral syndrome with hypopigmentation, J. Pediatr. **70:**398-406, 1967.

285. Drescher, E., et al.: Juvenile fibromatosis in siblings, J. Pediatr. Surg. **2:**427-430, 1967.

286. Houston, I. B., and Shotts, N.: Rutherford's syndrome: a familial oculodental disorder, Acta Paediatr. Scand. **55:**233-238, 1966.

287. Laband, P. F., et al.: Hereditary gingival fibromatosis: report of an affected family with associated splenomegaly and skeletal and soft tissue abnormalities, Oral Surg. **17:**339-351, 1964.

288. Murray, J.: On three peculiar cases of molluscum fibrosum in one family, Med.-Chir. Trans. Lond. **56:**235-238, 1873.

289. Puretic, S., and Puretic, B.: Clinical and histopathological observations on systemic familial mesenchymatosis, Proceedings of the 13th International Congress on Pediatrics, Vienna, **5:**373-381, 1971.

290. Puretic, S., et al.: An unusual form of mesenchymal dysplasia, Br. J. Dermatol. **74:** 8-19, 1962.

291. Rushton, M. A.: Hereditary or idiopathic hyperplasia of the gums, Dent. Pract. Dent. Rec. **7:**136-146, 1957.

292. Rutherford, M. E.: Three generations of inherited dental defect, Br. Med. J. **2:**9-11, 1931.

293. Witkop, C. J., Jr.: Heterogeneity in gingival fibromatosis, Birth Defects **7:**210-221, 1971.

Gorlin syndrome

294. Abrahams, I.: Basal cell nevus syndrome, Arch. Dermatol. **92:**747-748, 1965.

295. Anderson, D. E.: Linkage analysis of the nevoid basal cell carcinoma syndrome, Ann. Hum. Genet. **32:**113-124, 1968.

296. Anderson, D. E., and Cook, W. A.: Jaw cysts and the basal cell nevus syndrome, J. Oral Surg. **24:**15-26, 1966.

297. Anderson, D. E., Taylor, W. B., Falls, H. F., et al.: The nevoid basal cell carcinoma syndrome, Am. J. Hum. Genet. **19:**12-22, 1967.

298. Anderson, D. E., et al.: Genetics and skin tumors, with special reference to basal cell nevi. In Tumors of the skin, Seventh Annual Clinical Conference on Cancer, pp. 91-127, 1964.

299. Ashbury, H. E., et al.: Roentgenological reports of chest examination made of registrants at U.S. Army Induction Station No. 6, Third Corps Area, Baltimore, Md., May 1, 1941, to March 31, 1942, Am. J. Roentgenol. **48:**345-351, 1942.

300. Bang, G.: Keratocysts, skeletal anomalies, ichthyosis and defective response to parathyroid hormone in a patient with basal cell carcinoma, Oral Surg. **29:**242-248, 1970.

301. Bataille, R., et al.: Deux cas de naevomatose, Rev. Stomatol. **70:**305-306, 1969.

302. Batschwarov, B., and Minkov, D.: Naevo-

basiliom, Mesenterialzysten und Malignom, Derm. Wochenschr. **153**:1294-1302, 1967.

303. Bazex, A., et al.: Epitheliomatose multiple, multiforme generalisée (type Ferrari), Bull. Soc. Fr. Derm. Syph. **67**:72-74, 1960.

304. Beahrs, O. H., et al.: Chylous cysts of the abdomen, Surg. Clin. North Am. **30**:1081-1096, 1950.

305. Becker, M. H., et al.: Basal cell nevus syndrome: its roentgenologic significance: review of the literature and report of four cases, Am. J. Roentgenol. **99**:817-825, 1967.

306. Berlin, N. I., et al.: Basal cell nevus syndrome, Ann. Intern. Med. **64**:403-421, 1966.

307. Binkley, G. W.: Basal cell nevi with bone anomalies and dystopia canthorum, Arch. Dermatol. **9**:104-106, 1964.

308. Binkley, G. W., and Johnson, H. H., Jr.: Epithelioma adenoides cysticum: basal cell nevi, agenesis of corpus callosum and dental cysts, Arch. Dermatol. Syph. (Chic.) **63**:73-84, 1951.

309. Block, J. B., and Clendenning, W. E.: Parathyroid hormone hyporesponsiveness in patients with basal-cell nevi and bone defects, N. Engl. J. Med. **268**:1157-1162, 1963.

310. Bloom, R.: The metacarpal sign, Br. J. Radiol. **43**:133-135, 1970.

311. Bopp, C., et al.: Sindrome nevo baso celular, Rev. Assoc. Med. Rio Grande Sul. **12**:3-19, 1968.

312. Boyer, B. E., and Martin, M. M.: Marfan's syndrome: report of case manifesting giant bone of cyst of mandible and multiple (110) basal cell carcinomata, Plast. Reconstr. Surg. **22**:257-263, 1958.

313. Bramley, P. A., and Browne, R. M.: Recurring odontogenic cysts, Br. J. Oral Surg. **5**:106-116, 1968.

314. Browne, R. M.: The odentogenic keratocyst; histological features and their correlation with clinical behavior, Br. Dent. J. **131**:249-259, 1971.

315. Cairns, R. J.: Commenting on case of G. A. Caron, 1965.

316. Calnan, C. D.: Two cases of multiple naevoid basal cell epitheliomata? Porokeratosis of Mantoux, Br. J. Derm. **65**:219-221, 1953.

317. Carney, R. G.: Linear unilateral basal-cell nevus with comedones: report of case, Arch. Dermatol. Syph. (Chic.) **65**:471-476, 1952.

318. Caron, G. A.: Basal cell naevi with a neurological syndrome, Proc. R. Soc. Med. **58**:621-622, 1965.

319. Cawson, R. A., and Kerr, G. A.: The syndrome of jaw cysts, basal cell tumors and skeletal anomalies, Proc. R. Soc. Med. **57**:799-801, 1964.

320. Cernea, P., et al.: Naevomatose baso-cellulaire, Rev. Stomatol. **70**:181-226, 1969.

321. Clarkson, P., and Wilson, H.: Two cases of basal-cell congenital naevus, Proc. R. Soc. Med. **53**:295-296, 1960.

322. Clendenning, W. E., Block, J. B., and Radde, I. G.: Basal cell nevus syndrome, Arch. Dermatol. **90**:38-53, 1964.

323. Clendenning, W. E., Herdt, J. R., and Block, J. B.: Ovarian fibromas and mesenteric cysts; their association with hereditary basal cell cancer of skin, Am. J. Obstet. Gynecol. **87**:1008-1012, 1963.

324. Cook, W. A.: Family pedigree—cancer, cysts and oligodontia, Dent. Radiogr. Photogr. **37**:27-35, 1964.

325. Davidson, F.: Multiple naevoid basal cell carcinomata and associated congenital abnormalities, Br. J. Dermatol. **74**:439-444, 1962.

326. Davidson, F., and Key, J. J.: Multiple nevoid basal cell carcinomata and associated congenital abnormalities, Proc. R. Soc. Med. **57**:891, 1964.

327. Degos, R., et al.: Naevus Baso-Cellulaire, Bull. Soc. Fr. Dermatol. Syph. **73**:360-361, 1966.

328. Dyke, C. G.: Indirect signs of brain tumor as noted in routine roentgeno-examination: displacement of the pineal shadow: a survey of 3000 consecutive skull examinations, Am. J. Roentgenol. **23**:598, 1930.

329. Eisenbud, L., et al.: Klippel-Feil syndrome with multiple cysts of jawbones, Oral Surg. **5**:659-666, 1952.

330. Elejalde, B. R.: Personal communication, 1975.

331. Ellis, D. J., et al.: Nevoid basal cell carcinoma syndrome: report of case, J. Oral Surg. **30**:851-854, 1972.

332. Etter, L. E.: Osseous abnormalities of thoracic cage seen in 40,000 consecutive chest roentgenograms, Am. J. Roentgenol. **51**:359-363, 1944.

333. Ferrier, P. E., and Hinrichs, W. L.: Basal cell carcinoma syndrome, Am. J. Dis. Child. **113**:538-545, 1967.

334. Formas, I.: Naevobasaliom, Z. Haut. Geschlechtskr. **42**:131-140, 1967.

335. Gerber, N. J.: Zur Pathologie und Genetik des Basalzell-Naevus Snydroms, Humangenetik **1**:354-373, 1967.

336. Giansanti, J. S., and Baker, G. O.: Nevoid basal cell carcinoma syndrome in Negroes: report of five cases, J. Oral Surg. **32**:138-144, 1974.

337. Gilhous-Moe, O., et al.: The syndrome of multiple cysts of the jaws, basal cell carcinomata and skeletal anomalies, Br. J. Oral Surg. **6**:211-222, 1968.

338. Gorlin, R. J., and Goltz, R. W.: Multiple nevoid basal-cell epithelioma, jaw cysts and

bifid rib syndrome, N. Engl. J. Med. **262:** 908-912, 1960.

339. Gorlin, R. J., and Sedano, H. O.: The multiple nevoid basal cell carcinoma syndrome revisited, Birth Defects 7:140-148, 1971.

340. Gorlin, R. J., and Sedano, H. O.: Multiple nevoid basal cell carcinoma syndrome. In Vinken, P. J., and Bruyn, G. W., editors: Handbook of clinical neurology: the phakomatoses, vol. 14, New York, 1973, American Elsevier Publishing Co., Inc., pp. 455-473.

341. Gorlin, R. J., Vickers, R. A., Kellen, E., et al.: The multiple basal-cell nevi syndrome: an analysis of a syndrome consisting of multiple nevoid basal-cell carcinoma, jaw cysts, skeletal anomalies, medulloblastoma, and hyporesponsiveness to parathormone, Cancer 18:89-104, 1965.

342. Gorlin, R. J., Yunis, J. J., and Tuna, N.: Multiple nevoid basal cell carcinoma, odontogenic keratocysts and skeletal anomalies: a syndrome, Acta Dermatovener. (Stockh.) **43:** 39-55, 1963.

343. Graham, J. K., McJimsey, B. A., and Hardin, J. C., Jr.: Nevoid basal cell carcinoma syndrome, Arch. Otolaryngol. 87:72-77, 1968.

344. Graham, J. K., et al: Differentiation of nevoid basal-cell carcinoma from epithelioma adenoides cysticum, J. Invest. Dermatol. **44:** 197-200, 1965.

345. Gross, P. P.: Epithelioma adenoides cysticum with follicular cysts of maxilla and mandible: report of case, J. Oral Surg. **11:**160-165, 1953.

346. Gunderson, C. H.: The Klippel-Feil syndrome: genetic and clinical re-evaluation of cervical fusion, Medicine (Baltimore) ⟨6: 491-512, 1967.

347. Happle, R.: Neurofibroma and nevoid basal cell carcinoma, Arch. Dermatol. **108:**582-583, 1973.

348. Heidrich, R., and Kustner, R.: Über Falxverkalkungen, Fortschr. Roentgenstr. **107:** 402-405, 1967.

349. Hermans, E. H., et al.: Eine Fünfte Phakomatosis; Naevus Epitheliomatodes Multiplex, Hautarzt **11:**160-164, 1960.

350. Herzberg, J. J., and Wiskemann, A.: Die fünfte Phakomatose, Basalzellnaevus mit familiärer Belastung und Medulloblastom, Dermatologica **126:**106-173, 1963.

351. Holubar, K., et al.: Multiple basal-cell epitheliomas in basal cell nevus syndrome, Arch. Dermatol. **101:**679-682, 1970.

352. Howell, J. B., Anderson, D. E., and McClendon, J. L.: Multiple cutaneous cancers in children: the nevoid basal cell carcinoma syndrome, J. Pediatr. **69:**97-103, 1966.

353. Howell, J. B., and Caro, M. R.: Basal-cell nevus; its relationship to multiple cutaneous cancers and associated anomalies of development, Arch. Dermatol. **79:**67-80, 1959.

354. Howell, J. B., and Mehregan, A. H.: Pursuit of the pits in the nevoid basal cell carcinoma syndrome, Arch. Dermatol. **102:**583-597, 1970.

355. Hundeiker, M., and Petres, J.: Zur Klassifizierung und Differential-Diagnose multipler Basaliome, Dermatol. Wochenschr. **154:**169-176, 1968.

356. Jablonska, S.: Basaliome naevoider Herkunft (Naevo-Basaliome bzw. Basalzell-Naevi), Hautarzt **12:**147-157, 1961.

357. Jarisch: Zur Lehre von den Hautgeschwülsten, Arch. Dermatol. Syph. **28:**163-222, 1894.

358. Jones, J. E., et al.: The nevoid basal-cell carcinoma syndrome, Arch. Int. Med. **115:** 723-729, 1965.

359. Kahn, L. B., and Gordon, W.: Basal cell naevus syndrome, S. Afr. Med. J. **41:**832-835, 1967.

360. Kaufman, R. L., and Chase, L. R.: Normal stimulation of cyclic 3′,5′-AMP by parathormone, Birth Defects 7(8):149-155, 1971.

361. Kedem, A.: Basal cell nevus syndrome associated with malignant melanoma of the iris, Dermatologica **140:**99-106, 1970.

362. Keen, R. R.: Multiple basal-cell nevoid syndrome: report of two cases, J. Oral Surg. 27:404-408, 1969.

363. Kennedy, J. W., and Abbott, P. L.: Nevoid basal-cell carcinoma syndrome, Oral Surg. 26:406-414, 1968.

364. Kirsch, T.: Pathogenetische Beziehungen zwischen Kieferzysten und Hautveränderungen unter besonderer Berücksichtigung der Hautkarzinomatose, Schweiz. Monatsschr. Zahnheilkd. **66:**687-701, 1956.

365. Kopp, W. K., et al.: Basal cell nevus syndrome with other abnormalities, Oral Surg. 27:9-14, 1969.

366. Laugier, P., et al.: Syndrome naevique à prédominance baso-cellulaire (5e phacomatose), Ann. Dermatol. Syphiligr. (Paris) **93:** 361-372, 1966.

367. Lausecker, H.: Beitrag zu den Naevo-Epitheliomen, Arch. Derm. **194:**639-666, 1952.

368. Lehnert, K.: Multiple Kieferzysten bei Atherom der Mundschleimhaut und hyperkeratotischen Hautveränderungen; kasuistischer Beitrag zur Ätiologie der Kieferzysten, Dtsch. Zahnaertzl. Z. **10:**214-219, 1955.

369. Lile, H. A., et al.: The basal cell nevus syndrome, Am. J. Roentgenol. **103:**214-218, 1968.

370. Lipshutz, H., and Abramson, B.: Basal cell nevus syndrome in a Negro: case report, Plast. Reconstr. Surg. **47:**293-294, 1971.

371. Maddox, W. D.: Multiple basal cell tumors, jaw cysts and skeletal defects: a clinical syndrome, Thesis, Minneapolis, 1962, University of Minnesota.

372. Maddox, W. D., et al.: Multiple nevoid basal cell epitheliomata, jaw cysts and skeletal defects, J.A.M.A. 188:106-111, 1964.

373. Mason, J. K., et al.: Pathology of the nevoid basal cell carcinoma syndrome, Arch. Pathol. 79:401-408, 1965.

374. McEvoy, B. F., and Gatzek, H.: Multiple nevoid basal cell carcinoma syndrome: radiologic manifestations, Br. J. Radiol. 42:24-28, 1969.

375. McKelvey, L. E., et al.: Multiple hereditary familial epithelial cysts of jaws with associated anomaly of trichoepithelioma: report of case, Oral Surg. 13:111-116, 1960.

376. Meerkotter, V. A., and Shear, M.: Multiple primordial cysts associated with bifid rib and ocular defects, Oral Surg. 18:498-503, 1964.

377. Mills, J., and Foulkes, J.: Gorlin's syndrome: a radiological and cytogenetic study of 9 cases, Br. J. Radiol. 40:366-371, 1967.

378. Mordecai, L. R.: Basal cell nevus syndrome, J. Natl. Med. Assoc. 58:32-34, 1966.

379. Moynahan, E. J.: Basal cell nevus syndrome, Trans. St. John's Hosp. Dermatol. Soc. (Lond.) 50:187-188, 1964.

380. Murphy, K. J.: Subcutaneous calcification in the naevoid basal cell carcinoma syndrome: response to parathyroid hormone and relationship to pseudohypoparathyroidism, Clin. Radiol. 20:287-293, 1969.

381. Neblett, C. R., et al.: Neurological involvement in the nevoid basal cell carcinoma syndrome, J. Neurosurg. 35:577-582, 1971.

382. Nichols, L., and Solomon, L. M.: Basal cell nevi syndrome, Arch. Derm. 91:188-189, 1965.

383. Nicotra, A.: La calcificazione e l'osteoma della falce del cervello, al controllo anatomo-radiologico et clinico, Arch. Radiol. (Napoli) 5:794, 1929.

384. Nomland, R.: Multiple basal cell epitheliomas originating from congenital pigmented basal cell nevi, Arch. Dermatol. Syph. (Chic.) 25:1002-1008, 1932.

385. Noury, J. Y.: La naevomatose baso-cellulaire, Thesis, Paris, 1967.

386. Oliver, C. H.: Case of multiple dentigerous cysts, Br. Dent. J. 57:591-592, 1934.

387. Oliver, R. M.: Basal-cell nevus, Arch. Dermatol. 81:284-285, 1960.

388. Parnitzke, K. H.: Endokranielle Verkalkungen im Röntgenbild. Ihre Deutung und Bedeutung im Dienste der klinischen Hirndiagnostik, Leipzig, Germany, 1961, Georg Thieme Verlag.

389. Philipsen, H. P.: Om keratocyster (kolesteatomer) i kaeberne, Tandlaegebladet 60:963-980, 1956.

390. Pimenta, W. P., et al.: Sindrome do nevo-baso-cellular, Anais Bras. Derm. 40:190-191, 1965.

391. Pollard, J. J., and New, P. F. J.: Hereditary cutaneomandibular polyoncosis: a syndrome of myriad basal cell nevi of the skin, mandibular cysts, and inconstant skeletal anomalies, Radiology 82:840-849, 1964.

392. Pollitzer, J.: Eine eigentümliche Karzinose der Haut (Carcinoderma Pigmentosum-Lang) nebenher: punkt- und strichförmige Defekte im Hornstratum der Palmae und Plantae, Arch. Dermatol. Syph. (Berl.) 76:323-345, 1905.

393. Proposed guidelines for the classification, nomenclature, and naming of morphological defects, Syndrome Identification 3:1-3, 1975.

394. Rasmussen, P. E.: Follikulaere kaebecyster, basal-celle-tumorer og knogleanomalier som led i et hereditareret syndom, Nord. Med. 69:606-612, 1963.

395. Rater, C. J., et al.: Basal cell nevus syndrome, Am. J. Roentgenol. 103:589-594, 1968.

396. Readett, M. D., and Samuels, M. J.: Gorlin's syndrome, Br. J. Clin. Pract. 21:373-374, 1967.

397. Rebello, J. A., and Savatard, J. E. M.: Basal cell naevi with bony cysts, Trans. North Engl. Derm. Soc., 1960, pp. 53-56.

398. Reed, J. C.: Nevoid basal cell carcinoma syndrome with associated fibrosarcoma of the maxilla, Arch. Dermatol. 97:304-306, 1968.

399. Repass, J. S., and Grau, W. H.: The basal cell nevus syndrome: report of two cases, J. Oral Surg. 32:227-232, 1974.

400. Satinoff, M. I., and Wells, C.: Multiple basal cell naevus in ancient Egypt, Med. Hist. 13:294-296, 1969.

401. Schamberg, I. L.: Basal-cell nevi, Arch. Dermatol. 81:269, 1960.

402. Schønning, L., and Visfeldt, J.: The syndrome of jaw cysts–basal cell carcinomas–skeletal anomalies: clinical study with chromosomal analyses of a family, Acta Dermatovenereol. 44:437, 1964.

403. Schweisguth, O., et al.: Naevomatose baso-cellulaire associée à un rhabdomyosarcoma congénital, Arch. Fr. Péd. 25:1083-1093, 1968.

404. Shapiro, M. J.: Basal cell nevus syndrome: a case report with associated carcinoma of the maxilla, Laryngoscope 80:777-787, 1970.

405. Shear, M.: Primordial cysts, J. Dent. Assoc. S. Afr. 15:211-217, 1960.

406. Shear, M., and Welton, E.: Cytogenetic studies of the basal cell carcinoma syndrome, J. Dent. Assoc. S. Afr. **23:**99-104, 1968.

407. Slater, S.: The metacarpal sign, Pediatrics **46:**468-471, 1970.

408. Smith, N. H. H.: Multiple dentigerous cysts associated with arachnodactyly and other skeletal defects, Oral Surg. **25:**99-107, 1968.

409. Stanton, J. B., and Wilkinson, M.: Familial calcification of the petrosphenoidal ligament, Lancet **2:**736, 1949.

410. Stevanovic, D. V.: Nevoid basal cell carcinoma syndrome, Arch. Dermatol. **96:**696-698, 1967.

411. Stoelinga, P. J., Cohen, M. M., Jr., and Morgan, A. F.: The origin of keratocysts in the basal cell nevus syndrome, J. Oral Surg. **33:**659-663, 1975.

412. Stoelinga, P. J., Peters, J. H., van de Staak, W. J., et al.: Some new findings in the basal-cell nevus syndrome, Oral Surg. **36:**686-692, 1973.

413. Storck, H., et al.: Naevoid Basaliome mit Kieferzysten (Ward Syndrom); Icthyosis Vulgaris Palmo-Plantar Keratose; Kryptorchismus; Gespaltene Uvula, Dermatologica **133:**145-150, 1966.

414. Straith, F. E.: Hereditary epidermoid cyst of jaws, Am. J. Orthod. **25:**673-691, 1939.

415. Summerly, R.: Basal cell carcinoma: an aetiologic study of patients aged 45 and under with special reference to Gorlin's syndrome, Br. J. Derm. **77:**9-15, 1965.

416. Summerly, R., and Hale, A. J.: Basal cell naevus syndrome, Trans. St. John's Dermatol. Soc. (Lond.) **51:**77-79, 1965.

417. Swanson, A. E., and Jacks, Q. D.: An unusual propensity for odontogenic cyst formation, J. Can. Dent. Assoc. **27:**723-731, 1961.

418. Tamoney, H. J., Jr.: Basal cell nevoid syndrome, Am. Surg. **35:**279-283, 1969.

419. Taylor, W. B., et al.: The nevoid basal cell carcinoma syndrome, Arch. Dermatol. **98:**612-614, 1968.

420. Telle, B.: Multiple Basoliome bei einem jungen Mann, Dermatol. Wochenschr. **151:**1425-1431, 1965.

421. Thies, W., et al.: Zur Frage der Naevobasaliome, Arch. Klin. Exp. Dermatol. **210:**291-321, 1960.

422. Thoma, K. H.: Polycystoma, Oral Surg. **12:**273-281, 1959.

423. Thoma, K. H., and Blumenthal, F. R.: Hereditary and cysts formation, Am. J. Orthod. **32:**273-281, 1946.

424. Tobias, C.: Zum Basalzellnaevus-Kieferzysten Syndrome (Ward Syndrom) mit familiärem Auftreten, Schweiz. Med. Wochenschr. **97:**949-952, 1967.

425. Towns, T. M., and Lagattuta, V.: Basal cell nevus syndrome: 20 year follow-up, J. Oral Surg. **32:**50-53, 1974.

426. van Dijk, E., and Sanderink, J. F. H.: Basal cell syndrome, Dermatologica **134:**101-106, 1967.

427. van Erp, I. F. R.: Naevus epitheliomatodes multiplex, Dermatologica **136:**257-264, 1968.

428. Wallace, D. C., et al.: The basal cell naevus syndrome: report of a family with anosmia and a case of hypogonadotrophic hypopituitarism, J. Med. Genet. **10:**30-33, 1973.

429. Ward, W. H.: Naevoid basal cell carcinoma associated with dyskeratosis of palms and soles: new entity, Aust. J. Dermatol. **5:**204-208, 1960.

430. Worth, H. M., and Wollin, D. G.: The basal cell naevi and jaw cyst syndrome, Clin. Radiol. **19:**416-420, 1968.

431. Zackheim, H. S., et al.: Basal cell carcinoma syndrome, Arch. Dermatol. **93:**317-323, 1966.

Hallermann-Streiff syndrome

432. Blodi, F. C.: Developmental anomalies of the skull affecting the eye, Arch. Ophthalmol. **57:**593-610, 1957.

433. Falls, H. F., and Schull, W. J.: Hallermann-Streiff syndrome: a dyscephaly with congenital cataracts and hypotrichosis, Arch. Ophthalmol. **63:**409-420, 1960.

434. Francois, M. J.: A new syndrome: dyscephalia with bird face and dental anomalies, nanism, hypotrichosis, cutaneous atrophy, microphthalmia and congenital cataract, Arch. Ophthalmol. **60:**842-862, 1958.

435. Hoefnagel, D., and Benirschke, K.: Dyscephalia mandibulo-oculo-facialis (Hallermann-Streiff syndrome), Arch. Dis. Child. **40:**57-61, 1965.

436. Hopkins, D. J., and Horan, E. C.: Glaucoma in the Hallermann-Streiff syndrome, Br. J. Ophthalmol. **54:**416-422, 1970.

437. Hutchinson, M., et al.: Oral manifestations of oculomandibulodyscephaly with hypotrichosis (Hallermann-Streiff syndrome), Oral Surg. **31:**234-244, 1971.

438. Judge, C., and Chakanovskis, J. E.: The Hallermann-Streiff syndrome, J. Ment. Defic. Res. **15:**115-120, 1971.

439. Ponte, F.: Further contributions to the study of the syndrome of Hallermann and Streiff, Ophthalmologica **143:**399-408, 1962.

440. Schondel, A.: Two cases of progeria complicated by microphthalmus, Acta Paediatr. **30:**286-304, 1943.

441. Strivastava, S., et al.: Mandibulo-oculo-facial dyscephaly, Br. J. Ophthalmol. **58:**543-549, 1966.

442. Suzuki, Y., et al.: Hallermann-Streiff syn-

drome, Dev. Med. Child. Neurol. **12**:496-506, 1970.

443. Wolter, J. R., and Jones, D. H.: Spontaneous cataract absorption in Hallermann-Streiff syndrome, Ophthalmologica **150**:401-408, 1965.

444. van Balen, A. T. M.: Dyscephaly with microphthalmos, cataract and hypoplasia of the mandible, Ophthalmologica **141**:53-63, 1961.

de Lange syndrome

445. Beck, B.: Familial occurrence of Cornelia de Lange's syndrome, Acta Paediatr. Scand. **63**:225-231, 1974.

446. Beratis, N. G., et al.: Familial de Lange syndrome: report of three cases in a sibship, Clin. Genet. **2**:170-176, 1971.

447. Berg, J. M., et al.: The de Lange syndrome, New York, 1970, Pergamon Press.

448. Brachmann, W.: Ein Fall von symmetricher Monodaktylie durch Ulnadefekt, Jb. Kinderheilkd. **84**:225-235, 1916.

449. Daniel, W. L., and Higgins, J. V.: Biochemical and genetic investigation of the de Lange syndrome, Am. J. Dis. Child. **121**:401-405, 1971.

450. de Lange, C.: Sur un typ nouveau de degeneration (typus amstelodamensis), Arch. Méd. Enf. **36**:713-718, 1933.

451. Falek, A., et al.: Familial de Lange syndrome with chromosome abnormalities, Pediatrics **37**:92-101, 1966.

452. France, N. E., et al.: Pathological features in the de Lange syndrome, Acta Paediatr. (Scand.) **58**:470-480, 1969.

453. Kurlander, G. J., and deMyer, W.: Roentgenology of the Brachmann–de Lange syndrome, Radiology **88**:101-110, 1967.

454. Lee, F., and Kenny, F.: Skeletal changes in the Cornelia de Lange syndrome, Am. J. Roentgenol. **100**:27-39, 1967.

455. McArthur, R. G., and Edwards, I. H.: de Lange syndrome: report of 20 cases, Can. Med. Assoc. J. **96**:1185-1198, 1967.

456. Motl, M. L., and Opitz, J. M.: Phenotypic and genetic studies of the Brachmann-de Lange syndrome, Hum. Hered. **21**:1-16, 1971.

457. Pashayan, H.: Variability of the de Lange syndrome: report of 3 cases and genetic analysis of 54 families, J. Pediatr. **75**:853-858, 1969.

458. Ptacek, L. J., et al.: The Cornelia de Lange syndrome, J. Pediatr. **63**:1000-1020, 1963.

459. Rao, P. S.: Congenital heart disease in the de Lange syndrome, J. Pediatr. **79**:674-677, 1971.

460. Russell, B. G.: The Cornelia de Lange syndrome: Typus degenerativus amstelodamensis: histologic studies of the marginal gingiva, Scand. J. Dent. Res. **78**:369-373, 1970.

461. Schlesinger, B., et al.: Typus degenerativus amstelodamensis, Arch. Dis. Child. **38**:349-357, 1970.

462. Shear, C. S., et al.: Self mutilative behavior as a feature of the de Lange syndrome, J. Pediatr. **78**:506-507, 1971.

463. Shuster, D. S., and Johnson, S.: Cutaneous manifestations of the Cornelia de Lange syndrome, Arch. Dermatol. **93**:702-707, 1966.

464. Smith, G. F.: A study of the dermatoglyphics in the de Lange syndrome, J. Ment. Res. **10**:241-247, 1966.

465. Vischer, D.: Typus degenerativus amstelodamensis (Cornelia de Lange syndrom), Helv. Paediatr. Acta **20**:415-445, 1965.

Marfan syndrome

466. Adler, R. C., and Nyhan, W. L.: An oculocerebral syndrome with aminoaciduria and keratosis follicularis, J. Pediatr. **75**:436-442, 1969.

467. Allen, R. A., et al.: Ocular manifestation of the Marfan syndrome, Trans. Am. Acad. Ophthalmol. Otolaryngol. **71**:18-38, 1967.

468. Bowden, D. H., et al.: Marfan's syndrome: accelerated course in childhood associated with lesions of mitral valve and pulmonary artery, Am. Heart J. **69**:96-99, 1965.

469. Cartwright, E., et al.: Metachromatic fibroblasts in pseudoxanthoma elasticum and Marfan's syndrome, Lancet **1**:533-534, 1969.

470. Cross, H. E., and Jensen, A. D.: Ocular manifestations in the Marfan syndrome and homocystinuria, Am. J. Ophthalmol. **75**:405-420, 1973.

471. Estes, J. W., et al.: Marfan's syndrome, Arch. Intern. Med. **116**:889-893, 1965.

472. Grondin, C. M., et al.: Dissecting aneurysm complicating Marfan's syndrome (arachnodactyly) in a mother and son, Am. Heart J. **77**:301-306, 1969.

473. Hiragami, H., et al.: Marfan's syndrome accompanied by renovascular hypertension, Tokuko J. Exp. Med. **98**:13-20, 1969.

474. Keech, M. K., et al.: Familial studies of the Marfan syndrome, J. Chron. Dis. **19**:57-83, 1966.

475. Lehmann, O.: A family with Marfan's syndrome traced through an affected newborn, Acta Paediatr. (Scand.) **49**:540-550, 1960.

476. Loveman, A. B., et al.: Marfan's syndrome: some cutaneous aspects, Arch. Dermatol. **87**:428-435, 1963.

477. Lutman, F. C., and Neel, J. V.: Inheritance of archnodactyly, ectopia lentis, and other congenital anomalies (Marfan's syndrome)

in the E family, Arch. Ophthalmol. (Chic.) **41:**276-305, 1949.

478. Lynas, M. A.: Marfan's syndrome in Northern Ireland, Ann. Hum. Genet. **22:**289-301, 1958.

479. Macek, M., et al.: Study on fibroblasts in Marfan's syndrome, Humangenetik **3:**87-97, 1966.

480. McKusick, V. A.: Heritable disorders of connective tissue, ed. 4, St. Louis, 1972, The C. V. Mosby Co.

481. Murdoch, J. L., et al.: Parental age effects on the occurrence of new mutations for the Marfan syndrome, Ann. Hum. Genet. **35:**331-336, 1972.

482. Ramsey, M. S., et al.: The Marfan syndrome: a histopathologic study of ocular findings, Am. J. Ophthalmol. **76:**102-116, 1973.

483. Stinson, H. K., and Cruess, R. L.: Marfan's syndrome with marked limb-length discrepancy, J. Bone Joint Surg. **49A:**735-736, 1967.

484. Stone, J. H.: Ectopia lentis, cardiology and "the sign of the trembling iris," Am. Heart J. **72:**466-468, 1966.

485. Traisman, J. S., and Johnson, F. R.: Arachnodactyly associated with aneurysm of the aorta, Am. J. Dis. Child. **87:**156-166, 1954.

486. Wilner, H. I., and Finby, N.: Skeletal manifestations in the Marfan syndrome, J.A.M.A. **187:**490-495, 1964.

487. Wilson, R.: Marfan's syndrome: description of a family, Am. J. Med. **23:**434-444, 1957.

488. Young, D.: Familial dissecting aneurysm complicating Marfan's syndrome, Am. Heart J. **78:**577-578, 1969.

Mucopolysaccharidoses

489. Gorlin, R. J., Pindborg, J. J., and Cohen, M. M., Jr.: Syndromes of the head and neck, ed. 2, New York, 1976, McGraw-Hill Book Co.

490. McKusick, V. A.: Heritable disorders of connective tissue, ed. 4, St. Louis, 1972, The C. V. Mosby Co.

Neurofibromatosis

491. Baden, E., et al.: Multiple neurofibromatosis with oral lesions: review of the literature and report of a case, Oral Surg. **8:**268-280, 1955.

492. Benedict, P. H., et al.: Melanotic macules in Albright's syndrome and in neurofibromatosis, J.A.M.A. **205:**618-626, 1968.

493. Borberg, A.: Clinical and genetic investigations in tuberous sclerosis and Recklinghausen's neurofibromatosis, Acta Psychiatr. Neurol. (Suppl.) **71:**11-239, 1951.

494. Buntin, P. T., and Fitzgerald, J. F.: Gastrointestinal neurofibromatosis, Am. J. Dis. Child. **119:**521-523, 1970.

495. Canale, D., et al.: Neurologic manifestations of von Recklinghausen's disease of the nervous system, Confin. Neurol. **24:**359-403, 1964.

496. Chao, D. H.-C.: Congenital neurocutaneous syndromes in childhood. I. Neurofibromatosis, J. Pediatr. **55:**189-199, 1959.

497. Charron, J. W., and Gariepy, G.: Neurofibromatosis of the bladder: case report and review of the literature, Can. J. Surg. **13:**303-306, 1970.

498. Christensen, E., and Pindborg, J. J.: A rare case of neurofibromatosis Recklinghausen (plexiform type), Acta Odontol. Scand. **14:**1-10, 1956.

499. Crowe, F. W.: Axillary freckling as a diagnostic aid in neurofibromatosis, Ann. Intern. Med. **61:**1142-1143, 1964.

500. Crowe, F. W., and Schull, W. J.: Diagnostic importance of café-au-lait spot in neurofibromatosis, Arch. Intern. Med. **91:**758-766, 1953.

501. Crowe, F. W., et al.: Multiple neurofibromatosis, Springfield, Ill., 1956, Charles C Thomas, Publisher.

502. Davidson, K. C.: Cranial and intracranial lesions in neurofibromatosis, Am. J. Roentgenol. **98:**550-556, 1966.

503. Fienman, N. L., and Yakovac, W.: Neurofibromatosis in childhood, J. Pediatr. **76:**339-346, 1970.

504. Freeman, M. J., and Standish, S. M.: Facial and oral manifestations of familial disseminated neurofibromatosis, Oral Surg. **19:**52-59, 1965.

505. Grant, W. M., and Walton, D. S.: Distinctive gonioscopic findings in glaucoma due to neurofibromatosis, Arch. Ophthalmol. **79:**127-134, 1968.

506. Halpern, M., and Currarino, G.: Vascular lesions causing hypertension in neurofibromatosis, N. Engl. J. Med. **273:**248-252, 1965.

507. Hankey, G. T.: Von Recklinghausen's disease with local tumors of the palate, Proc. R. Soc. Med. **26:**959-961, 1933.

508. Harkin, J. C., and Reed, R. J.: Tumors of the peripheral nervous system, 2nd ser., fasc. 3, Washington, D.C., 1969, Armed Forces Institute of Pathology.

509. Hayes, D. M., et al.: Von Recklinghausen's disease with massive intraabdominal tumor and spontaneous hypoglycemia: metabolic studies before and after perfusion of abdominal cavity with nitrogen mustard, Metabolism **10:**183-199, 1961.

510. Holt, J. F., and Wright, E. M.: The radiologic features of neurofibromatosis, Radiology **51:**647-663, 1948.

511. Hunt, J. C., and Pugh, D. G.: Skeletal le-

sions in neurofibromatosis, Radiology **76**:1-20, 1961.

512. Izumi, A. K., et al.: Von Recklinghausen's disease associated with multiple neurilemomas, Arch. Dermatol. **104**:172-176, 1971.

513. Jacobs, M. H.: Oral manifestations in von Recklinghausen's disease (neurofibromatosis), Am. J. Orthod. (Oral Surg). **32**:28-33, 1946.

514. Jaffe, H. L.: Tumors and tumorous conditions of the bones and joints, Philadelphia, 1958, Lea & Febiger, pp. 242-255.

515. Johnson, B. L., and Chormeco, D. R.: Café-au-lait spot in neurofibromatosis and in normal individuals, Arch. Dermatol. **102**:442-446, 1970.

516. Kaufman, R. L., et al.: Family studies in congenital heart disease. IV. Congenital heart disease associated with neurofibromatosis, Birth Defects **8**(5):92-95, 1972.

517. Knight, W. A., et al.: Neurofibromatosis associated with malignant neurofibromata, Arch. Dermatol. **107**:747-750, 1973.

518. Koblin, I., and Reil, B.: Changes in the facial skeleton in cases of neurofibromatosis, J. Maxilolfacial Surg. **3**:23-27, 1975.

519. Kragh, L. V., et al.: Neurofibromatosis of the head nad neck, Plast. Reconstr. Surg. **25**:565-573, 1960.

520. Mertin, H., and Graves, C. L.: Plexiform neurofibroma (von Recklinghausen's disease) invading the oral cavity, Am. J. Orthod. **28**:694-702, 1942.

521. Meszaros, W. T., et al.: Neurofibromatosis, Am. J. Roentgenol. **98**:557-569, 1966.

522. Norman, M. E.: Neurofibromatosis in a family, Am. J. Dis. Child. **123**:159-160, 1972.

523. Preston, F. W., et al.: Cutaneous neurofibromatosis (von Recklinghausen's disease): clinical manifestations and incidence of sarcoma in sixty-one male patients, Arch. Surg. **64**:813-827, 1952.

524. Reese, A. B.: Tumors of the eye, ed. 2, New York, 1963, Paul B. Hoeber, Inc.

525. Rittersma, J., et al.: Neurofibromatosis with mandibular deformities, Oral Surg. **33**:718-727, 1972.

526. Rosenquist, G. C., et al.: Acquired right ventricular outflow obstruction in a child with neurofibromatosis, Am. Heart J. **70**:103-108, 1970.

527. Rosman, N. P., and Pearce, J.: The brain in neurofibromatosis, Brain **90**:829-838, 1970.

528. Ross, D. E.: Skin manifestations of von Recklinghausen's disease and associated tumors (neurofibromatosis), Am. Surg. **31**:729-740, 1965.

529. Saxena, K.: Endocrine manifestations of neurofibromatosis in children, Am. J. Dis. Child. **120**:265-271, 1970.

530. Smith, C. J., et al.: Renal artery dysplasias as a cause of hypertension in neurofibromatosis, Arch. Intern. Med. **125**:1022-1026.

531. Spencer, W. G., and Shattock, S. G.: Macroglossia and neurofibromatosis, Proc. R. Soc. Med. **1**:8, 1908.

532. Stein, K. M., et al.: Neurofibromatosis presenting as the epidermal nevus syndrome, Arch. Dermatol. **105**:229-232, 1972.

533. Stillman, F. S.: Neurofibromatosis, J. Oral Surg. **10**:112-117, 1952.

534. von Recklinghausen, F.: Über die multiplen fibroma der Haut und ihre Beziehung zu den multiplen neuromen, Berlin, 1882, A. Hirschwald.

535. Weber, F. P.: Neurofibromatosis of the tongue in a child, together with a note on the classification of incomplete and anomalous cases of Recklinghausen's disease, Br. J. Child. Dis. **7**:13-16, 1910.

536. Whitfield, A.: Cutaneous neurofibromatosis in which newly formed nerve fibres were found in the tumours, Lancet **1**:1230-1232, 1903.

537. Whitehouse, D.: Diagnostic value of the café-au-lait spot in children, Arch. Dis. Child. **41**:416-419, 1966.

538. Winters, S. E., et al.: Neurofibromatosis (von Recklinghausen's disease) with involvement of the mandible, Oral Surg. **13**:76-79, 1960.

Oculodentoosseous dysplasia

539. Eidelman, E., et al.: Orodigitofacial dysostosis and oculodentodigital dysplasia, Oral Surg. **23**:311-319, 1967.

540. Gorlin, R. J., et al.: Oculodentodigital dysplasia, J. Pediatr. **63**:69-75, 1963.

541. Kurlander, G. J., et al:. Roentgen differentiation of the oculodentodigital syndrome and the Hallermann-Streiff syndrome of infancy, Radiology **86**:77-85, 1966.

542. Meyer-Schwickerath, G., et al.: Mikrophthalmussyndrome, Klin. Monatsbl. Augenheilkd. **131**:18-30, 1957.

543. Pfeiffer, R. A., et al.: Oculodento-digitale dysplasia, Klin. Monatsbl. Augenheilkd. **152**:247-262, 1968.

544. Rajic, D. S., and de Veber, L. L.: Hereditary oculodentoosseous dysplasia, Ann. Radiol. **9**:224-231, 1966.

545. Reisner, S. H., et al.: Oculodentodigital dysplasia syndrome, Am. J. Dis. Child. **118**:600-607, 1969.

546. Sugar, H. S., et al.: The oculo-dento-digital dysplasia syndrome, Am. J. Ophthalmol. **61**:1448-1451, 1966.

Osteogenesis imperfecta

547. Becks, H.: Histologic study of tooth structure in osteogenesis imperfecta, Dent. Cosmos **73**:437-454, 1931.

548. Berggren, L., et al.: Intraocular pressure and excretion of mucopolysaccharides in osteogenesis imperfecta, Arch. Ophthalmol. (Kbh.) **47:**122-128, 1969.

549. Bethge, J. F. J., et al.: Biochemische Untersuchungen bei Osteogenesis imperfecta, Bruns Beitr. Klin. Chir. **214:**448-458, 1967.

550. Blumcke, S., et al.: Histochemical and fine structural studies on the cornea with osteogenesis imperfecta congenita, Virchows Arch. (Zellpathol.) **11:**124-132, 1972.

551. Bolletti, M., and Disertori, A.: Su di un caso di osteogenesi imperfecta tipo Lobstein associata a sindrome di Ehlers-Danlos, idrocefalia, e piedi torti, Pediatria (Napoli) **75:**310-330, 1967.

552. Caniggia, A., et al.: Fragilitas ossium hereditaria tarda (Ekman-Lobstein disease), Acta Med. Scand. (Suppl.) **340:**172, 1958.

553. Carey, M. C., et al.: Osteogenesis imperfecta in twenty-three members of a kindred with heritable features contributed by a nonspecific skeletal disorder, Q. J. Med. **37:**437-449, 1968.

554. Chawla, S.: Intrauterine osteogenesis imperfecta in four siblings, Br. Med. J. **1:**99-101, 1964.

555. Chowers, I., et al.: Familial aminoaciduria in osteogenesis imperfecta, J.A.M.A. **181:**771-775, 1962.

556. Eddowes, A.: Dark sclerotics and fragilitas ossium, Br. Med. J. **2:**222, 1900.

557. Falvo, K. A., and Bullough, P. G.: Osteogenesis imperfecta—a histometric analysis, J. Bone Joint Surg. **55A:**275-286, 1973.

558. Francis, M. J. O., et al.: Instability of polymeric skin collagen in osteogenesis imperfecta, Br. Med. J. **1:**421-424, 1974.

559. Freda, V. J., et al.: Osteogenesis imperfecta congenita: a presentation of 16 cases and review of the literature, Obstet. Gynecol. **18:**535-547, 1961.

560. Godfrey, J. L.: A histological study of dentin formation in osteogenesis imperfecta congenita, J. Oral Pathol. **2:**85-111, 1973.

561. Gussen, R.: The stapediovestibular joints: normal structure and pathogenesis of otosclerosis, Acta Otolaryngol. (Suppl.) (Stockh.) **248:**1-38, 1969.

562. Haebara, H., et al.: An autopsy case of osteogenesis imperfecta congenita—histochemical and electron microscopical studies, Acta Pathol. Jap. **19:**377-394, 1969.

563. Heller, R. H., et al.: The prenatal diagnosis of osteogenesis imperfecta congenita, Am. J. Obstet. Gynecol. **121:**572-573, 1975.

564. Heys, F. M., et al.: Osteogenesis imperfecta and odontogenesis imperfecta: clinical and genetic aspects in eighteen families, J. Pediatr. **56:**234-245, 1960.

565. Ibsen, K. H.: Distinct varieties of osteogenesis imperfecta, Clin. Orthop. **50:**270-290, 1967.

566. Janke, D.: Klinische und blutchemische Untersuchungene bei der Osteogenesis imperfecta, Z. Orthop. **105:**423-430, 1968.

567. Jett, S., et al.: Bone turnover and osteogenesis imperfecta, Arch. Pathol. **81:**112-116, 1966.

568. Kosoy, J., and Maddox, H. E.: Surgical findings in van der Hoeve's syndrome, Arch. Otolaryngol. **93:**115-122, 1971.

569. Lancaster, G., et al.: Dominantly inherited osteogenesis imperfecta in man: an examination of collagen biosynthesis, Pediatr. Res. **9:**83-88, 1975.

570. Langness, U., and Behnke, H.: Biochemische Untersuchungen zur Osteogenesis imperfecta, Dtsch. Med. Wochenschr. **95:**213-221, 1970.

571. Maroteaux, P., and Gilles, M.: Étude radiologique de l'osteogenesis imperfecta, Ann. Radiol. **8:**571-583, 1965.

572. McKusick, V. A.: Heritable disorders of connective tissue, ed. 4, St. Louis, 1972, The C. V. Mosby Co., pp. 390-454.

573. Mehregan, A. H.: Elastosis perforans serpiginosa, Arch. Dermatol. **97:**381-393, 1968.

574. Niemann, M. W.: Aminoacid composition of bone collagen in osteogenesis imperfecta, J. Bone Joint Surg. **51A:**804, 1969.

575. Pindborg, J. J.: Dental aspects of osteogenesis imperfecta, Acta Pathol. Microbiol. Scand. **24:**47-64, 1947.

576. Remigio, P. A., and Grinvalsky, H. T.: Osteogenesis imperfecta congenita, Am. J. Child. **119:**524-528, 1970.

577. Riley, F. C., et al.: Osteogenesis imperfecta: morphologic and biochemical studies of connective tissue, Pediatr. Res. **7:**757-768, 1973.

578. Roberts, E., and Schour, I.: Hereditary opalescent dentin, Am. J. Orthod. **25:**267-276, 1939.

579. Rushton, M. A.: Structure of the teeth in late cases of osteogenesis imperfecta, J. Pathol. Bacteriol. **48:**591-603, 1939.

580. Rushton, M. A.: Anomalies of human dentine, Br. Dent. J. **98:**431-444, 1955.

581. Schroder, G.: Osteogenesis imperfecta, Z. Menschl. Vereb. Konstit. Lehre **37:**632-676, 1964.

582. Scott, D., and Stiris, G.: Osteogenesis imperfecta tarda: a study of three families with special reference to scar formation, Acta Med. Scand. **145:**237-257, 1953.

583. Seedorff, K. S.: Osteogenesis imperfecta: a study of clinical features and heredity based on 55 Danish families comprising 180 affected persons, Copenhagen, 1949, Thesis Munksgaard, pp. 1-229.

584. Solomons, C. C., and Styner, J.: Osteogene-

sis imperfecta: metabolism, Calcif. Tissue Res. **3**:318-326, 1969.

585. Spurway, J.: Hereditary tendency to fracture, Br. Med. J. **2**:844, 1896.

586. Stein, R., et al.: Brittle cornea: a familial tract associated with blue sclerae, Am. J. Ophthalmol. **66**:67-69, 1968.

587. Stevenson, C. J., et al.: Skin collagen in osteogenesis imperfecta, Lancet **1**:860, 1970.

588. Witkop, C. J., Jr., and Rao, S.: Inherited defects in tooth structure, Birth Defects **7**: 153-184, 1971.

Prader-Willi syndrome

589. Brissenden, J. E., and Levy, E. P.: Prader-Willi syndrome in infant monozygotic twins, Am. J. Dis. Child. **126**:110-112, 1973.

590. Cohen, M. M., Jr., and Gorlin, R. J.: The Prader-Willi syndrome, Am. J. Dis. Child. **117**:213-218, 1969.

591. de Fraites, E. B., et al.: Familial Prader-Willi syndrome, Birth Defects **11**(4):123-126, 1975.

592. Dubowitz, V.: A syndrome of benign congenital hypotonia, gross obesity, delayed intellectual development, retarded bone age, and unusual facies, Proc. R. Soc. Med. **10**: 1006-1008, 1967.

593. Dunn, H. G.: The Prader-Labhart-Willi syndrome: review of the literature and report of nine cases, Acta Paediatr. Scand. (Suppl.) **186**:1-38, 1968.

594. Evans, P. R.: Hypogenital dystrophy with diabetic tendency, Guy's Hosp. Rep. **113**: 207-222, 1964.

595. Forssman, H., and Hagberg, B.: Prader-Willi syndrome in boy of 10 with diabetes, Acta Paediatr. Scand. **53**:70-78, 1964.

596. Hall, B., and Smith, D. W.: Prader-Willi syndrome, J. Pediatr. **81**:286-293, 1972.

597. Hoefnagel, D., et al.: Prader-Willi syndrome, J. Ment. Defic. Res. **11**:1-11, 1967.

598. Jancar, J.: Prader-Willi syndrome, J. Ment. Defic. Res. **15**:20-29, 1971.

599. Juul, J., and Dupont, A.: Prader-Willi syndrome, J. Ment. Defic. Res. **11**:12-22, 1967.

600. Landwirth, J., et al.: Prader-Willi syndrome, Am. J. Dis. Child. **116**:211-217, 1968.

601. Laurance, B. M.: Hypotonia, mental retardation, obesity, and cryptorchidism associated with dwarfism and diabetes in children, Arch. Dis. Child. **42**:126-139, 1967.

602. Parra, A., et al.: Immunoreactive insulin and growth hormone responses in patients with Prader-Willi syndrome, J. Pediatr. **83**: 587-593, 1973.

603. Prader, A., and Willi, H.: Das Syndrome von Imbezillität, Adipositas, Muckelhypotonie, Hypogenitalismus, Hypogonadismus

und Diabetes mellitus mit 'Myotonie'-Anamnese, Proceedings of the Second International Congress of Psychic Developmental Defects in Children, Vienna, 1963, pp. 353-357.

604. Prader, A., et al.: Ein Syndrom von Adipositas, Kleinwuchs, Kryptorchismus und Oligophrenie nach myotonieartigem Zustand im Neugeborenenalter, Schweiz. Med. Wochenschr. **86**:1260, 1956.

605. Prader, A., et al.: Ein Syndrom von Adipositas, Kleinwuchs, Kryptorchismus und Idiotie bei Kindern und Erwachsenen, die als Neugeborene ein Myotonieartiges Bild geboten haben, Proceedings of the Eighth International Congress of Pediatrics **10**:13, 1956.

606. Ridler, M. A. C., et al.: A case of Prader-Willi syndrome in a girl with a small extra chromosome, Acta Paediatr. Scand. **60**:222-226, 1971.

607. Stolecke, H., et al.: Prader-Labhart-Willi Syndrom, Monatschr. Kinderheilkd. **122**:10-17, 1974.

608. Zellweger, H., and Schneider, H. J.: Syndrome of hypotonia-hypomentia-hypogonadism-obesity (HHHO) or Prader-Willi syndrome, Am. J. Dis. Child. **115**:588-598, 1968.

Pycnodysostosis

609. Braun, J. P., and Peterschmitt, J.: L'aspect radiologique de la pycnodysostose, J. Radiol. Electrol. **46**:508-512, 1965.

610. Dusenberry, J. F., and Kane, J. J.: Pycnodysostosis: report of three new cases, Am. J. Roentgenol. **99**:717-723, 1967.

611. Elmore, S. M., et al.: Pycnodysostosis with a familial chromosome anomaly, Am. J. Med. **40**:273-282, 1966.

612. Giedion, A., and Zachmann, M.: Pyknodysostose, Helvet. Paediat. Acta **21**:612-621, 1966.

613. Kajii, Y., et al.: Pyknodysostosis, J. Pediat. **69**:131-133, 1966.

614. Maroteaux, P., and Lamy, M.: La pycnodysostose, Presse Méd. **70**:999-1002, 1962.

615. Maroteaux, P., and Lamy, M.: The malady of Toulouse-Lautrec, J.A.M.A. **191**:715-717, 1965.

616. Sedano, H. O., et al.: Pycnodysostosis: clinical and genetic considerations, Am. J. Dis. Child. **116**:70-77, 1968.

617. Shuler, S. E.: Pycnodysostosis, Arch. Dis. Child. **38**:620-625, 1963.

618. Soto, R. J., et al.: Pycnodysostosis: metabolic and histologic studies, Birth Defects **5**(4): 109-116, 1969.

Rubinstein-Taybi syndrome

619. Berg, J. M., et al.: On the association of broad thumbs and first toes with other physi-

cal peculiarities and mental retardation, J. Ment. Defic. Res. **10**:204-220, 1966.

620. Coffin, G. S.: Brachydactyly, peculiar facies, and mental retardation, Am. J. Dis. Child. **108**:351-359, 1964.

621. Coffin, G. S.: Three retarded children with unusual face and hands: a variant of the wide-thumbs syndrome? In Richards, B. W., editor: Symposium of the International Association for the Scientific Study of Mental Deficiency, Montpellier, France, 1967, A. A. Fauve Co., pp. 600-605.

622. Davison, B. C. C., et al.: Mental retardation with facial abnormalities, broad thumbs and toes and unusual dermatoglyphics, Develop. Med. Child Neurol. **9**:588-593, 1967.

623. Filippi, G.: The Rubinstein-Taybi syndrome: report of 7 cases, Clin. Genet. **3**:303-319, 1972.

624. Giroux, J., and Miller, J. R.: Dermatoglyphics of the broad thumb and great toe syndrome, Am. J. Dis. Child. **113**:207-209, 1967.

625. Herrmann, J., and Opitz, J. M.: Dermatoglyphic studies in a Rubinstein-Taybi patient, her unaffected dizygous twin sister and other relatives, Birth Defects **5**:22-24, 1969.

626. Jancar, J.: Rubinstein-Taybi's syndrome, J. Ment. Defic. Res. **9**:265-270, 1965.

627. Jeliu, G., and Saint-Rome, G.: Le syndrome de Rubinstein-Taybi: à propos d'une observation, Union Med. Can. **96**:22-29, 1967.

628. Job, J. C., et al.: Études sur les nanismes constitutionnels. II. Le syndrome de Rubinstein et Taybi, Ann. Pédiat. **11**:646-650, 1964.

629. Johnson, C. F.: Broad thumbs and broad great toes with facial abnormalities and mental retardation, J. Pediat. **68**:942-951, 1966.

630. Kroth, von H.: Cornelia de Lange-Syndrom I bei Zwillingen, Arch. Kinderheilkd. **173**:273-283, 1966.

631. Kushnick, T.: Bradydactyly, facial abnormalities and mental retardation: Rubinstein-Taybi syndrome, Am. J. Dis. Child. **111**:96-98, 1966.

632. Lamy, M., et al.: Le syndrome de Rubinstein-Taybi, Arch. Fr. Pediatr. **24**:472, 1967.

633. McArthur, R. G.: Rubinstein-Taybi syndrome: broad thumbs and great toes, facial abnormalities and mental retardation: a presentation of three cases, Can. Med. Assoc. J. **96**:462-466, 1967.

634. Neuhauser, G.: Pneumoencephalographic findings in the Rubinstein-Taybi syndrome symposium 10: Rubinstein-Taybi syndrome. In Richards, B. W., editor: Proceedings, First Congress of the International Asso-

ciation for the Scientific Study of Mental Deficiency, Montpellier, France, 1967, A. A. Fauve Co., pp. 615-617.

635. Padfield, C. J., et al.: The Rubinstein-Taybi syndrome, Arch. Dis. Child. **43**:94-106, 1967.

636. Robinow, M.: A familial syndrome of mental deficiency and broad thumbs, Birth Defects **5**(2):42, 1969.

637. Robinson, G. C., et al.: Broad thumbs and toes and mental retardation: unusual dermatoglyphic observations in two individuals, Am. J. Dis. Child. **111**:287-290, 1966.

638. Rohling, B., et al.: Rubinstein-Taybi syndrome, Am. J. Dis. Child. **121**:71-74, 1971.

639. Roy, F. H., et al.: Ocular manifestations of the Rubinstein-Taybi syndrome: case report and review of the literature, Arch. Ophthalmol. **79**:272-278, 1968.

640. Rubinstein, J. H.: A syndrome of broad thumbs and first toes, mental retardation, and characteristic facial features—a follow-up report: symposium 10: Rubinstein-Taybi syndrome. In Richards, B. W., editor: Proceedings, First Congress of the International Association for the Scientific Study of Mental Deficiency, Montpellier, France, 1967, A. A. Fauve Co., pp. 589-595.

641. Rubinstein, J. H.: The broad thumbs syndrome—progress report 1968, Birth Defects **5**:25-41, 1969.

642. Rubinstein, J. H.: Broad thumb–hallux syndrome. In Bergsma, D., editor: Birth defects compendium and atlas, Baltimore, 1973, The Williams & Wilkins Co., pp. 218-219.

643. Rubinstein, J. H., and Taybi, H.: Broad thumbs and toes and facial abnormalities, Am. J. Dis. Child. **105**:588-603, 1963.

644. Salmon, M. A.: The Rubinstein-Taybi syndrome: a report of two cases, Arch. Dis. Child. **43**:102-106, 1968.

645. Smith, G. F., and Berg, J. M.: Dermatoglyphics in Rubinstein-Taybi syndrome: Symposium 10: Rubinstein-Taybi syndrome. In Richards, B. W., editor: Proceedings, First Congress of the International Association for the Scientific Study of Mental Deficiency, Montpellier, France, 1967, A. A. Fauve Co., pp. 606-612.

646. Spencer, D. A.: Partial Rubinstein-Taybi syndrome, Lancet **2**:713-714, 1971.

647. Takeuchi, M.: Rubinstein's syndrome in two siblings, Gann J. Med. Sci. **15**:17, 1966.

648. Taybi, H., and Rubinstein, J. H.: Broad thumbs and toes, and unusual facial features: a probable mental retardation syndrome, Am. J. Roentgenol. **93**:363-366, 1965.

649. Taybi, H.: Broad thumbs and great toes, fa-

cial abnormalities, and mental retardation syndrome: symposium 10: Rubinstein-Taybi syndrome. In Richards, B. W., editor: Proceedings, First Congress of the International Association for the Scientific Study of Mental Deficiency, Montpellier, France, A. A. Fauve Co., 1967, pp. 596-599.

650. True, C. W., and Rubinstein, J. H.: Pathological findings in a case of the Rubinstein-Taybi syndrome: Symposium 10: Rubinstein-Taybi syndrome. In Richards, B. W., editor. Proceedings, First Congress of the International Association for the Scientific Study of Mental Deficiency, Montpellier, France, 1967, pp. 613-614.

651. van Gelderen, H. H., et al.: Trisomy G/normal mosaics in non-mongoloid mentally deficient children, Acta Paediatr. Scand. **56:** 517-525, 1967.

652. Wilson, M. G.: Rubinstein-Taybi and D₁ trisomy syndromes, J. Pediatr. **73:**404-408, 1968.

Russell-Silver syndrome

653. Curi, J. F. J., et al.: Elevated serum gonadotrophin in Silver's syndrome, Am. J. Dis. Child. **114:**658-661, 1967.

654. Ganner, E., and Schwingshackl, A.: Neigung zu Chromosomenbrüchen bei Russell-Syndrom, Monatschr. Kinderheilkd. **48:**629-632, 1970.

655. Gareis, F. J., et al.: The Russell-Silver syndrome without asymmetry, J. Pediatr. **79:** 775-781, 1971.

656. Girard, J., and Kaufman, H. J.: Der Russell-Zwerg, Monatschr. Kinderheilkd. **113:**696-702, 1965.

657. Lässker, G., and Reich, J.: Das Russell Syndrom—eine Form des kindlichen Zwergwuchses, Arch. Kinderheilkd. **178:**303-315, 1969.

658. Moseley, J. E., et al.: The Silver syndrome: congenital asymmetry: short stature and variations in skeletal development, Am. J. Roentgenol. **97:**74-81, 1966.

659. Reister, H. C., and Scherz, R. G.: Silver syndrome, Am. J. Dis. Child. **107:**410-416, 1964.

660. Russell, A.: A syndrome of "intra-uterine" dwarfism recognizable at birth with craniofacial dysostosis, disproportionately short arms, and other anomalies (5 examples), Proc. R. Soc. Med. **47:**1040-1044, 1954.

661. Schumacher, G., and Niederhoff, H.: Die Syndrome nach Russell und Silver, Helv. Paediatr. Acta **22:**404-421, 1967.

662. Silver, H. K.: Congenital asymmetry, short stature and elevated urinary gonadotropin, Am. J. Dis. Child. **97:**768-773, 1959.

663. Silver, H. K.: Asymmetry, short stature and

variations in sexual development: a syndrome of congenital malformations, Am. J. Dis. Child. **107:**494-515, 1964.

664. Silver, H. K., et al.: Syndrome of congenital hemihypertrophy, shortness of stature, and elevated urinary gonadotropins, Pediatrics **12:**368-376, 1953.

665. Spranger, J., and Friedrich, I.: Primordialer Zwergwuchs: Typ-Russell-Silver, Pediatr. Praxis **4:**507-518, 1965.

666. Stool, S., and Cohen, P.: Silver's syndrome, Am. J. Dis. Child. **105:**199-203, 1963.

667. Szalay, G. C.: Pseudohydrocephalus in dwarfs: the Russell dwarf, J. Pediatr. **63:** 622-633, 1963.

668. Szalay, G. C.: Intrauterine growth retardation versus Silver's syndrome, J. Pediatr. **64:** 234-240, 1964.

669. Szalay, G. C.: Russell dwarf versus Silver syndrome, J. Pediatr. **80:**1066, 1972.

670. Tanner, J. M., and Ham, T. J.: Low birthweight dwarfism with asymmetry (Silver's syndrome): treatment with human growth hormone, Arch. Dis. Child. **44:**231-234, 1969.

671. Tulinus, H., et al.: 45,X/46,XY chromosome mosaic with features of the Russell-Silver syndrome, Dev. Med. Child Neurol. **14:**161-172, 1972.

672. Vestermark, S.: Silver's syndrome, Acta Paediatr. Scand. **59:**435-439, 1970.

Sturge-Weber dysplasia/Klippel-Trénaunay-Weber syndrome

673. Alexander, G. L., and Norman, R. M.: The Sturge-Weber syndrome, Bristol, England, 1960, John Wright & Sons, Ltd.

674. Andriola, M., and Stolfi, J.: Sturge-Weber syndrome: report of an atypical case, Am. J. Dis. Child. **123:**507-510, 1972.

675. Arrighi, M. F.: Hamartose ecto-medodérmique: un cas d'angiomatose diffuse avec fusion de maladie de Sturge-Weber-Krabbe et de maladie de Parkes Weber, Bull. Soc. Fr. Dermatol. Syph. **67:**562-563, 1960.

676. Arrighi, M. F.: Hamartose ecto-mesodérmique: un cas de fusion de maladie de Recklinghausen (avec éléphantiasis névromateux de Virchow) et de maladie de Klippel-Trénaunay-Parkes Weber, Bull. Soc. Fr. Dermatol. Syph. **67:**564, 1960.

677. Baer, P. N., et al.: Gingival hemangioma associated with Sturge-Weber syndrome, Oral Surg. **14:**1383-1390, 1961.

678. Bentson, J. R., et al.: Cerebral venous drainage pattern of the Sturge-Weber syndrome, Am. J. Roentgenol. **101:**111-118, 1971.

679. Bereston, E. S., and Roberts, D.: Congenital hypertrophy of extremities, South. Med. J. **58:**302-307, 1965.

680. Bonse, G.: Röntgenbefunde bei einer Phakomatose (Sturge-Weber Kombiniert mit Klippel-Trénaunay), Fortschr. Roentgenstr. **74:** 727-729, 1951.

681. Brooksaler, F.: The angioosteohypertrophy syndrome (Klippel-Trenaunay-Weber syndrome), Am. J. Dis. Child. **112:**161-164, 1966.

682. Brushfield, T., and Wyatt, W.: Sturge-Weber disease, Br. J. Child. Dis. **24:**98-106, 209-213, 1927; **25:**96-101, 1928.

683. Buchanec, J., and Galanda, V.: Polymalformačný Klippelov-Trenaunayov-Weberov syndróm s progresívnou lipodistrofiou u 6-ročného chlapca, Cesk. Pediatr. **24:**228-232, 1969.

684. Caplan, D. B., et al.: Angioosteohypertrophy syndrome with protein-losing enteropathy, J. Pediatr. **74:**119-123, 1969.

685. Chao, D. H.-C.: Congenital neurocutaneous syndromes of childhood. III. Sturge-Weber disease, J. Pediatr. **55:**635-649, 1959.

686. Cigiati, L.: Klinischer und pathologischer Beitrag zum Studium der halbseitigen Hypertrophie, Dtsch. Z. Nervenheilkd. **32:**282-293, 1907.

687. da Silva, M., and Neves, H.: Über einen Fall von Klippel-Trénaunay-schem Symptomkomplex, der Erfolgreich mit Röntgenstrahlen behandelt wurde, Fortschr. Roentgenstr. **90:**475, 1959.

688. Dimitri, V.: Tumor cerebral congenito (angioma cavernoso), Rev. Med. Argent. **36:**1029, 1923.

689. el Mostehy, M. R., and Stallard, R. E.: The Sturge-Weber syndrome: its periodontal significance, J. Periodontol. **40:**243-246, 1969.

690. Furukawa, T., et al.: Sturge-Weber and Klippel-Trénaunay syndrome with nevus of Ota and Ito, Arch. Dermatol. **102:**640-645, 1970.

691. Gyarmati, I.: Oral change in Sturge-Weber's disease, Oral Surg. **13:**795-801, 1960.

692. Hall, B. D.: Bladder hemangiomas in Klippel-Trénaunay-Weber syndrome, N. Engl. J. Med. **285:**1032-1033, 1971.

693. Inceman, S., and Tangun, Y.: Chronic defibrination syndrome due to a giant hemangioma associated with microangiopathic hemolytic anemia, Am. J. Med. **46:**997-1002, 1969.

694. Inui, M., et al.: An autopsy case of Klippel-Trénaunay-Weber's disease, Acta Pathol. Jap. **19:**251-263, 1969.

695. Ippen, H.: Systematisierte Angiektasie mit Gliedmassenatrophie (ein Beitrag zum "Klippel-Trénaunay-Syndrom"), Hautarzt **8:**317-320, 1959.

696. Kalischer, S.: Demonstration des Gehirns eines Kindes mit Teleangiectasie der linkseitigen Gesichts-Kopfhaut und Hirnoberfläche, Berl. Klin. Wochenschr. **34:**1059, 1897.

697. Klippel, M., and Trenaunay, P.: Du naevus variqueux ostéo-hypertrophique, Arch. Gén. Méd. **185:**641-672, 1900.

698. Koch, G.: Zur Klinik Symptomatologie, Pathogenese und Erbpathologie des Klippel-Trénaunay-Weber'schen Syndroms, Acta Genet. Med. (Roma) **5:**326-370, 1956.

699. Krabbe, K. H.: Facial and meningeal angiomatosis associated with calcifications of brain cortex: clinical and anatomo-pathologic contribution, Arch. Neurol. Psychiatr. **32:**737-755, 1934.

700. Krabbe, K. H., and Wissing, O.: Calcifications de la pie-mère du cerveau (d'origine angiomateuse) démonstrée par la radiographie, Acta Radiol. **10:**523-532, 1929.

701. Kuffer, F. R., et al.: Klippel-Trenaunay syndrome, visceral angiomatosis and thrombocytopenia, J. Pediatr. Surg. **3:**65-72, 1968.

702. Lamar, L. M., et al.: Klippel-Trénaunay-Weber syndrome, Arch. Dermatol. **91:**58-59, 1965.

703. Lindenauer, S. M.: The Klippel-Trénaunay syndrome: varicosity, hypertrophy and hemangioma with no arteriovenous fistula, Ann. Surg. **162:**303-314, 1965.

704. Lindenauer, S. M.: Congenital arteriovenous fistula and the Klippel-Trenaunay syndrome, Ann. Surg. **174:**248-263, 1971.

705. Miller, S. J. N.: Ophthalmic aspects of the Sturge-Weber syndrome, Proc. R. Soc. Med. **56:**419-421, 1965.

706. Morgan, G.: Pathology of the Sturge-Weber syndrome, Proc. R. Soc. Med. **56:**422-423, 1963.

707. Nellhaus, G., et al.: Sturge-Weber disease with bilateral intracranial calcifications at birth and unusual pathologic findings, Acta Neurol. Scand. **43:**314-347, 1967.

708. Noriega-Sanchez, A., et al.: Oculocutaneous melanosis associated with the Sturge-Weber syndrome, Neurology **22:**256-262, 1972.

709. Parkes Weber, F.: Angioma formation in connection with hypertrophy of limbs and hemi-hypertrophy, Br. J. Dermatol. **19:**231-235, 1907.

710. Peterman, A. F., et al.: Encephalotrigeminal angiomatosis (Sturge-Weber disease): clinical study of thirty-five cases, J.A.M.A. **167:** 2169-2176, 1958.

711. Poser, C. M., and Taveras, J. M.: Cerebral angiography in encephalotrigeminal angiomatosis, Radiology **68:**327-336, 1957.

712. Protzel, M. S.: Sturge-Weber syndrome, Oral Surg. **10:**388-399, 1957.

713. Rademacher, R.: Über einen Fall einer Kombination von Sturge-Weber und Klippel-Trénaunay Syndrom mit konstitutioneller Neurodermitis, Dermatol. Wochenschr. **143:** 381-386, 1961.

714. Roizin, L., et al.: Congenital vascular anomalies and their histopathology in Sturge-Weber-Dimitri syndrome (naevus flammeus with angiomatosis and encephalosis calcificans), J. Neuropathol. Exp. Neurol. **18:**75-97, 1959.

715. Rose, L. M.: Hypertrophy of the lower limbs with cutaneous naevus and varicose veins, Arch. Dis. Child. **25:**162-169, 1950.

716. Schirmer, R.: Ein Fall von Telangiektasie, Albrecht von Graefes Arch. Klin. Ophthalmol. **7:**119-121, 1860.

717. Shepherd, J. A.: Angiomatous conditions of the gastro-intestinal tract, Br. J. Surg. **40:** 409-421, 1953.

718. Sturge, W. A.: Case of partial epilepsy apparently due to lesion of one of vasomotor centres of brain, Trans. Clin. Soc. London **12:**162-167, 1879.

719. Thoma, K. H.: Sturge-Kalischer-Weber syndrome with pregnancy tumors, Oral Surg. **5:**1124-1131, 1952.

720. Weber, F. P.: Right-sided hemi-hypertrophy resulting from right-sided congenital spastic hemiplegia, with morbid condition of left side of brain, revealed by radiograms, J. Neurol. Psychopathol. **3:**134-139, 1922.

721. Wohlwill, F. J., and Yakovlev, P. I.: Histopathology of meningofacial angiomatosis (Sturge-Weber's disease); report of four cases, J. Neuropathol. Exp. Neurol. **16:**341-364, 1957.

Tuberous sclerosis

722. Ackermann, A. J.: Pulmonary and osseous manifestations of tuberous sclerosis, Am. J. Roentgenol. **51:**315-325, 1944.

723. Berland, J. I.: Roentgenological findings in tuberous sclerosis, Arch. Neurol. Psychiatr. **69:**669-683, 1953.

724. Bourneville, D.: Sclereuse tubereuse des circonvolutions cerebrales: idiotie et epilepsie hemiplegique, Arch. Neurol. (Paris) **1:**81-91, 1880.

725. Bundey, S., and Evans, K.: Tuberous sclerosis: a genetic study, J. Neurol. Neurosurg. Psychiatr. **32:**591-603, 1969.

726. Butterworth, T., and Wilson, M., Jr.: Dermatologic aspects of tuberous sclerosis, Arch. Dermatol. Syph. (Chic.) **43:**1-41, 1941.

727. Chao, D. H.-C.: Congenital neurocutaneous syndromes in childhood. II. Tuberous sclerosis, J. Pediatr. **55:**447-459, 1959.

728. Crichton, J. V.: Infantile spasms and skin anomalies, Develop. Med. Child. Neurol. **8:** 273-278, 1966.

729. Dawson, J.: Pulmonary tuberous sclerosis and its relationship to other forms of the disease, Q. J. Med. **23:**113-145, 1954.

730. Dickerson, W. W.: Characteristic roentgen changes associated with tuberous sclerosis, Arch. Neurol. Psychiatr. **65:**683-702, 1951.

731. Fitzpatrick, T. B., et al.: White leaf-shaped macules, Arch. Dermatol. **98:**1-6, 1968.

732. Gold, A. P., and Freeman, J. M.: Depigmented naevi: the earliest sign of tuberous sclerosis, Pediatrics **35:**1003-1005, 1965.

733. Gorlin, R. J., et al.: Oral manifestations of the Fitzgerald-Gardner Pringle-Bourneville, Robin, adrenogenital and Hurler-Pfaundler syndromes, Oral Surg. **13:**1233-1244, 1960.

734. Hawkins, T. D.: Radiological bone changes in tuberous sclerosis, Br. J. Radiol. **32:**157-161, 1959.

735. Holt, J. F., and Dickerson, W. W.: The osseous lesions of tuberous sclerosis, Radiology **58:**1-7, 1952.

736. Hurwitz, S., and Braverman, I.: White spots in tuberous sclerosis, J. Pediatr. **77:**587-594, 1970.

737. Jervis, G. A.: Spongioneuroblastoma and tuberose sclerosis, J. Neuropathol. Exp. Neurol. **13:**105-116, 1954.

738. Jordan, W. M.: Familial tuberous sclerosis, Br. Med. J. **2:**132-135, 1956.

739. Kirby, T. J.: Ocular phakomatosis, Am. J. Med. Sci. **222:**227-239, 1951.

740. Lago, J. C., and Gomez, M. R.: Tuberous sclerosis: reappraisal of a clinical entity, Mayo Clin. Proc. **42:**26-49, 1967.

741. Lebrun, H. I., et al.: Renal hamartoma, Br. J. Urol. **27:**394-407, 1955.

742. MacCarthy, W. C., and Russell, D. G.: Tuberous sclerosis: report of a case with ependymoma, Am. J. Roentgenol. **71:**833-839, 1958.

743. Nevin, N. C., and Pearce, W. G.: Diagnostic and genetical aspects of tuberous sclerosis, J. Med. Genet. **5:**273-280, 1968.

744. Nickel, W. R., and Reed, W. B.: Tuberous sclerosis, Arch. Dermatol. **85:**209-226, 1962.

745. Pagenstecher, W. J.: Tuberous sclerosis: historical review and report of two cases, Am. J. Ophthalmol. **39:**663-676, 1955.

746. Pringle, J. J.: A case of congenital adenoma sebaceum, Br. J. Dermatol. **2:**1-14, 1890.

747. Reed, W. B., et al.: Internal manifestations of tuberous sclerosis, Arch. Dermatol. **87:** 715-728, 1963.

748. Reese, A. B.: Tumors of the eye, New York, 1951, Paul B. Hoeber, Inc.

749. Rushton, M. A.: Some less common bone lesions affecting the jaws: tuberous sclerosis with jaw lesions, Oral Surg. **9:**289-304, 1956.

750. Singer, K.: Genetic aspects of tuberous

sclerosis in a Chinese population, Am. J. Hum. Genet. **23**:33-40, 1971.

751. Smith, T. K., et al.: Orthopaedic problems associated with tuberous sclerosis, J. Bone Joint Surg. **51A**:97-102, 1969.

752. Thibault, J. H., and Manuelidis, E. E.: Tuberous sclerosis in a premature infant, Neurology **20**:139-146, 1970.

753. Whitaker, P. H.: Radiological manifestations in tuberose sclerosis, Br. J. Radiol. **32**:152-156, 1959.

754. Zaremba, J.: Tuberous sclerosis: a clinical and genetical investigation, J. Ment. Defic. Res. **12**:63-80, 1968.

Williams syndrome

755. Anim, V. G., and Engel, P.: Mental retardation related to hypercalcaemia, Dev. Med. Child Neurol. **6**:366-377, 1964.

756. Anita, A. U., et al.: Pathogenesis of the supravalvular aortic stenosis syndrome, J. Pediatr. **71**:431-441, 1967.

757. Beuren, A. J.: Supravalvular aortic stenosis: a complex syndrome with and without mental retardation, Birth Defects **8**:45-56, 1972.

758. Beuren, A. J., Apitz, J., and Harmjanz, D.: Supravalvular aortic stenosis in association with mental retardation and a certain facial appearance, Circulation **26**:1235-1240, 1962.

759. Beuren, A. J., Schulze, C., Eberle, P., et al.: The syndrome of supravalvular aortic stenosis, peripheral pulmonary stenosis, mental retardation and similar facial appearance, Am. J. Cardiol. **13**:471-483, 1964.

760. Blancquaert, A., et al.: Stenoses pulmonaires et aortiques postvalvulaires avec facies particulier et retard intellectuel, Acta Cardiol. (Brux.) **21**:611-643, 1966.

761. Chantler, C., et al.: Cardiovascular and other associations of infantile hypercalcaemia, Guy's Hosp. Rep. **115**:221-241, 1966.

762. Char, F.: Williams facies with portal vein aplasia and mental retardation, Birth Defects **8**(5):262-263, 1972.

763. Char, F., and Rowe, R. D.: Infantile hypercalcemia syndrome with mitral regurgitation and hypoplasia of aorta, Birth Defects **8**(5):258-261, 1972.

764. Dupont, B., et al.: Idiopathic hypercalcemia of infancy: the elfin face syndrome, Dan. Med. Bull. **17**:33-46, 1970.

765. Ebeling, J., et al.: Ein weiterer Beitrag zu den kardiovaskulären Veränderungen und der Klinik defektgeheilter infantiler Hyperkalzämien, Arch. Kinderheilkd. **180**:1-14, 1969.

766. Faivre, G., et al.: Le rétrécissement aortique sus-valvulaire avec malformations multiples, Arch. Mal. Coeur **58**:977-996, 1965.

767. Fanconi, G., and Girardet, P.: Chronische Hypercalcämie, kombiniert mit Osteosklerose, Hyperazotämie, Minderwuchs und kongenitalen Missbildungen, Helv. Paediatr. Acta **7**:314-334, 1952.

768. Forbes, G. B., et al.: Impaired calcium homeostasis in infantile hypercalcemic syndrome, Acta Paediatr. Scand. **61**:305-309, 1972.

769. Frank, R. M., et al.: Aspects odonto-stomatologiques de la stenose aortique susvalvulaire, Rev. Stomatol. (Paris) **67**:223-232, 1966.

770. Friedman, W. F.: Vitamin D and the supravalvular aortic stenosis syndrome, Adv. Teratol. **3**:85-96, 1968.

771. Friedman, W. F., and Mills, L. F.: The relationship between vitamin D and the craniofacial and dental anomalies of the supravalvular aortic stenosis syndrome, Pediatrics **43**:12-18, 1969.

772. Friedman, W. F., and Roberts, W. C.: Vitamin D and the supravalvular aortic stenosis syndrome: the transplacental effects of vitamin D on the aorta of the rabbit, Circulation **34**:77-86, 1966.

773. Gorin, R., et al.: Un nouveau cas d'hypercalcémie idiopathique grave, Ann. Pediatr. **13**:20-42, 1966.

774. Harris, L. L., and Nghiem, Q. X.: Idiopathic hypercalcaemia of infancy with interruption of the aortic arch, J. Pediatr. **73**:84-88, 1968.

775. Härtel, G., et al.: Supravalvular pulmonic stenosis, abnormal facial appearance and mental retardation, Am. Heart J. **75**:540-544, 1968.

776. Heinemann, M. R., and Cohen, M. M., Jr.: Personal observations, 1974.

777. Jones, K. L., and Smith, P. W.: The Williams elfin facies syndrome: a new perspective, J. Pediatr. **86**:718-723, 1975.

778. Jorgensen, G., and Beuren, A. J.: Genetische Untersuchungen bei supravalvularen Aortenstenosen, Humangenetik **1**:497-515, 1965.

779. Joseph, M. C., and Parrott, D.: Severe infantile hypercalcemia with special reference to the facies, Arch. Dis. Child. **33**:385-395, 1958.

780. Jue, K. L., et al.: The syndrome of idiopathic infancy with associated congenital heart disease, J. Pediatr. **67**:1130-1140, 1965.

781. Kivalo, E., et al.: Mental retardation, typical facies and aortic stenosis syndrome, Ann. Med. Intern. Finn. **54**:81-87, 1965.

782. Levy, E. P.: Infantile hypercalcemia facies and mental retardation associated with atrial septal defect and anomalous pulmonary venous return, Birth Defects **8**:(5):73-74, 1972.

783. Murgeon, —.: Anomalies dento-maxillo-faciales et stenose aortique susvalvulaire, Thesis, Paris, 1970.

784. Myers, A. R., and Willis, P. W., III.: Clinical spectrum of supravalvular aortic stenosis, Arch. Intern. Med. **118:**552-561, 1966.

785. Ottesen, O. E., et al.: Peripheral vascular anomalies associated with the supravalvular aortic stenosis syndrome, Radiology **86:**430-435, 1966.

786. Page, H. L., et al.: Supravalvular aortic stenosis, Am. J. Cardiol. **23:**270-277, 1969.

787. Rashkind, W. J., et al.: Cardiac findings in idiopathic hypercalcaemia of infancy, J. Pediatr. **58:**464-469, 1961.

788. Roberts, N. K., and Moes, C. A. F.: Supravalvular pulmonary stenosis and unusual facial appearance, Birth Defects **8**(5):57-59, 1972.

789. Roy, F. H., et al.: Infantile hypercalcemia and supravalvular aortic stenosis, J. Pediatr. Ophthalmol. **8:**188-193, 1971.

790. Schlesinger, B. E., Butler, N. R., and Black, J. A.: Severe type of infantile hypercalcaemia, Br. Med. J. **1:**127-134, 1956.

791. Schlesinger, B. E., et al.: Chronische Hypercalcämie mit Osteosklerose, Helv. Acta **7:** 335-349, 1952.

792. Schmidt, R. E., et al.: Generalized arterial fibromuscular dysplasia and myocardial infarction in familial supravalvular aortic stenosis syndrome, J. Pediatr. **74:**576-584, 1969.

793. Singleton, E. B., et al.: The radiographic features of severe idiopathic hypercalcemia of infancy, Radiology **68:**721-726, 1957.

794. Sutcliffe, J.: Severe infantile hypercalcaemia and stenosis of major arteries, Ann. Roentgenol. **8:**277-278, 1965.

795. William, J. C. P., et al.: Supravalvular aortic stenosis, Circulation **24:**1311-1318, 1961.

Index

DATE DUE